Cancer Is One Big Pain-In-The-Neck!

(And Many Other Body Parts)

What I Learned During My Three+–Year Head-and-Neck Cancer Journey From Diagnosis to "Cancer-Free" Survivor

Ron "Butch" Sickler

9+-Year Survivor of Stage IV Head-and-Neck Cancer

INFINITY PUBLISHING

ISBN 978-0-7414-9925-7 Paperback
ISBN 978-0-7414-9926-4 Hardcover
ISBN 978-0-7414-9927-1 eBook

Printed in the United States of America

Published June 2014

INFINITY PUBLISHING
1094 New DeHaven Street, Suite 100
West Conshohocken, PA 19428-2713
Toll-free (877) BUY BOOK
Local Phone (610) 941-9999
Fax (610) 941-9959
Info@buybooksontheweb.com
www.buybooksontheweb.com

Also By Ron "Butch" Sickler

Out of My Mind, From My Heart, & Off My Chest!

My Thought-Provoking Quotes, Opinions, and Commentary
about <u>Almost</u> Everything
to Enlighten, Inspire, Amuse, and Rouse Your Brain

(Infinity Publishing - 2009)

A Time for Rhyme – Parts I and II

An Autobiographical Journey
Through a Lifetime of Poetic Verse

(Watermark Press – 2005)

Hope Wins!

©

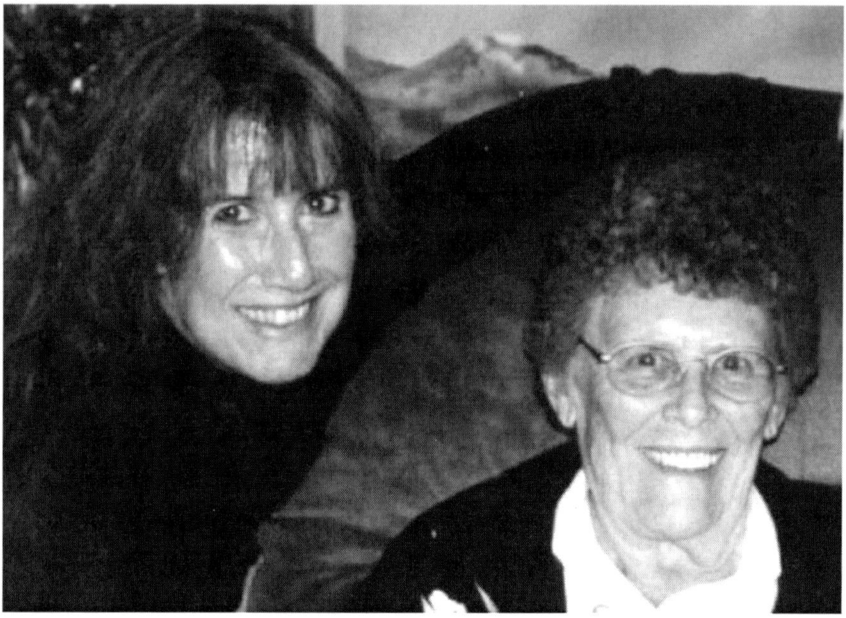

Our Beloved Sister, Vikki, and Our Beautiful, Loving Mom, Betty

Sir John Bowring, the Nineteenth Century Linguist, Writer, and Member of British Parliament, was quoted as saying, *"A happy family is but an earlier heaven."* That is a wonderful thought, and I believe captures perfectly the heavenly feelings of sanctity and love that can be shared by members of close, cheerful families. Certainly, there are no greater blessings in the entire universe than the heartfelt love, forgiveness, security, and understanding that devoted mothers, fathers, sons and daughters can provide to one another in both good times, and bad. In this regard, our supportive family had fortunately been blessed with the pure, unconditional love that our Mom, Betty, and our Sister, Vikki, shared with each of us throughout their lives. It's been said that when a nice person passes away, it is because God is in need of more Angels. Without a doubt, I know that both Mom and Vikki are now happily serving in that capacity, and that they are unselfishly spreading their divine love far-and-wide, just as they did when they were with us here on earth. Our kind, thoughtful Vikki—my Kid-Sister and Best Buddy—passed away in 2005 at 55 years of age. And, regrettably, in April of 2012, just thirteen days after her 84th birthday, we lost our incredible Mom due to natural causes, but not because of Cancer, which she overcame her entire adult life. We miss them both dearly, but their heavenly love is always with us.

Dedications

This book is dedicated to my lovely Wife, Jayni, my Best Friend, Soul Mate, and dedicated Partner, who helps me realize each and every day just how wonderful and how fulfilling this life can be. Jayni is the sunshine that lights my life and warms my heart.

I also dedicate this book to our Mom, Betty, who was a 38+ year Survivor of Breast Cancer before she passed from her Earthly dwelling to her Heavenly resting place on April 13, 2012. Mom was always our brave Heroine, and she had been put through the ringer, physically, for many years. Her health problems began with her first Breast Cancer Mastectomy in 1974, and persisted until her loss. But, no matter the obstacle or the discomfort that she experienced during those many years, she always made the best of her situation, and did it with the biggest smile on her face. Mom passed away due to non-Cancer-related natural causes, so, the fearless Warrior that she was, she did show her Cancer who was "boss." Mom has always been an inspiration to our family, and to all those who know her. Now, she, thankfully, rests happily and peacefully in her new Heavenly home. Mom will always continue to inspire us with her bravery and Love.

This book is also dedicated to my terrific Brothers, Buz and Rich—who graciously shared their love and support with me during my Cancer ordeal—and to the memories of our Dad, Rudy, and our kind, beautiful, and selfless Sister, Vikki. Both Dad and Vik passed from this Life with so much more love and happiness to share. And, also to our gracious Grandmothers—Mom's Mother, Ellen, and our Dad's Mother, Kathryn—and our Aunt Connie. All of these brave women fought their own courageous battles against Cancer, but, in the end, they each, regrettably, lost their personal conflicts with the disease. These wonderful women were guiding lights in each of our lives, and even with their passing, they continue to show us the way.

Additionally, this book is gratefully dedicated to my Miracle Workers—my skilled Physicians and Nurses, and all the other health care professionals on my Cancer Treatment Medical Team—without whose intelligence, care, and helpful, positive attitudes, I may not be alive today. My appreciation especially goes out to my Oncologist, Dr. Ahuja, my Radiation Oncologist, Dr. Hetelekidis, my Surgeon, Dr. Sater, and to each member of their thoughtful staffs. And to my Caregiver, Joanne, who gave so much of her life to help save mine.

I further thankfully dedicate this book to Mr. Larry Blossom, my Psychotherapist, and the person with whom I entrusted my very delicate emotional state after surviving my battle with Cancer. He reassured me that it was safe to laugh again, and that it was okay to open my eyes once more to the world. He also helped to convince me that I could once again trust and believe in my body and mind.

It is, likewise, to the roughly six million men, women, young children and teenagers, worldwide, who are diagnosed with Cancer each year—including over one-and-a-half-million in the U.S.—that I also dedicate this book. And, likewise, to their loved ones, families, Caregivers, Medical Teams, and friends, who love, encourage, and support these brave souls in the fights of their lives.

And, to finish, I dedicate this book to the lives of the far-too-many courageous mothers and fathers, brothers and sisters, sons and daughters, and grandparents, aunts, uncles, cousins and friends who have perished at the hands of Cancer after doing everything possible to beat and survive their disease. With the love, help, and support of their families, physicians, and friends, these brave warriors gave it their best. But, sadly, in the end, their best just wasn't quite enough. The special memories of these devoted relatives and friends will be forever locked in our hearts and minds. And, the love, strength, and wisdom that they shared with us during *their* lives will always serve as an inspiration to those of us who would follow in their footsteps.

Hope Wins!

©

An Open Letter to Cancer, From Those Diagnosed

Following the receipt of a Cancer Diagnosis, the affected person, and their family, Caregiver, and health care specialists, will have much to do to prepare for the all-important Treatments that will be researched, decided upon, and ultimately employed in an effort to safely and completely remove Cancer from the patient's body while inflicting as little damage as possible to their healthy bodily tissues. Finally, after every one of the pre-Treatment preparations have been successfully completed, the patient's Cancer Treatment will begin.

The commencement of a patient's vital Cancer Treatment(s) communicates a very powerful statement to the cancerous trespasser that is shortly to be addressed and hopefully annihilated. But, more importantly, the Treatment speaks to the courage and toughness of the valiant patient-warrior who will be combating their Cancer on a daily basis, sometimes for weeks, months, or maybe even years.

Just prior to the beginning of their Cancer Treatments, the Cancer-patient-turned-warrior-turned-hopeful-Survivor may want to convey a very personal and heartfelt message to their Cancer just to make sure that it thoroughly understands the reasons for the ensuing battle. Additionally, the brave patient may want to communicate to their Cancer that there is no question in their heart or mind about the optimistic and anticipated final outcome: ***The patient's survival!***

Such a letter to one's Cancer may go something like this:

"My Cancer, My Nemesis,

Yes, I admit it – you are very good at what you do. You certainly succeeded in shocking me at first with your clever ambush, which I fortunately found out about when my doctor handed me my fateful Diagnosis some time ago. What a horribly devastating surprise that you orchestrated at my expense! That is something for which I will never forgive you. I am, however, very grateful that my doctors did expose you silently lurking inside me, for had they not, you and I may never have had the opportunity to meet each other on the battlefield. Nor, would I be contacting you with this letter on the eve of what I expect to be the most challenging, but rewarding, fight of my life. I cannot express in words how upset that would have made me.

But, getting back to the discovery of you within my body, you also successfully frightened me with the malicious reputation that you have acquired over the years by indiscriminately attacking not only adult men and women, but also, by being so low, and so despicable, that you actually have the nerve to prey upon innocent young boys and girls and teenagers who are just beginning their life's journey. That is simply unforgivable! But, that's what you do isn't it? Without warning, you sneakily evolve within our bodies, multiply, and feed, and spread, and ravage—no matter our gender, our age, or our health status—and you keep on doing so until you are found out and the tables are turned on you. I will tell you that you angered me to no end with your cowardly intrusion and vicious violation of my body! I mean, you didn't even knock or announce your arrival – you just barged right in as though you owned the place!

And, don't even get me started on how nonchalantly, but abusively, you took it upon yourself to interrupt my career or my schooling. And, as self-serving as you are, you did so without even the slightest regret whatsoever, not caring how important they are to me. You waltzed right in to my life and demanded that I put everything on-hold, just so that I could deal with the unwelcome, nasty wrath of your presence within my body. For, if I don't make you the center of attention for the next few weeks or months, you know full-well what could possibly happen to me. Yes, your devious plan could succeed, while my plan for my own life could... well... you know the rest.

Additionally, what were you thinking that you would be so bold as to enter into my relationship with my loved ones, family, and friends, in a brazen attempt to come between them and me? It's one thing to attempt to catch me off-guard in some dark alley, and to try to mess with my body and mind. But, you couldn't just let it go at that, could you? No. You have to be so scary, so persistent, and so lethal, that you will do everything you can to not only rob me of my good health and peaceful life, but, you must also see how many of my family and friends you can frighten, intimidate, and take along with me. That is not just terribly mean and greedy – it is reprehensible and unforgiveable.

And finally, but, most offensively, you not only had the audacity to attempt to lay waste to my health, but, much worse than that, you saw it as your primary objective to slowly and methodically destroy my body from within—to devastate my life-sustaining systems and organs, and, to continually wear me down both physically and emotionally—until ultimately, after you've thoroughly accomplished your selfish, destructive mission, you would simply take that which is dearest to me: my Life. Yes, MY life, which is not yours to take, no matter how powerful, how devious, or how deadly you think you are. How dare you even assume that I would let that happen at your hands!

Well, my Cancer, those <u>WERE</u> your plans. Yes, WERE. But, now, it's <u>MY</u> turn to give <u>YOU</u> a big surprise! Yes, that's right. During the last few weeks, after I found out that you had chosen me to be your victim and host, I, and my family and Caregiver, have been meeting with the best and brightest doctors to devise a treatment plan aimed at completely destroying you and removing you from my body. And, the great part is, now that we know exactly where you are hiding and where you may have spread to do your dirty deeds, there is very little that you can do to escape. To paraphrase the words of Commodore Oliver Perry during the War of 1812, "I have met the enemy, and you are mine."

To give you an idea of what to expect during our upcoming battles, first of all, I want for you to know that I have my own strength and will to survive, not to mention a ton of faith and hope. Then, you will also be up against the love and devotion of my loved ones, and my family and friends, who will be supporting me from start to finish. And, finally, you will be challenged non-stop by the determined and skilled doctors I just mentioned to you, as well as the state-of-the-art equipment, medicines, and techniques that they have in their arsenal, all of which being designed for one purpose, and one purpose only: TO ELIMINATE CANCER!

Basically, for lack of a better way of putting it, once we hit you with this 1-2-3 punch in the very near future, you will be history; finito!; kaput! Yes, my Cancer, your glory days are over. I will see you in battle, my unworthy and soon-to-be-exterminated, adversary."

Humbly Signed,

Author's Disclaimer

I have utilized the daily journaling notes that I wrote during my Cancer experience, and materials provided to me by my Medical Team, as a foundation for relating much of the information included in this Book. However, I've also researched Cancer, in general, and Head and Neck Cancers, specifically, using the very informative and reliable U.S. Government materials and websites. As such, much of the information for this book has also been legitimately and legally derived and then adapted from the U.S. National Cancer Institute Internet Resources (www.cancer.gov), and accurately incorporated in accordance with "Web Policies for the National Cancer Institute (NCI)."

Below, for the Reader's perusal, are the "NCI Web Policies," which I have taken directly from the NCI website, (www.cancer.gov):

> ***"Copyright and Reuse of Graphics and Text***
>
> ***You May Reuse Information from the National Cancer Institute (NCI) Web Site***
>
> ***Most of the information on the National Cancer Institute (NCI) Web site, Cancer.gov, is in the public domain and is not subject to copyright restrictions. No special permission is required to use or reproduce public domain material. NCI's public domain information includes health professional and patient information in NCI's Physician Data Query (PDQ®) cancer information database and patient education brochures, booklets, and fact sheets. However, any reproduced material should acknowledge NCI as the originator and the NCI Web site, www.cancer.gov, as the source. The source can be cited as: the National Cancer Institute (www.cancer.gov)***
>
> ***You Do Not Need Permission to Use text from NCI information products in your own materials.***
>
> ***However, you cannot use the registered trademark logos for NCI, National Institutes for Health (NIH), or PDQ in your materials because NCI has not reviewed or approved your product."***

Contents

"Many medical maladies strike in a very swift and decisive way. But, Cancer is slow and determined, and, therein lie both its strength and its weakness. We can either let this sly and sluggish killer have its way with us, or, we can commandeer Cancer's own lingering timetable to prepare and unleash our own plan-of-attack, aimed precisely at its demise."

-- Butch Sickler

Prologue

"I'm sorry, but you have Cancer"

This concise but uncompromising phrase may be the most feared in the English language. I *will* say that those words definitely scared the *you-know-what* out of me when my doctor delivered the unexpected news of my Head and Neck Cancer diagnosis to me at age 52, on June 7, 2004. As I write this, that was over 9 years ago.

Even to this day, I'm still not quite sure what frightened and upset me more when I first heard the physician utter that matter-of-fact statement to me: That the diagnosis was so sudden and without warning; that it was utterly unbelievable because I had always lived an extremely healthy and fit lifestyle; or, if it was the scary thought that my own immune defenses had permitted this deadly parasite to assault my otherwise healthy body that I had worked so assiduously for over thirty years to fortify. All three of these concerns were very hard for me to bear, but, I think it was my own body's *betrayal-of-self* that was the most difficult and puzzling for me to comprehend.

"There has to be a mistake - this can't happen to me!" I kept saying to myself and pleading to the doctor when he initially shared my fate with me. For the first few moments after the physician told me the news, I was in disbelief, and I didn't know what to say or do. I had a difficult time breathing, and, although I had many questions I wanted to ask, I could not reason or think clearly, much less speak with any lucidity. Nothing that had just occurred in that exam room made any sense to my rational brain. I sobbed, I denied the claim, I asked, *"Why me?"* and, *"How could this happen?",* and, as people will often do when suddenly surprised with such heart-stopping and frightening information, I immediately thought the worst.

No one "deserves" to receive a Cancer diagnosis, regardless of their health habits or lifestyle behaviors, and, certainly, no person can ever anticipate how they will respond when such a disconcerting revelation is initially presented to them by their physician or other health care professional. However, as many recent Cancer statistics indicate, the experience that I just described with my own surprising Cancer diagnosis will be replicated in some form or another by over one-and-a-half million Cancer victims in the U.S. in 2013, and, by over six million men, women, children, and teenagers, worldwide.

Cancer, in all of its many forms, is the second most common life-threatening disease in America today, right after Heart Disease – or Cardiovascular Disease. This medical menace can screw up the health and lives of anyone, be they young or older, male or female, rich or poor, royalty or average Joe, or healthy or not. Yes, Cancer is a very indiscriminate disease, able and willing to strike anyone at any time. But, the *real unfair advantage Cancer has* is that in many cases, it doesn't give its victim the slightest inkling that it is lurking within their body, uncontrollably feeding, spreading, and growing, and destroying the very tissue upon which it depends to live.

While Cancer is a serious disease, the Treatments to cure or to hold the disease at-bay can be almost as devastating and painful. As such, an individual's journey through Treatment, Recovery, and Aftercare can be a very challenging one, and the patient may want to pack for a very long haul. Thankfully, however, the traveler will not be alone. The road through Cancer treatment and on to hopeful triumph is well-travelled by the millions of bold patients who have made this long and arduous trip before. Along the way, these brave men, women, and children have been supported by their loved ones and friends and aided by the best that science and modern medicine have to offer. And, in the end, millions of these strong, courageous fighters have survived their wearisome journeys, overpowered their destructive Cancers, and reclaimed their precious lives. The most noteworthy take-away here is that receiving a Diagnosis of Cancer should *never* be confused with being handed a Sentence to Die.

Yes, this insatiable intruder *can possibly be conquered if it is* ***detected early*** *through screening tests, or due to Cancer-related or other symptoms, and, if it is* ***treated as quickly as possible***. Cancer can be treated thru the use of conventional Surgery, Chemotherapy, Radiation Therapy, Immunotherapy, Bone Marrow Transplantation, and other modalities, and also via Alternative Medicine. In several cases, and especially in early Stages, Cancer can be cured forever.

Thanks to years and years of far-reaching Cancer testing and Research Studies, modern medicines and equipment, greatly skilled medical professionals, and several state-of-the-art technologies, the survival rates for multiple types of Cancers have not only increased a great deal in recent years, but the quality of life for Survivors after Cancer has also been radically enhanced. Add to these factors, the will, the faith, and the strength of the patient, the power of prayer, and the love and support of caring family and friends, and you will have all of the right ingredients to transform a potentially negative outcome into one that can be constructive, strengthening, and life-renewing. Some dark clouds do, indeed, have silver linings!

I was very fortunate to have been blessed with a magnificent Caregiver, and family, friends, and many others who supported me from beginning-to-end, after I was diagnosed in 2004 with *Stage IV Cancer at the Base of the Tongue***.** Yes, despite a lifetime of regular exercising, very healthful eating, nominal wine drinking, and never smoking, Cancer still managed to lock me in its sights. The saying, *"No good deed goes unpunished"* comes instantly to mind, as does the good ole' reliable adage, *"Shit happens." Que sera, sera...*

After the initial shock of my Cancer diagnosis, I gave up on asking the, *"how?"* and the, *"why?"* questions, and I started devoting a majority of my time to the development of a plan-of-attack to kill the disease. I and my Caregiver had done extensive research to learn about Cancer in general, and to identify the most effective treatment options for my form of Cancer, specifically. My Medical Team and I then designed my Treatment Plan accordingly. It was after I started formulating my treatment strategy with my physicians that I initially knew that ***I—not the Cancer***—would be the one in command of the situation and *my* fate. Knowledge is power, and power kills Cancer.

My customized Cancer treatment plan consisted of Radiation Therapy every day, which I received in tandem with Chemotherapy infusions on a weekly basis. This was then followed by Surgery to remove any leftover traces of the Primary Tumor on my tongue. My entire course of treatments lasted approximately 2 ½ months. While I did win a bet by holding on to all of the hair on my head during my Chemo, I also fell prey to many of the nasty Side-Effects of both the Chemotherapy and Radiation Therapy, which ***did*** take their toll.

But, as difficult and distressing were the relentless, burning mouth, tongue and throat pain, weight loss, and continuous nausea to endure during and after my Chemotherapy and Radiation Therapy treatments, what I had an ***extremely difficult*** time dealing with was the unanticipated deep, dark depression that followed, as well as my unforeseen dependency on the narcotic prescription painkillers used during my treatments. But, just as I went to hell-and-back with the pain and conquered my Cancer, I also eventually beat the depression and prescription painkiller dependency demons as well. Thankfully, during my Cancer Treatment and Recovery Phases, I found help at every turn from the professionals on my Medical Team, a Support Group, and, from my family and Caregiver, and my friends.

Without a doubt, the completion of one's Cancer Treatment is a well-earned relief and an extremely momentous achievement. But, after the day-to-day and the week-to-week treatment schedule has finally finished, the Recovery and Aftercare Phases are equally as essential in helping the patient to reclaim their pre-Cancer life. It is for this reason that Cancer patients will not ever drop off of the "medical radar screen" when they finish their treatments. Instead, all Cancer survivors—youthful, old, and everyone in-between—are constantly examined, tested, and monitored by physicians, closely, for life, following the completion of their courses of treatment.

During this vital time of Recovery and Aftercare, with each hopeful, encouraging test result, the patient will gain faith that their Cancer is gone. And, with every favorable check-up and exam, the *Cancer Patient* could find themselves journeying one step closer to becoming a *Cancer Survivor.* While I am definitely blessed to be a Cancer Survivor, myself, our Mother, Betty, who first contracted Breast Cancer in the 1970s, continued to be a Cancer Survivor for more than 35 years. It was on April 13, 2012, that our lovely Mom unfortunately passed away because of Pneumonia and other natural causes. *But, our Mom did survive her Cancer!* She was the ultimate Cancer Warrior, and she courageously continued to beat the disease during her entire adult life. If all of us could only be as blessed.

Without question, the major focus of any Cancer Treatment Program, including Recovery and Aftercare, is on the *patient*, right where it should be. But, of equally critical significance through the patient's Cancer-fighting program is an unsung hero that should not be overlooked: the ***Cancer Caregiver*** – a family member, a loved one or a friend, who has kindly taken it upon themselves to provide whatever level of time, assistance, comfort, and support their patient may need along their journey. While these unselfish Caregivers may not experience the same physical torment that some Cancer patients endure, the emotional anguish that they bear in taking good care of their impacted loved one, family member, relative, or friend, can be equally as distressing, and should never be taken for granted. When praying for, and encouraging, the Cancer patient, please also do the same for the patient's Caregiver. It truly does make a difference.

That you are now holding this book in your hands may mean that you have been diagnosed with Cancer yourself, or, that you may be a family member, friend, or a Caregiver of a person who has been diagnosed with this despicable disease. Or, possibly, you and yours have not been negatively impacted by Cancer, but you have chosen to read this book for the purpose of gaining knowledge about Cancer in general, or Head and Neck Cancer, specifically. In either case, I have written this book—which is based upon those many things that I experienced during my own Cancer journey, lessons that I learned along the way, and, beneficial information which I researched from bona fide sources—so that it will hopefully assist others whose lives have been suddenly upended by this harmful, but treatable, disease.

If any of the above scenarios happen to fit your own personal situation, I hope that you will find this book useful and uplifting as you forge your journey ahead. But, whatever you do, always look to the Heavens as you travel, and focus *only* on the Silver Linings. The dark, dreary clouds have no place in your plans.

My prayers, positive thoughts, and best wishes are with you. Be well, and above all…always have Hope. *Hope Wins!*

Butch Sickler
December 2013
Edgewood, New Mexico
www.headandneckcancerbook.com

"Every individual is different; every individual's type of Cancer is different; and, every individual's response to Cancer treatment is different. What all Cancer patients do share in common, however, is the never-ending Hope, and the undying Faith, that good will triumph over bad, and, that Life will continue to hold for them, their place."

— Butch Sickler

Introduction

My Dear Reader: I have Authored this Book in an attempt to provide enlightening, inspirational, and beneficial information to individuals that have been impacted in different ways by Cancer — whether it is as a Patient, a Loved One, a Family Member, a Friend, or a Caregiver. As a person can very easily visualize, the volume of information available today about the topic of Cancer is endless. As such, it can all be mind-boggling for first-time patients, family, and Caregivers to attempt to learn what they might about this formidable foe, and, to try to figure out how in the world their loved one, family member, or friend, will possibly ever get from Diagnosis to hopeful Survivorship. With this Book, it is my goal to attempt to distill and summarize information about Cancer, in general, and the form of the disease that I had—*Head and Neck Cancer,* in particular—into one helpful, easy-to-read-and-understand resource that focuses on those subjects that I found to be of the greatest importance during my own Cancer experience. It is my sincere hope that these same topics will be just as meaningful and beneficial to the Readers of this Book.

I learned quite alot during my approximate three-year Cancer ordeal, from Diagnosis to a *"Cancer-free"* outcome, but, I did have to acquire much of the information the hard, old-fashioned way – I had to work for it. This is because, in many instances, I found that relevant "layperson-friendly" information about my form of Cancer (i.e., ***Cancer at the Base of the Tongue***) was not readily available in libraries, bookstores, or on the Internet. In such cases, I ultimately had to search for, locate, and learn most of it on my own. I did find that most of the books on the subject of Head and Neck Cancer were written by doctors—for doctors—and, that there were absolutely no books written by Head and Neck Cancer patients or survivors for the benefit of others "in the same boat" as they. As an outcome of those futile initial explorations for *layperson* books about Head and Neck Cancer, I realized that the lessons, pitfalls, and best practices that I learned during *my own* Cancer experience may prove beneficial to others. And, that is just why I decided to transform my own research and journal notes into this book: To hopefully help others who have been affected by this disease as they chart their own, brave journeys ahead. ***As of 2013, This Book is one of only two or three*** available *about Head and Neck Cancer, written from a survivor's perspective.*

I would like to make it clear, up-front, that I am not a doctor, therapist, psychologist, counselor, or other health professional, and, that it is not my intent with this book to dispense medical advice or recommendations. That being said, I am rather knowledgeable of human anatomy and physiology thanks to my BS Degree in Biology, 30+ years of Bodybuilding, and my prior certification as a Personal Fitness Trainer. I also am a 9+-Year Survivor of Stage IV Head and Neck Cancer, and a Writer who is trying to turn his own bittersweet Cancer experience into an optimistic springboard of sorts – A means by which others affronted by this disease can possibly benefit from the information contained within these pages as they kick-off their own, hopefully, safe and successful Cancer-killing journeys through Treatment, Recovery, and Aftercare. If nothing else, it would be my desire that the Reader of this Book would acquire some knowledge about Cancer and how to deal with its occurrence, and that this book would inspire meaningful dialogue between the patient and doctor.

A bulk of the information contained within this book I have drawn from my own Cancer experience and journaling notes, as well as advice and materials that I received from my Cancer Treatment Medical Team. Additionally, some materials in this book represent the accumulation of applicable information and statistical data that I have researched in many trustworthy and respected medical sources, especially, the reliable and reputable online Cancer resources of the U.S. Government websites for the National Institutes for Health, the National Cancer Institute (http://www.cancer.gov), and the Centers for Disease Control. Finally, at the ending of this book, I've included an Index that I trust will assist the Reader in finding any specific topics within these pages. Locating, gathering, learning, and documenting the information within this book has been a true *labor of love*. I am honored to pass along the fruits of my labors to benefit others.

From the instant that my doctor first delivered the stark news of my Cancer diagnosis to me on that unforgettable day in 2004, and throughout my roughly 3-year-long ordeal with assorted aspects of Treatment, Recovery, and Aftercare, I maintained a daily journal in which I jotted down just about everything that took place during my Cancer journey that I thought to be of significance. This journaling process included my taking of notes during all of the meetings I had with members of my Medical Team and other health care providers, as I wanted to be sure that I had such information for historical and future reference purposes. Additionally, my daily journaling entries consisted of methodical explanations of the particulars of my actual treatments, including any Side Effects and my reactions to those; my emotional and physical states; the levels of pain I was experiencing (on a scale of 1 to 10+++); and the medications that I was prescribed to counter the pain. And, finally, my daily recordings included other information, including my nutritional regimen, calorie counts, body weights, and basic descriptions of my daily "highs and lows," etc.

During the many months of my Cancer journey, both during my Treatment and Recovery phases, the physicians on my Medical Team and other health care professionals provided me with a litany of hard copy materials pertaining to Cancer, Head and Neck Cancer, Cancer Treatment, Recovery, and Aftercare, Treatment Side Effects, nutrition, psychotherapy, and, many other topics relating to Cancer, coping with Cancer, and survivorship. Over nine years after I began receiving this considerable quantity of information from my doctors, capturing it in my extensive journaling notes, and assembling a large magnitude of ***non-copyrighted*** materials from government websites, I felt compelled to put pen to paper and write a book that may serve as an inspirational informational resource—a "one-stop-shop" if you will—for the benefit of those whose lives have been unduly beset by this terrible disease. This book that you are holding, ***Cancer Is One Big Pain-In-The-Neck!***, is a compilation of my Cancer experiences, and the information that I have gathered via those various sources.

While I have done my best to incorporate as much pertinent information in this book as I think will be informative and useful to the Reader, I did not want to provide so much that it would cause the individual to experience "information overload." The millions upon millions of websites on the Internet, and the numerous other books and materials available on the topic of Cancer, will do an extremely decent job of that on their own. Likewise, while I have attempted to apply responsible due diligence in conducting extensive research for much of the material contained herein, because I am just a "regular

Joe" Cancer survivor, and not a scientist, physician, or other health care professional, I have authored this book, and provided the results of my research, in easy-to-read, non-technical, everyday language. Other than my necessary references to common medical terms used in the scientific classifications and treatment of Cancer, the Reader will not find too much "medical-speak" contained within this book.

What the Reader *will* find in this book, however, is a basic introduction to the ubiquitous disease that is Cancer, and, additional information on Head and Neck Cancers, specifically, of which there are many unique forms. This book will also provide a brief synopsis of my own Head-and-Neck Cancer journey—from Diagnosis to me becoming a *Cancer-Free* Survivor—in which I disclose "insider" information on the subject of my Cancer Treatment preparations, the Treatments I received, the Side Effects I experienced, my Recovery and Aftercare outcomes, and things—both planned and unplanned, good, and not-so-good—that happened during these multiple phases of my Cancer journey. In this regard, I have included lessons that I learned during my Cancer experience, and, I have also provided my insight as to those actions that I would take differently, or, those that I would repeat, if I had to do it all over again *(no thanks!)*. Further, I make suggestions—based on good and poor experiences during my 3+-year journey—regarding what a patient might do to avoid many traps that I fell into, and/or, how they can take better control of their Cancer treatment, their recovery, their aftercare, and their outcome. Again, these are *my* own suggestions based on *my* experiences, and while they are offered for the patient's benefit, they are not meant to replace the medical advice of competent health care professionals.

As I mention multiple times within this book, much of the information incorporated within these pages is based upon my own journaling notes that I captured every single day during my 3+-year-long Head-and-Neck Cancer experience. Yes, no matter how crappy I felt—physically or mentally—I consistently took the time to write. That said, I did not make those daily journal notations so that I could one day author a book about my Cancer experience – truthfully, that was actually the last thing on my mind when I was keeping track of each of my day's activities, meeting outcomes, and so many actions related to my Cancer treatments and Side Effects. But, in retrospect, my copious and very comprehensive journal notes have provided me with the perfect foundation on which I could "build" a book; a book to hopefully assist others who might be feeling, thinking, worrying, and rejoicing, much the same as I did when I was walking the same challenging path a few short years ago. Not only did my journaling ***help me*** immensely during my own ordeal, but I can only hope that my notes will also ***benefit others*** via the words on these pages.

On the topic of journaling, because of my generally positive, helpful, note-taking experiences, I would heartily recommend that the Cancer patient keep a daily diary or a calendar to chronicle his or her feelings or thoughts of the day. Also, a personal Cancer Diary is a perfect mode to record the outcome of discussions with physicians during their conferences and others', of which there could be quite a few. Capturing important information on paper not only frees up the patient's already-burdened mind from having to remember the many details of each day's activities—thus alleviating any accompanying anxiety—but it also documents reference points from which one can measure their forward-progress and document any possible setbacks during their therapy, recovery, and aftercare. Moreover, and maybe most importantly, keeping a journal provides the patient with a very therapeutic experience by allowing them to express their feelings—positive or negative—in writing. I found that journaling was a great way of recording my thoughts—good and bad, happy and sad—and the perfect means of getting all my frustrations "off my chest" every day, so that I could attempt to *start each day with a clean, new slate.*

As I alluded to previously, my principal objective in writing this book is to provide the Reader—who could be a Cancer patient, a family member, or a Caregiver—with a resource that might help to empower and enlighten him, or her, or them. Specifically, with this book, it is my purpose to assist the patient and their family, and/or, Caregiver, in taking the following positive and responsible actions:

1) Becoming more knowledgeable about Cancer, and *their* form of Cancer, to learn what it is, and the best and safest ways to fight it
2) Making well thought-out decisions prior to, during, and after treatment, in conjunction with the Medical Team
3) God-willing, enjoying and building on the positive moments and successes that are so important, both physically and emotionally, during treatment and recovery, to forge a favorable outcome

4) Prompting the patient to ask questions of his or her health care providers that they may not have thought of, or asked, otherwise
5) Answering questions that the patient may have about a variety of issues related to the Cancer experience
6) Avoiding unforeseen pitfalls and obstacles, prior to, during, and after Treatment, Recovery, and Aftercare
7) Maximizing the useful application of newfound knowledge and best practices about Cancer treatment to the patient's benefit

The above seven objectives of this book being specified, it is understood that all Cancer patients differ from each other physically, mentally, emotionally, and spiritually, and, that their backgrounds and family histories are not the same. It is also totally apparent that each individual's race, Cancer type or location, and their physicians, treatment modalities, responses to treatment, and recoveries may not be similar. But, what all Cancer patients *do* share, and what I have attempted to capture within this book, are the similarities that *most* Cancer patients would come to anticipate following their diagnosis: That they should be able to acquire the finest, and the most effective and timely medical counsel, treatment, care, and outcome possible. As the factual saying goes, *"The devil is in the details."* and it is the details—such as the questions not asked nor answered, responsible due diligence not performed, or, a necessary action not taken by the patient or health care professional—that I am attempting to address and preclude with this work. With several things in life we only get one shot, so, *we had better make damn sure that single shot counts!*

As all Cancer patients will quickly realize after being blind-sided by the intimidating disease, one's experience with Cancer will test and challenge several things about them, not the least of which will be their mental strength, physical endurance, and, perhaps, even their religious faith and spiritual fortitude. But, this is not all a grim thing, because every Cancer patient—being a Human Being—has an intrinsic will to survive. However, while the predisposition to endure that which places a person in life-or-death circumstances does come naturally, the ability to survive a hazard is not necessarily automatic. Essentially, for lack of a better way of putting it, *the Cancer patient must want to survive*. And, in wanting to continue living, the Cancer victim should take any and all necessary steps that will enhance their chances of conquering their disease in the best shape possible. Make no mistake about it, ***all Cancers,*** no matter their forms, Stages, or locations within the body, are potentially deadly, and they should be swiftly and effectively addressed "as if there is no tomorrow." And, it is precisely because of this austere actuality that I have written this book in an honest endeavor to enlighten and inspire those unfamiliar with Cancer to do all they can to know it, battle it, and survive it.

With that in mind, and, from my perspective as the Author of this book, I will feel satisfied that this book has achieved its primary goal and has fulfilled its intended motive, if it has prompted *just one* Cancer patient or survivor to understand:

1) That he or she *should* make every proactive attempt to educate themselves as much as possible about the disease and the best Treatment(s) in their personal case to remove it from their body
2) That he or she *must* assume responsibility for their own Cancer treatment(s) and recovery, which may include being assertive in making requests of their Medical Team members
3) That he or she *should* obtain Second, Third, and, perhaps, Fourth Opinions from different physicians as circumstances may dictate (and from *outside* their HMO, with approval, if a member)
4) That he or she *must* conduct due diligence in the development of their Medical Team, and, as applicable, must "fire" those health care practitioners who do not provide the best, most professional and compassionate *(good "Bedside Manners")* service possible
5) That he or she *must* continue to ask questions, and must not take "no" for an answer. *"There is more than one way to skin a cat"*
6) That he or she *must* never stop learning and achieving corrective adjustments as necessary during Treatment and Recovery
7) That he or she *must never* discontinue battling their Cancer until it is vanquished; and, perhaps, most importantly:
8) That he or she *must always* have <u>Hope</u> that they will defeat their Cancer and Survive in the best, viable physical and mental shape

As you continue to read on in this book, you must know that *the information provided on these pages is meant to **supplement** the care and guidance of competent medical professionals. At no time do I, the Author, suggest that the information contained herein take the place of conventional medical treatment.* In all instances, do not attempt a self-diagnosis, and, do not embark upon self-treatment of a serious illness without seeking support and guidance from a trusted, qualified, medical professional. Today, there are a growing number of informed health care professionals who will work with patients to integrate the Body, Mind, and the Spirit into their Cancer Treatment, Recovery, and Aftercare Programs. Attempt to find these health care professionals and form healing partnerships with each. And, please rest reassured that the patient's Medical Team, in conjunction with the Cancer patient, their loved one, family, Guardian, and Caregiver, will establish a safe and effective Treatment and Recovery/Aftercare plan that is best-suited to the patient's specific needs.

Readers must also understand that the story and explanations of my personal Cancer journey that I've written within this book are an anthology of *my own experiences.* Please consider this important point, because, just as every individual is different from me, so, too, will their Cancers differ, as, possibly, will their Cancer treatment(s), their responses to their treatment(s), their possible Side Effects, and, the ultimate outcomes of their very personal Cancer experiences.

In late 2007, approximately three-and-a-half years after my Cancer diagnosis, a good friend of mine in Virginia who knew that I was a Cancer survivor asked me, *"What benefit, if any, do you think has come out of you getting Cancer? What I mean is – have there been any 'silver linings' to go along with the 'dark clouds?'"*

My friend posed two appropriate and introspective questions to me. I contemplated his inquiries and I thought for a few moments before responding. I then said to him, *"I learned a lot about myself, and I learned a lot about Cancer during my experience."*

"As for myself," I continued, *"I know now that I can't take my life or my good health for granted. I once thought that I was invincible because I took such great care of myself, but my Cancer made me well aware that 'just like that,' our lives can be yanked out from under us, no matter how healthy or strong we may be."*

Finally, I added, *"My Cancer made me realize that I must be grateful for, and make the most out of, every moment in life that I can." "Surviving Cancer,"* I told him, *"will force a person to think twice about life, and about everything and everyone in their life."*

Regarding my self-taught education about Cancer, I paused briefly to inwardly reflect. I then told my friend, *"During my entire Cancer experience, I did tons of research, and took notes every day for over three years about what I went through and what I learned."*

"One day," I continued, *"it would be my wish that I will be able to write a book about my experiences that will help others with Cancer, and give them hope during their own journeys. If I can do that,"* I concluded, *"everything I went through with my own Cancer will have been worth it."* This book, ***Cancer Is One Big Pain-In-The-Neck!,*** is that long-awaited wish of mine finally coming true.

Some Readers may wonder why it took me over 9 years after my diagnosis, and about 6 years after being told that I was *"Cancer-free,"* to write this book. The truthful answer is that I have actually been working away on a book about Cancer, and continuing to learn about Cancer, since 2005 – one year after my diagnosis. I've come up with no fewer than three partly finished manuscripts during that time, all of assorted book sizes and layouts, with different titles, and similar, but diverse objectives. Finally, with this book, as hefty as it may be, I've managed to squeeze everything between the covers that I've wanted to include for the benefit of others touched by this nasty medical menace. That is: general information about Cancer; specific information about Head and Neck Cancer; and, a summary of my own Head and Neck Cancer experience. That's 9 years well spent!

With these thoughts in mind, I must mention that it is not my intention with this book to profit money-wise from my own Cancer experience, or, from the misfortune of persons who have Cancer, or, who know someone who does. I am offering my thoughts from my own Cancer journey to others with the hope that me sharing what I experienced, endured, and learned during my Treatment, Recovery, and Aftercare, will assist all Cancer patients, Caregivers, family and friends to better understand, cope with, fight, and hopefully survive, this nasty, unwelcome disease that has abruptly invaded their lives.

If I am fortunate enough to sell any copies of this book, I can honestly say that I will donate the Royalties from book sales to one or more of the Childhood Cancer and Breast Cancer Research and Support Organizations to which I have already been contributing for many, many years. I feel a need to give back to others in return for all of the love, encouragement, prayers, and support that I received during my own protracted Cancer experience. If this book is able to "pay forward" to assist other Cancer patients and survivors in some small way, the proceeds I receive from the book will help yet others, and, it will also serve to repay the debt of gratitude I feel that I owe.

I will close by mentioning that the total prevention of Cancer is a very ambitious objective, and one for which both the scientific and medical communities are continually striving. Unfortunately, at this time, it does not exist, basically, because Cancer becomes all the more ruthless as time passes by, and, it seems to always be one step ahead of scientific capabilities and efforts to control and prevent its occurrence in human beings completely. Nonetheless, scientists will relentlessly endeavor to develop better and safer means of doing so.

Individual Cancers *are treatable and many can be eliminated from patients* if they are detected, identified, and treated early-on in the process. Considering the immense significance of early detection and treatment of Cancer in battling and beating the disease, it would be my desire that the Reader would endeavor to use the information throughout this entire book for the exact reasons that I have included it in these pages: To learn all that they can about their Cancer; to use what they have learned to steadfastly combat their Cancer and safely overcome any harmful Side Effects; and, most importantly, to defeat their Cancer and become a Survivor. There are several factors that must come together at the same time to produce Cancer, and, it takes just as many others, if not more, to fully remove it from our bodies.

Sir Francis Bacon, a Sixteenth Century Renaissance author and the Father of Deductive Reasoning, aptly avowed that, ***"Hope is the most beneficial of all the affections and doth much to the prolongation of life, it be not too often frustrated; but entertaineth the fancy with an expectation of good."*** From one fearless Cancer patient and Survivor to another, here is to hope, to the prolongation of life, and to an expectation of good!

May your Cancer journey be as lengthy as it needs to be, and your life as long as you want it to be. And, may this book hopefully help you in some small way to achieve both.

Cancer Is One Big Pain-In-The-Neck!

(And Many Other Body Parts)

What I Learned During My Three+-Year Head-and-Neck Cancer Journey From Diagnosis to "Cancer-Free" Survivor

"Cancer flies no flag and knows no bounds. It is a gluttonous pirate that travels the world and attacks six million each year who would cross in its path – young and old, rich and poor, and healthy and sick. But, this evil demon underestimates the courage, the faith, and the will of the Cancer Warrior. That, in the end, is what sinks its ship."

- Butch Sickler

Chapter One

Cancer 101 - Part 1 – *An Introduction to This Most Despicable Disease*

"The worst kind of enemy is indiscriminate, torturous, silent, deadly, devious, and concealed, and, although controllable at times, can never be completely conquered. So is Terrorism."

- Butch Sickler

As we all know, there are several things that we can do in our lives to control our own destinies and to reduce risks to our well-being, such as ***not*** jumping right in front of an oncoming train, *not* drinking and driving, and, *not* abusing our bodies with the multitude of ever-present temptations that exist. But, there are also many other acts—some of them random and uncontrollable—that can, likewise, impact our lives in an unfavorable way. For example, a strong wind could blow a huge tree down on a house, or, a person's genes could mutate, possibly due to heredity, advanced age, or a fragile Immune System compromised by multiple risk factors. The fallen tree may cause serious injury to the home's occupants, and, the mutated genes may result in the formation of irregular cells. These abnormal cells may, in turn, lead to the genesis of Cancer in a man, woman, teen, or young child. And just like that, a person's life can change forever.

"Good" Cells vs. "Evil" Cells

Very simply put, all Cancers begin in *cells*, the body's basic unit of life and the building blocks of all living things. At last count, the human body is comprised of approximately 75,000,000,000,000 (*trillion!)* cells of millions of different types. Normal cells grow and divide in a controlled way to produce more cells as they are needed to help keep the body healthy. When "everyday" cells become old or damaged, typically they die and are automatically replaced with new cells. Sometimes, however, this orderly process goes awry. In such cases, and with any unsafe internal or external catalysts, the genetic material (Deoxyribonucleic Acid (DNA)), that transmits instructions for all cell activities (both good and bad) can become damaged.

When the normal cells become "abnormal" or mutated due to any measure of causes and risk factors, the cellular DNA produces and replicates irregular mutations that affect normal cell growth and division. As a direct outcome, the mutated cells don't die when they should, and new, damaged, abnormal cells form when the body does not need them. Say *Hello* to Cancer. Cancer appears to occur when the growth of cells within the body is too fast and out of control, and when cells simply "forget" how to pass on. These "forgetful" Cancer cells do, however, know one thing for sure: They know how to feed, multiply, and spread within one's body, and they will continue to do so until they are stopped by a force much more powerful than they.

"Go Ahead – Make my Day"

During our lives, our bodies naturally produce thousands of abnormal, genetically faulted and mutating cells, all of which being brutally similar to the dastardly, no-good-for-nothing "Bad Guys" in any Hollywood portrayal of *"Good vs. Evil."* To take this cinematic comparison one step further, our bodies, equally, make White Blood Cells—our body's "Dirty Harry-esque" Good Guys—that typically patrol our bodily systems, 24 / 7 (even on holidays!), in an effort to detect and destroy any inward or outward threats that they sense to our health and well-being. This "dragnet" includes, by the way, the White Blood Cells' efforts to subdue genetically altered, potentially cancerous cells. Occasionally, however, despite the valiant efforts of our body's "Cops" to ward off attackers, our immunological defense systems become vulnerable and permit the "villains" to move on in. Certainly, all of us have experienced this when we have caught the Common Cold, or come down with the Flu or other minor illnesses.

Unfortunately, though, just as with real-life malcontents, not all bodily "Bad Guys" come and go after inciting negligible damage.

Some "terroristic" bodily trespassers put down roots, cover up out of sight, and wreak as much mayhem as possible until they are stopped. The name that *this* rebellious gang goes by is, *"Cancer."* Should an individual happen to have a destabilized Immune System that could have been compromised by one or more environmental or other risk factors, the mutating Cancer cells may find conditions perfect within the body to break into one or more of the person's bodily systems to form Primary Tumors. From these "Cancer hubs," rogue cancerous cells could begin spreading through the person's Circulatory (blood) and Lymphatic (Lymph Node) Systems, and, then, may metastasize, or establish colonies, in other areas and organs of the body. And, as if that's not enough, one's age, inherited Cancer genes, and "random chance," can also play a role in causing the formation of the disease.

Cancer's Insatiable Appetite

Almost every tissue within our bodies gets blood from small capillaries that intertwine throughout each of our internal systems. It is through these tiny capillaries *(country roads)* in our Circulatory Systems *(Interstate hiways)* that life-sustaining nutrients (vitamins, minerals, fats, proteins, sugars, oxygen, chemicals, etc.), and other critical elements disperse into our cells. These ongoing mechanisms typically maintain our health, fight off diseases, and they permit our bodies to flourish, develop, and heal themselves. In essence, these critical, blood-delivering systems are an imperative network of "life lines," upon which our vital organs and other bodily systems depend to remain strong and properly function. In a healthy man, woman, or child where *all systems are go,* the individual's body and mind will normally operate at optimum, functional, and life-sustaining levels – naturally – as a matter of course. However, the moment that Cancer is thrown into the mix, the affected bodily systems and organs may slowly begin to lose their functionality. Ultimately, if the Cancer is not quickly and properly addressed, they will shut-down altogether.

Cancer Tumors have their beginnings without any dedicated vascular (blood) circulation to sustain them. In their initial stages of development, the tumors are limited to nutrients that they can "rob" from any nearby capillaries. At a specific time after their formation, however, these parasitic tumors begin to stimulate healthy tissues to generate thousands of new blood vessels to maintain the cancerous growth itself. This process, along with Cancer's insatiable appetite for Glucose (body blood sugar), is what enables Cancer to succeed. Without the capability to nourish itself and develop, a Tumor cannot enlarge. If the blood supplies can be minimized or cut off, the tumor will shrink or die. Unfortunately, however, all too often, because of the unremitting, voracious cravings of Cancer cells, just the opposite occurs: The greedy Cancer cells continue to take and take from the healthy tissue, thus starving it of the life-sustaining nutrients that ***it*** needs to live. The result, of course, is tissue death. This devastating outcome perfectly justifies the constant battle-cry for early detection and appropriate treatment: ***Kill the Cancer before it kills you!***

Garden Weeds and Cancer – A Comparison of Two "No-Good-for-Nothing" Invaders

Our dear old friend, Sir Francis Bacon, the Sixteenth Century English philosopher, statesman, scientist, lawyer, jurist, author and pioneer of the *Scientific Method,* was once quoted as remarking, *"A man's nature runs either to herbs, or to weeds; therefore, let him seasonably water the one, and destroy the other."* Indubitably, Mr. Bacon was referring to the desirability of one vegetative form of life over another—nourishing, visibly appealing, aromatic, palpable, and edible *Herbs*, vs. determinedly invasive, objectionable, irksome, and potentially harmful *Weeds*—but, his words could also aptly apply to another appalling organism that can flourish where it's not welcome: ***Cancer.*** Yes, the premise espoused by Mr. Bacon for the salvation of desirable plants, while simultaneously removing unpleasant ones, would also equate to the protection of the healthy bodily tissues of a Cancer patient by very cautiously eliminating the destructive Cancer presence from its human host. Both are delicate processes, indeed.

To Better Understand Noxious Cancer, Consider Obnoxious Weeds

Keeping in mind that Cancer is an exceedingly merciless and potentially deadly disease, and that the common, everyday weed, is, for the most part, merely, an unwelcome, unsightly, and sometimes, pricey annoyance, it might assist the Reader—who may be new to a

Cancer occurrence—to better understand Cancer by comparing it to the "garden-variety" weed, with which they may be more familiar.

With that in mind, weeds and Cancer, when looking at their bare essentials, do have quite a lot in common with one another. For example, let's consider the fact that both can, and do—unprovoked and unsolicited—overrun, overwhelm, and suppress fertile earth or perfectly healthy body tissue, respectively. Additionally, they both will rob life-sustaining nutrients from the earth or human body to the potential detriment of the desirable vegetation or healthy body tissue already situated in-place; they both will continue forming, growing, reproducing, and spreading, unhindered, unless they are stopped and removed by some outside force, be it natural, physical, chemical, or otherwise; they both can induce either temporary or permanent harm to the vigorous, pleasing plant life, or, to the healthy bodily systems with which they are closely associated; and, finally, they both will occasionally be deadly to the very hosts upon which they depend for their own sustenance and life support. Basically, they're suicidal.

Weeds and Cancer: Similarities in Occurrence, Spread, Treatment, and Removal

To take the likenesses of garden weeds and Cancer one step further, just think about this: Both weeds and Cancer can spring up when many conditions are favorable to support their emergence and growth. For example, weeds can occur almost anywhere *(seemingly growing out of solid concrete, in 100° temperatures, with no water for months!),* while Cancer can form in almost any tissue in the body if the Immune System is weakened, and, if one or more risk factors come into play. As for their spreading, weeds can relocate from one plant to other areas via seeds scattered by the wind, swept away in water, or on the fur or in the waste of animals and birds. Cancer, on the other hand, can metastasize from the Primary Tumor site to other areas of the body by being carried through the patient's Circulatory (blood) or Lymphatic Systems. In either case, as haphazard as the process of seed dissemination in weeds and the metastasis of Cancer cells in Human Beings may seem to the unaware, both processes, by nature, are very systematic and *extremely good* at what they do. One Law of Nature states, *"The Fittest Will Survive."* How true it is.

Finally, both obnoxious weeds and noxious Cancers can be treated and hopefully destroyed through some curiously comparable methods. Specifically, both weeds and most Cancers can usually be controlled and eliminated through physical removal (hoeing/pulling or Surgery); chemical annihilation (herbicides and Chemotherapy); and, through the use of intense heat (propane torches and Radiation Therapy). But, while weeds and Cancer may be alike in some ways, they do have one extremely important distinction: Whereas weeds are usually just a royal pain-in-the-ass, Cancer, in all of its varieties, can be royally painful to the patient's entire body, and, regrettably, can sometimes be lethal. So, just as weeds should be tended-to early in the Spring in an effort to control and prevent their further growth, reproduction, and spread, so too, is it critical to the patient that any Cancer be detected, identified, and treated, as quickly as possible.

Cancer Causes and Risk Factors

In today's pressure-packed, industrialized, and quickly-paced world, it is no shocker that the integrity of our Immune Systems is often compromised, and that diseases such as Cancer are allowed to establish a foothold. Ironically, this lapse can occur despite our best efforts to strengthen and fortify our Immune Systems by indulging only in healthful, non-risky habits, but, that is surely a rarity. Ruling out inheritance or random chance when it comes to Cancer invading our healthy tissues, there is absolutely no shortage of other reasons why our Immune Systems—and thus our bodily systems—become weak and especially vulnerable to attack by Cancer and lots of other diseases. And, unfortunately, there is also no deficiency of Cancers that can develop in humans due a variety of causes and risk factors. Likewise, there is certainly no lack of humans on which it can prey.

Cancer: A Medical "Perfect Storm"

There are well-over 200 known varieties of Cancer, and they can materialize in any type of body tissue, no matter the age, sex, or other factors affecting each individual that Cancer chooses to serve as its host. However, per www.cancer.gov, a Cancer that affects one body tissue may not affect another. For example, non-smokers that breathe in others' risky second-hand tobacco smoke may prompt the formation of Lung Cancer in the non-smoker. And, a person that's overexposing their skin to the sun could result in the development of a Melanoma (Skin Cancer) on the person's body. But, the sun won't necessarily cause Lung Cancer, and smoking won't unilaterally lead to Melanoma. With this being said, there is typically not one single cause of Cancer. Cancer, like many other illnesses, may result from the interactions of numerous risk factors, all coming together in the same person, place, and time. For lack of a better way of putting it, a Cancer occurrence is the medical equivalent of a, *"Perfect Storm."*

Many forms of Cancer are preventable, but a person would have to have a pretty good idea of what causes Cancer, and what the risk factors are, to know to steer clear of them. Also, several Cancer risk factors can be avoided, thus reducing the likelihood of a person developing the disease. But, each individual's habits, lifestyles, job requirements, work or play environments, and other factors, all-too-often clash with these "preventive" measures. So, when considering Cancer risk factors, it is also very important to understand that while some Cancer risk factors are controllable and can be avoided, others, such as one's age, their genetic family history, and, random chance, are not, and can not. In this day and age, with the multiple things in this world to which we are all (over)exposed, it would be extremely difficult for a person to dodge 100% of all potential Cancer causes. That being said, the secret to effective Cancer prevention is that all individuals, young and old, male and female, should attempt to ***steer clear of as many risk factors as possible*** in their daily lives.

Cancer Risk Factors – "The Cards That Life Deals Us"

According to the National Institutes for Health (NIH) and the National Cancer Institute (www.cancer.gov), following are some of the causes of Cancer (in no particular order) and their associated risk factors, most of which, if avoided, could help to reduce one's risk of contracting Cancer. For the millions of existing Cancer patients and Cancer survivors, steering well-clear of the following Cancer risk factors may help to prevent a recurrence of the survivors' respective diseases, or, might preclude completely new Cancers from forming:

- **Use of tobacco (including smoking, dipping, chewing, etc.)**

- **Getting older** ***(Sorry, but not too much we can do about this one – "age happens!")***
- **Poor oral (dental) hygiene**
- **Exposure to sunlight (without protection)**
- **Exposure to some viruses (i.e., HPV), and bacteria**
- **Certain hormones**
- **A family history of Cancer** ***(Sorry again, but we can't choose our own birth parents or ancestors – at least not yet!)***
- **Use (or abuse) of alcoholic beverages**
- **Poor diet, lack of physical activity, and/or, being overweight**
- **Environmental factors such as exposure to radiation, certain chemicals, pollutants, asbestos, etc.**
- **Random chance** ***(i.e., Good ole' fashioned, "Shit happens")***

☛***Authors Note:*** If a person believes that they may be at risk for developing Cancer due to some of the aforementioned or other risk factors, they should discuss their concerns with their doctor or health care provider. There also are innumerable other professional medical resources available today that can educate individuals about ways to decrease their Cancer risk factors. Likewise, services are available through medical facilities and organizations that promote a proactive approach to Cancer detection through regular medical checkups, and thru the utilization of Cancer screening tests such as Mammograms for women, and the Prostate Specific Antigen (PSA) exam for men. The participation of women and men in these two Cancer screening programs has had a noteworthy outcome on the lives of those many individuals whose Cancers were found because of the testing. Early identification of the disease leads to quicker therapy, which, in-turn, can make these patients' Breast Cancers and Prostate Cancers much more treatable and survivable. In fact, there are well over 2.5 million women and 2 million men alive in the U.S. today as a result of their Cancers being discovered earlier with these screening tests. Dentists and Oral Surgeons are trained, as well, to recognize signs of Cancer, so regular oral exams are also crucial in the identification of disease.

Random Chance and Cancer

Let's assume that a person somehow manages to steer clear of all of the primary Cancer risk factors through their life, including each of those referenced previously, with the exception of their age and heredity, which they cannot control *(at least, not as I write this in 2013!).* Now, if such a person was fortunate enough to be able to do this (which, by the way, would be virtually impossible), it would logically mean that they might have a 100% likelihood of avoiding Cancer completely – correct? Well, perhaps in a perfect world. But this is life, and, as we all know, life always seems to have a wildcard of some sort hidden up its sleeve. In the case of Cancer, that devious Wildcard is none other than *Random Chance* – otherwise known as *"Shit happens."* Some people will win the Lottery thanks to random chance, while others develop Cancer due to random chance. Just my luck! – I would be in that latter group, along with countless others.

The concept of "Random Chance" can be loosely defined as a state in which there may be a number of potential outcomes for a given situation, some of which that are likely, some of which that are unlikely, and one of which that will ultimately transpire, despite, any other factors or influences. The mathematics of probability will often be used in predicting, but not determining, the outcome of a random event. Applying Random Chance to adult women and their incidence of Breast Cancer as an example, per www.cancer.gov, over 70% of women with Breast Cancer have ***absolutely no risk factors at all, other than being female.*** The other 30% might exhibit one or more Cancer risk factors, ***but so do millions of other women that never get Breast Cancer.*** In these specific instances and numerous others like it, we will most likely have Random Chance to thank (or blame?) for this irrational inconsistency. But then, of course, all of us have heard the stories about someone's "Uncle Charley," who has guzzled moonshine every day since he was 14 years old, or, another person's Grandmother who has smoked 5 packs of cigarettes per day since she was a young teenager – and they both lived to be over 100 years old! Please, whatever you do, don't try to figure out this *Game of Chance called Life.* Believe me, it *will* drive you crazy.

Sorry - The "Smoking Gun" Doesn't Exist

If you have been diagnosed with Cancer, or if a loved one or a friend have been confirmed by medical laboratory testing to have malignant Cancer, it is relatively possible that your Cancer, or theirs, may have developed over time as an outcome of one or more of the aforementioned Cancer causes and risk factors. While reviewing the information in this Chapter, perchance you remembered and became aware of a singular incident or multiple occurrences during your life that may have put you in harm's way from a Cancer standpoint. In some circumstances, a person may believe that they can estimate the approximate times and places that specific Cancer risk factors could have come into play. The truth of the matter, however, is that there may be no definite way of determining the exact cause of a person's weakened immune state that may have precipitated their Cancer. In these circumstances, any endeavors to search for the "smoking gun" can be futile, frustrating, and speculative at best. In some instances in Life—with this being one—it's just best to *let sleeping dogs lie.*

Definitely, one need only take a look at young, innocent, and otherwise healthy children who have been diagnosed with Cancer to wonder how, when, and why their infant Immune Systems may have become compromised. This is particularly disconcerting when one considers the fact that these babies, and youngsters and teens, have most likely had very little, if any, exposure to many of the unhealthy environmental or lifestyle threats that adults might have encountered during their much longer lives. Environmental causes of childhood Cancer have long been suspected by several scientists, but have been difficult to pin down, partly because Cancer in children is rare, and also because it is very difficult to quantify previous exposure levels in children, particularly during potentially important periods such as pregnancy, or, even prior to conception. The worst irony here is that these young Cancer victims' Immune Systems must first be exposed to life's many risky impurities—including Cancer—before they can develop any sort of resistance to them. This is one more example of another "Catch 22" situation that Life has chosen to lob our way.

A Suppressed Immune System –The Weak Link

It is a scientifically well-known and medically proven reality that an individual's weakened immunological state is the "lowered drawbridge" that allows Cancer to enter one's "castle." But, despite many years of science behind Cancer research, per www.cancer.gov, doctors and medical scientists often cannot decipher why one person will develop Cancer and another does not, ***even when they are both exposed to identical risk factors.*** However, research *does* noticeably indicate that certain risk factors can significantly increase a person's chances of developing the disease. While various Cancer risk factors are avoidable, some, such as one's age, race, and genetics, are not.

All Cancers form as a disease at the cellular level within the body. When a cell's Deoxyribonucleic Acid (DNA) (which contains a cell's genetic guidelines) becomes damaged by influences such as ultraviolet radiation, toxins, pollutants, or other risk factors, the cell will often enter a senescent state (it stops dividing as people age) as a precautionary measure against the cancerous growth that can result from such damage. A healthy Immune System will normally remove dormant cells from tissues. But as a person ages, their tiring Immune Systems begin to falter in the fight against these "cellular zombies." As a consequence, senescent cells begin to accumulate in the older person's body, gaining strength in numbers. Then, you guessed it.

DNA – Can't Live With it - Can't Live Without it

Normal human cells replicate or divide in a very predictable manner. But, normal cells in which the DNA has been damaged due to internal or external stimulus can become cancerous and undergo cellular division in a very random and uncontrollable fashion. These cells are termed "genetically mutant." A person produces thousands of mutant cells during their life that could, potentially, be cancerous. In a majority of these situations, however, the individual's vigorous Immune System, which is comprised of millions of protective White Blood Cells, is there to fortify the body and to attack and destroy the invaders before they have an opportunity to gain any traction and do damage to healthy tissue. However, if, due to environmental factors or other reasons, the body's Immune System has become weakened, the renegade Cancer cells could find just the window of opportunity that they need to exploit the vulnerability and to take up residence in one or more of any dozens of potential sites within a person's body.

Dr. Otto Warburg, a two-time Nobel Prize recipient for his research work with human cells, discovered that Cancerous cells are damaged in their chemical makeup—compared to healthier normal cells—and that they feed on the fermentation of Blood Sugar known as Glucose, which is where these cells get all of their energy. If left unchecked by the body's Immune System, a solitary Cancerous cell will multiply independently and soon get out of control. Some of the unchallenged cells will gather to form localized tumors, while others will be carried by the Circulatory or Lymphatic Systems to different parts of the body to form colonies of secondary tumors known as Metastases. All of this occurs without the person having any idea.

Cancer - An "Inside Job"

Regarding the modes and means of Cancer, perhaps Virginia Livingston-Wheeler, MD., author of the ***Conquest of Cancer***, put it best when she wrote, "Cancer is a disease of the Immune System. Or, more accurately, it is a disease of a weak Immune System. Your immunity must drop to a very low level before Cancer can grow, and when it drops to an extremely low and weak level, the Cancer cells start to spread. Your body has no defense against them, or what small defense it has is not enough." Despite the numerous inherent safeguards found within our bodies (i.e., White Blood Cells) that are supposed to defend our bodies against "all enemies, both foreign and domestic," Cancer incidence statistics indicate that cancerous cells, still, are able to successfully compromise the immunological defense systems of over 6 million people worldwide on an annual basis. As life would have it, there are countless risk factors that can contribute to destabilized immunological circumstances in an individual, which could then lead to that person developing some form of Cancer.

If you, or a loved one, or a friend, have been diagnosed with Cancer and are part of this select group of Cancer victims, there is a very strong possibility that one or more causes and risk factors may have played a part in the formation of your or their Cancers. Minus any remembrance of a direct exposure to manmade or environmental toxins, deadly bacteria, or noxious viruses, and, ruling out any links to inherited cancerous genes, there may be a possibility that Random Chance *("shit happens,")*, may also come into play as a contributing factor leading to the development of one's disease. Quite honestly, it would be extremely difficult for an individual with Cancer to be able to pin down, with any certainty, how, when, and why their Immune System was compromised to permit the occurrence of Cancer. It *is* safe to say, however, that if opportunistic Cancer sees an opening, it will sometimes take it, much to the bewilderment of the individual, and, despite the health state of the person's immunological defenses.

Good-to-Know Cancer Facts

Over time, numerous risk factors may operate together, or by themselves, to spur healthy, normal cells to mutate and then become cancerous. However, when considering Cancer risk factors, one may want to think about the following scientifically proven facts, which I have adapted from the National Cancer Institute, (www.cancer.gov):

- ***Having one or more risk factors does not mean that a person will automatically develop Cancer. And, a person <u>not</u> having risk factors does not mean that they will <u>not</u> develop Cancer.*** So, that makes it clear: It's darned if you do, darned if you don't
- Cancers can be caused by *by-products of our own body's normal processes* known as ***Free Radicals.*** Free Radicals are extremely reactive, natural, oxygen-free compounds that our bodies create during normal bodily functions (think of them as the detrimental exhaust produced by a lawn mower). The unstable Free Radical molecules can damage important cell proteins and enzymes, and can even cause DNA changes at the cellular level that can result in the formation of Cancer. ***Antioxidants,*** though, interact with, and stabilize, Free Radicals, and may prevent some of the injury Free Radicals might otherwise cause. Examples of Antioxidants include Beta-carotene, Vitamins C, E, and A, some Amino Acids herbs and mushrooms, Lycopene, Selenium, and Bioflavonoids
- Not everything in life causes Cancer (despite what it may seem), but some people are more sensitive than others to known Cancer risk factors, and thus are at greater risk of developing the disease
- Cancer is not caused by an injury, such as a bump, bruise, skin cut, abrasion, puncture, broken bone, burns, or other *boo-boos*
- Cancer is not contagious. However, being infected with certain viruses or bacteria *may increase the risk* of some types of Cancer through sexual or further human contact. But, speaking literally, no one can "catch," or give, Cancer, from, or to, another person
- Most people who have Cancer risk factors never develop Cancer because their Immune Systems (White Blood Cells) are healthy and sufficiently robust enough to identify and destroy any threats

to the body before they have an opportunity to move in and take hold. In other words, the person's Immune System will, "raise the drawbridge" before the Cancer can "cross the moat"

Types of Cancer and Tumors

Cancer is not just a single disease, per se. Actually, the term "Cancer" constitutes several diseases, of which there are *more than 200 known varieties* that have been identified to-date. Most Cancers are named for the organ, system, or cell-type where they begin. For example, Cancer that develops in the Colon is called Colon Cancer; Breast Cancer first forms in the Breast, etc. The type of Cancer with which I was diagnosed was categorically termed as a *Head and Neck Cancer.* Medically speaking, however, my particular form of Cancer was classified as *"Cancer at the Base of the Tongue,"* because that's where the Primary Tumor was located, even though the Cancer had spread to, and metastasized in, the Lymph Nodes in my neck.

Cancer types are, in general, grouped into broader categories, which are typically based on the organs, tissues, systems, or the cells in which they originate. According to the National Cancer Institute, www.cancer.gov, the main categories of Cancer are:

- **Carcinoma** - Cancer that begins in the skin or in tissues that line or cover internal organs *(This is the type of Cancer that I had)*
- **Sarcoma** - Cancer that commences in bone, fat, blood vessels, cartilage, muscle, or other connective and supportive tissues
- **Leukemia** - Cancer that starts in blood-forming tissue such as in the Bone Marrow, and induces large numbers of abnormal blood cells to be produced and to enter the Circulatory System
- **Lymphoma** and **Myeloma** - Cancers that form in the cells of the Immune and Lymphatic Systems
- **Central Nervous System Cancers** - Cancers that develop in the tissues of the Brain and the Spinal Cord

Some Cancers do not create actual tumors, but materialize in other tissues. For example, Leukemias are Cancers of the Blood and Bone Marrow. And, Tumors can be either Benign (non-Cancerous), or Malignant (Cancerous). Following are their descriptions:

- **Benign Tumors** – Benign Tumors are not cancerous. They can usually be removed, and, in most cases, they will not come back. Cells in benign tumors do not spread to other parts of the body

- **Malignant Tumors** – Malignant Tumors are cancerous. Cells in these tumors can invade adjacent tissues and can migrate to, and metastasize in, other bodily locations via the Lymphatic (Lymph Node) System and the Circulatory or Vascular (blood) System

Most Frequent Cancer Diagnoses

Of the approximate six million individuals globally that will be diagnosed with Cancer in 2013, it is estimated that more than 1.7 million of them will be American men, women, and children. And, included within those anticipated 1.7 million U.S. Cancer diagnoses, could be ten (10) Cancers (excluding Non-melanoma Skin Cancers) that Studies point out may be diagnosed with greater frequency than others. According to the U.S. Cancer Incidence Statistics developed and published by the National Cancer Institute (www.cancer.gov), the most common "adult" Cancers that are predicted to be diagnosed in the United States in 2013 are (*in alphabetical order*):

Bladder Cancer
Breast Cancer
Colon and Rectal Cancer
Endometrial Cancer
Kidney (Renal Cell) Cancer
Leukemia
Lung Cancer
Melanoma
Non-Hodgkin's Lymphoma
Pancreatic Cancer
Prostate Cancer
Thyroid Cancer

<u>Out-of-the-Ordinary Symptoms to be Watchful For</u>

When a man, woman, teen or child feels, sees, or senses that something new, and/or, abnormal, is taking place either within or on their body, and/or, if that abnormality persists for an unusual period of time, hopefully, that person will take it upon themselves to go get medical attention at the earliest possible time. According to the U.S. Government National Cancer Institute, (www.cancer.gov), *unusual and unexplained* symptoms that could be caused by Cancer include:

- Severe chest pain
- Shortness of breath (*not* caused by exercise)
- New, localized pain in the body
- Onset of chills or fever
- Swelling of Lymph Nodes or other areas
- Continuous fatigue
- Lack of function of certain body parts
- Unplanned, unwanted weight loss
- New lack of appetite
- General malaise or pessimism about life
- New skin growth, rash
- Blood in the stool

Cancer and the Family Tree

We all know the maxim, *"The apple doesn't fall far from the tree,"* or, we have heard someone described as a, *"Chip off the old block,"* or, being, *"Cut from the same piece of cloth."* As many of us can most likely relate simply by observing ourselves and our own families, some things we inherit from Mom and Dad are wonderful, while others—such as our big schnoz, our bald head, or God-forbid, a propensity to develop Cancer—we can all most likely live without. That said, "inheritance" is what it is, and, as I write this in 2013, no one—with the probable exception of Hollywood screenwriters—has figured out a mode for children to pre-select their biological parents, or, to be conceived *without any parents at all.* Until that capability exists, every person's risk of contracting some variety of Cancer will continue to be influenced to some extent by their genetic make-up.

In rare instances whereby certain hereditary influences might provoke a cancerous response, something may happen to chemically modify the genetic programming of a normal cell, thereby disrupting its harmony with the rest of the body. According to the words of Dr. Otto Warburg—the two-time Nobel Prize recipient for his research with human cells—"Cancerous cells have lost all of their genetically programmed instructions, therefore becoming genetically faulted. These genetically-mutated cells no longer know how to contribute properly to the body of which they are a part. The only property these cells retain is the useless one of growth." As the genetically-faulted Cancer cells divide and attach themselves to the body's vital organs, the healthy tissues become oxygen- and nutrient-starved, the organ shuts down, and the inevitable can possibly occur.

Cells and Genes "Gone Wild"

Each individual has two copies of each *Gene* (and, we're not talking *denim*) – one from each parent. Basically, genes contained in a person's *DNA* are the "blueprints," that program our cells, and thus our bodies, to grow-up, develop, and function in specific, distinctive ways throughout our lives. Every cell envelopes these exact copies, which, throughout the *normal* development and division phases of cellular replication tells them exactly what to become. For example, a blood cell becomes another blood cell, or a muscle cell replicates into another muscle cell, and so-on within the body. This process of cellular division, which, incidentally, is known as *Mitosis,* transpires millions of times each day and night without us having the slightest clue that it is taking place. Now, that's what I call efficiency!

When changes, called mutations, occur in the cell as a result of internal or external risk factors that hold back our body's Immune System defenses, *this can prompt certain cells to, literally, grow out of control.* Per www.cancer.gov, mutations or abnormal cells occur when a part of the gene in the person's DNA is damaged and cannot be repaired. These cells then multiply themselves (think *Copy and Paste)* and do not die. In Hereditary Cancer, the person has inherited the mutation from either one of their parents. If one of the genes is already damaged due to inheritance, this may cause the person to be at higher Cancer risk, or, in medical-speak, "genetically susceptible" to developing Cancer. However, just because a person has damaged inherited genes doesn't necessarily mean that it is automatic that he or she will develop, or be diagnosed with, Cancer. There have been *countless cases of people in multiple generations of Cancer-stricken families who have lived their entire life without ever receiving the fateful diagnosis of Cancer.* Can anyone say, ***"Random Chance?"***

Cancers Linked to Heredity

Not all 200 forms of Cancer are hereditary (thankfully), but genetic experts are beginning to see a pattern in various Cancers. Per most recent Studies conducted by the U.S. National Cancer Institute (www.cancer.gov), it is now believed that "moderate risk" or "low-risk" genes might be responsible for Cancer in families where there are fewer cases or where the disease skips generations. These genes could be guilty of contributing to Cancer without an apparent family history. Recent Studies indicate that a small number of Cancers (5-10%) are caused by faulty genes in children that were inherited from one or the other parent. These genetically-faulted cells will increase the risk of their offspring developing certain types of Cancer.

Inherited faulty genes that can cause occurrences of Cancer in successive generations of a family are rare, and are referred to as "high risk" genes. Scientists have acknowledged many of the "high-risk" faulty genes that can be so uncomforting to some families. Per www.cancer.gov, those genes can produce familial Breast, Thyroid, Ovarian, and Colorectal Cancers. It is estimated that roughly 10% to 15% of Breast, Ovarian, and Colorectal Cancers are the result of hereditary risk factors. Melanoma Skin Cancer also sometimes runs in families. Having two or more direct relatives who have had this form of disease is a risk factor. About 10 percent of all patients with Melanoma have had a family member that has been diagnosed with this type of the disease. ***When Melanoma Cancer runs in a family, all family members should be checked regularly by a doctor.***

Heredity Happens – Don't Blame Mom or Dad

With over one-and-a-half million Cancer diagnoses of men, women, and children anticipated annually within the U.S. in 2013, it stands to reason that dozens of risk factors—such as those specified by the National Cancer Institute (www.cancer.gov), and referenced elsewhere in this Book—will contribute in some means or another to the weakening and compromise of these individuals' immunological system. And, when that happens, the absence of a speedy and deadly immune response by their White Blood Cells *(They've gone fishin')* to the cancerous menace may ultimately help contribute to the cause and development of these people's respective Cancers. Somewhere in this extensive mixture of individuals, Cancer types, and causative factors, will be a relatively small number of cases (5-10%), in which genetic inheritance may end up playing a role in the incidence of the disease. In any case, there probably will be no way of knowing for sure if a person has inherited a genetic predisposition for Cancer.

Children will inherit countless genes from both parents that will dictate several developmental factors within each child in the family – some that are similar within any of their siblings and some that are not. We need only to look within our own families to realize in some situations, that, indeed, *"The apple doesn't fall far from the tree."* Whether it is in the contour of our nose, the color of our eyes, the appearance of our bodies, or, in the ways we walk, talk, perform, speak, or live our life in general, there are indeed some unmistakable habits, appearances, behaviors, and other factors that genetically link us—for better or for worse—to good ole' Ma and Pa.

In some situations, however, children from the same parents will look, act, and develop surprisingly differently than their parents or any of their siblings. How and why these disparities transpire is a function of genetics, *or the Postman (sorry, that's my futile attempt at humor),* and the frequency or regularity with which dominant and recessive genes will manifest themselves in members of family from generation to generation. You may have always wondered why you are the only one who got Great-Grandma's bright blue eyes!

Mom, and/or, Dad, may also pass along genetically mutated Cancer cells to the children as part of the entire inheritance package. But, there is obviously nothing that they can do to prevent this from occurring, short of the parents not having any children in the first place. If you are an individual who has been diagnosed with Breast, Ovarian, Thyroid, Colorectal, and/or Melanoma Cancer, and, if your Mother and/or Father, had been diagnosed before with one of these Cancers, there is a possibility—based on scientific verification—that your Cancer ***could*** be the result of a hereditary link, in combination with other risk factors. But, please do keep in mind, that inheritance also ***may not*** be the guilty party, so please don't hold Mom or Dad responsible for "giving" you Cancer. They *did* give you life, and the last thing they would want to do would be to subject you to anything that would cause you any pain and suffering. Well, that's with the possible exception of dear ole Dad wearing his plaid Bermuda shorts with black dress shoes and white socks on a family outing in public. In that case, you *do* have a right to feel just a little uncomfortable!

Children and Cancer

Where is it written that blameless, untainted young children *must* suffer much of the same fate with Cancer, as do adults, most of whom have been exposed to several of life's destructive health risks during their much longer lives? And, just where does it state that a wholesome, passionate older child or teenager who is just gathering speed on his or her expedition through life, *must* have their forward progress brought to a screeching halt by this destructive, dangerous disease? Well, unfortunately and pragmatically, it is all right there, documented in the proverbial *"Handbook of Life."* That's correct. In stark black and white, the "book of life's rules" states very clearly, that no human being, regardless of their age, size, gender, religious preference, ethnicity, health condition, education level, employment position, looks, or, their social, political, or economic status, will be excused from contracting Cancer, or, any other medical condition, if all circumstances are favorable for such an occurrence, and, if it is meant to be. Unfortunately, this exact rule-of-life also applies to all children—young and old, girl and boy—even if that person happens to be a fragile one-year old boy, a 19-year-old girl, or, any youngster in between. It certainly isn't right, but, regrettably, it is what it is.

Life Interrupted

The dreadful reality of childhood Cancer is that it *does* strike approximately 1 out of every 300 children in the U.S. before the age of 19, according to www.cancer.gov. When the Cancer patient is a young child or teenager, the family's life as they knew it, will all but cease after the diagnosis has been delivered. Parents will need to be away from work, the child patient will have to leave school, siblings might be separated from one another, and, the family's days may be packed with one appointment after another – for weeks, months, or years on-end. For lack of a better means of putting it, a diagnosis of Cancer in a child will quickly turn the family's world upside-down.

For the parent(s) or Caregivers of children with Cancer, the diagnosis will be altogether shocking and numbing. Parents, family members, friends, classmates, and those who know the child or teen may become frightened and bewildered upon hearing the news. And, although a childhood Cancer diagnosis may originally seem to bring life to a standstill for people closest to the affected child, important decisions *do need to be made quickly by the parent(s), Guardian or Caregiver,* about the childhood Cancer patient's treatment and care.

If the parents don't want to agree to the child's or teenager's Cancer diagnosis, or, if they react to it by retreating into denial or by getting irritated, questioning their spiritual faith, feeling betrayed by life, or, by doing all of the above, that is just fine – these are normal first reactions and defense mechanisms that can help parents cope with the initial surprise of such an alarming revelation. But, parents should also be well aware of the fact that their child's Cancer, being what it is, will require them to respond quickly to the situation, and to take positive medical action on the child's behalf. Accepting the facts of the situation, and, reacting to the child's Cancer diagnosis—sooner rather than later—will greatly enhance their child's chances for a successful Cancer treatment experience and overall outcome.

In a Child's Perfect World **...**

In some children's perfect world, puffy, fluffy white clouds would be made of cotton candy, mountains would be molded of ice cream, and chocolate-syrup rivers would flow in the valleys below. To other kids, youngsters or teenagers, their ideal life might include never-ending days full of video games, candy, soccer, music, sodas, bicycles, texting, toy trucks, movies, popcorn, hanging out with their "BFFs," awesome rides at the carnival, and, of course, sharing fun, loving, and exciting times with Mom, Dad and their family. And, then, for still many other children—especially those living in some impoverished nations—their thoughts of fulfillment may be defined, simply, by them and their family members having ample food to eat, clothes to wear, water to drink, or, perhaps, having the security of a solid roof over their heads at night. Forget all the toys, sweets, and electronic gadgets for *these* courageous souls – these individuals are simply doing everything they can to *survive life* from one day to the next. But, all things being considered, these assorted children from around the globe do all share the same, simple fact that they are very precious, unique, and unassuming individuals from several different countries, diverse cultures, and, possibly, with varying expectations and opportunities in life. They're similar in a dissimilar sort of way.

Despite the apparent distinctions, and the significant physical expanses connecting most of the Children of the World, however, all children—from Alabama to Africa, and from Jordan to Japan—are interconnected to one another by extremely similar needs and wants, comparable hopes and dreams, and, the same unbridled zest for life. And, unfortunately, as it turns out, all of the world's youth are also united with each other in another, far less virtuous way: All of these precious and modest youngsters, through no faults of their own, are susceptible to becoming the unlikely victims of childhood Cancers.

It would certainly be a perfect world if all kids could just be kids, and, if scary, wicked health problems, such as Cancer, could be postponed, or, even better than that, done away with entirely before they become adults. But, thanks to life's many inequitable surprises, the reality for many of these youthful children is that *their* lives, and the lives of their families, will be affected by medical circumstances, including Cancer, at an innocent time in their lives when their main worries should be regarding the "monsters" hiding underneath their beds at night. The good news is that there are no monsters concealed beneath their beds at night. The bad news, at least for some of these young, brave kids, is that the *actual* monster—Cancer—is obscured within their pure, vulnerable bodies, both day *and* night.

Childhood Cancer Causes – Still Searching for Answers

According to the National Cancer Institute (www.cancer.gov) and the U.S. Centers for Disease Control, many causes of childhood Cancers are still largely not known. Over the last several years, there has been widespread research on causative risk factors for childhood Cancer, but, unfortunately, the definite causes of childhood Cancers, for the most part, continue to be a great mystery to the scientific and medical communities. That said, scientific research *has* found that some children who are born with specific genetic conditions *do have* an increased likelihood of forming Cancer later in life. These genetic conditions are Down's syndrome and Neurofibromatosis (A genetic condition of the child's Nervous System that principally affects the development and growth of neural (or nerve cell) tissues, that causes cancerous tumors to develop on nerves, and that may produce other abnormalities). However, Scientific Studies do indicate that only a small percentage of children having these two conditions will end up contracting Cancer through their lifetimes. In fact, only one to two new Cancer patients out of 100 have one of these genetic conditions.

Childhood & Teen Cancers vs. Adult Cancers

Among the twelve (12) foremost types of childhood Cancers, the National Cancer Institute (www.cancer.gov) reports that Cancers of the Brain and Central Nervous System, and Leukemias (White Blood Cell Cancers), account for more than half of the new cases in children. Roughly one-third of all childhood Cancers are Leukemias. Of those, Acute Lymphoblastic Leukemia (ALL) is the most typical type, and ALL is the most prevalent childhood Cancer, overall. The second and third most common childhood Cancers are Brain Tumors (Gliomas and Medulloblastomas), and Lymphatic System Cancers (Lymphomas). These three Cancers encompass approximately 75% of all Cancers that are diagnosed in children. The remaining 25% of childhood Cancers are comprised of Kidney tumors (Wilms' tumor), Bone tumors (Osteosarcoma, Ewing's tumor), Rhabdomyosarcoma (a disease in which Cancer cells grow in muscle tissue), Cancers of the Testis and Ovary (Germ Cell tumors), Neuroblastoma (a form of Cancer that starts in certain types of very primitive nerve cells found in an embryo or fetus), and other, less common forms.

In contrast to childhood Cancers, the most common Cancers in adults include Skin Cancers, Prostate Cancer, Colorectal Cancers, Breast Cancer, and Lung Cancer. The Stage (level of progression) of the Cancer, and its location in the body, are noteworthy differences between adult Cancers and childhood Cancers. The immaturity and fragility of a child's organs, systems, and tissues, will usually dictate the types of Cancer treatment that will be prescribed to eradicate the disease, as well as the dosages, frequencies, and the durations of the protocol(s). This typically is not an issue with adult Cancer patients, although there are numerous factors that are taken into consideration relative to both the Cancer *and* the patient when the adult's Cancer treatment plan is being developed by the patient's Medical Team.

While childhood Cancers are much rarer than several "adult" Cancers and do occur less regularly by comparison, medical Studies have indicated that childhood Cancers do tend to be more aggressive than adult Cancers. More aggressive Cancers tend to proliferate and metastasize faster and deeper throughout the body, which can make the treatment opportunities more challenging and limited, the further advanced that the child's Cancer becomes. It is for this justification, alone, that it is *extremely significant* for children to be taken to their Pediatrician or Primary Care Physician for an exam ***at the first signs that the child or teenager is experiencing any abnormal symptoms or signs connected to any unexplained health problem(s) the child might be having.*** The earlier that childhood Cancers are detected—just as with adult Cancers—the quicker the Cancer can be properly treated, and, the higher the probability will be for a positive, healthy post-Cancer treatment prognosis, and, for long-term survivorship.

Children's Cancer Treatment Centers

After physicians on the child Cancer patient's Medical Team discuss potential treatment options—and the possible benefits, risks, and prognoses of each—with the child patient (as applicable), and their parent(s), Guardian, and/or, Caregiver, and, when they all have ultimately decided on the child's Treatment Plan, another extremely important decision will have to be made: To find the best Childhood Cancer Treatment available. The methodology for treating Cancer in children is different from treating adults with Cancer. In roughly all cases, the best treatment available for children will be conducted at a Children's (or Pediatric) Cancer Center. Children's Cancer Centers are specialized centers designed for children (and their families) and are often members of the Children's Oncology Group (COG).

All of the COG Children's Cancer Centers are coupled with a university, and most are connected with a children's hospital. The American Cancer Society and the U.S. Government National Cancer Institute (www.cancer.gov) both recommend the Children's Cancer Centers because they provide a cohesive team approach to meet the needs of childhood Cancer patients, as well as the child's parent(s), and their family members. The Medical Team at Children's Cancer Centers is always comprised of Oncology Physicians and Oncology Nurses who have specialized training and skills in treating Cancer in children and teens, as well as Social Workers, Teachers, Dieticians, Psychologists, and others, all of whom will be available to assist the child patient, and the patient's parent(s), Guardian, or Caregiver.

Children's Cancer Centers are aware that when a child is the Cancer patient, their whole family is affected. While the parent(s) or Caregiver may think that their world is spinning out of control after receiving their child's Cancer diagnosis, aid and support are offered to families of children with Cancer to help them make it through the initial shock and fear, so that they will be in a clearer frame-of-mind to play a part in making their child's treatment and care judgments. The child patient's family will benefit from the education, support, and counseling help offered at the Children's Cancer Center. Many treatment centers offer Support Groups for families of child patients.

Coping with a Childhood Cancer Diagnosis

As discussed in materials developed by the National Cancer Institute, (www.cancer.gov), anger in a parent whose child has been diagnosed with Cancer is a perfectly ordinary reaction for a Mother, and/or, Father, who knows that their child did absolutely nothing to invite their wicked Cancer – other than simply *being a child.* Quite honestly, the parent(s) may feel that life has paradoxically turned its back on them and betrayed their undeserving youngster or teenager. The fact that Cancer has formed in their child's body and that it may threaten *their child's life* can often make the parent(s) livid at life in general, and at its unfair and haphazard inequality – especially when the sufferer is a young and blameless child. When an individual we love—regardless of their age—is assaulted, and especially by an evil and random disease such as Cancer, it is very easy to want to blame someone or something else, or to ask the *"Why me?"* or *"Why us?"* questions. For some parents, God or another Supreme Being may be the target of parents' wrath, as they may question their own faith and beliefs. The parent(s) may also wonder what manner of world would allow kind, loving, helpless children to become not well, suffer, and possibly die, while known, vicious criminals in society are permitted to live, and in many instances, tolerated to roam freely on this earth. When it comes to Cancer diagnoses in individuals—and, especially in young kids—life may not be fair, but it is definitely inequitable!

Some parents might also feel upset because of the upcoming experiences they know their child will face, including the diagnostic tests, and the potentially painful procedures, treatments, and Side Effects. It is normal for all individuals, including parents of children diagnosed with Cancer, to feel disturbed, stressed, and fearful when facing unfamiliar events and outcomes over which they have little or no control. And, with the possible exception of Superman, virtually everyone is frightened by the despicable Cancer and the bodily harm of which it is very capable. *But, then, of course, even Superman has his Kryptonite!* Seriously, though, compounding these fears may be what the child's parents or family members have heard or seen about the potentially dangerous and hurtful Cancer treatment Side Effects, or, that a diagnosis of Cancer, is, in itself, a "Death Sentence."

While it is true that some Side Effects from Cancer treatment can be very uncomfortable, and at times, rather distressing, a Cancer diagnosis is *certainly not a Sentence to die.* There are several actions that the patient, their parents, and their Caregiver or Guardian will take, in conjunction with the patient's Medical Team, in an effort to help the gallant child patient navigate successfully though treatment and to hopeful survivorship. During the length of the child's Cancer journey, the parent(s), family members, and/or, Caregiver, may also need assistance to help them better cope with any of the physical or emotional issues. The diagnosis of Cancer in a child or a Teenager is serious business, not only for the patient, but for all concerned.

The Good News about Childhood Cancers

The diagnosis and the treatment of childhood Cancers takes time, and there are both short-term and longer-term Side Effects that can affect the child. Thankfully, however, the child patient, and their parents and family members, will be directed by skillful health care professionals every step of the way so that nothing is left to chance. When it comes to any person having Cancer—but especially young children—life is absolutely not reasonable. However, just as life can discourage us with its bleak things, so too, can life turn right around and raise our hearts with happiness, and bless us with the optimistic opportunity for renewal. Undoubtedly, Cancer scientists and medical researchers and practitioners are determined each and every day to transform childhood Cancer victims into healthy Cancer survivors.

As disheartening as childhood Cancer diagnosis information might be, there is, fortunately, also some ***very great news*** to go right along with it. Specifically, according to the National Cancer Institute (www.cancer.gov), the ability to quickly detect, diagnose, and treat childhood Cancers has greatly improved in the last fifty years, which has had a very positive impact on the outcomes of Cancer incidences in most children. The major improvements in survival rates are due to early diagnosis and considerable advances in treatment (thanks to large-scale research efforts), and have resulted in a cure or long-term remission for a substantial proportion of children with Cancer.

Alas! More and more children with Cancer are now finishing their treatments successfully, leaving hospitals, clinics, and Cancer Care Centers, and are growing up strong, bright, and active, just like most of the kids around them. The *Big Story* here is that childhood Cancer *is not* a Death Sentence. Nor, does the horrible disease carry with it the same negative stigma that it has in past decades. Instead, most Cancers are very treatable, and, in fact, some current statistics have indicated that the ***survival rate for some childhood Cancers is now over 90%!*** I say that we take that number and run with it!

Following is a comparison of the five-year (or greater) survival rate averages of childhood Cancers between 1962 and today, which have been adapted from the National Cancer Institute (www.cancer.gov) materials. These childhood Cancers are in alphabetical order):

Childhood Cancers and Body Locations (Alphabetized)	**1962 Survival Rate**	**2013 Survival Rate**
Acute Lymphoblastic Leukemia (Blood)	4%	94%
Ewing Sarcoma (Bone)	5%	65%
Hodgkin's Lymphoma (Lymph System)	50%	95%
Medulloblastoma (Brain)	10%	85%
Neuroblastoma (Peripheral Nervous Tissue)	10%	75%
Non-Hodgkin's Lymphoma (Immune System)	7%	80%
Osteosarcoma (Bone)	20%	70%
Retinoblastoma (Eye)	75%	95%
Rhabdomyosarcoma (Muscle)	30%	65%

As is apparent from this Study data, the outlook for young childhood Cancer patients—including teenagers—is very favorable indeed. We have modern medicine, and brave parents and children, to thank.

"These are the definitive ironies of life, that we must first know war to appreciate peace; loathing, to be grateful for love; depression, to value contentment; and, darkness, to welcome the light. So, too, when life serves one Cancer, does it prompt them to give thanks for better health when they have it, and, for their Life when they finally reclaim it."

- Butch Sickler

Chapter Two

Cancer 101 - Part 2 – *An Introduction to This Most Despicable Disease*

"Cancer is that silent, scary neighbor who moves in and speaks with no one, but huddles behind their dark, dirty secrets, until one day they are discovered and flushed out, leaving the neighborhood at peace once again."

- Butch Sickler

As most of us have discovered, either in our personal lives, our professional lives, or both, screw-ups do happen, and, when they do, there is typically more than enough blame to go around. In fact, there is so much misdirected blame today, particularly in American politics, that one could logically wonder who, if anybody, ever does anything wrong. Well, let us get past this finger-pointing mess as it pertains to this wacky life in general, and relate the subject of *blame* specifically to the occurrence of Cancer. When speaking of a Cancer diagnosis, the first rule-of-thumb that all Cancer patients have got to remember is: ***Don't hold themselves responsible for their Cancer!***

Don't Blame Yourself for Your Cancer

Like many things in life, when something goes awry, one of the first things that many individuals do is attempt to figure out why it happened, or, what could have been done to prevent its occurrence in the first place. The second thing that some individuals or groups have a proclivity to do is to attempt to hold someone responsible for the oversight. In some circumstances the culprit may, in fact, be "the other guy," and, they may or may not take ownership of their gaffe.

Or, the problem could have simply been caused by a force beyond our control – in other words, "stuff happens," to put it nicely. But, in still other life situations, we may have a propensity to hold *ourselves* personally accountable for a perceived or an actual mistake, and, in the process, we will often punish ourselves severely in repentance.

In some cases when we self-flagellate for an error that we've committed (or believe we have), this can be a useful and therapeutic process (assuming that we live through whatever took place). This is because it could provide us with an opportunity to learn from our (or others') oversights and their catalysts, so that we, hopefully, will not commit the same, or a similar, *faux pas* again. Oftentimes, however, the unfortunate "casualty" of such introspection and self-assessment is the unjustified assignment of blame to oneself, followed up by the probable feelings of guilt, regrets, anger, and self-recrimination. All of these negative responses, of course, are counter-productive, and could be very injurious to one's health and well-being. For a Cancer patient, it is especially critical that a majority of their thoughts and actions are of the optimistic, constructive, and healthy variety.

Only One Person Knows for Sure, and He's Not Sharing

When it comes to the occurrence of any of the 200 or more known forms of Cancer, as I have attempted to describe within this Book, the causative factors could be few or several, and, they could be the result of one's incidental exposure to environmental toxins, risky personal habits or lifestyle behaviors, heredity, gender, and/or, age, or, a personal and fateful combination thereof. And, as if these likely Cancer-causing candidates aren't enough, let's throw in some good old-fashioned *random chance* to round out the mix. Given all of these possible risk factors that can likely suppress one's Immune System and facilitate the formation of Cancer, it should be evident to most that it would be exceedingly difficult, if not impossible, for one to hang the cause of their Cancer on any one responsible hook.

Even if one was able to unequivocally determine how, when, and where they "got Cancer," there would be absolutely no benefit of assigning blame to themselves for contracting their disease. The deed has already been done – the, *"cow is already out of the barn."*

As such, it could be very emotionally and physically damaging for a Cancer patient to blame them self for their disease, for them to feel guilty or regretful, or, for them to adopt a non-productive, *"shoulda, coulda, woulda,"* frame-of-mind. That being said, I will admit that Life sure would be great if it came with some sort of "Undo" key, or "Back Arrow" button. Unfortunately, though, that is not the case.

No, Nobody Deserves or "Earns" Their Cancer

Certainly, no individual deserves to "get Cancer," and no one "earns" their Cancer by doing "wrong" things, or by not doing all of the "right" things in their lives. Perhaps a person's religion preaches "an eye for an eye," and they may feel that their Cancer is their *just punishment* for some previous transgression or *sin.* Or, maybe one's guilt from a past experience in their life will cause them to believe that Karma—*"What goes around, comes around"*—is paying them back with Cancer for some preceding slip-up because they think that *they have it coming.* To these two absurd possibilities, I ask that you please permit me to insert my own unvarnished opinion – ***Bullshit!!*** Yes, Cancer is unfortunate; yes, Cancer can be devastating; and, yes, Cancer will ruin a person's day in a heartbeat. But, not unlike a bolt of lightning, *Cancer happens,* and when it strikes, we should do our utmost to contain and kill it so that it doesn't strike in the same place twice. In a perfect world, there would be no Cancer. Or, it would be just our luck that in a perfect world, the Cancer would, likewise, be perfect. But, in either case, like everything else we encounter in life, there are some things we can control, and some that we cannot.

Cancer – the Great Equalizer

It really doesn't matter if the individual diagnosed with Cancer practiced excellent health habits prior to their Cancer diagnosis, or, if the individual diagnosed may have assumed that they were "asking for trouble" with their risky voluntary or involuntary exposures to Cancer risk factors before receiving their fateful news. Either way, know this: a Cancer diagnosis is always undeserved and invariably very sobering (literally and figuratively!). Yes, regardless of every Cancer patient's personal circumstances, a Cancer diagnosis will, invariably, make for a very bad day. For many people (and I will modestly include myself in this bunch), their Cancer occurrence and diagnosis were like a 2 x 4 up alongside the head, and the unashamed message that it deposited on us victims was: *"You are not as invincible as you think you are. You are vulnerable; you are susceptible; you are human. Now, deal with it!"*

Yes, it's rather true. The dose of reality that a Cancer diagnosis serves up will humble and neutralize even the most well-known, self-confident, best looking, intelligent, accomplished, or cocky individual. Cancer is, without a doubt, a *great equalizer*. At the very least, one's diagnosis will definitely compel the individual to take pause from what may have been a very busy, fun, and successful family, work, or social life. And, it will also force them to think long and hard about this life-threatening occurrence that, without warning or apology, has suddenly taken center-stage in their life. The Bi-Monthly Financial Spreadsheet due to the manager on Thursday; the manicure and lunch with friends on Wednesday; and the child's Christmas pageant on Saturday, will all have to take a back seat – at least for awhile. There's a new priority in town, and it goes by the name of *Cancer.* The delivery of the Cancer diagnosis to the patient and their family will soon transform into a new way of life for numerous weeks, months, and sometimes, years, for the Cancer patient, their family, and their Caregiver, and friends.

While the revelation of a Cancer diagnosis may not *completely* turn the patient's world upside down, it will definitely throw it off-axis for a period of time. Over the next few months (or maybe longer) after the diagnosis, the Cancer patient, and their family and Caregiver, will travel a long and arduous journey together, continually focused on one difficult, but very achievable goal: To survive their Cancer in the best physical, emotional, and mental state possible. Having overcome what could undoubtedly be one of the most challenging—yet conquerable—obstacles in most of their lives, it would be the definitive hope of these brave men, women, and children that they will one day be able to stand atop the lofty summit and announce to the world that they are *Cancer Survivors!* Over 13.7 million Americans have done that very thing.

The "Bad" News about Cancer *(Optional reading for patients)*

Cancer, as with most things in nature, loves the path of least resistance. It can raise its ugly head at any time, and can do it within anyone. And the nastiest part, is that it can sometimes be so stealth, and so devious, as to not induce any symptoms or send up any "red warning flags" until it has already become solidly entrenched in the finely-tuned and complicated, but masterfully designed, systems that are our bodies – a very scary proposition to say the least. Whether a person be young or elderly, man or woman, nobleman or brick layer, celebrity or regular Joe, healthy or not – it doesn't matter; Cancer is an indiscriminate disease, and, if the conditions are favorable for its occurrence and growth, then occur and grow it will. The keys, then, to decreasing Cancer's opportunities for incidence and development, are prevention, early detection, and safe, appropriate treatment.

☛***Author's Note:*** In the Section below, I have incorporated the "bad" news that is associated with the omnipresent Cancer problem: gloomy, but eye-opening statistics pertaining to Cancer occurrences, diagnosis, and mortality. This data is based on the most current and accurate information available from the dependable resources of the National Cancer Institute (www.cancer.gov), and other government health organizations. Please be aware that I did not incorporate the forbidding numbers in this Book to overwhelm, to discourage, or to frighten the reader. To the contrary, I have provided the information, both to inform and to enlighten the reader, as if he or she may have any uncertainties as to the scope and severity of this unrelenting and ubiquitous disease. ***Cancer patients may wish to skip this Section.***

Cancer Occurrence, Diagnosis, and Mortality Statistics

With more than 200 known types of Cancers and billions of people around the world, there is more than enough of the disease to go around, and, there are an abundance of hosts around the world to fall victim to its nasty assaults. Globally, around 6 million males and females of all ages will fall prey to this cruel medical threat in 2013. According to more recent scientific Cancer analyses, the number of occurrences is anticipated to more than double by the year 2020, and may even jump to approximately 15 million men, women, teens, and young children, worldwide. *Good grief! What's going on here?*

Specifically within the U.S., according to the most up-to-date National Cancer Institute (www.cancer.gov) statistics, it is estimated that in 2013, approximately 1,729,560 new cases of Cancer will be diagnosed in men, women, children, and teens. Of the projected 1.7 million Cancer diagnoses in the U.S., it is estimated that there will be 889,620 males, and 810,380 females of all ages. These statistical totals *do not include* non-Melanoma Skin Cancers, including Basal Cell Carcinomas (BCCs), and Squamous Cell Carcinomas (SCCs).

While Heart Disease is now the leading cause of health death in the U.S. (28%), Cancer comes in a close runner-up at 23%, with 1 out of 4 American fatalities resulting from the disease. Presently, the United States is No. 9 in the world in numbers of Cancer deaths per year. Approximately 1,500 Americans die *each day* due to various forms of Cancer, which translates to over 580,350 U.S. deaths per year. Of these regrettable mortalities, it is likely that 260,577 will be females, young and old, and over 319,733 will be males. Some groups of populations appear to have higher or lower rates of Cancer incidence and deaths than others, but no one completely understands why. Possible explanations may include the problems of poverty and racism, nutrition and physical fitness, habits and lifestyle behaviors, environmental exposures, inequitable access to healthcare, disparate treatment within the health care system, genetic factors, and others.

Although Cancer is the leading cause of mortality by disease amongst American children aged one to nineteen, Cancer diagnoses are still relatively rare in this age group. On average, 1 to 2 children develop the disease each year for every 10,000 children in the U.S. Over the past twenty years, there has been a slight increase in the incidence of children diagnosed with all forms of invasive Cancer, from 11.5 cases per 100,000 children in 1975 to 14.8 per 100,000 children in 2004. Looking on the bright side, however, during this same period of time, *mortality rates for children due to Cancer have decreased, and survival rates have showed a steady increase.*

Anticipated Percentages of Common Cancer Diagnoses

According to the National Cancer Institute (www.cancer.gov), it is anticipated that the most prevalent forms of Cancer that will be diagnosed in the United States during 2013, along with their relative percentages of estimated occurrence in *adult men and women*, will be the following:

Adult Males		**Adult Females**	
Cancer Type	**%**	**Cancer Type**	**%**
Prostate	25	Breast	26
Lung/Bronchus	15	Lung/Bronchus	14
Colorectal	10	Colorectal	10
Urinary/Bladder	7	Uterine Corpus	6
Non-Hodgkin's Lymphoma	5	Non-Hodgkin's Lymphoma	4
Melanoma – Skin	5	Thyroid	4
Kidney/Renal	4	Melanoma – Skin	4
Oral Cavity	3	Ovary	3
Leukemia	3	Kidney/Renal	3
Pancreas	3	Leukemia	3
All Other Sites	20	All Other Sites	23

Of the total projected 1.7 million Cancer diagnoses in the United States in 2013, it is estimated that approximately 30% will be caused by smoking and other tobacco use, a principal risk factor for the cancerous disease. Researchers found that alcohol use is a risk factor for Breast, Liver, Colon, and Head and Neck Cancers, and it results in about 20,000 Cancer deaths annually, accounting for about 3.5 percent of all Cancer deaths in the U.S. per year. Even minimal use of alcohol can be dangerous: 1.5 drinks per day result in 30% of all alcohol-related Cancer deaths. The remaining Cancers, including Prostate, Breast, Colorectal, Head and Neck and others, will run the gamut, both in terms of their types and their causative factors.

Anticipated Numbers of New Diagnoses By Cancer Type – Men, Women, and Children

Of all of these new Cancer diagnoses anticipated in the U.S. in 2013, Lung Cancer will be the most prevalent diagnosed in both men and women, with more than 228,190 new cases being expected. The Cancer with the lowest incidence will be Leukemia in all of its forms. It is estimated that over 43,050 new cases of Leukemia will be diagnosed in the U.S. in 2013, including in younger children and teens, with Chronic Lymphocytic Leukemia being the most common type, with just over 14,990 new instances. Breast Cancer is the most frequently diagnosed Cancer in women. It is estimated that 234,580 new cases of Breast Cancer will be diagnosed in women in 2013. In the U.S., a woman is diagnosed with Breast Cancer every 2 minutes.

Unbeknownst to many people, men can also contract Breast Cancer. In 2013, in the U.S., it is estimated that 2,190 men will be diagnosed with this variety of the disease. The most common Cancer diagnosed in American men, as anticipated, is Prostate Cancer, with approximately 238,590 new cases projected during 2013. Colon and Rectal Cancers are often referred to as "Colorectal Cancers," and in 2013, 143,460 new incidences of Colorectal Cancer are estimated to be diagnosed. Kidney Cancers are separated into two groups. 53,581 new cases of both forms of Kidney Cancer are anticipated in 2013.

Male Cancer Diagnoses

Recent Cancer Studies indicate that men are more likely than women to contract some form of Cancer throughout their lifetimes. Specifically in the U.S., the lifetime probability of a man developing some type of Cancer will be 1 out of 2 (women's odds are 1 out of 3), with Prostate Cancer having the greatest likelihood of occurrence (25%). Lung and Bronchus Cancers, at 15%, are the second most prevalent for men, while Colorectal Cancer comes in third, at 10%. Nationally, male Cancer rates are highest among African Americans (689 men out of 100,000), followed by Caucasians (556 men per 100,000), Hispanics, Asians, American Indian/Alaska Natives, and Pacific Islanders. Cancer deaths among men are higher for African Americans than they are for Caucasians, Hispanics, and Asians, and for American Indian/Alaska Natives than Asian/Pacific Islanders.

Female Cancer Diagnoses

With respect to the diagnosis of Cancer in American women, most recent statistics indicate that 1 out of 3 will develop some form of Cancer during her lifetime. As might be projected, Breast Cancer will represent the highest occurrence rate of female Cancers at 26% (1 out of 8 likelihood), followed by Lung and Bronchus Cancers at 14%, and Colorectal Cancers at 10%. Nationally, Studies do indicate that Caucasian women are most likely to form Cancer, with African American women at second in probability, followed by Hispanics, Asian/Pacific Islanders, and American Indian and Alaska Natives. Studies find that Cancer deaths among American females are most common in African Americans, followed by Caucasians, American Indian/Alaska Natives, Hispanics, Asians, and Pacific Islanders.

Childhood Cancer Diagnoses

Regarding occurrence of Cancer in children aged 0 to 14 in the U.S., most recent statistics show that 16 boys and 14 girls out of 100,000 will develop some form of Cancer. Leukemia (Blood Cell Cancer) accounts for approximately 30% of all childhood Cancers, with Acute Lymphocytic Cancer being the most common form of Leukemia in children. Among the twelve major types of childhood Cancers, Leukemias and Cancers of the Brain and Central Nervous System account for over 50% of the cases. In the U.S. in 2013, it is estimated that 10,400 children under age 15 will be diagnosed with Cancer, and that an anticipated 70,000 individuals between their late teens and early 30s will contract the disease. Studies also have found that approximately 1,545 children will die from the disease in 2013. Blood Cancers combined—Leukemia, Myeloma, and Lymphoma—will regrettably, cause one child to pass away every 10 minutes.

Head and Neck Cancer Diagnoses (My Cancer Type)

The form of Cancer with which I was diagnosed—Head and Neck Cancer—is quite uncommon, comprising only about 3% of all Cancers in the United States. Head and Neck Cancers encompass many forms, and comprise those tumors that are situated in the Oral Cavity (i.e. Mouth, Teeth, Gums, Lips, Cheeks, etc.), the Throat, the Tonsils, the Tongue (Anterior and Base - *my type*), the Nasopharynx (back behind the Nose), the Salivary Glands, and, within the Larynx (Voice Box, Windpipe), but exclude Cancers of the Brain, the eyes, the Esophagus, the Thyroid Gland, and the skin, muscles, and bones of the head and neck, which have their own medical classifications.

In a typical year in the U.S., research Studies have revealed that approximately 55,000 males and females, generally over the age of 50, will develop some form of Head and Neck Cancer. Of those patients, for every one woman who develops the disease, three men will become Cancerous. As one might anticipate, a great majority of Head and Neck Cancers are caused by the lengthy and excessive use of tobacco products, and/or, alcoholic beverages. This stark reality makes *my own* Head and Neck Cancer diagnosis—and the Cancer diagnoses of other non-tobacco users and non-alcohol drinkers such as myself—all the more mysterious and "difficult to swallow" – pun definitely intended! Regrettably, each year in the U.S., about 13,000 courageous Head and Neck Cancer warriors will lose their conflicts with Cancer, and will eventually succumb to their disease.

"Prevention" is the Name of the Game

The Cancer statistics referenced in this section of the Book—which, again, have all been gleaned from the Government National Cancer Institute (www.cancer.gov), and Centers for Disease Control online resources—broadcast a very austere and telling message to all who will notice: That Cancer in all of its many forms is very serious business, and that if one takes it lightly, they will be doing so at their own risk. Simply stated, the occurrence of Cancer in each one of us can be only a few Risk Factors away, some of which we can control, and some of which—such as our age and our heredity—we cannot.

Hopefully, these disturbing numbers will serve to encourage all individuals—whether they are male or female, young or old—to obtain all their periodic Cancer Screening Exams and their annual Medical Check-Ups. Additionally, for those individuals engaged in high-risk lifestyle behaviors such as excessive smoking and alcohol consumption; not exercising or not eating a healthy diet; and/or, not taking proper steps to avoid environmental toxins or overexposure to sunlight, perhaps these alarming statistics will function as a wake-up call, and will strongly encourage them to alter their dangerous ways. Whatever the case, the "handwriting is on the wall" and has been for years—each and every one of us must be aware of, and prepared for, the potential that this parasitic disease may materialize in our own bodies, or in those of our families or friends. Based on the foregoing historical data, chances are very likely that during the course of our lifetimes and theirs, it will. This is all the more reason for each of us to take actions to minimize our risks. *For example, if obese women lose 5% of their weight, it may reduce Breast Cancer risk by 22%.*

Turning Negatives into Positives

I would ask the Reader to please realize that I have included the aforementioned, up-to-date statistical figures concerning Cancer occurrences, diagnoses, and mortalities, for informational purposes only. There is no question that Cancer is a dire, monumental health problem around the world and in the U.S. And, it is equally as well known that all of us stand a very good chance of contracting Cancer at some point during our lifetimes. Regrettably, we are also only too aware that some Cancer warriors will loose their courageous battles with the disease. But, even though these "bad" statistics do provide a somewhat raw and disheartening picture about Cancer, on a more constructive note, they also communicate to all Cancer patients and their loved ones that they are not alone with their diagnosis, or, in their personal struggles with this common enemy. When it comes to overcoming many obstacles and challenges in life, including Cancer, there truly is "strength in numbers." It is in these numbers of fellow Cancer patients to whom a person can look for inspiration, hope, and a "one-for-all-all-for-one" type of attitude. This may serve to guide each brave warrior ever-forward in their respective Cancer battles.

In the ubiquitous realm of Cancer, despite all of the negative information associated with its occurrence, diagnosis, and mortality statistics, a Cancer patient, their family, and their Caregiver should not ever lose sight of the fact that countless of these occurrences and diagnoses ***will be transformed over time into the positive outcomes of patients who have reclaimed their precious lives after surviving the disease***. As such, my hope is that one will view the information in the above Sections simply for what it is: Scientifically researched and factual figures pertaining to the actuality of Cancer incidence in America that is not necessarily reflective of the potential outcomes of each Cancer patient's efforts to rightly address their own disease. In other words, all of the Cancer incidence, diagnosis, and mortality statistics speak for themselves, and they make no other claims as to an individual's post-Cancer prognosis, notwithstanding their form of Cancer. As I have discussed in other Chapters within this Book, the ultimate results of each Cancer patient's instance will be contingent upon the health status of the individuals, themselves, their responses to the Cancer treatment(s), and several other factors associated with the patients' respective treatments, recoveries, and aftercare.

The "Good" News about Cancer *("Must" reading for patients)*

"I'm sorry to have to tell you this, but you have Cancer." Some of the most dreaded words in the English language, to say the least. But, thanks to early detection and the magnificent strides that have been achieved during more recent years in Cancer research and treatments for some types of Cancer, those disarming words do not necessarily carry with them the same gloomy stigma as they have in days gone by. Nor are those words necessarily an automatic *"death sentence,"* as has been perceived by many people when they receive the devastating news of their Cancer diagnosis from their physician *(which is what I feared with mine!).* So instrumental are many tools being utilized for early detection, and, so effective are several of the treatment modalities for treating various forms of Cancer these days, that there are presently 13.7+ million Cancer survivors in the U.S. Survivorship is destined to increase as research continues to uncover enhanced preventive measures and treatments, and, as all health care providers continue to improve their recovery, aftercare, and regular monitoring programs. Much evolution has been made in this regard in recent years for child Cancer patients, and, ongoing research and developmental efforts continue to be directed toward improving the treatment and aftercare of adult Cancer patients and survivors.

Surviving Cancer - The Ultimate Goal

"Any individual that has been diagnosed with Cancer, from the time of discovery, and for the balance of life." This would be the detailed definition of "Cancer Survivor" that is furnished on the canceradvocacy.org website. On wikipedia.org, "Cancer Survivor" is succinctly classified as, *"An individual with Cancer of any type, current or past, who is still alive."* Further, usoncology.com simply exemplifies a "Cancer Survivor" as, *"Anyone living with a history of Cancer, including newly diagnosed survivors as well as long-term survivors."* Then, to finish, in its "Dictionary of Cancer Terms," the

Government National Cancer Institute (www.cancer.gov) defines a Cancer Survivor as follows: *"One who remains alive and continues to function during and after overcoming a serious hardship or life-threatening disease. Regarding Cancer, a person is considered to be a survivor from the time of diagnosis until the end of life."*

Regardless of how the phrase, "*Cancer Survivor,*" is defined, just as long as the operative words, *"life," "living,"* and *"alive,"* are in there somewhere, that's all that really matters. Yes, regardless of how you slice-and-dice it, being alive-and-kicking definitely trumps the avoid-at-all-costs alternative. And, that is specifically why early recognition, accurate diagnosis, immediate and successful treatment, and attentive aftercare, are the critical keys to achieving the ultimate objective – a healthy and lengthy Cancer Survivorship.

Overestimating Cancer – Underestimating Patients

Many Cancer patients who were told by their physician that they were, *"terminally ill,"* or, that they had, *"six-or-so months to live,"* are now entirely enjoying and celebrating life—and several of them writing about their stories of survival—ten, twenty, thirty years or longer—after the doctor provided them the medical equivalent of a "Death Sentence." Physicians are in the business of saving lives, not planning deaths, but in their defense, they are professionally and ethically compelled to inform the Cancer patient of their *most-likely* prognosis, as grim and upsetting as it may be. One can rest-assured, however, that *most* physicians do take this momentous and difficult responsibility very seriously. In delivering their assessments to the patient, perhaps the conscientious physician will provide the Cancer patient, their loved one, family or the Caregiver, with "worst-case," "best-case," and "most-likely" possibilities concerning the patient's overall prognosis. Or, the physician may give the patient and family the most probable prospects for the patient's future after treatment.

In any event, should the patient's doctor provide the patient, and family or Caregiver, with his or her predictive estimates on the patient's survivability of their Cancer, these projection(s) *should* be based, not on guesses, speculation, or conjecture, but, will take into consideration many known factors surrounding the patient and their Cancer. Typically, the individual medical facts that the responsible member of the patient's Medical Team will take into account when approximating the Cancer patient's probabilities of longevity and survival will include: The patient's type of Cancer and its magnitude (its location, and/or, its advancement within the body); the patient's general health condition and age; the safest, and most applicable and effective treatment options available for that individual; the patient's probable, or actual, responses to their treatment(s); and, other factors that are considered on a case-by-case, patient-by-patient basis.

To be perfectly forthright, though, no health care provider—even with the best, most reliable data at their disposal—will be able to accurately anticipate how a patient will react to any given Cancer treatment procedure. And, of course, there are the unquantifiable (or "anecdotal" in medical phrasing) considerations, such as the power of the patient's faith and hope, the patient's uncompromising will to live, and, the patient's mental, physical, and spiritual life-forces, that should be factored into the "survivor" equation. And, finally, as we all know (though most Cancer physicians will not acknowledge this concept), there is always room at the table for the incomprehensible miracles to come to pass – which they sometimes do! Many people, including several in the "Medical establishment" will downplay the importance of these "immeasurable" factors. That's *their* problem.

Taking all of this into account, thankfully, not all *most-likely* predictions of Cancer prematurely ending a survivor's life will come true. In fact, I dare say, that a lot of "terminal" Cancer patients have outlived the very physicians who delivered to them their fateful (and inaccurate) prognosis. Statistically speaking, there are *a whole host of very promising and encouraging outcomes* associated with earlier Cancer detection, diagnosis, treatment, and recovery. Statistics do specify that Cancer survivors are living longer, experiencing a better quality of life than Cancer survivors were only a few years ago, and, that many people have not only conquered their disease completely, but have reclaimed their lives, and are surviving it in the long-term.

Decreased Cancer Mortality Rates

According to the most current Cancer Survivability Studies published by the U.S. National Cancer Institute (www.cancer.gov), scientific researchers have determined that ***mortality rates from the***

dreaded disease have decreased by 3% over the last few years! That might sound small, but it's actually major! In the 1940s in the U.S., Studies found that only ***one patient in four*** survived their Cancer on the average. By the 1960s, that figure improved to ***one survivor for every three*** patients. According to the latest research and data from the American Cancer Society (www.cancer.org), ***over three out of four American Cancer patients—or >75% of those diagnosed—will survive their disease.*** In fact, for the first time since the 1930s, the numbers of American deaths caused by Cancer has decreased. In particular, during the years 1990 to 2005, Cancer mortality rates had dropped 21% among men, and 12% among women. Mortality rates for Breast Cancer, the most widespread form of Cancer in American women, have been decreasing by about 2% per year, since 1999.

Increased Cancer Survival Rates

Keeping pace with the significant decreases in the mortality rates due to many types of Cancers in recent years, the ***survival rates of patients diagnosed with some forms of Cancer have also steadily increased*** during the same period of time. For example, according to the National Cancer Institute (www.cancer.gov), the survival rates for the most common Cancers in women and men—Breast Cancer, and Prostate Cancer, respectively—have increased incrementally in more recent years. Specifically, the Breast Cancer survival rate has risen from 75% in 1975, to 88% in 2008, while the survival rate of men having Prostate Cancer has improved from 67% to 99% during the same time period. Survivorship kicks mortality's butt every time.

Survival rates have also increased markedly for several other common Cancers in both men and women in more recent years. For example, the survival rate for Colorectal (Colon and Rectal) Cancer has improved to 55%; Ovarian Cancer to 70% in women aged 15 to 44 years old; Testicular Cancer to 95%; and, Skin Melanoma to over 85%. Hodgkin's Lymphoma also realizes an increased recovery with survival rates greater than 92% amongst younger patients. However, in older people, the survival rates decrease to less than 50%.

Childhood Cancer survival rates have also experienced some promising increases in the last few years. Specifically, from 1975 to 2004, deaths from Childhood Leukemia declined dramatically, and

5-year survival rates have increased for most childhood Cancers. For example, the 5-year survival rate for all childhood Cancers together, increased from 58.1 percent in 1975, to 77 to 79.6 percent in 1996 to 2003. This improvement in survival rates is unquestionably due to significant advances in treatments, resulting in a cure or a long-term remission for a significant number of childhood Cancer patients.

Likewise, just as positive, the survival rate among Head and Neck Cancer Patients has improved for both men and women ***if the disease is detected and treated early enough.*** Studies have shown that when a Head and Neck Cancer does reoccur in a victim, 80% of the time it will happen within the first two years following effective Treatment, and/or, Surgery. If a Head and Neck Cancer Patient can make it successfully through the first two years—and hopefully, past the first five—chances are, and statistics do support, that the person will most likely survive the disease in the long-term. *Please be true!*

A Brief History of Cancer

From an historical perspective, Cancer is not the new kid on the block. Generally thought of as a "modern" disease, Cancer has apparently always been with us – at least based on historical records. Yes, believe it or not, Archaeologists have made nearly 200 possible Cancer discoveries that date as far back as *prehistoric* times. So, if the Saber-toothed Tiger or a Caveman didn't get you, *Cancer did!*

Cancer Through the Ages

In one example of a prehistoric Cancer occurrence unearthed by scientists just a few years ago, Archaeologists excavated a large burial mound in Russia and discovered the skeletons of a man and a woman crouched on the floor of a dark inner chamber. The two were surrounded by royal garb adorned with gold paraphernalia that has been dated to roughly 2,700 years ago. While the excavation of the Russian man was a very important Archaeology find, it was also an extremely extraordinary scientific discovery from a Paleopathology standpoint. Paleopathologists, or scholars of ancient disease, found that almost every bone within the man's body had been pierced with tumors. Following the laboratory evaluation of the specimen, it was confirmed that what these Pathologists had actually discovered was the oldest known case of metastasizing Prostate Cancer. The man's Prostate, itself, had disintegrated years ago, but malignant cells from the Gland had migrated according to a recognizable pattern, and had metastasized to his bones, where they left identifiable scars. Proteins extracted from the man's bones tested positive for PSA, or Prostate Specific Antigen. Being the first known victim of Prostate Cancer is one title that I'm sure this unlucky man could've lived without!

Approximately twenty-five hundred years ago, or about 200 years after our aforementioned Russian friend perished with Prostate Cancer, Hippocrates, the Greek Father of Western Medicine, firstly identified and described Cancer as an illness. Hippocrates called the disease, *karkinos,* which is Greek for "crab," possibly because of the unfettered crablike movements of the disease through the body. The term "Cancer" was later anglicized from the Greek *karkinos.* During Hippocrates' time, Cancer was a particularly rare illness and, based on history, probably occurred in only a small fraction of the world's population. However, beginning in the 1600s, during the Industrial Revolution, Cancer first began to appear in Western civilization.

By the early Twentieth Century, Cancer was responsible for approximately 4% of the overall deaths in the U.S. As recently as a generation ago, many forms of Cancer that are common today were rare or non-existent. Fast-forward to the present time, however, and, unbelievably, there are now over 200 identified forms of the disease. Statistical Studies indicate that in 2013, an estimated 6 million men, women, and children throughout the world will be diagnosed with one or more of these forms of Cancer. 1.7 million of these Cancer cases are predicted to impact American men, women, and children.

The Costs of Cancer

According to the government National Institutes for Health, and the National Cancer Institute (www.cancer.gov), in 2010, it was estimated that the overall costs associated with Cancer were $263.8 billion, of which $102.8 billion was for direct medical costs (total of all health expenditures); $20.9 billion for the loss of job productivity due to the disease (being off of work to go to medical appointments, exams, treatments, recovery, etc.); and, $140.1 billion for the cost of lost productivity due to premature death. In 2011, the Journal of the National Cancer Institute estimated that the total cost of Cancer care in the U.S. will rise between $158 billion and $173 billion in 2020, a 27% increase from 2010, due to an aging population. Specifically regarding Head and Neck Cancers, it is estimated that approximately $3.1 billion is spent each year on the treatment of the disease.

Common Myths Associated with Cancer Causes

Preceding in this Chapter, the true and medically established risk factors and causes associated with many Cancer diagnoses were listed briefly and explained to provide the Reader with information that will perhaps answer some questions that they may have, or, that will hopefully serve as helpful warnings about specific things in life that a person may want to avoid if at all possible. However, with life being what it is, along with truths will invariably come untruths and myths. I will finish this Chapter with some thoughts about a few of the "wives' tales" that periodically swirl about regarding the topic of Cancer. Most of these myths are responsible for causing confusion and unnecessary fears among those unaware of Cancer realities.

According to the dictionary, a "myth" is *"Any invented story, idea, or concept, with or without a determinable basis of fact or a natural explanation."* Cancer, as everybody is aware, can be a very deadly adversary, which is probably why many people cite a Cancer diagnosis as one of the most frightening concerns in their life – and rightly so. Cancer can be one mean SOB! And, perhaps, because of those justifiable suspicions and lack of understanding on the part of so many individuals, is why several widespread myths, untruths, and rumors have been unjustly generated about this disreputable disease. Unfortunately, these falsified beliefs—some prompted by erroneous claims, others as products of public fear, and still others reported by careless organizations in the news about specious, non-scientifically controlled "Cancer Studies"—do nothing to calm people's nerves or to help them to think rationally about the topic. Unfortunately, most Cancer Myths do serve to unreasonably increase one's anxieties and doubts about the disease. I refer to Cancer Myths as, ***"Rumors about Tumors,"*** because, that, essentially, is what they are.

Whatever their source, Cancer myths, not unlike Cancer the disease, can be very damaging if they are not contained and stopped, and, if they are allowed to multiply and spread out-of-control. False beliefs about Cancer could unnecessarily distract an individual from taking precautions to protect themselves from known Cancer causes, instead drawing their attention to "false alarms" – things that have no impact on increasing, or decreasing, their chances of contracting Cancer. Additionally, untruths or "wives' tales" about Cancer could very well have a rather disruptive effect on Cancer patients' chances of defeating the disease by initiating a sense of hopelessness in their minds, or, by enticing them to pursue unproven remedies that would leave them disillusioned and discouraged with the results.

The U. S. National Cancer Institute (www.cancer.gov) has identified nine well-known Myths associated with Cancer. Following are the nine Myths, accompanied by substantiated information that refutes the rumors, and attempts to explain the truth behind the false beliefs:

Myth 1. The Chance You'll Die of Cancer Increases Every Year – *False*

It is true that one of the recognized risk factors for Cancer in individuals is them aging. And, yes, it is factual that more people are being diagnosed with Cancer these days than has taken place in prior years. Much of this increase, though, is due to enhanced awareness thru education, and, as a result of improved screening techniques – meaning that *more people are submitting to early testing*, which, in-turn, is resulting in more Cancer *being detected* now that may have been missed in the past. Advances in Medicine have also improved survival rates and the overall quality of life for Cancer patients. As a result, the five-year survival rate for all Cancers, combined, (there are over 200 known forms) has shown steady improvement over the past three decades. In fact, more than 80% of people diagnosed with Cancer are still living five years after a diagnosis. Conversely, there has been a constant decrease in the Cancer-related mortality, even as the overall population of the United States has increased. So, while the potentiality of a person *getting* Cancer might increase with their age—because "getting older" is a scientifically proven risk factor for the disease—the ***likelihood of them dying from Cancer does not.***

Myth 2. A Person is More Likely to Develop Lung Cancer from Air Pollution than from Smoking Cigarettes – *False*

Anyone who has ever lived in an overpopulated urban area, a traffic-clogged town, or an industrialized region, is well aware of the ugly grayish or brownish haze that typically frequents the air in such areas. In these types of environments, folks are also just as familiar with the stinking stench and horrible caustic taste of such "air" when attempting to breathe. However, it is proven that breathing the air of a polluted city—while admittedly, is probably not a healthy thing to do—is much less likely to initiate Lung Cancer in individuals than is smoking cigarettes, or, even the people being frequently exposed to secondhand smoke of cigarette smokers. In this regard, the numbers speak for themselves: Nearly 9 in 10 Lung Cancers, or about 87 %, are the result of individuals smoking tobacco in its various forms, or, being repetitively exposed to secondhand cigarette smoke. ***Beware:*** *Both first- and second-hand cigarette smoke kills!* That's no Myth!

Myth 3. Using Certain Antiperspirants, Shampoos, Hairsprays, Hair Colors, or other Personal Toiletries Can Increase Breast Cancer Risk – *False*

In many developed countries in the world, men, women, and teenagers utilize thousands upon thousands of different self-care and grooming products in an effort to look, smell, and feel their best (an American woman will spend an average of $12,000 a year on these products, and, all men in the U.S. annually contribute approximately $217 million to the industry). As most of us realize, when one reads the list of ingredients on many of these self-care products (including even some found in "health" or "natural food" stores), the chemicals and other things specified on these product labels read more like the ***Periodic Table of Elements***, than simply a list of additives that will help the user with keeping their *flyaway* hair in place, keeping their armpits from reeking, or, helping them get that *50-going-on-20* look.

That being said, the real basis of this particular rumor is that some of the chemicals and the other potentially injurious substances found in these products might be absorbed through the skin, or enter the body through nicks or cuts. In such instances, the main concern is that the use of such products can increase the chances of a woman contracting Breast Cancer. However, medical Studies have found no substantiation to support this assertion. Frankly, one scientific Study compared women using toiletries who developed Breast Cancer with women using the same toiletries who *had not* contracted the disease. Researchers found no certifiable link between the affected women's use of toiletries, and their incidences of Cancer. *So…spray away.*

Myth 4. Cell Phones Can Cause Brain Cancer – *False*

Show me someone who doesn't have a cell phone nowadays and I'll show you a child still in the womb. Everywhere all of us go, people—young and old alike—are using some form of cell phone or communicative device that enables them to stay in-touch with others – sometimes annoyingly so, as in the case of "loud talkers" in public who want to try to impress ***everybody*** with ***their*** business. However, with all of the millions of cell phone users that have squashed these electronic gadgets to their heads for the last 30 years, there has been no credible evidence to prove that exposure to electromagnetic fields released from cell phones, or from other personal electronic devices, can incite Cancer, including Brain Cancer. One recent Study found that cell phone users had no increased risk for a number of different Cancers, even if they'd been using the phones for a decade or more. While the risk seems minimal, please do us a favor: *Keep it down.*

Myth 5. Fluoridated Water Increases One's Cancer Risk – *False*

Whenever a "new" chemical is introduced into products that we use, eat, or drink—even if it is naturally occurring (as are many chemicals), and even if it is intended for a purpose to promote good health or prevent health problems—some people have a tendency to become very suspicious about the possible Side Effects of doing so. In some ill-fated cases, based on past histories, these apprehensions are justifiable. However, concerning fluoride in municipal drinking water, rumors that it causes Cancer have existed for decades, but no evidence has ever been found to support this myth. A recent survey carried out by the U.S. Centers for Disease Control and Prevention found no scientific data to support a claim of increased Cancer risk in people who drink fluoridated water, as does half of the U.S.

Myth 6. There IS a Cure for Cancer, but the Medical Establishment is Hiding it – *False*

The probable basis for this falsehood is that skeptical people may want to believe that were cures for Cancer to be discovered and administered to Cancer patients, it would put many physicians, drug manufacturers, hospitals, health care-type corporations, and similar operations out of business. This thought process suggests that were a cure to be found (there would have to be cures for the 200+ forms of known Cancer), no more people would *get Cancer* and the problem would disappear, together with the need for Cancer doctors, clinics, medicines, and other treatments. However, to relate this sort of logic to the epidemics of Polio and Syphilis—both of which being awfully lethal or harmful conditions in their day—no doctors, hospitals, drug companies, or health care providers had to close their doors after the vaccinations for both outbreaks were developed and administered to the general population in the 1940s and 50s – thus effectively curing those diseases. Thankfully, the vaccinations did kick the butts of the diseases, but, as one would wisely suspect, all of the medical entities who had been treating the conditions, just basically moved on to the next health concern in need of tending. The same would hold true if the scientific and medical establishment was able to create a much-needed cure for Cancer, which, as stated previously, is not only one disease, but a medical malady with over 200 known types, each with their own characteristics, treatments, and responses to treatment.

Another valid point worth thinking about is that people who research and treat Cancer—such as doctors and nurses, pharmacists, and scientists who develop the medications, as well as the engineers who design the medical equipment—is that they, and their family members, friends and relatives, also contract Cancer at the same rate as do all other individuals. In other words, just because these people help remove Cancer from others' bodies, doesn't mean that they are not susceptible to a Cancer diagnosis themselves. Presumably, were there to be a definite cure for Cancer, these individuals would be the first to know about it, and, would be the first to use it on themselves or their family members who were diagnosed with the disease. That just does not happen, quite frankly, because there is no general cure for the 200+ forms of the disease. With all this being said, however, several Cancer patients, especially those whose Cancer is identified, diagnosed, and treated at the earliest, may have successful outcomes in which all follow-on tests and exams indicate that they are *Cancer-Free.* In such instances, at least for these specific individuals, their respective Cancers could be considered as being "cured."

Myth 7. Cancer is Always a Painful Disease, so if a Person Feels Fine, They Don't Have Cancer – *True and False*

As this myth is presented, it can be *both true and false.* It can be ***true***, because, thankfully, a vast number of people who feel fine physically and emotionally *do not* have Cancer. That said, however, these people, like all men, women, teens, and children in this world, do embody the *potential* for developing the destructive malady if all conditions are optimal, and, if it is meant to be. Statistics do support, though, that most individuals will never contract any form of Cancer during their lifetime. This myth as written, though, can also be ***false.*** This is because Cancer, being the surreptitious, silent, and scheming potential destroyer that it is, will often assault a person and continue to feed, multiply, and disperse throughout the person's body without sending up any "red flags," or, without causing any apparent inward or outward signs or symptoms, such as pain, discomfort, or swelling.

In such instances, the person may feel terrific, and eat, sleep, work, and play as if nothing is untoward, but, all the while, they will have Cancer growing and advancing within their body. This could be especially true in the early Stages of many Cancers, because their parasitic and gluttonous methods have not yet had an opportunity to debilitate, destroy, or "shut down" other crucial tissues and systems within the body. Some Cancers, however, such as Lung Cancer and Pancreatic Cancer, are so secretive, and so non-disruptive for such a long period of time during their development in the body, that these Cancers, unfortunately, are typically discovered much too late in the program to be treated successfully, or, with little hope of a favorable prognosis. One need only look at the Cancer occurrences of the late

Senator Edward Kennedy, Apple CEO Steve Jobs, and actor Patrick Swayze, to realize just how devastating these silent killers can be.

In many cases, these slow-working, clandestine Cancers, and others, are accidentally or serendipitously detected by a physician or during an exam, not necessarily due to signs or symptoms associated with the Cancer's existence, but, because the patient saw the doctor for a medical issue completely not related to the Cancer occurrence. Typically, however, when the destructive means of Cancer *do* begin wreaking havoc in a person's body, some types of Cancer will begin "revealing themselves" to the individual host. In such instances, the body's *"check engine light"* may *"light up"* to notify the person that something unhealthy or very unusual may be occurring within their body. Such symptoms could consist of sudden and unexplained pain or discomfort, loss of weight, lack of functionality of a specific area, loss of appetite, and other indicators that things "aren't right." If and when such signs or symptoms occur, it is incumbent upon the person to *seek medical assistance as early as possible* so that the probable cause of the medical condition can be identified, and so appropriate actions can be taken. Thankfully, during my own Cancer experience, my tumor did put up such *warning signs* in the form of a non-stop, throbbing sore throat on one side of my neck, which prompted me to seek medical attention. This, unquestionably, helped save my life.

Myth 8. If Mom or Dad Had Cancer, their Child Will Have it One Day – *False-'ish'*

Much has been discussed of the prospect that prior ancestors of a person's family, or their biological Mother, and/or, Father, may contribute to the manifestation of a Cancer in their child or children. Some of this argument may be reasonably founded on scientific fact. However, a considerable amount of the information concerning the role of heredity in Cancer formation may be somewhat exaggerated. Specifically, Studies have indicated that some forms of Cancer, like Breast Cancer, Ovarian Cancer, Thyroid Cancer, Colorectal Cancer, and Melanoma *can be* passed on genetically from parents to the next generation. However, these genetic links have been proven to occur only approximately 5 to 10 percent of the time. While the potential varies depending on the forms of Cancer, a family history of Cancer doesn't necessarily mean that a child will *automatically* develop the disease. Therefore, this myth is false based on that (un)likelihood.

Myth 9. Female Smokers Get Lung Cancer More than Male Smokers – *False*

A few Cancer Studies performed in the early-1990s may be responsible for this myth, and might have led some people to believe that a woman, simply being a woman, increases her risks of getting Lung Cancer. But, recent research shows that women are no more vulnerable to tobacco-smoke carcinogens than men. Recent Studies have also found that non-smoking women are also no more likely to get Lung Cancer than non-smoking men, and, further, that there isn't any evidence that women are more susceptible to Lung Cancer from secondhand smoke than are men. *But, these findings are certainly no reason for women to celebrate*. The cold reality is that cigarette-induced Lung Cancer *does* kill more women than any other kind of Cancer – Breast Cancer included. In both women and men, current smokers of two or more packs each day are generally ***50 times more likely to develop Lung Cancer*** than those who have never smoked. Additionally, women who smoke are almost 20 times more prone to developing Lung Cancer than are non-smoking women. Exposure to secondhand smoke increases a non-smoker's risk of Lung Cancer by 30 percent. ***If a person doesn't smoke, they should not start, and if a person does smoke, they should stop – Now!*** – and reduce their risk of Lung Cancer, Heart Disease, and Bladder and Throat Cancer.

Conclusion: Leave the Myths to the "Big Foot" and "Nessie" Hunters

Without a doubt, it can be very hard for Cancer patients and survivors—not to mention the medical and scientific establishments as a whole—to attempt to determine precisely how, why, and where some individuals—young and old, male or female, healthy or not—came down with their respective Cancers. However, science *is very clear* and verifiable when it comes to several of the causative factors that induce the development of Cancer in individuals, in general, as was discussed in a prior Section in this Chapter. Further, physicians and scientists are persistently conducting research in an enterprise to identify any other potential Cancer risk factors that, heretofore, have been undiscovered. Amid all of this extensive research, science also has overwhelming proof about what *does not* cause Cancer, such as the false beliefs or myths stated in the Section just above. As such, an individual would be well-advised to stick with the *realities* about Cancer, and to dedicate these *myths* to those individuals in search of Sasquatch or the Loch Ness Monster. They *do exist,* don't they??

Live to Survive – Survive to Live

It goes without saying that most people in the world cannot avoid all of the many risk factors that can provoke the occurrence of Cancer, basically, because their lives, their work, and their behaviors and lifestyles—not to mention their ages and heredity—can position them directly in the crosshairs of the disease. Even if an individual is young, with no family history of Cancer, and, if they were somehow able to do everything possible to diminish or eliminate most of their exposure to Cancer risk factors, there is still a chance (i.e., a *random chance*) that the relentless disease would hunt them down anyway.

Based on my own Cancer experience, I am living proof that a person can dedicate their life to doing most of the "right" things to protect themselves from serious health conditions such as Cancer—by eating healthy, not using tobacco or alcohol, exercising regularly, and limiting exposure to pollutants—but, can still become a hapless victim nonetheless. I will say, though, that such random incidences of Cancer are rare (as scientific Studies have shown, and, as my own Medical Team would attest), and that most Cancer incidences *can be reduced* if potential victims would do their part to pitch in and help.

Truthfully, if each individual—young and elderly, male and female—would try to make a determined effort to reduce or alleviate as many Cancer risk factors as possible in their lives that are within their control (obviously, one's age and heredity, cannot be altered – *yet!*), and, assuming that that everyday nuisance, *"random chance,"* doesn't crash the party in the meantime, each of us—in conjunction with many physicians and health care providers—will, hopefully, be able to help decrease the excessive numbers associated with Cancer diagnoses and mortality. Likewise, it is significant that both women and men participate in periodic and regular medical screenings and physical exams—such as Mammogram screenings for women, and Prostate Specific Antigen (PSA) screenings for men—as they both have been scientifically proven to help save many people's lives. By accomplishing this lofty, but achievable goal, not only would fewer men, women, and children become afflicted with, and perish from, this terrible disease, but, those who do fall victim could dramatically increase their probabilities of defeating their respective Cancers and becoming *Survivors* – the one Cancer statistic that truly matters!

When one considers the totality of everything that a Cancer patient, and their loved one, family members or Caregiver may have to accomplish during what can be a potentially lengthy, challenging, and, hopefully, rewarding Cancer journey, it would be very easy to understand how they could feel overwhelmed, and wonder how they will ever be able to accomplish the assorted actions – especially with the gloomy cloud of Cancer looming overhead. Well, to be perfectly honest, just like with any good plan or strategy, preparations for the Cancer journey are all carried out and completed one step at a time, one appointment and meeting at a time, and, one day at a time.

Thankfully, the patient and their family or Caregiver will not be alone in setting the stage to prepare for their Cancer journey, the treatment(s), the Side Effects, and anything that may be encountered along the way. They will have an entire Medical Team and support staff comprised of physicians, nurses, dentists, social workers, HMO employees, medical specialists, lab technicians, dieticians, and other health professionals helping them along their way. Additionally, of course, the patient will also have their extremely strong and reliable support network comprised of their loved ones, any family members and friends, and, of course, their helpful, encouraging, and devoted Caregiver, who may be one of those individuals already listed.

In the end, what really matters—actually, the ***only*** thing that matters—is that the patient receive the fastest, finest, and safest care possible; that all Cancer is completely eliminated from their body; and, that the patient not only survives their Cancer, but, survives in the best shape possible – physically, mentally, and emotionally. Let us never forget that the ultimate goal of this entire Cancer mess is to help the patient reclaim their life. That's Job One, pure and simple.

"Cancer is a prolific and indiscriminate disease. I found out how much so during a conversation that I had in 2004 with an African American woman at the Cancer Clinic. The 50+ year old grandmother of two and I were "chair neighbors" while we received our respective Chemotherapy treatments. She told me that she had just been diagnosed with Breast Cancer, and that of her family of 17 children, 9 of her brothers had been diagnosed with, and treated for Prostate and Colorectal Cancer. In that particular family, 10 out of the 17 children had developed some form of the disease—an unbelievably harsh and unfair statistic, but, that's Cancer. Thankfully, at the time of our conversation, the woman told me that all 9 of her brothers had survived their respective Cancers and were living normal lives."

- Butch Sickler

Chapter Three

The Cancer Journey Explained – *Steps 1 thru 4 on the Journey:*

Pathology; Staging; Diagnosis; Caregiving

"Wisdom teaches one not how to walk, but how not to walk through a Minefield."

- Butch Sickler

Every journey, no matter how brief or how prolonged, has to commence somewhere. For the Cancer patient, their journey will normally start with the fateful delivery of the Diagnosis to them by their physician or other health care professional. From that shocking and unsettling beginning, the patient's adventure thru "Cancer-land" will take them on numerous paths—many of them wide and straight, some of them winding, steep and narrow—but all of them ultimately leading to the same magnificent, warranted, and hopeful destination: *Cancer Survivorship.* To achieve the ultimate objective—a ***Cancer-Free*** or ***Cancer-in-Remission*** conclusion—will require the strength, the will, the faith, and the hope of the patient; the support, prayers, and encouragement of family, Caregivers, and friends; the skills of health professionals; and, the safe use of state-of-the-art technology and medicine. Many planets must align to make this all possible.

A Brave New World

While the Cancer journey might be a long and difficult one, it can also be a triumphant and life-renewing experience for the man, woman, or child who safely and successfully conquers their Cancer. As all Cancer patients, and their loved ones, families and Caregivers will soon discover, after the patient initially receives their diagnosis, their world as they knew it, will be abruptly transformed into what could be a seemingly non-stop flurry of activity for days, weeks, and even months, on-end. The clean daily calendars and schedules of all involved can become extremely busy as they attempt to juggle their personal and family lives, and, possibly, even their work and school obligations, with the plethora of medical meetings, exams, tests, and other commitments that will suddenly consume much of their time.

For those individuals that have not been intimately involved with a Cancer occurrence in their lives previously, the suddenness of the diagnosis and the, *"what do I do now?"-type* feelings, will create an absolutely new and unfamiliar world for them. As such, for these individuals—whether they are the patient, their loved one, or family member or friend—it will doubtless take some time for the shock of the Cancer revelation, and their fear of the unknown, to give way to feelings of self-confidence, hope, and "being in control." Then, as each person involved with this "new" Cancer journey becomes more informed, knowledgeable, and reassured about the steps ahead—as steep and challenging as they may be at times—their world, which, without any warning, was one day unexpectedly turned upside-down with the Cancer Diagnosis, will become their new world – a *Brave New World.* It is within this startling world rudely thrust upon them that the courageous patient—supported by those around them—and their Caregiver, will hunker down and do all that they need to do to battle and beat their Cancer, and to, hopefully, become a Survivor.

A Journey Worth Taking to Reclaim One's Life

After a Diagnosis, but prior to the commencement of Cancer Treatment(s), the proactive, able Cancer patient should take valuable steps to prepare themselves for what can be a lengthy, taxing battle with their Cancer by learning all they can about their new opponent, and, by educating themselves on the best and most effective means that they can carefully and effectively eradicate it from their bodies. Then, after successfully making it through Treatment and safely past any Side Effects that may develop, the patient will need the time to recuperate during the Recovery phase, and then, in Aftercare, will be regularly monitored and tested by doctors for the remainder of their lives to confirm that their Cancer is gone…and gone…and gone…

Ultimately, the Cancer-patient-turned-survivor will, perhaps, get their "old," pre-Cancer life back, or, possibly, will move on to a *"new normal"* approach to living, all the wiser, and all the stronger, because of their humbling Cancer experience. Some Cancer patients occupied in their Cancer journey will both reconnect with their pre-cancerous life, while at the same time committing to transform some things during their post-Cancer survivorship that they may not have done otherwise. No two Cancer survivors will respond identically. The survival of Cancer can be a very useful motivator, and can serve to rejuvenate, strengthen, and humble those individuals who happen to cross in its path. Regardless of who the individual is, however, a diagnosis of Cancer will typically encourage them to take pause, to reexamine life and the people, places, and things in their life, and, to realize just how vulnerable and fragile this life—their life—truly is.

Because a Cancer occurrence will motivate most patients to rethink many things about their lives, it can also serve as a "wake-up call" – a helpful means of urging people to set new priorities in their lives. It will usually encourage them to better appreciate the people, places, and things that they might have taken for granted prior to the onset of their Cancer. Equally, one's Cancer may help them actually "see" things that they were much too busy to view before. The life-threatening impact of Cancer can also motivate Cancer patients and survivors to finally start doing some of those things on their "Bucket Lists" that they've been putting off for years. Undeniably, how each Cancer patient responds to their personal situation will be dissimilar for many reasons. But, *it is* safe to say that *all* patients—no matter their ages, genders, Cancers, or anything else—will do everything they can to battle and beat their disease, and to live as long of a life as possible. It is, after all, human nature to want to survive.

A Path Well-Worn by the Feet of Millions

Millions of Cancer patients take the same, or similar, Cancer journeys every year, and millions of these fearless warriors survive their Cancers, and are able to eventually recapture their lives. If you are a Cancer patient yourself, or, if your loved one, family member, or friend has been stricken by the disease, you, and they, must know that as each Cancer patient embarks on their individual journey, they will not be walking this zigzag path alone. There will be loved ones, family, friends, the Caregiver, and healthcare professionals, at every point along the way to support, encourage, and assist the patient, and to ensure that both they, and their Cancer, are properly treated.

As is frequently the case with most travels worth taking, the journey that one follows with their Cancer can, in the end, be very fulfilling, exhilarating, and triumphant. But, in all honesty, to get to that point, there may be many challenges, with some discomfort and distress along the way. Survival of most things in life typically does not come without paying some sort of price. But, I assure you, as a Cancer survivor, myself, the objective of Cancer survivorship is well worth any amount of toll that a patient is asked to pay to get there.

☛ ***Authors Note:*** Much of the information that is provided in the following Chapters in this Book was obtained from my daily journal notes that I kept during my prolonged Cancer experience, and, from materials provided to me by my Cancer Treatment Medical Team. Additionally, some of the material in these Chapters is based on data contained within the National Institutes for Health and the National Cancer Institute (www.cancer.gov) Internet resources. Information within this Chapter may be explained in greater detail in subsequent Chapters in this Book. Please understand that the material provided in these Chapters is only for educational and informational purposes. Every Cancer patient is dissimilar, as are the circumstances of their respective Cancers. Likewise, the patients' responses to treatments and any Side Effects will vary, as will each patient's prognosis.

Finally, the Reader ought to consider that the Cancer journey steps provided here are simply a fundamental guide I've prepared to hopefully assist the Cancer patient, and their family and Caregiver, in planning and preparing for the Cancer journey ahead. While much of the following material is based upon my own Cancer experience, Readers should understand that other Cancer patients' journeys may include some, or all, of the "steps" that I've described below. Some Cancer patients may even experience some added junctures that I've not incorporated herein. Because all Cancer patients are different, as are factors associated with their Cancers, treatments, and recoveries, the milestones that they encounter on their respective journeys—and their sequence—may differ from those that I have suggested below. Cancer patients, and their families and/or, Caregivers, should always consult their Medical Team for information regarding their specific Cancer situation, or, if they should have any questions or concerns.

"Steps" Along the Cancer Journey Explained

In the following Sections of this Chapter, and in Chapters 4 thru 8 of this Book, detailed summaries of the various "steps" on the patient's Cancer journey are furnished in an attempt to make clear to the patient, and their loved ones, family members, Caregiver, and/or, Guardian, on what they can possibly (emphasis on ***possibly***) expect to experience after receipt of the Diagnosis, then through Treatment, Recovery, and Aftercare, and, ultimately, to the hopeful destination of Survivorship. ***Please note:*** *Some of the following "steps" might occur in succession, or simultaneously with others, or not at all.*

➢ *Cancer Pathology – Step 1 on the Journey*

During the course of an individual's life, there is a possibility that cancerous cells, and/or, a malignant tumor, may be suspected in one's body due to the realization of specific symptoms, and/or, via discovery (accidental or intended) during a medical examination. In such situations, the person will generally be asked to submit to some form of diagnostic test or procedure. In most instances of suspected Cancer, the doctor will order a Computed Tomography (CT) Scan or another form of image of the suspected area in an effort to obtain a pictorial representation that will further help facilitate the diagnostic process. Based on the results of the scans and perhaps other tests, a Surgical Biopsy of the suspected area(s) will typically be performed via the removal of body tissue samples, be they internal, or external.

The tissue samples will then be microscopically examined in a lab to determine if Cancer exists, and if so, whether the Cancer is ***Benign*** (not harmful and doesn't spread) or ***Malignant*** (harmful and can metastasize). The Biopsy results will be assessed and confirmed by a Pathologist, who will release a Pathology Report that details the laboratory findings. The Pathology Report will identify any Cancer presence, and, if known, its form, its location, its Stage (its level of progression within the body), and other data pertinent to the medical findings. This will assist physicians and other health care providers in assessing the individual Cancer patient's case, and, in developing and recommending an all-inclusive treatment strategy. Patients can obtain 2nd and 3rd diagnostic opinions (or more) from doctors that are "outside" their HMO, but, must first receive approval to do so.

Per www.cancer.gov, the Pathology Report will stipulate the location of the Cancer cells taken from the body during the Biopsy procedure(s), but may not necessarily identify the precise location of the Primary Tumor, from which additional cancerous cells may have spread or metastasized in other areas of the body. It is the Pathology Report—which will contain either favorable or poor news from the patient's perspective—that is generally what the physician will have in their hand and read to the patient when they deliver the diagnosis during the post-Biopsy follow-up meeting. If malignant Cancer is present, the diagnosis results will surely distress, scare, confuse, and possibly anger the patient, who will need to be comforted, consoled, and encouraged by the physician, and/or, by loved ones, family, and friends. Such support of the patient is crucial, especially early-on in the process, as the patient will be attempting to do their very best to emotionally process this new development in their life, and, will be busy taking positive steps to better understand their Cancer, and how they and their doctors will go about ridding it from their body.

➢ *Cancer "Staging" – Step 2 on the Journey*

Preparations for a bulk of life's happenings, including one's Cancer treatment, will generally call for a given number of steps that should be completed—often in a particular order—to ensure that all important issues are proactively addressed and that nothing is left to chance. Of course, life is life, so mistakes are made and some things may "slip through the cracks." This can happen, sometimes, due to human error; sometimes, because of occurrences that are beyond our control; and, sometimes, due to that failsafe, age-old equalizer, *"Shit happens."* With this being the case, a high amount of due diligence *is* carried out by the patient's health care professionals to ensure that the Cancer patient's individual needs are being met, their Cancer is being properly addressed, and, that any risks are being managed and minimized in an effort to maximize the potential for overall success.

When thinking of the planning process in general, how many times have you heard the phrase, ***"You don't go after Grizzly Bear with a BB Gun"***? Chances are that you never have. But, even if you are not familiar with that quirky aphorism, its meaning is still pretty straightforward. What these words attempt to convey is that prior to taking on a particular adversary (and especially **BIG** ones), one will want to learn all they can about their foe so that they can prepare and arm themselves appropriately, just in case things happen to go from bad to worse. And, so it also goes with Grizzly Bears and Cancer. Bear Hunters will know from the very get-go precisely what sorts of firepower, maps, and other necessary survival tools they will require prior to stepping one foot into the woods. When it comes to "Cancer hunting," however, doctors must depend upon a medical assessment "weapon," referred to as ***Cancer Staging***, for them to be able to gain any insight as to the size, location, and breadth of *their* nemesis.

What is Cancer Staging?

The process of assessing or "grading" a malignant tumor is referred to as *"Cancer Staging."* According to the National Cancer Institute (www.cancer.gov), Staging is a logical means of describing the severity of a person's Cancer based on the characteristics of the original (Primary) Tumor, and whether or not the Cancer has spread to (or metastasized in) other locations of the body. If a malignancy (harmful Cancer) is identified during diagnosis and confirmed in a Medical Lab by Pathological assessment, efforts are undertaken by medical professionals to "Stage" (i.e., to "grade" or assign a "rating" to) the patient's Cancer. The Staging of Cancers is a by-product of the Cancer diagnostic process, which, itself, typically consists of CT Scans, MRIs, X-Rays and other imaging techniques, Biopsy Surgery tissue samples, laboratory examination of the Cancer by experienced Medical Pathologists, and, confirmation of the Cancer form (and its location, if identified) on the Pathologist's Report. The standardized Staging of Cancer is a vital tool used by physicians to help "level the playing field" for the patient's upcoming battle with their Cancer.

Cancer Staging is based on awareness of the way that Cancer progresses. Cancer cells mature and divide without control or order, and they do not die when they should. As a result, they often form a mass of tissue called a *Tumor*. As the tumor develops, it can invade adjoining tissues and organs. Cancer cells can also break apart from the tumor and go into the Bloodstream or the Lymphatic System. By travelling through the Bloodstream or Lymphatic system, cancerous cells can spread from the Primary Tumor and metastasize in Lymph Nodes or other organs, where they could form new tumor colonies.

How are Cancers Staged?

The Cancer Staging Systems are explained in more detail in numerous other Cancer resource materials, and in Chapter 9 of this Book. But, basically stated, Cancer Stages are based on a “scoring” system that’s usually numbered from 0 to IV, with additional data to indicate other factors about the Cancer incidence. And, just as in the game of Golf, the lower the Cancer Staging “score” the better. For example, Stage 0 is for *potential* Cancers; Stage I denotes *localized* tumors—the least invasive and the most treatable—while Stage IV Cancers are still treatable, but are the *most severe and challenging*. The Stage takes into account the size of a tumor, how deeply it has penetrated surrounding tissue, whether it has invaded nearby organs, and to how many Lymph Nodes it has metastasized (if any).

Staging Systems for Cancer have evolved over time, and as scientists and physicians continue to learn more about the over 200 known forms of Cancer, Staging Systems will be adapted as deemed necessary to better accommodate the new findings and data. Some Cancer Staging Systems actually cover many forms of Cancer, while others are more specific and tend to center on a particular type of the disease. That being said, there are some elements common to most Staging Systems that are utilized to evaluate and document Cancer progression and severity, regardless of the form of Cancer.

Why is Cancer Staging Important?

According to the National Cancer Institute (www.cancer.gov), one of the most noteworthy purposes of Cancer Staging is to provide a universally understood definition of the progress of Cancers. Once the baseline Staging level has been determined, it helps the Medical Team in planning the treatment protocols for that particular Cancer, and helps them in determining the patient's prognosis. In this regard, Staging is probably the most powerful predictor of survival. That is, the lower the Stage of one's Cancer, the higher the prospects of their survival. After the Cancer Stage has been medically assessed for the patient's specific form of Cancer, the Medical Team, in concurrence with the patient and their family, and/or, Caregiver, will employ the diagnosis and Staging information to help design a Cancer treatment plan that is best suited to the patient's particular situation.

Just as a General or Admiral utilize intelligence and proven military tactics to innovate a strategy for battle, or, the sportsman (or woman) uses their outdoor survival skills and knowledge to prepare for an adventure into the wild, physicians will utilize Cancer Staging information to help them design the most appropriate treatment for a patient's particular form of Cancer. One of the benefits of assigning Stages to Cancers is that it enables physicians, health care providers, and researchers to communicate with one another in a standardized "language" about information that would otherwise be discussed in diverse and subjective terms. This advantage not only speeds up the treatment planning and implementation process, but, precludes any potential misinterpretations or any confusion on the part of multiple health professionals who may be involved in treating the patient.

From a less individual perspective, but just as significant, is that the Cancer Staging process facilitates governmental and private Cancer research institutions' abilities to track Cancer records, and to maintain a statistical database for each type of Cancer. For example, several of the Cancer statistics that I've cited in this Book from the National Cancer Institute (www.cancer.gov), were available, thanks to the Cancer Staging System. Ultimately, these statistics benefit the medical community and patients, both in research and in treatment.

➢ *Cancer Diagnosis – Step 3 on the Journey*

It all begins with a Cancer Diagnosis – the uncertainties, the treatments, the tests, the generally, inconvenient, uncomfortable, and stressful Side Effects, the seemingly non-stop schedule, the worries, questions, and uncertainties about survival – the list goes on, and on, and on. Considering all of this, it would be rather easy for a Cancer victim to place any and all of their fear, self-loathing and self-doubts squarely on the shoulders of the Diagnosis. Without the Diagnosis, there would be no awful news, and, if there were no bad news, there would be no feelings of hurt, or anguish, or anger. Isn't this correct? Well, literally, that may be true, but, realistically, nothing could be further from the truth. Sadly, it is Cancer, the Disease—not Cancer, the Diagnosis—that is the lone offender responsible for invoking the pain, worry, and suffering in those affected by this medical menace. And, the Diagnosis? – Well, it is the best thing that could possibly ever happen to a victim of Cancer. If a person has Cancer brewing inside their body, believe me, ***they DO want to know about it!***

The Cancer Diagnosis - A Blessing, Not a Curse

"I'm sorry, but you have Cancer." When an individual first hears that dreaded term, "Cancer," come out of their doctor's mouth, especially when it is aimed at the individual with whom the doctor is speaking, there, frankly, is no means of capturing in mere words the multitude of thoughts, emotions, concerns, and questions that come instantly to the patient's mind. Even though the patient, the doctor, or both, might have had an inkling that the Biopsy laboratory results could come back positive for malignant Cancer, when one hears the actual word spoken, or reads proof-positive of its incidence on their Pathology Report, it imparts a stark reality to the moment that—not unlike a blazing Howitzer shot—is altogether shocking, threatening, fear-provoking, and bewildering. This unavoidable disquietude is to be anticipated, however, for both the cannon and one's Cancer can cause considerable damage, unless they are silenced first.

There is no question about it – a Diagnosis of Cancer is very serious business, especially to the individual on the receiving end of such a medical finding. And, definitely, such information can be just as devastating to their loved one, family members, and friends. But, a Cancer diagnosis is not <u>all</u> bad – it truthfully can be a blessing-in-disguise. Rather than one viewing a Cancer diagnosis as a threat or *hazard* to their lives, those diagnosed with the disease might want to think of their diagnosis as a positive, and very important "highway warning sign," that could actually help them *save* their lives.

That's correct – metaphorically speaking, a Cancer diagnosis is really no different than a big, bright *"Bridge Out Ahead"* warning sign posted on the shoulder of the road – both serve as precautionary notices to alert individuals that very hazardous conditions lie ahead. And, each warning, in its own way, strongly suggests that corrective actions be taken as urgently as possible to prevent a harmful, if not fatal, disaster. The benefit of signs is that they do the thinking for a person, and they notify them what they should do to avoid a perilous situation – that is, *if the people wish to read and heed.* If you, or a family member, a loved one, or a friend has received a Diagnosis of Cancer, do endeavor to consider it to be a blessing, and not a curse. Definitely, the Diagnosis is not a blessing because one *has* Cancer, but, because it enables one ***to know*** that they have Cancer.

The Ideal Cancer Diagnosis - Early and Accurate

The bottom line in the race against time in properly treating a Cancer is that any unfortunate miscalculations and setbacks for any reason can result in the Cancer's unremitting, risky advance within a person's body. This can place the individual's health and prognosis in much greater jeopardy should it spread within the bodily systems, organs, and tissues. Considering this, it is apparent just how critical are both timing and accuracy in promptly and correctly identifying, evaluating, and Staging the Cancer, so that an appropriate treatment plan can be developed and implemented at the earliest opportunity. Once a confirmed Cancer diagnosis has been delivered, the next act will be to generate the plan-of-attack to safely remove the disease.

Strength in Numbers

Without question, a Cancer diagnosis is not an easy thing for a doctor to deliver, and, speaking from a patient's perspective, it is a much more difficult thing to receive. Hopefully, however, when the news is conveyed to the patient for the first time, the *doctor does so compassionately and in-person for the patient's sake, vs. indirectly, such as over the telephone or some other impersonal means* (believe me, I have heard some horror stories of doctors actually doing that!). This person-to-person interaction is vital to the process, for there is no knowing how the patient will react, or, how much consoling they will require. If the physician is the only person in the room with the patient at the time the diagnosis is delivered, the doctor, by default, will become the patient's instantaneous "support system." He or she will be the first person to whom the bewildered patient will look for reassurance, strength, answers to questions, and a shoulder to cry on.

However, if a loved one or a friend is with the patient when the doctor provides the diagnosis, that person will be able to be the patient's *Rock,* and should be able to offer whatever level of comfort and assurance the patient might need. This person will definitely be just as overwhelmed and saddened by the news of the diagnosis, but, hopefully, they will retain their self-control, and will remain strong and determined on behalf of, and in front of, the patient. This is very important, especially right after receiving the diagnosis, because the patient may experience and display a combination of uncontrollable emotions while their mind may be in a bit of a fog, preoccupied with trying to make sense of the 2 x 4 that just smacked them between the eyes. More than anything in this tough situation, however, what the patient *really* needs is someone to hold them close, to look them in the eyes, and to tell them that everything is going to be alright.

Patient Quiet Time

Whether the patient is alone with the doctor or accompanied by a loved one, a family member, or a friend when the diagnosis is handed down, the doctor could offer to the patient some "quiet time" alone in the room, so that the patient, and any others, can attempt to gather their thoughts and try to assimilate and process the entirety of what has just transpired. Following the receipt of the shocking and troublesome diagnosis, there will be much to think about, and it may be difficult for one to form any sensible thoughts about what has just occurred. This peaceful and private setting is important—even if the patient is by themselves—as it will provide the individual(s) with an opportunity to express their true emotions without feeling judged or interrupted by other commotions, or, weighted down by the dull and sterile medical environment in which they are left to sit and ponder.

Some patients may respond to this sad moment in their own way by sobbing or bawling out loud (it's likely for one to be scared and cry upon receiving the news), while others may internalize their strife and remain hushed. Still others may seek spiritual intervention to pray or meditate and reflect inwardly upon their destiny. Clearly, every patient's reaction and rejoinder to such news will be as varied as the individuals, themselves. Unlike the bombshell of winning the lottery and wondering what one will do with all of that money in the future, the shock of getting Cancer will cause one to question if they will even have a future. In either event, it is a lot to think about and to process, both emotionally and physically. However, the sadness and fear that can accompany a Cancer diagnosis will dictate that *this* life-altering event be handled with the utmost compassion and care.

Discussing Next Steps with the Doctor

At some point after the diagnosis is delivered, and when the patient feels that they are emotionally and mentally strong enough to discuss particulars, the doctor will, typically, sit with the patient and will try their best to address any questions and concerns the patient may have. Additionally, the doctor may describe the specifics of the diagnosis in greater detail by telling the patient what form of Cancer they have, its mass or Stage (severity and progression in the body, if known or indicated on the Pathology Report), and the site where the Primary Tumor is located, if that is known. Sometimes, the Primary Tumor is not initially apparent or obviously noticeable to physicians (as was the situation with my own Cancer), and may require further follow-up testing and examination to be positively located.

The physician may also discuss treatment options that will possibly be pursued, and, they may provide as much information as is appropriate to basically familiarize the patient with the Treatment, Recovery, and Aftercare processes, including any possible timelines, possible benefits and risks, and potential expectations. Additionally, depending upon the form of Cancer with which the patient has been diagnosed, the doctor may refer the patient to one or more medical specialists—such as an Oncologist, a Radiation Oncologist, and/or, a Cancer Surgeon—so that each of them can meet with the patient to discuss, make clear, and plan their respective treatment strategies. In such cases, the specialists will contact the patient to schedule visits.

Post-Diagnosis Support

Part-and-parcel of any process to properly address a Cancer patient's post-diagnosis needs would include any efforts that can be taken—or any tools that can be used—that will help to provide the patient, their family members, and their Caregiver, with the support, information, and relevant resources that they may need to help them "weather the storms" during their Cancer journey. For each patient diagnosed, Cancer is a distinctive and personal experience. No two people will travel the same, precise journey prior to, during, or after their treatment(s). How people will cope after being diagnosed, and, how they will respond physically and emotionally, both during their treatment(s) and afterward, is also very different for each individual. However, despite the overt variations in people and their respective Cancers and treatment plans, there *is* one common thread that links all people together who are diagnosed with Cancer: The need for an accessible, helpful, encouraging, and continuous support system.

Coping with Cancer Post-Diagnosis Stress

When individuals initially receive the report of their Cancer diagnosis, of course, their worst thoughts and worries will typically come to mind. Mine definitely did. This is because almost everyone in America is related to, is friends with, or knows, someone who has Cancer now, or who has had Cancer in the past. As such, people are well aware of the battles to be fought, the possible Side Effects to be experienced, and, the potential outcomes to be had. Along with the initial fright, anxiety, shock, and sense of bewilderment that can be experienced by the Cancer patient, will also come some stress – ***lots*** of stress, to be exact. In the first place, if the patient is anything like me upon initially receiving their Cancer diagnosis, they will likely be asking themselves, and perhaps their doctor, many unanswerable questions, such as, *"Why me?," "How could this have happened to me?," "What did I do to deserve this?,"* and, *"Am I going to die?"*

Of course, all of the various, *"Why?" "When?" "What?"* and *"How?"* questions are reasonable inquiries, but, the answers are not simple; nor, will they be forthcoming anytime soon, if at all. It is the patient not knowing the cause(s) of their Cancer, and, the patient not being able to envision their Cancer outcome, that perhaps causes the most distress and fear of all, especially early-on in the process. But, thankfully, there are some coping mechanisms and resources that are available to all Cancer patients to help them get past the initial shock of their diagnosis, and, to assist them in preparing their bodies and minds for their upcoming long journeys thru Treatment, Recovery, Aftercare, and ultimately—hopefully—Cancer survivorship.

After a person receives a shocking diagnosis of Cancer, it is to be expected that they will feel terribly worried and overwhelmed. Many individuals may even feel that they have just been handed the equivalent of a "Death Sentence," unsure of what their future holds, while others will handle the report with a more optimistic approach, having every intention of defeating the disease at its own game and turning a negative circumstance into a positive and constructive life-renewing outcome. Still other patients may be equally as worried, if not more so, about their families, finances, and other factors in their lives than they will be about their own fates. In any event, there is a high likelihood that all Cancer patients—no matter how mentally or physically weak or strong they may be—will realize some negative responses to the Cancer diagnosis news, not the least of which will be anxiety, fright, and stress. *"Fear of the unknown"* is probably the worst kind of anguish, but rest-assured, it should go away over time.

Seeking Help for Cancer Post-Diagnosis Stress

One of the main problems with Stress—and we all know this because we have certainly suffered from it at some point during our lives—is that it can be ***very*** stressful. *Duh!!* But, seriously speaking, prolonged occurrences of this downhearted mental state can lead to hopelessness, frustration, anger, and, at times, deep, dark depression. Individuals might have difficulty sleeping, they may feel exhausted, their body may have aches and pains, and/or, they may be suffering from a lack of confidence or low self-esteem. Each of these factors on its own is extraordinary, but, when combined with one or more of the others, it can be increasingly overwhelming to a person who has just suffered the devastating surprise of a Cancer diagnosis. And, as would be anticipated, the individual with Cancer is not the only one affected by the diagnosis and ensuing aftermath – loved ones, family members, friends, and others near to the patient are also impacted by the emotional and physical changes of a person with Cancer.

If left unchecked, prolonged stress and depression can spiral out of control. But, thankfully, there are things that a patient can do, early-on, to help themselves cope with the veracity of their diagnosis and their fears of not knowing what awaits. Not knowing what lies beyond the fog can be very scary. But, there are many means to deal with the stress and fear associated with Cancer, including education and supportive care, which will help to better equip a patient to cope with the diagnosis and the follow-on treatment of their Cancer.

There are also a host of self-help-type actions and behaviors that a Cancer patient can adopt and pursue on their own in an effort to help them make the best of what can be an otherwise non-optimal situation. However, if "going it alone" isn't helping the patient cope with their personal circumstances, and, if they feel that they require additional or professional support, they should certainly consult with their Medical Team or other health care professionals, as there may be a need for more extensive counseling and assistance. ***Remember: It is a strength, not a weakness, to seek professional help.***

Post-Diagnosis Stress-Coping Strategies

Every Cancer patient is an individual unto themselves. As such, even though a patient may share a Cancer type common with others, the circumstances of their specific case are very personal and varied, as are the abilities of the person to cope with the big, massive weight that just dropped out of nowhere and landed on their head. Some people might have faced adversity in their past, and, therefore, may be better-conditioned and more prepared to deal with bouts of stress. Others, however, may have lived a more "sheltered life," and, through no fault of their own, have not had the experience with life-trauma; nor are they already "equipped" to cope with adversities and any associated stress – especially that which comes on the heels of a life-threatening medical revelation such as Cancer. No matter how seasoned an individual may be when it comes to dealing with stress, however, there are a few tips for better coping with this mental and emotional menace that should apply to all patients across the board.

Suggested ideas for coping with stress following a Diagnosis of Cancer, which have been adapted from the online resources of the National Cancer Institute (www.cancer.gov), include:

- Maintain a journal, and if possible, try to make daily entries. Journaling can be an extremely therapeutic means of privately expressing one's feelings, worries, set-backs, joys, and triumphs, and, it allows one to externalize any pent-up frustrations and to "get them off their chest." During my own Cancer experience, I found journaling to also be an excellent method of maintaining a chronology of everything that I experienced each day through my Treatments, Recovery, and Aftercare. My journaling notes, which I maintained from the day I received my Cancer diagnosis until over 3 years later, are the primary basis of each Chapter in this Book, and a source of the information contained within
- Meditate for at least 15 minutes every day in a peaceful, private setting if at all possible. While meditating, practice taking deep breaths, and allow the mind to travel to a tranquil destination
- Exercise regularly, if the physician and time will permit. Some form of physical activity, be it swimming, bicycling, stretching, jogging or running, yoga, walking, weight-training, and others, will help to stimulate *Endorphins,* the stress-reducing hormones. Remember, *a strong body yields a strong mind – and visa versa*
- Adopt and try to maintain an optimistic, positive mental attitude, and, as difficult as it may be, attempt to laugh, despite all that is happening around you, and any negativity you may see or hear
- Accept the fact that things occur in life that we cannot control – In other words, "Stuff happens," to put it nicely
- Don't count on drugs, alcohol, cigarettes, or binge-eating to help reduce stress. These "temporary fixes" usually just make matters worse, and, in the long term, one will eventually have to pay the price for these "bad habits" in more ways than one
- Get and nurture a pet, no matter or big or small, if circumstances and schedule and health status will allow. Pets can be consoling
- Make a concerted effort to relax, free of as many responsibilities as possible, if only for a few minutes at a time. Softer, soothing music and a good book may assist, including optimistic books about faith and hope, and those written by Cancer survivors
- Don't be too proud or "shy" to request professional assistance with a Mental Therapist who is trained to help patients cope

- Eat nutritious, well-balanced meals, devoid of "bad" fats, sugar, and salt, if possible, and try to consume water – lots of water to be exact, each day, as well as a multi-vitamin, if permitted
- Find comfort, reassurance, hope, and strength in one's spiritual and religious faith and convictions, if so-inclined. Ask the leader of the church, synagogue, mosque or other religious center if he or she—as well as members of the congregation—can pray for the patient's good health and recovery
- Be assertive but not aggressive. "Assert" your feelings, opinions, or beliefs—including to your physician(s) as necessary—instead of becoming angry, combative, submissive, or passive
- Share companionship with a Loved One or a friend in whom you can confide, and with whom you can speak, listen to, and ask for advice, or, for a shoulder to lean on every now and then
- Perhaps, most significantly of all, get plenty of rest and sleep. A person's body and brain require time to "recharge," so that they both have the strength and the endurance to face, and to recover from, stressful events. One's Cancer Treatments and associated Side Effects will unquestionably fall into this dubious category

Post-Diagnosis Protection of the Immune System

Realizing all the information in this Book about Cancer, and, considering the millions of other books, articles, internet sites, and other media and materials pertaining to the disease, it may cause one to wonder how in the world we are able to ever live and function at all in this life without all of us falling prey to this ubiquitous medical menace. By the looks of things, Cancer—or potential causes of the disease—could be loitering around every corner, hiding under every rock, and cowering in every alley, be it light or dark. But, while it may seem that way, fortunately for us, it is not necessarily the case. But, what *is* true, is that the knowledge of this information regarding Cancer and what an individual chooses to do about it, and with it—*after learning of the diagnosis*—are of paramount importance.

Honestly, a Cancer patient's understanding of their Cancer, its treatments and Side Effects, the advantages of a healthy Immune System, and the steps they can take to protect it *after receiving their diagnosis*, will be critical in the patient's decision to do all they can to help them conquer and recover from their disease. It definitely is very important for the patient to do everything possible to strengthen their Immune System after their Cancer diagnosis. But, ***it is just as fundamental that the patient not feel guilty or blame themselves or their parents*** for contracting this nasty disease. By the way, this rule pertains to ***every*** Cancer patient, regardless of any potential genetic links, environmental exposures, or personal behaviors, lifestyles, or "bad" habits that they believe may have caused their illness. For lack of a better way of putting it, "it is what it is," and nothing can be done to get rid of the diagnosis, or, to modify any of the causative factors that may have led up to the disconcerting medical findings.

However, it is when the, *"Cow is out of the barn,"* and after the consequential diagnosis has been delivered to the patient by their doctor, that everything promising that can be achieved by the Cancer patient to care for their body should be done. This might include the patient's need to modify any past risky habits or lifestyle behaviors going forward (such as using tobacco, drinking alcohol, eating fatty foods, not exercising, going into the sun without protection, etc.) as well as minimizing their exposures to any avoidable environmental threats. But, perhaps, most importantly, the post-diagnosis emphasis will be completely on the patient focusing all of their future efforts, thoughts, and energies towards fighting and conquering their disease during their Treatment, Recovery and Aftercare phases. Ultimately, however, what *truly* matters, is meeting, treating, and beating one's Cancer, and, turning that nasty diagnosis into a healthy, fruitful life.

Not unlike a terrorist out to do some damage, Cancer can be undetectable, mobile, and deadly. But, *exactly like* a terrorist, it *can be* identified, outgunned, and eliminated. For any outward or inward hazard to be conquered, however—whether in a military battle zone or in one's body—the enemy must first be discovered, identified and confirmed. In the war that is Cancer, the diagnostic tests are the first critical weapons to be used in fighting and defeating the disease, and ultimately, in reclaiming one's life. It takes detection to precipitate a Cancer diagnosis; it takes a diagnosis to instigate treatments; and, it takes the treatment(s), and the will of the patient and expertise of the physicians, to eliminate one's Cancer. Then, finally—confidently—after everything is said and done, the fearless Cancer-patient-turned-Survivor, will be able to look back at their hard-fought war, and will look forward to their opportunity to live, once again.

➢ *Adopting a Cancer Caregiver – Step 4 on the Journey*

Gratefully, I, and almost 13.7 million other Cancer Survivors currently alive in the U.S., have been blessed with a Second Chance at Life. A few of the survivors I know have been granted three or more opportunities to reclaim their lives after they have successfully survived the awful attack, damage, and recovery from more than one Cancer tumor or metastasis. In a great majority of these cases, I dare state that most of the Cancer patients and survivors were surrounded by an extremely close-knit network of caring, compassionate family members, friends, religious acquaintances, business associates, and others, who offered their prayers, good wishes, encouragement, and positive thoughts during the Cancer patient's time-of-need.

I definitely am grateful for the expressions of love and caring with which my "network" of family, friends, and Caregiver blessed me through my own Cancer experience. Without question, the love, prayers, and support that I received from these kind souls was, in my opinion, just as powerful, and just as critical to my fight for survival, as were my many Cancer Surgeries, Radiation Therapy sessions, and the Chemotherapy medications that coursed throughout my body.

The Cancer Caregiver – An Unsung Hero

Following the diagnosis and Staging of the patient's Cancer, and, after the patient has been told of the medical findings by their physician or health care professional, things begin getting very busy, very fast. One of the initial things that usually happens after a person receives a diagnosis of Cancer and the news is shared with others, is that someone will, naturally, either come forward and volunteer, or, will be asked by the patient to help support them during their Cancer journey. This kind, selfless person could be the patient's significant other, a family member, a friend, or another person who has stepped up to do what they can to assist the patient during their conflict with the disease. This self-sacrificing, unsung hero of the Cancer Wars is none other than the patient's ***Caregiver.*** In rare situations where the Cancer patient has no loved one, family members or friends that can help, the patient's Medical Team will appoint a volunteer to assist.

The Cancer Caregiver will be the kind, thoughtful individual who will take it upon themselves to contribute their own life to help save the patient's. The Caregiver will encourage, support, help out, comfort, and, otherwise, aid the gutsy Cancer patient in making their way safely, steadfastly, and, hopefully, successfully, thru their entire Cancer journey. It has been mentioned that when an individual gets Cancer, so does the person charged with their care. Not literally, of course, but in the sense that both people will be taking the same long journey together, side-by-side, from start to finish, come what may.

Throughout the complete length of their combined travels on this journey, both the patient and Caregiver will be apt to experience the same sorrow and joy, the same set-backs and achievements, and, the same stress and serenity. Opportunely, when the dust has settled, and, if all of the Cancer-killing treatments have accomplished their objectives, the brave Cancer patient—that is, the Cancer *Survivor*—and their Caregiver, will hopefully be able to share with one another the greatest gift of all: That precious, Second Chance at Life.

During my own three+-year Cancer journey, from Diagnosis and Treatment, thru Recovery and Aftercare, my Caregiver was my girlfriend at the time, Joanne, which was convenient. In most of my experiences with other adult Cancer patients, I've noticed that their Caregivers have tended to be their "significant others" as well, such as their spouses, or their boyfriends or girlfriends. And, while it did break my heart to see the young and teenage children courageously fighting their respective Cancers in the clinic, the harshness of their plight was softened considerably when I observed the outpouring of love, support, and hugs provided by *their* Caregivers—their parents, grandparents, Guardian, and often, their siblings and friends.

Roles of the Cancer Caregiver

It is estimated that 44 million Americans care for somebody with an illness or a disability at home. Out of this astonishing total, I would venture a guess that an exceedingly substantial percentage of these Caregivers are those individuals who are looking after a family member or a friend who has been diagnosed with Cancer. Whether the Cancer patient is a man, woman, teenager, or a young child, their Caregivers all share the same selfless desire to provide their patients with their love, support, counsel, compassion, hugs, encouragement, assistance, and their physical and emotional strength, often on a 24/7 basis, for several months at a time. These helpful individuals serve in several capacities throughout the entire Cancer ordeal, from being the patient's primary health advocate, and perhaps their legal Power of Attorney, to functioning in the role of ad-hoc Cancer researcher, appointment scheduler, chauffer, cook, and strong, wise companion. And, of course, all Cancer Caregivers also become the patient's all-important-warm-person-to-hug, or their strong-shoulder-to-cry-on.

Perhaps one of the most vital responsibilities of a Caregiver, however, is that of a participant on the Cancer Treatment Medical Team, which may also be comprised of the patient, family members, and health care professionals of multiple disciplines. In this setting, amongst other responsibilities, the Caregiver will help to ensure that the patient is provided with, and completely comprehends, all of the information that will aid them in determining the treatment plan that is best personalized for the patient's Cancer situation. Because the Cancer patient's Caregiver will be *riding shotgun* beside the patient for the duration of the journey, it is significant that the Caregiver is involved with, and knowledgeable of, most elements of the patient's care. As one can imagine, this is especially necessary for parents and Caregivers of young or elder patients who need to be steadily aided.

Information that could be disclosed, evaluated, talked about, and agreed upon among the patient's Medical Team may include the following: The most suitable and effective Cancer treatment options available and their frequency of administration; any potential pain or other Side-Effects to be encountered during the Treatment(s) and the prospective tactic to safely address them; and, the probable expected outcomes of the Treatment(s) and Recovery, based on the patient's physical state and the form, site, and severity of their Cancer. In this regard, the Caregiver will assist the patient—and, thus, the Medical Team—in arriving at a decision as to the courses of treatment to be followed that all estimate will yield optimal Cancer-killing benefits, while best minimizing risk to the remainder of the patient's body.

Just as all Cancer patients are different from one another, so too could there be distinctive variations in the circumstances of their respective Cancers, their personal treatment plans, their responses to their individual treatment(s), and, ultimately, to their recoveries and final outcomes. Considering this, it stands to reason that the roles of individual Caregivers would also differ somewhat, depending on the specific needs of their respective patients and the circumstances of a given situation. Certainly, all Cancer Caregivers will respond to the personalized requirements of their patients on a day-to-day basis and they will do what is required as conditions dictate. But, even though each Caregiver's specific roles and responsibilities may differ from person to person depending on individual patients, all Cancer patient Caregivers do share some common and fundamental duties that may apply in all cases, regardless of their individual states-of-affairs.

Potential Responsibilities of the Cancer Caregiver

Specific responsibilities that active Cancer Caregivers could potentially perform on behalf of their Cancer patients (depending on the patients' ages, forms of Cancer, types of treatments, responses to the treatments, and other factors) may include, but are not limited to:

- Accompanying the patient to their meetings with physicians, and during their exams, tests, treatments, etc.
- Taking notes, as is necessary, during meetings with physicians to ensure that discussion highlights and answers to any questions are captured for future reference purposes
- Serving as the patient's Power of Attorney in medical and other matters, as necessary, and if legally entitled to do so
- Scheduling the patient's doctor's appointments, as necessary
- Being the patient's primary health advocate in interacting with medical staff, and helping to determine the best treatment for the patient that will help them fight and hopefully defeat the disease
- Assisting the patient with the conduct of research on Cancer, its possible treatment options, potential Side-Effects and strategies to minimize or eliminate them, and anticipated therapy outcomes
- Encouraging the patient to continually remain strong, rested, and optimistic thru the Treatment and Recovery phases, and to never give up hope that the journey and efforts will be successful
- Taking care of the patient's household chores, as necessary, to include doing laundry, feeding pets, watering plants, etc.
- Reading a good book to the patient, or sharing a movie together

- Taking the patient out for a short drive or to sit at a nearby park or on the beach if the patient is getting "cabin fever" in the house and is emotionally and physically able, and cleared by the doctor to take such "mini-getaways" during the day
- Helping the patient take their at-home medications at prescribed dosages, times, and frequencies, and as needed, to ensure that all symptoms and any Side Effects of the Cancer and treatments—especially any pain and nausea—are being effectively managed
- Driving the patient to and from Dr. appointments, as applicable
- Visiting the patient in the hospital, as necessary, and interacting with medical staff to make sure that the patient's needs are being met, and, if not, that staff is aware and takes proper steps to help
- Accompanying the patient to their meetings with physicians, and during their exams, tests, treatments, etc.
- Helping to look after the patient's financial and other business-related responsibilities, as applicable
- Preparing and serving food to the patient, including special diets if one is indicated
- Shopping for the patient for food, beverages, medications, and other household or health care supplies, as needed
- Giving the patient time to themselves, as requested
- Being a good listener, and giving the patient honest feedback, as needed, and compassionate counsel, as requested
- Being the "voice of reason" and providing sound, rational, and prudent advice and intervention should circumstances dictate
- Providing the patient with support, companionship, and things (that the doctor will permit and that are legal), that will help to bring the patient comfort, reassurance, self-confidence, strength, and a feeling of well-being
- Laughing and crying right alongside the patient during the ups and downs of treatment and recovery
- Being the patient's "rock" by maintaining a strong and positive outward appearance and attitude (when and where possible), and being the "beacon" on that rock that the patient can turn to when the going gets rough
- If the patient is a young child or a teenager, meeting with the school officials to notify them about the child's or teen's Cancer situation, and interfacing with the school and the young patient to help them keep up with schoolwork, as applicable

One could take a look at the above listing and easily ask how in the world any person could ever possibly accomplish all of these Caregiver roles and responsibilities, often in addition to maintaining their own family, personal, and job commitments. Well, to be totally truthful, when dealing with one's Cancer, and, when considering the potentially difficult journey, it is actually remarkable the things that people can step up and accomplish that they never dreamed possible of themselves. Oftentimes, it takes a horrifying thing like Cancer to literally bring out the best, most miraculous, qualities in people.

This resolve, resilience, and "rising to the occasion" applies uniformly to both the Cancer patient *and* the Caregiver. While only one of the two people must experience the actual treatments, both of the individuals—in their own ways—must try to muster the strength to persevere, and, each will feel both the pain and the joy of having done so. Ultimately, when all is said and done, and after the healing process has begun, it is hopeful that both individuals will realize the positive fruits of their exhaustive labors. That aspiration, of course, would be that both the patient and, indirectly, the Caregiver, will be blessed with a ***Cancer-Free,*** or ***Cancer-in-Remission*** outcome.

Cancer Caregiver Stress – Signs and Suggestions for Coping

It goes without saying that a Cancer patient obviously does not volunteer or sign up to get their disease – that is one *freebie* that they can certainly live their life without. Their Cancer Caregiver, on the other hand, will typically take it upon themselves to step forward and assist the Cancer patient in-need. This will happen naturally, out of love, kindness, necessity, or, a feeling of familial responsibility or friendship. And, just like the Cancer patient when they first receive their diagnosis, the new Cancer Caregiver will, most likely, also be a "*Cancer Virgin*" – potentially unknowledgeable of, unfamiliar with, and unprepared for, the unavoidable wild-and-wooly Roller Coaster ride that awaits. But, despite the forthcoming uphill battles, and the probable lengthy and wearisome journey marked with hours of pain, joy, uncertainty, achievement, frustration, progress, and discomfort, the Cancer Caregiver will stand by their courageous patient from the rocky but promising start, to the, hopefully, favorable finish.

The patient's Cancer journey, however, will, sometimes, take its toll, not only on the patient, but also on their dedicated Caregiver. Caregiver Stress is an all-too-common Side Effect of being a Cancer Caregiver. Because of the steady physical and emotional energy and continuous attention that the Caregiver devotes to the Cancer patient throughout their ordeal, the Cancer Caregiver will, in many cases, basically, "run out of gas in their *own* tank," which, of course, can severely limit their abilities to take care of themselves, much less the patient. Likewise, the Cancer Caregiver must often put their own life on-hold while they tend to the patient's, which can potentially cause issues with *their own* familial responsibilities, financial obligations, work commitments, and other such activities that have had to take a "back seat" when their lives were abruptly interrupted by Cancer.

Thankfully, the more intensive and time-consuming care of a Cancer patient will normally be in the first few weeks or months of the Cancer journey. This is all because for days and weeks following the Cancer diagnosis, it will seem that there is one meeting or exam after another, and there will be quite a lot that has to be done to learn about the patient's form of Cancer and to prepare for their upcoming treatment and other medical commitments. After this initial flurry of activity, the seemingly non-stop timetable *will* diminish (but will not disappear completely), and both the patient and Caregiver can "catch their breath," and take the time to begin healing. But, however brief or long-lasting the Caregiver's "tour of duty" may be, the pressures associated with caregiving can cause valid and significant emotional and physical issues that must be recognized and properly addressed.

Warning Signs of Cancer Caregiver Stress

Cancer Caregivers are not always aware of, or prepared for, the physical and emotional impact that caregiving can have on them, especially when they are busy trying to manage all of the numerous caregiving responsibilities for the Cancer patient, while at the same time, doing their best to keep their own life in order. As a result, the Caregiver's health, both physically and mentally, can suffer, as may other portions of their own life. Should this occur, it can also have considerable consequences for the Cancer patient receiving the care. Some anguish resulting from Cancer caregiving is unavoidable. It is also very customary to feel mentally and physically exhausted when taking care of Cancer patients – the process can be challenging, and the hours may be lengthy and distressing. Therefore, if the Caregiver experiences some of the warning signs of Caregiver stress, their own health may be at-risk and they should talk to their doctor about ways to minimize, cope with, or, eliminate the debilitating problem.

Below are typical indicators of Cancer Caregiver Stress that Caregivers should be aware of in an effort to recognize and avoid any physical and emotional impacts to their health. The information below is based on my journaling notes, from materials provided by my Medical Team and obtained during many Cancer Support Group meetings that I attended, and, as adapted from www.cancer.gov:

- **Caregiver Physical Wellness**

Many Cancer Caregivers are so busy "caring," that they may sometimes not take the time to do things in their own lives that they would generally do, such as eating right, regularly, and sufficiently, and/or, devoting time to exercise, and getting satisfactory sleep. As such, Caregivers can, themselves, suffer from multiple health issues such as exhaustion, headaches, or digestive problems. Some Studies have confirmed that Cancer Caregivers have increased rates of high blood pressure, heart disease, and mortality, when compared to non-Caregivers of the same ages. For these reasons, it is necessary that Cancer Caregivers try to maintain as "normal" of a life as is possible during their Caregiving responsibilities, so that they don't disregard *their* personal desires too. Cancer Caregivers are in no shape to care for others if they don't take the time, and make a conscious effort, to take care of themselves. They must also look after their own health.

- **Caregiver Emotional Wellness**

For many feasible reasons, some Cancer Caregivers are often overwhelmed emotionally. Many people complain of feeling lonely, drained, worried, and helpless. Some may have feelings of regret for having taken on the intense Caregiver role, while others may harbor excessive anger directed toward the Cancer patient for needing their constant or intermittent care. Still others might have their own health problems to worry about. If Caregivers permit their anxiety levels to build up, their emotional issues may then lead to serious mental and physical conditions of their own. Should the Caregiver's own health problems then start hindering the quality of care that they are able to provide, it could cause negative consequences for the patient.

- **Caregiver Depression**

Studies show that between 40 to 70 percent of Caregivers, in general, have exhibited symptoms of major Clinical Depression. As such, Cancer Caregivers may lose interest in things that they enjoy, and, they may withdraw socially, or have a tough time concentrating and making decisions. In some cases, Cancer Caregivers might have excessive feelings of guilt or worthlessness, and they may entertain suicidal thoughts, which *must* be addressed – ***fast!*** If the Caregiver, themselves, or the patient, family members, friends, or members of the Medical Team observe that the Caregiver is being overwhelmed, physically or mentally with their caregiving duties, it is essential that someone step in and "care" for the Caregiver. The Caregiver must receive professional help and counseling, as deemed appropriate.

- **Caregiver Financial Costs**

Cancer Caregivers, aside from sometimes not managing their own financial affairs as religiously as they should when tending to a patient, will often utilize their own money or credit to procure food, medications, and other patient needs, in addition to paying for fuel expenses to chauffer the patient to and from their numerous medical appointments. For obvious reasons, this extra and unbudgeted load can put the Caregiver's own financial obligations in jeopardy, which could clearly prompt unforeseen and very detrimental consequences with the Caregiver's personal life and responsibilities. Were this to occur, it could also lead to feelings of anger, resentment, or regret on the part of the Caregiver for "footing the bill" for the patient, at the expense of addressing their own financial obligations.

Suggestions for Coping with Caregiver Stress

Being a Caregiver to a Cancer patient can be one of the most significant, challenging, and rewarding things an individual can do.

It may give the person a chance to find a new meaning in their life, and it should enrich the life of the Cancer patient as well. But, it is vital—both for the patient and the Caregiver—that the Caregiver do everything they can in an effort to strike a healthy balance between taking care of the patient *and* looking after themselves. If a Cancer Caregiver doesn't take care of him or herself, it could be difficult for them to provide proper and attentive care for the patient – something that is extremely imperative to help ensure a positive overall Cancer outcome. Being well aware of the causes of Cancer Caregiver stress, and also knowing how to set realistic limits, can mean the difference between experiencing a productive caregiving relationship with the patient, and having one that is less than optimal for either party.

Below are suggested steps—drawn from my journal notes, materials provided to me by my Medical Team, from Cancer Support Group meetings that I attended, and from www.cancer.gov—that a Cancer Caregiver can take in an effort to circumvent the potential physical and emotional pitfalls of providing care to a Cancer patient:

- **Become Educated About Cancer – Know the Enemy**

A Cancer Caregiver, not unlike a commander in the military, should make a concentrated endeavor to "get to know the enemy" in advance of battle – why it occurs; how and where it functions; and, what it will take to remove it from the patient's body. The more the Cancer Caregiver becomes familiar with their patient's Cancer, the Cancer treatments, any potential Side Effects and remedies, and the patient's physical condition and their anticipated health care needs, the more "comfortable" the Caregiver becomes, and, the better they will understand and cope with the complete process. This could help them be better able to assist in the decision-making process, and will help them to foresee possible problems so that they can take steps in advance to avoid them. Partnering with the Medical Team to help plan for the patient's treatments, and to prepare for, and deal with, potential issues as they happen, will serve to reduce the Caregiver's anxiety levels, and will help give them some sense of control during the ordeal. It also allows the Caregiver to become a more informed and active advocate for their patient during meetings with members of the Medical Team, and in addressing the patient's personal needs.

• Make the Most of Available "Me" Time

Being a Cancer Caregiver can be a very time-consuming and labor-intensive investment in one's life, as there will be a seemingly endless quantity of medical appointments, tests, meetings, and other such commitments to go to. And, in some instances, especially if the patient starts experiencing damaging Side Effects from their Cancer treatments, the Caregiver will be nearby the patient's side, or will be "on-call" on a 24x7 basis for days, to make sure that the patient is as comfortable as possible, and that their needs are being met. Because of this very challenging and wearisome schedule, the Caregiver will need to prioritize and balance both their caregiving responsibilities and their other personal activities to the best of their abilities. This is crucial so that there will be sufficient "me" time for the Caregiver to take care of *their own* needs. This would include taking the time for their eating, sleeping, exercising, having fun, working or pursuing a hobby, and visiting with family and friends outside of the hospital or Caregiver environment. If the Caregiver doesn't manage their time well, time will manage them, and it will *not* be sympathetic.

• Don't Suppress Emotions – Talk With Others

Believe it or not, feelings of fear, guilt, regret, frustration and anger are actually normal for Cancer Caregivers. Cancer Caregivers might also feel weighed down and under-appreciated with all of the time and effort that they are devoting to the patient, while sacrificing many of their own life's activities for the duration. The significant thing to remember is that "Cancer Caregiver" is not a profession, per se, but it is a role typically filled by family members, and/or, friends who have volunteered to care for the patient. They, themselves, may not have any medical, psychological, nutritional, or other health care training; yet, the Caregiver will receive a "crash course" in these and other subjects, and, may be called upon to act on some of what they have learned at some point during the patient's Cancer journey.

As mentioned in this Book, there are various responsibilities and expectations of Cancer caregiving that can translate into a lot of pressure on the first-time Caregiver. This, in-turn, can cause anxiety and other emotional problems, and also physical health concerns. It, therefore, is vital that the Caregiver stay in-touch with their feelings at all times, and, as is necessary, seek the ear and the assistance of a family member, friend, counselor, or a Psychotherapist. The worst thing a Cancer Caregiver can do is to withhold all of their emotional feelings – be they positive or negative. If a preponderance of those Caregiver's feelings are pessimistic and woeful, at some point in the journey, something may trigger the unstable release of all emotions, which could cause a major "meltdown" on the part of the Caregiver. Before this occurs, Caregivers should seek help from others.

- **Participate in a Cancer Caregiver Support Group**

Cancer caregiving can be difficult work, and, it can be rather time-consuming. Few people can deal with it alone, especially those with other personal commitments of their own. A Caregiver asking for assistance is not a signal of weakness or insufficiency, but, is an honorable and honest admission that the work, the schedule, or other factors associated with the caregiving could be just too much for one person to handle alone – at least at that point in time. A Caregiver must know their limitations, and they must request the assistance of other people if their responsibilities become too overwhelming. One beneficial, enlightening, and uplifting resource available to Cancer Caregivers is a Cancer Caregiver Support Group.

Such support groups are networks of Cancer Caregivers who voluntarily share their own experiences about Cancer care, including any emotional issues with which they're coping, successes they have realized, tips for coping with stress, educational materials on Cancer and treatment, and other resources and advice from people just like them, who can empathize and understand. Several Cancer Treatment Centers have Caregiver Support Groups, or, one can partake online. We have all heard the sayings, *"There is strength in numbers,"* and, *"Been there and done that."* Cancer Caregiver Support Groups are made up of people, who, just like others in that group, have possibly faced the same or similar problems, and can lend not only their ears, but their advice, based on their own experiences. This can be very beneficial for both the "veteran" Caregivers, as well as for the newer Caregivers who have just begun to perform in their new role. Cancer Caregivers, just like Cancer patients, do not have to go it alone.

Give Care to the Cancer Caregiver

The long and tedious journey to a, hopeful, *Cancer-Free* or *Cancer-in-Remission* health status can be a very dark and foggy one in the beginning. But, the longer the road is traveled by the patient, their family, and their Caregiver, the brighter and clearer it becomes. Along the entire route, the patient will be cheered and supported by their Caregiver, family members, the Medical Team, and others, all of whom will be anxiously and patiently waiting at the "Finish Line" to congratulate them for their achievement. In my own experience, the outpouring of love, support, encouragement, and expertise with which I was blessed, made my long, painful, joyful, and, ultimately, successful journey, well worth every step along the way.

While family and friends of a Cancer patient are contributing their love, prayers, and support to the patient, they should also take the time to offer just the same—and their *"Thanks"*—to the patient's Caregiver. The Caregiver is similarly invested in the Cancer-fighting process as is the patient, and this person is, perhaps, one of the most significant individuals in helping the patient to succeed through their Diagnosis, Treatment, any Side Effects, and, through Recovery and Aftercare. But, more importantly, it is the Caregiver—whether he or she is the patient's loved one, family member or friend—who will share, most intimately with the patient, the final outcome of the long and convoluted war. And, it is the Caregiver who will humbly stand side-by-side with their patient in their hopeful, well-earned victory.

No Cancer patient can fight Cancer alone, and no Caregiver will let them. Neither one of these people would have ever dreamed that a wicked thing such as Cancer would suddenly enter their lives one day, and then consume their time, energy, physical strength and emotional endurance for the next few weeks, months, or even years. But when it does, the patient and the Caregiver will come together, and they will simply do what must be done. So, when sharing your love, support, and encouragement with the Cancer patient, please be sure to do the same for their Caregiver, who is experiencing much of the same physical and emotional ups and downs as the patient. They both certainly have earned it, and they both will become all the more optimistic, encouraged, and hopeful because of it.

Chapter Four

The Cancer Journey Explained – *Steps 5 and 6 on the Journey:*

The Medical Team; Treatment Preparations

"The strength of a Team dwells not only in the minds of its members, but also in their hearts and souls."

- Butch Sickler

Have you ever known anyone who has volunteered to sign up for an *All-Expenses-Paid Cancer Diagnosis?* Okay, how about someone who has entered a *Sweepstakes to win from six-month's- to a year's-worth of the discomfort and distress that is often associated with some of the Side Effects from Cancer Treatment?* Chances are pretty good that you have not in either case, any more than you have heard of an individual hoping to get in a serious vehicle accident, or, wishing to see their home and possessions being engulfed in flames. And, while a sound, reasonable, and clear-thinking individual would never wish these, or similar, unspeakable occurrences on themselves or others, Cancer *does* force itself upon 1.7 million Americans each year; Americans *do* find themselves in about 5.25 million vehicular accidents annually; and, sadly, greater than 4 million families in the U.S. *do* watch their homes go up in smoke on an annual basis.

Life-Saving First Responders

Much of the catastrophe in life can be prevented and some of it cannot. But, because life is life, these things—and much worse—

do, and will, happen. When these types of emergency "911" events take place, however, it is extremely reassuring to know that trained, skilled, and knowledgeable professionals will respond to the scene, and, that they will try to do everything within their power to provide comfort and aid to those-in-need. In the instance of vehicle accidents and house fires, these brave teams of emergency "First Responders" are typically comprised of Police Officers, Firemen and Women, and Emergency Medical Technicians, or Paramedics.

When speaking about the rescue of a man, woman, or child, whose life has suddenly suffered a serious "head-on collision" with Cancer, however, the responsive Medical Team will be comprised of Cancer physicians and nurses, and a large group of other health-care professionals. This multi-disciplined team—known as the patient's Cancer Treatment Medical Team—will be responsible for taking all necessary precautions to ensure that the Cancer is correctly treated, and, that the patient is as secure and as comfortable as possible. It is these skilled, knowledgeable, and dedicated professionals that will respond to the "911 call" from the Cancer patient-in-need.

➢ *Assembling the Patient's Cancer Treatment Medical Team – Step 5 on the Journey*

The planning for, and administration of, a patient's Cancer treatment program can be a comprehensive, somewhat stressful, and time-consuming process. As such, there are several things that will need to be accomplished, and several people that may be involved—at relatively the same and time and place—to successfully carry out the patient's treatment regimen. This is where, potentially, the third most critical and significant post-diagnosis activity comes in – the formation of the patient's Cancer Treatment Medical Team.

The medical, scientific, and health care disciplines that will be represented on the patient's Medical Team—Cancer physicians nurses, pharmacists, and other medical specialists—will typically be determined by the form of Cancer the patient has, the Stage (severity or spread) of their Cancer, any unique healthcare requirements and personal needs of the patient, the treatments that will be best suited for the patient, for the patient's age, *and,* for the patient's Cancer.

Formation and Objectives of the Medical Team

There is no doubt about it – the Cancer Medical Team that is accumulated to assist and provide support for the Cancer patient and their family and Caregiver through the Cancer journey will be made up of several professionals, each well-trained and highly skilled in their respective fields. This said, not all Team members will "join" the team at the exact same time during the outset, and, some "early" members may eventually depart the Team because their services are no longer required. So, while the Cancer Treatment Medical Team may be thought of as being "dynamic" and ever-changing, there will always be a main cluster of professionals who will be on the Team, working and meeting with the patient, their family members, and/or, the Caregiver. The core group will be with the patient throughout.

Each of these health care providers on the patient's Medical Team, depending on their individual roles and responsibilities, will make it their principal objective to correctly, safely, and effectively treat both the patient, *and* the patient's Cancer. The Medical Team members will meet with the patient and their Caregiver prior to the start of therapy for the purpose of developing a personalized Cancer Treatment Plan. In so doing, their goal will be to make sure that the patient is as safe, comfortable, and vigorous as possible during their treatments, while also taking all appropriate precautions, and doing everything possible, to eliminate Cancer from the patient's body.

For the Patient – For the Duration

Once the Treatment portion of the patient's Cancer journey has been completed, the Medical Team doesn't just "go away" and abandon the patient. Applicable members of the Medical Team will continue to interrelate with, and provide guidance to, the patient and their family, or Caregiver, as the patient is shepherded through the Recovery and Aftercare phases of the program. The vital follow-on processes after the cessation of treatments are fundamental to ensure a successful, overall conclusion for the patient's Cancer experience. Both the Recovery and Aftercare phases offer an opportunity for the patient to heal—physically, emotionally and mentally—from their potentially long and challenging battle with the disease.

Additionally, both post-treatment periods are also when the patient will continue to be regularly monitored by medical personnel extremely closely to make sure that the Cancer has been completely eradicated from the patient's body. But, in a worst-case scenario, if follow-up tests or examinations reveal that some of the nasty culprit, *A.K.A. Cancer*, still resides within the patient's body, the tests will provide the Team Members with the information they will need to readdress the Cancer in an attempt to *completely* remove it from the body. In such cases, the Medical Team will develop another plan of attack, if appropriate, and will remain with the patient throughout.

The Patient's Right to "Select" Medical Team Members

It is generally known that most Physicians, Nurses, Dentists, Psychotherapists, Dieticians, and the other health care professionals involved with the treatment and care of Cancer patients will be very thoroughly educated, knowledgeable, and skilled in their respective fields of proficiency. The ambitious and continuous training, testing, and certifications that they achieve and obtain as prerequisites to the evaluation, treatment, and care of patients, are admirable, and speak highly of both the individuals, themselves, as well as of the medical and health care professions and organizations to which they belong.

There is no stone left unturned when it comes to health care organizations making sure that their respective providers deliver the most advanced, professional, ethical, and effective medical care and services possible to their patient "customers." But, while all of this does sound great on paper, there *is* a minor glitch with this premise: All doctors, dentists, nurses, and other health care professionals are Human Beings. And, as humans, they, like the rest of us, can have good days and bad days, can work wonders and make mistakes, and, (this is a *big* one), they can also embody either pleasurable, personal attitudes, or disrespectful, condescending, and unprofessional ones – otherwise known in medical jargon as "*Bad Bedside Manners.*"

It's all About "Respect" and Saving the Patient's Life

Because the safe, rapid, and successful treatment of a Cancer patient's disease is possibly one of the most significant undertakings of the patient's entire life, and because the individual's life, literally, is hanging in the balance, there is an obvious need for the patient to ensure that those entrusted with their care—and their *life*—are not only qualified to accomplish their professional responsibilities, but, that they do so in agreement, and in confidence, with the patient, and their family, and/or, Caregiver, as applicable. Because the patient will be meeting with applicable members of the Medical Team quite frequently throughout the patient's Cancer journey, both prior to and during Treatment, and for several months after during the Recovery and Aftercare phases, it is very important that the patient, and their family, and/or, Caregiver, feel at-ease and comfortable in speaking with, and asking questions of, those charged with the patient's care.

The requirement for patient / family member / Medical Team compatibility pertains not only to all of the Medical Team members' abilities to deliver the fastest, safest, most effective Cancer-removal treatments and health care possible. It also applies to the prerequisite that the health care professionals dedicate satisfactory time with the patient to plainly clarify information, and to answer questions so that the patient absolutely understands what the professionals are saying. Likewise, the professionals must speak to, and treat, the patient, and their family and Caregiver, with compassion, dignity, and reverence. Effective communications are always a two-way street, but, a large responsibility for accurately, promptly, and professionally providing information to the Cancer patient, their family, or Caregiver, rests squarely on the shoulders of the Medical Team members. It is only when this repartee is mutually accomplished that all parties will feel comfortable that the patient's Cancer program is being administered in the best possible manner. That is, after all, what all of this mess is about: *Safely and completely removing the patient's Cancer.*

"Firing" and "Hiring" Medical Team Members

If any members of the patient's Medical Team fail to deliver on one or more of their professional responsibilities to offer the most appropriate, professional, timely, and compassionate medical service possible—including practicing and displaying respectful "Bedside Manners"—the patient is well within their rights to talk about their complaint honestly with the health care professional in question, or, to raise their issues to the Head of the Department at the health care organization, or to any other supervising office. If nothing changes after the patient has communicated their apprehensions and concerns to either the Medical Team member or a responsible authority, the patient should strongly consider “firing” or “letting go” the doubtful health care professional, no matter if it is an expert Cancer doctor, a dentist, nurse, or any other highly-trained and skilled individual.

In instances where the patient or their family want to change a health care professional on their case or Medical Team, the patient can request that that individual be replaced with another professional of the same discipline who has equitable knowledge and expertise to perform their duties, but, *who is also graced with the very important interpersonal skills* that will enable this new member of the Medical Team to interact more personably, and with compassion and respect, to the patient and their family or Caregiver. With the “hiring” of a new, receptive, respectful, and professional Team Member, comes a constructive change that will help to put all persons at-ease. A more responsible and accountable health professional will help to promote a very communicative and productive environment that is critical to the successful treatment and recovery of the Cancer patient.

A Life’s at Stake – “Shop” for the Best Team Possible

When one considers that the Cancer patient’s life can hang in the balance during their Cancer journey, the patient and their family and Caregiver, must be aware that there is absolutely no disgrace or embarrassment on the part of the patient in letting a doctor or other health-care professional on their Medical Team go, and asking that they be replaced with another – if the provider’s below-par behavior or actions warrant. As is true in most other business relationships in life, we consumers typically have alternatives to choose one product, service, company, or individual over another, and, this practice most certainly applies to something as important as one’s Cancer care.

If a person is going to shop around for the perfect cell phone, the ultimate pair of high heels, or, the best-performing 4-wheel drive pick-up truck, why then, should they not dedicate just as much due diligence and a watchful thought process in selecting the health care professionals that they will be trusting with their life? The very clear answer to this is that they should. Please keep in mind, however, that in some circumstances, such as with hospitals or medical clinics in some remote, rural, or smaller cities, the numbers of medical Cancer specialists may be limited. As such, an individual may not have the option of choosing one physician over another. In such cases, it is in the best interest of all represented parties that a mutually-respectful, compassionate, communicative, and professional patient / physician relationship be fostered early-on in the process to help facilitate the most constructive and successful Cancer outcome possible.

The Patient's Right to Obtain Additional Dr. Opinions

The lessons to be learned regarding Cancer diagnosis are that all Cancer patients must be able to have faith and to confide in well-intentioned physicians and the health professionals assigned to their case. Secondly, all involved should initially discuss, understand, and concur with the lab-reported Cancer diagnosis prior to the planning and employment of possible treatment alternatives moving forward. Likewise, the patient, their loved one, family, and Caregiver should have complete confidence in the initial diagnosis of Cancer that has been given to them by their doctor before they will feel comfortable proceeding with Cancer treatment(s). If there are any apprehensions on the part of the patient upfront, it could cause issues down the line.

The bottom line is that while all the members of the patient's Medical Team will provide the Cancer patient with their health care knowledge, expertise, and skills to help conduct them safely through Treatment, Recovery, and Aftercare, it will be the patient, and their family or Caregiver, who will generally be the ones making many of the significant decisions regarding the patient's care following their Cancer diagnosis. Such decisions might include patients *requesting and obtaining confirmation of the diagnosis from 3rd-party medical professionals.* If a patient, a family member, or Caregiver does not feel convinced with the medical findings on the patient's Pathology Report when the Cancer diagnosis is delivered by their physician, or, if those concerned desire to confirm the diagnosis with a third-party doctor, it is suggested that patients get second or third opinions from other physicians. Cancer patients are encouraged to get second opinions from knowledgeable Cancer specialists outside the Health Management Organization (HMO), ***but, with prior HMO approval.***

☛ ***Author's note***: Patients, family members, Caregivers, and all those responsible must be advised that most ***HMOs/PPOs must first approve any medical interface with an "out of plan" physician*** or health provider, including obtaining a physician's diagnosis opinion, before the transaction will be covered by the patient's insurance. It is advisable that a Cancer patient first check with their HMO/PPO for approval prior to seeking medical assistance outside their health plan. Not obtaining HMO/PPO approval for "outside tests" or doctor visits could result in the patient being liable for charges incurred.

➢ *Preparing for Cancer Treatment – Step 6 on the Journey*

There is a term often thrown around in business circles these days—and I have definitely heard it used in my government job on a few occasions—that, pretty much, sums up the potential risks of not properly preparing for any sort of project or effort. The expression I'm speaking of, *"If you fail to plan, you plan to fail,"* squarely hits the nail on the head, and, it really lends itself perfectly to almost any undertaking in life, no matter how seemingly large or small it might be. I'll be the first one to admit that spontaneity and the element-of-surprise can be fun and exciting happenings in life, if circumstances will allow. But, there are other, more serious times in life, when one must sit down, think, and deal truthfully with the situation-at-hand.

Whether a person is rehearsing for a Grade School Christmas Pageant, practicing to play in the NFL Super Bowl ®, designing and building a house, arranging a Wedding, or preparing for a week-long camping trip into the wilderness, there is much in advance that has to be scheduled, planned, and accomplished if the endeavor is going to have any opportunity for success. And, as one might reasonably expect, the premise for organizing, preparing, and doing, is also very applicable—as to the actions one should take and the strategies one should make—prior to the commencement of the patient's Cancer Treatment program. *With Cancer planning, no one wants to fail!*

After the patient's Cancer has been assessed and Staged and the Pathology Report issued, the diagnosis will be transmitted to the patient by their doctor. And, following the assignment of a Cancer

Caregiver and the preliminary assemblage of the patient's Medical Team, a new set of gears will begin turning in an attempt to put the vital diagnostic outcomes to good use thru the creation of a patient's Treatment Plan. The doctor who conveys the Cancer diagnosis to the patient might possibly be the one who initially informs the patient of the potential Cancer-removal/killing treatment option(s) that may be employed in the individual's personal situation. This physician may also take the time to address any concerns and questions the patient may have, and to briefly clarify the treatment methods, how they are performed, and any Side Effects that may be realized by the patient.

Getting the "Cancer Ball" Rolling

Ultimately, if one or more Cancer-killing treatment therapies are being considered for the patient, the physician who had initially requested the patient's diagnostic examinations, and, who, possibly, had transmitted the Cancer diagnosis to the patient, will—if they are not the treating specialist—typically refer the patient to one or more health care professionals that specialize in Cancer treatments such as Surgery, Chemotherapy, Radiation Therapy, Immunotherapy, and/or others. Finally, this central nucleus of health care professionals will comprise the patient's Medical Team, who will shepherd the Cancer patient through their respective courses of treatment, and, thereafter, throughout the Recovery and Aftercare phases of their program.

The Medical Team doctors, in accord with the Cancer patient and their family and Caregiver, will meet early-on in the process to discuss, develop, and agree on a Cancer treatment regimen that will maximize the potential for eradicating the disease, while minimizing the unfavorable effects on the patient. However, before the Medical Team meetings begin taking place, and, prior to the commencement of Cancer treatments, there are some activities that the patient will want to accomplish, if possible, and if time permits. These suggested actions are covered in the following Sections of this Chapter.

How Soon After Diagnosis Will Treatments Begin?

Typically, there is no "normal" time period as to how promptly a patient's respective treatment regimen will begin after their Cancer is initially diagnosed. For obvious reasons, however, sooner is better than later. As I talk about in subsequent Sections within this Chapter and elsewhere in this book, several planning meetings may typically take place with the Medical Team and their respective staffs, and, it may take a period of time to incorporate a patient into the clinic's or hospital's Surgery, and/or, Cancer treatment scheduling docket. For the most part, though, the urgency in administering Cancer treatment can depend on many factors. Typically, such significant criteria will include the form, Stage, location, and severity of one's Cancer, the overall health condition of the patient, and any pain, functionality, or other life-threatening or disabling symptoms being experienced.

In most Cancer treatment programs, several processes and activities may occur before treatment begins. But, in some patient's cases, due to a multiplicity of reasons, their Cancer treatment(s) may be put on the fast-track by the patient's Medical Team in an effort to immediately address their Cancer before it can do more bodily harm. In such situations, there could be insufficient time for accomplishing all or some the suggested pre-treatment activities. In the case of my own Chemo and Radiation Therapy treatments, they both kicked off approximately five to six weeks after I first received my diagnosis.

Pre-Treatment "Need to Do," and "Nice to Do" Activities

To say that the Cancer patient has a few things to do after the delivery of their diagnosis and the Staging of their Cancer, but prior to the commencement of the Treatment segment of their program, is just a *wee bit* of an understatement. Pragmatically speaking, the type and severity of one's Cancer, the emotional and physical state of the patient, and the variety of potential Cancer treatment(s) that a patient may undergo—Chemotherapy, Immunotherapy, Surgery, Radiation Therapy, or an incorporation thereof—will all have a say in dictating the amounts and types of pre-treatment prep that may be necessary.

It is safe to say that all Cancer patients, irrespective of their personal situation or their form of Cancer, and, despite the type(s) of treatment they may be due to receive, can stand to benefit from their accomplishment of some elemental and universal things prior to the "show getting on the road." And, while there will be many potential considerations that the patient may want to take into account before their treatment begins, there are quite a few of the more significant activities that the Cancer patient (along with their loved one, family, or Caregiver) should try to accomplish in an effort to improve their chances of overall success. Such dealings could take place one after the other, or simultaneously, in conjunction with some of the others. Such Cancer pre-treatment activities will, or may, include:

- Requesting that a loved one, family member or friend become their Caregiver—if such an individual doesn't voluntarily come forward—to help support the patient during their Cancer journey
- Conducting research on, and learning about, Cancer, in general, and the patient's form of Cancer, specifically, including possible treatment options, and jotting down questions for the doctor(s)
- Attending meetings with physicians and many other health care professionals that will comprise the patient's Medical Team, to discuss the treatment options and other related information, and to develop the patient's treatment, recovery, and aftercare plan
- Ensuring that everything is completely understood during meetings with the Medical Team health professionals, and if not, to ask the doctor(s) to explain in "layperson"-type language
- Keeping a daily journal to record thoughts, feelings, happenings, meeting notes, etc., to ease stress, and to use for future reference
- Requesting a different physician or health care professional if the current doctor does not meet the patient's needs, or exhibits a lack of patience or compassion, or has poor "bed-side manners"
- For children or teen patients, informing the school and making necessary arrangements to keep up with school work, even while the child is undergoing treatment (as circumstances will allow)
- Meeting with a Registered Dietician or Nutritionist on the Team (who is familiar with the Cancer patient's needs), as necessary, to adjust the quality and quantity of the patient's food intake
- Submitting to necessary screening tests, exams, scans, and other preparatory procedures, etc., as scheduled, and as applicable
- Getting any necessary dental, and/or oral surgery work done, and taking proactive steps to prepare the mouth, gums, and teeth for Cancer treatment-related Side Effects, as necessary

- Taking steps to get a wig or head coverings (specially made for Chemo patients), per personal preference, and as needed
- Ensuring that all health insurance needs are in order
- Getting ample rest and relaxation before treatments commence
- Participating in exercise, including, stretching, walking, biking, yoga, swimming, etc., if possible, and as permitted by doctors
- Taking a loved one or family on a pre-Cancer treatment vacation or night out to that special restaurant and hotel they've always loved, but told themselves they could never afford (If physicians approve, and if health, family, and other circumstances permit)
- Arranging to have a family member or a close friend take care of any children, pets, the yard, house plants, etc., as necessary
- Informing the employer, as applicable, of the upcoming need to use Sick Leave to obtain tests, attend meetings with physicians, undergo treatments, and to recover and heal *(could take months)*
- Getting all personal obligations, including finances, in-order, or requesting the assistance of another to help with this, as needed

Preparing to Meet with the Medical Team – A Summary

After the patient has been delivered the news of their Cancer diagnosis, and has been provided with the Pathology Report by their physician or other health care professional, there will be numerous important tasks that will need to be accomplished in preparation for the treatment of the disease. One of the original activities the Cancer patient might want to embark on will be to ask a loved one, a family member, or a good friend, if they would want to be their "right-hand person," or their Caregiver, upon whom the patient will rely for their support, encouragement, and assistance during their Cancer journey.

In most cases, one of these individuals will step up and offer to care for the patient from start to finish. But, if not, the patient may have to "volunteer" someone to take up this role. Perhaps the second important thing that the patient might do following diagnosis will be to accomplish research on Cancer in general, and on their type of the disease, in particular. One must know their Cancer well before they will know which treatment(s) will be the most effective in removing it from their body. And, they should be familiar with the variety of

Treatment-related Side Effects that they may possibly encounter as well as any steps they can take to try to reduce or eliminate them.

With the patient holding the Pathologist's Report in-hand—that provides the Cancer diagnostic results and other information—the focus of their treatment program will next shift to the third most important juncture in the Cancer patient's journey: Formation of the patient's Cancer Treatment Medical Team. The Medical Team will be comprised of those physicians and other health care professionals who specialize in individual areas of Cancer medicine, be it Surgery, Oncology, Radiation Oncology, Dentistry, and assorted medical and health care disciplines. It is this alliance of health care professionals that will be consulting with the patient and their family/Caregiver to develop the comprehensive Cancer treatment plan, and, who will be facilitating the delivery of the respective courses of treatments from launch to finish. Members of this inter-disciplinary cluster of health care professionals will be knowledgeable and trained in all facets of safe, effective, and, hopefully, kind Cancer patient comfort and care.

- **Get Down to Business**

The patient, and their loved one, and/or, their Caregiver, will eventually meet separately with each one of the medical and health care specialists to talk about the pertinent therapies in detail, as well as potential Side Effects of those treatments, actions to mitigate any Side Effects, and the follow-on activities that will take place through the Recovery and Aftercare phases of the patient's Cancer program. After the patient has had satisfactory opportunity—however long it may take—to deal with the reality of their diagnosis, and, when they consider themselves to be emotionally and physically equipped and able to proceed to the next step, it might be beneficial for the patient to start preparations for their upcoming meetings with their Medical Team, and ultimately, for the commencement of their treatments.

In essence, the patient and the Caregiver, having been duly informed of the Cancer diagnosis and the form of Cancer the patient has, will be well-advised to learn about their enemy so that they will be fully prepared when they meet with the Medical Team to discuss and begin drawing up battle plans to prevail over the Cancer that has ruthlessly invaded the patient's body. There will likely be numerous activities that will take place prior to first meeting with the Medical Team members and before beginning Cancer therapy. But, one of the first things the patient and their Caregiver may want to do would be to learn more about Cancer in general, and, preferably, about the specific form of Cancer with which they have been diagnosed.

- **Learn About the Diagnosed Cancer**

In life, when faced with any sort of a challenge, it is always beneficial to learn ahead of time what one may be up against, or, any potential issues one may expect to come across during the process of facing whatever the test might be. Nobody likes to be blind-sided by things—with the possible exception of a "Bumper Car" driver at the County Fair—so, preparing in advance, and doing one's homework *prior to* undertaking an activity, can often yield noteworthy rewards. However, as one might expect, with many quandaries in life, such as unexpected disasters and some medical occurrences, there often isn't sufficient time or information to enable one to plan ahead before the unforeseen "bolt of lightening" strikes. In such instances, it might be one's intuition, faith, physical or emotional strength, or, maybe, just plain ole' common sense, that will see them through to the end.

When speaking of an individual's Cancer, however, there is a tremendous amount to be gained—and, probably, even more to be saved—by the patient, should they devote sufficient time to learning about their newfound enemy, and what it might take to defeat it. To prepare for their upcoming meetings with members of their Medical Team, the patient might want to search for, locate, read, and absorb information about Cancer in an effort to enlighten themselves about the disease in general, and/or, about the specific form of Cancer with which the patient has been diagnosed. If at all possible, some of the Cancer patient's family members, and/or, Caregiver, may also want to be involved in this pre-meeting, Cancer-education process. This will especially be the case if the patient is too elderly, too young, or, emotionally or physically incapable of doing such activities on their own. Likewise, this would apply if the patient can't use, or doesn't have any access to the Internet, or, if they can't drive to libraries or bookstores. Knowledge is only useful if a person can obtain it.

The learning process is extremely significant for those close to the Cancer patient for a very good reason: Some individuals in the patient's *inner circle* will, by default, become the patient's eyes and ears, and, their sounding-board, memory bank, voice of reason, and filter, thru which a large bulk of the information and decisions about the patient's Cancer treatment(s) should be processed and discussed. Because of this, it obviously would be of great benefit to the patient, and to their ultimate success, if their family members and Caregiver were to have even just a basic understanding of the, *"how's, when's, what's, why's, and wheres"* of Cancer, and of the Cancer treatment process, including any potential Side Effects that may arise.

As the patient, and their family, and/or, Caregiver, become more involved in their searches for materials on the topic of Cancer, they will speedily come to the realization that information about the disease is seemingly ceaseless. They will also ascertain that much of the material will be crammed with "medicalese" (overly scientific or technical information meant for *physicians' use*, not patients'), and intricately complex to comprehend. What this might advocate to the average Cancer patient and their Caregiver is that they may not only become overwhelmed with the unreal quantity of materials, but, that they also might not understand some of the more technical, scientific explanations being presented. In such instances, it may be best for the person to give in to the old-fashioned notion that "less is more," and, they should only attempt to read and assimilate the amount and level of information that both their mind and their time will allow.

- ## Locate Cancer Information Resources

When trying to determine where a person should go to obtain information on Cancer in general, or, about their form of diagnosed Cancer, specifically, there are few practical *"resource sources"* that will come to mind. In addition to reading the book that you are now holding—which I have written to be an easy-to-read-and-understand resource for Cancer patients, their families, and Caregivers—I also heartily recommend other reliable sources for Cancer information.

I found the following resources to be useful in my research and knowledge-gathering efforts during my own Cancer experience:

- Medical Team / Health Care Professional-provided materials
- Bookstores, both online and actual "brick and mortar" stores
- Government websites for the National Institutes for Health, and Centers for Disease Control
- National Cancer Institute government website (www.cancer.gov), Fact Sheets, Booklets, and other materials
- American Cancer Society website, and materials
- Cancer Research organizations' websites, and materials
- Medical information websites like pubmed.com and webmd.com
- University and clinical websites, and materials
- Cancer research magazines and journals

Should the Cancer patient and the Caregiver choose to learn a little or plenty from one or more Cancer resources prior to meeting with the members of their Medical Team, their actions could be well worth the time and the effort devoted. It can be a very advantageous confidence-booster for the patient to prepare themselves with a basic understanding of Cancer and its potential Treatments, Side Effects, and probable outcomes. Not only will such knowledge regarding the disease help the patient in asking relevant questions of their Medical Team, but the patient's basic comprehension of the information will better prepare them to discuss with their physicians many aspects of their case going forward. An informed patient is a strong patient.

The doctors and other professionals on the patient's Medical Team will be the *Subject Matter Experts* who will be developing and administering the patient's personally-customized Cancer treatment program. As such, the knowledge, expertise, and recommendations of these health care professionals will be where the patient will want to place their trust. But, as crucial as the physicians, medicines, and technology are in treating the patient and hopefully eradicating their Cancer, the actual, eventual success of the Cancer treatment process will essentially come down to the Cancer patient, and their family or Caregiver, giving it their all – physically, mentally, and emotionally.

Certainly, a Cancer patient, family, and/or, Caregiver, are not expected to know a great deal about Cancer, in general, or about the patient's form of Cancer, specifically (that is, unless they are Cancer doctors, health professionals or scientists, themselves, who are very accustomed with the disease). However, when the patient has a basic understanding of how Cancer functions, how the selection of Cancer treatments work, and what one may experience during treatment and recovery, this information will not only serve them well during the meetings with their Medical Team, but, could, ultimately, pay them back one-hundred-fold in the form of a successful outcome.

Attend Planning Meetings with the Medical Team

The patient, their loved one, family, and/or, Caregiver, will typically have one or more scheduled meetings with each member of their Medical Team prior to the actual commencement of any of the patient's anti-Cancer treatments or therapies. The goals of these pre-treatment meetings are many-fold, but the central focus of the initial consultation is on all parties getting to know one another – not only on a professional doctor-patient basis, but also in a friendly person-to-person manner. These individuals will, after all, be seeing quite a lot of one another during the course of the next several months, and throughout this journey, will often become very close acquaintances. Most doctors and nurses don't like to be called "heroes," but I assure you, when they help a patient successfully battle and overcome their Cancer, these miracle workers will always hold a special place in the patient's heart. There is a very close bond that develops between the Oncologist(s) and their staff and the person being treated, that only a Cancer patient, and their family or Caregiver, can truly understand.

If the patient's prescribed Cancer treatment plan will call for conventional Cancer Surgery, Chemotherapy, Radiation Therapy, Immunotherapy, or a combination of all these, the patient, and their family or Caregiver, will be meeting individually with each treating physician, and/or, their staffs, preceding the commencement of their treatment(s). During these meetings, the patient and their Caregiver (who, hopefully, will have accomplished their "homework," and will have accumulated *some* level of knowledge about Cancer, and *their* Cancer) will discuss with the respective health care professionals, all of the, *"what's, when's, where's, how's, and why's,"* regarding their specific treatments, including any prospective Side Effects, possible risks and benefits, and, the estimated outcomes. These pre-treatment Medical Team meetings are also perfect opportunities for the patient and their Caregiver to express any concerns and fears that they may have about their upcoming journey throughout Cancer treatment and recovery, and, to ask the health professionals any questions that they may have about any aspect of the forthcoming process.

- **Take Notes During Medical Team Meetings**

Based on my private journaling experiences during meetings with members of my Medical Team both prior to, during, and after my treatments, it is strongly recommended that the patient, and/or, the Caregiver, take notes during their many meetings with their own physicians. This is suggested so that either one or both individuals can capture the highlights of the meeting discussions, as well as the physicians' responses to any questions that might have been raised. Because the quantity of the information that will be discussed at the individual Medical Team meetings may be significant and, perhaps, somewhat scientific in nature, the journaling notes may prove to be very valuable for a couple of notable reasons: First, the patient's or Caregiver's notations will be available for reference purposes should they ever be necessary. Secondly, the notes will also free one's mind from having to remember the important specifics of everything that was discussed, and the questions answered, in each of the meetings.

With all of the information, questions, thoughts, and feelings that may be swirling around in the patient's brain for weeks on-end during the Treatment Phase, they will need all the help they can get in terms of not being seriously overburdened with *TMI* (Too Much Information). Daily note-taking will certainly be a big benefit in this regard. Plus, there is always that possibility that the patient might desire to author a book about *their* Cancer journey some day. If that endeavor *does* transpire, as it did for me and my Cancer experience, such journaling notes will provide the perfect fodder and facts that will help the Cancer survivor to precisely recall and share their story (especially if it's several years later, as is the case with this Book!).

- **Understand What the Doctor is Saying – If Not: Ask**

If the patient does not understand what their doctor is telling them during their pre-Treatment meetings, or at any stage during the process, the patient, and/or, Caregiver, *must* tell the doctor that they don't understand, and ask the doctor to re-explain. Doctors are well-versed in the services and information that they have been trained and educated to provide, so, most can probably do so automatically, *(including in their sleep!)* and without giving either a lot of thought. As a result, some physicians may have a tendency to explain briefly, play down, or rapidly cover important information because it is very well-known to them. In other words, the physician may go on "auto-pilot," failing to take into consideration that he or she may be *flying way above the patient's, family's, or Caregiver's heads.* As a "new" Cancer patient who might have limited or no knowledge of Cancer, Cancer treatments, and other Cancer-related information, the patient must take it upon themselves to let their physician know when they are talking too hurriedly, not totally explaining what they are saying, or, speaking beyond the patient's capability to comprehend.

If any of these dynamics, or others, are preventing the patient from comprehending, learning, or vocalizing about the information being presented by the doctor, the patient, or their family member or Caregiver, *must speak up and tell the physician to slow down*, better explain the information, and/or, to restate it in simple, non-technical language, until all of the parties can fully comprehend. Patients and families should not permit the doctor—or his or her conduct or level of knowledge—to intimidate them in any manner. The bottom line is that the Cancer patient must be entirely aware of what is to occur at each juncture of their treatment, including all of the options ahead of them. And, it is up to the health care professionals to provide them with this information in an understandable, "layperson" fashion.

As stated previously, having a Caregiver at all the meetings with the patient can be extremely helpful, as they will be able to act as a second set of eyes and ears, as well as to be an advocate on the patient's behalf. This is especially beneficial for younger and elderly patients. Also, as was suggested previously, the patient should write down any questions ahead of time that they will want for the doctor to answer. The patient is also free to tape record all of their meeting discussions, and then make notes from the recordings. Whatever the strategy that is utilized to capture the outcomes of the meetings, it is extremely important that the patient completely comprehend all that their physician is telling them, and that the doctor is aware when the patient does not understand. Patients should always be honest with their physicians. They should never hold back any information, even when answering questions about how the patient feels, physically or emotionally, or, how well the patient or Caregiver understands what the doctor says. ***Remember: Fighting Cancer is a Team Effort!***

Attend Preparatory Medical Tests and Procedures

As has been explained in this Chapter and elsewhere in this Book, there is great deal of due diligence that must be performed by members of the Medical Team to work with the patient (and their family or their Caregiver, as applicable) to develop the personalized, comprehensive Treatment Plan, which is determined by the patient's specific form of Cancer and its Stage and location, as well as on the patient's age and their general state of health. But, just as important as the efforts to design the plan, are the actions that must be taken in advance of the treatment(s) to ensure that the patient meets all of the minimum health requirements to safely receive the treatment(s).This is necessary so that the treatments can be delivered to the patient in appropriate doses, frequencies, and durations, and with minimal risk to their health, while maximizing the Cancer-killing benefits of the respective therapies. Before a Cancer patient submits to their initial round of Cancer treatment—whatever it may be—the patient may be referred by the Medical Team for a variety of blood tests, scans, or other procedures. The following test descriptions have been adapted from the National Cancer Institute (www.cancer.gov) resources:

- ### Pre-Treatment Medical Tests to Ensure That the Patient Qualifies for Treatment

The pre-treatment tests, exams and procedures to which the patient will submit will provide the physician with the vital wellness information that they will need vis-à-vis the patient's health status to verify if Cancer treatment is practicable in the first place. Also, they will help see if any precautions must be taken, or adjustments made, prior to proceeding with the therapy(ies). The pre-Cancer treatment tests are also significant because they will enable the Medical Team to establish a "baseline" of health data on the patient, including their body weight, blood cell counts, assorted organ function test results, and other compulsory factors, that the Medical Team members can compare with the results of tests taken after treatment begins.

The pre-treatment baseline results, and the test results taken during treatment, will be utilized by the doctors to chart the patient's progress or regress over time. These tests are critical to the success of both the patient's *and the Cancer's* response to the therapies. As such, the results of the many tests, exams, and scans will enable the physicians to make any in-course corrections to the treatment(s), and to fine-tune any number of variables that could enhance the patient's level of comfort, while simultaneously doing everything possible to make the *Cancer's* life just as miserable as possible.

In addition to the Cancer patient participating in a battery of pre-treatment tests, exams, and imaging scans, the patient's Medical Team doctors and their staff will also frequently examine the patient to ensure that all "conditions are go." Chemotherapy drugs are very powerful, and their use can aggravate a patient's Bone Marrow from producing sufficient levels of Red Blood Cells, White Blood Cells and Platelets. As a result, the Chemo patient will need to have blood tests taken prior to each Chemotherapy drug infusion to confirm that their blood cells are being naturally maintained at normal levels.

This is important, of course, to make sure that the individual is producing a sufficient level of White Blood Cells in their Immune System so that their body can fight off any potential infections that may arise before, during, and after treatment. If the patient's White Blood Cell count drops beneath a pre-defined threshold, the treating Oncologist might temporarily postpone the patient's Chemotherapy infusions and prescribe a medication *(as happened with me)* that will help to facilitate the formation of the necessary blood cells. Once the patient's blood cell counts return to a normal or allowable level, the Oncologist may order the Chemotherapy sessions to resume.

- **Pre-Treatment Screening Tests**

The types of pre-treatment tests, exams, and procedures that some of the Medical Team members will order for the patient will be contingent upon the patient's specific needs, including their form of Cancer, the prescribed course of treatment(s), and other personal factors. Based on my own journaling notes, and materials provided to me by my Medical Team, following are examples of the types of tests, exams, procedures, and scans that a Cancer patient's Medical Team physician(s) may order to prepare for the start of treatment:

- ***Chemotherapy and Radiation Therapy Prep***

If the patient is slated to receive a course of Chemotherapy, and/or, Radiation Therapy, there may be some additional procedures that will be ordered by the Medical Team physician(s) to accomplish some important pre-treatment business, as specified below. Both of these procedures are described in greater detail within this book.

  - ***Prep For Chemotherapy – Mediport Placement***

If the patient will be administered Chemotherapy medicines intravenously, the doctor may prescribe the surgical placement of a Mediport in the patient, which is a small, sterile fixture implanted in the chest area, just beneath the skin next to the patient's collarbone. The plastic / metal device is surgically connected to one of the larger veins in the chest via a catheter tube. The objective of the fixture is to permit the convenient, sterile, and recurrent drawing of blood and the infusion of medications into the port via a special needle. This prevents the patient from having to always undergo the possible fear and pain (not to mention bruises) of being repeatedly "stuck" with a standard needle in the arms or hands. To use a "car tire" analogy, the Mediport could be viewed as a "valve" in which needles are inserted to permit the flow of fluids, both into, and out of, the body.

  - ***Prep For Radiation Therapy – Mask, Tattoo***

Should the patient be scheduled for Radiation Therapy, there will usually be significant background work that must be performed at the Radiation Oncology Clinic in advance of the first treatment to design the patient's personalized therapy plan. Likewise, for patients with Cancer that will necessitate Radiation Therapy to the ***head and neck area***, treatment preparations will include the development of a custom stabilization mask that will be utilized to secure the patient's head to the treatment table. The mask—designed to allow airflow to the patient's head and the infiltration of radiation waves to the target location—prevents the patient's head from moving during treatment. The patient's chest is also tattooed with a small dot to help precisely and safely align the radiation machine during each therapy session.

- ***Pre-Treatment Tests to Check the Lungs***

Some Chemotherapy medications can influence the way that a Cancer patient's lungs function. If the patient is going to be having Chemotherapy treatments, their physician will recommend that they obtain a Lung Function Test before they initiate their Chemotherapy sessions. Lung Function Tests measure how much air the Lungs can hold, and how well the Lungs are absorbing oxygen.

- ***Pre-Treatment Tests to Check the Heart***

The Cancer patient's physician may request that the patient undergo an Electrocardiogram or ECG or EKG, which is a recording of the patient's heartbeat. Or, the Medical Team physician(s) may order an Ultrasound Echocardiogram. Some Chemo medications can result in temporary damage to the muscles of the Heart, which might change the rhythms of the heartbeat. In most patients, the heartbeat will return to normal after the treatment has ended. But, in all cases prior to beginning Chemotherapy treatments, the patient will need to have their Heart evaluated to confirm a normal heartbeat before they can begin treatment. Another test that can be ordered by the Medical Team physician(s) is the Cardiac Ejection Fraction. This is an exam conducted to measure the force with which the Heart is pumping.

- ***Pre-Treatments Tests to Check the Liver***

Most Chemotherapy medications are tremendously powerful, and while they are busy doing their job by killing the "bad" Cancer cells, they also can incite "collateral damage" to the normal, "good" cells throughout the body, including those in the Liver – the body's vital clearinghouse for filtering and ridding the body of toxins. With this risk in mind, the patient's Medical Team physician(s) may order blood tests for the patient in an effort to verify how well the Liver is functioning. Many medications and other chemicals in the body are broken down by the Liver—including Chemo drugs—so it is critical that this vital organ is working in perfect form to assist in efficiently removing the residual Chemotherapy medications from the body.

- ***Pre-Treatment Tests to Check the Kidneys***

A Cancer patient's Kidneys can be susceptible to the damage that can be precipitated by some Chemotherapy drugs. In an effort to monitor and track the medicine's impact on the patient's Kidneys, the Medical Team doctor(s) will order blood, and/or, urine tests for the patient. The Kidneys share the joint responsibility with the liver of filtering and eliminating the toxic residue from the Chemotherapy medications after they have been broken down in the body. For this reason, it is extremely important that the Cancer patient's Kidneys are functioning properly before, during, and after, treatment.

- ***Pre-Treatment Tests for HIV and Hepatitis***

There is some possibility that the Medical Team physician(s) may request that the Cancer patient have their blood tested for HIV and Hepatitis. If this occurs, the physician will thoroughly explain this need to the patient, and the patient will first have to sign a form to consent to the HIV / Hepatitis test before their blood is drawn.

Meet with a Dentist - Have Dental Work Done

Even though dental or oral health can be one of the neglected components in properly preparing for Cancer therapy, it is extremely significant, and it should not be overlooked by the patient and their Caregiver – regardless of the form of Cancer with which the patient has been diagnosed. Honestly, the patient's Oral Surgeon or Dentist should be an active and participating member of the patient's multi-disciplinary Cancer Treatment Medical Team who interacts with the Surgeon, Oncologist, and/or, Radiation Oncologist, as applicable.

Following are pre-Cancer treatment guidelines adapted from materials of the National Cancer Institute (www.cancer.gov), which pertain to measures that Cancer patients—adults, children, and Head and Neck Cancer patients, especially—should take when preparing to receive treatment for their Cancer, and after therapy is completed:

- **Pre-Treatment Dental Care - All Patients**

Regular visits to see the Dentist, and scheduling a dental visit well before the beginning of Cancer treatment, are critical steps in preparing for Cancer treatment, especially if the patient's treatment plan includes the administration of Chemotherapy, and/or, Radiation Therapy. In this instance, common infections of the teeth and gums can produce significant negative effects when the White Blood Cell count is low, as it may be at times during Cancer therapy.

According to the National Cancer Institute (www.cancer.gov), and material given to me by my Medical Team, when receiving anti-Cancer therapy, severe problems can be experienced with the Cancer patient's oral cavity (mouth), including their tongue, mouth linings, lips, and teeth. As a result, the patient's capability to consume adequate quantities of food and beverages can be impacted. This, in-turn, can drastically affect the patient's consumption of essential nutrients and calories, and, ultimately, could impact their quality of life, and, the body's natural ability to heal, during and after treatment. Oral issues may even cause the Medical Team to temporarily interrupt treatment if the problems are severe enough. *That is definitely a big no-no!*

Many medications and special Cancer treatments affect parts of the body that are not directly associated with the specific disease, as systemic Chemo medications travel throughout a patient's blood system. Likewise, bacteria and infections in other parts of the body can have a magnified impact at critical times during Cancer therapy when the patient's Immune System is in a weakened state due to powerful Cancer-killing medications, and thru the use of Radiation. Health of the mouth, gums, and teeth is not often the first thing that comes to mind when preparing for Cancer treatment, but treatments like Chemotherapy and Radiation Therapy can have consistent and potentially harsh impacts on the dental health of most patients who receive these forms of Cancer treatment. For these reasons, *prior to* any dental work is to be performed, the patient's White Blood Cell counts should be checked to be sure that their levels are high enough to ward off any potential infections or bleeding. Low White Blood Cell counts can lead to infections, and a low Platelet count may lead to bleeding. Therefore, ***any periodontal or dental work to be done prior to the initiation of Cancer treatment HAS to be coordinated with the patient's Oncologist and Radiation Oncologist.***

If the Cancer patient's teeth are healthy, they shouldn't have to have any pulled prior to the beginning of Chemotherapy, and/or, Radiation Therapy. The majority of Cancer patients will be able to retain most, if not all, of their teeth during the treatments. However, if there is remaining dental work still to be done, such as a tooth that needs to be yanked, a Root Canal done, bridgework that needs to be performed, or, a crown that needs to be fitted and placed, the patient will want to bring their impending Cancer treatment to the attention of their Dentist. Equally as vital, the patient will also want to inform their Cancer Medical Team about any unfinished dental work.

Typically, dental procedures such as the removal of decayed, broken, or loose teeth should be performed before Cancer treatment begins. However, the patient's Dentist, along with their Oncologist, Radiation Oncologist, and other specialists as necessary, will make a determination as to whether the dental work should be done prior to Cancer treatment, or if it should be postponed until after treatment at some point in the future. In pre-treatment cases where the extraction of teeth is necessary, two to three weeks should elapse, if possible, prior to starting Radiation Therapy. This period will allow sufficient healing of gum tissue to occur prior to beginning treatment.

In my own Cancer experience, my pre-treatment dental exam revealed a bad tooth that needed to have a Root Canal, a procedure which I subsequently scheduled and had completed per my Dentist's and Radiation Oncologist's instructions. This painful process ended up delaying my Cancer treatments for a short while, but, that small interruption was deemed necessary by my Medical Team to prevent any further problems down the line. Where dental extractions are not indicated or necessary, a few days should elapse to allow for some preparation of dental services, or for further procedures by the dental provider. Responsible and proactive dental hygiene is always a very important consideration for all people. But, for Cancer patients, its importance cannot be overstated. In such instances, emphasis must be placed on daily prevention strategies, including the maintenance of conscientious oral hygiene, daily applications of topical fluoride, and, the consumption of a healthy, nutritious, Cancer treatment diet.

Those Cancer patients having Chemotherapy must tell their Dentist and then make an appointment for a dental exam at least two to three weeks prior to their first Chemotherapy session. Patients, or their loved one, family, Caregiver, or Guardian must make sure that the patient's dental health is completely up-to-date before beginning Chemotherapy. If the patient's mouth and teeth are awfully healthy before Chemotherapy, they will possibly have fewer and milder oral Side Effects both during and after treatment. Patients should have a regular dental exam and cleaning, be current on their X-rays, and get any fillings or other maintenance done *prior* to the commencement of treatment. The patient should also ask for any special instructions regarding mouth care that they will need during Chemotherapy.

If the Cancer patient wears dentures, they should have their gums and jaws examined, and/or, should have the dentures adjusted if they don't position right. Patients should always use an extra-soft toothbrush and ***alcohol-free*** mouthwash to decrease any pain while brushing and rinsing what can become a ***very*** sensitive mouth during treatment(s). Patients should brush their teeth gently two times a day and floss regularly. The bottom line is that practicing acceptable and responsible dental hygiene is one of the more significant preparatory and preventive activities that a Cancer patient can do entering in to their Cancer treatment. Not only should their proactive diligence and efforts help to possibly mitigate the potential pain and discomfort of any Cancer treatment-related Side Effects both during the therapies and after, while recovering, but, they will also provide longer-term benefits to the patients as they look forward to hopeful survivorship.

- **Pre-Treatment Dental Care - Head and Neck Cancer Patients**

Patients who are diagnosed with Oral Cancers and Head and Neck Cancers—the variety of Cancer with which I was diagnosed—are commonly treated with Surgery, Chemotherapy, and Radiation Therapy, or, a mixture of two, or all three of these therapy protocols.

Chemotherapy, and/or, Radiation Therapy, may be components of a patient's treatment(s), prior to, or subsequent to, surgical removal of the Primary Tumor. Radiation Therapy and Chemotherapy—which are generally given together—are used to treat Cancer because they both effectively kill Cancer cells. However, in addition to destroying Cancer cells, radiation to the head and neck area, and Chemotherapy via intravenous infusion, can also injure normal cells, including the vital, rapidly dividing cells in the mouth, Salivary Glands, Jawbones and Oropharynx (the part of the *Pharynx* that is just beneath the Soft Palate and above the Epiglottis and is continuous with the mouth).

Patients receiving Radiation Therapy to the head and neck areas will be at risk for developing specific oral problems, including *Xerostomia* (dry mouth), alterations in tastes, extensive tooth decay, increased susceptibility to, and development of, cavities, *Mucositis* (any inflammation of a mucous membrane, such as the linings of the mouth and throat), and, oral and systemic infections. Each of these Side Effects on their own are really significant, but, one or more in combination with the others can be devastating, both from a physical and an emotional standpoint. Each of these Cancer treatment-related mouth conditions might have an extremely detrimental influence on the ability of the Cancer patient to consume the requisite numbers of calories, and the varieties and quantities of food that they will need each day. Sound nutrition is essential as it provides the patient with the emotional and physical energy, and the strength and endurance, to get through treatment, and to eventually heal in its aftermath.

In an effort to mitigate risk, Head and Neck Cancer patients are advised to have a meticulous dental check-up and any necessary dental work completed ***before their treatment begins.*** The patient's Radiation Oncologist may recommend that the patient see a Dentist who has experience in treating individuals who have Head and Neck Cancers—and who are commonly treated with Radiation Therapy—rather than visiting their own Dentist, prior to the commencement of treatment. The Dentist or Dental Hygienist will provide the person with advice on how to care for their mouth, teeth and gums, and will perform an exam to ensure that their teeth are healthy. This is very important because Cancer treatment could make the patient's mouth much more sensitive and prone to infection, particularly if Radiation Therapy is prescribed in the patient's comprehensive treatment plan.

Necessary oral dental care that includes diligent adherence to proper dental treatment planning strategies prior to, during, and after Cancer treatment may prevent or reduce the incidence and severity of some oral problems. By seeing their Dentist a few weeks prior to starting Radiation Therapy, and/or, Chemotherapy, the patient might be able to prevent some of the more serious mouth Side Effects that could arise as a result of their treatment(s). It is very critical that the patient's mouth and teeth are as healthy and strong as possible prior to beginning Chemotherapy, and/or, Radiation Therapy. Taking just a few preparatory steps prior to Cancer treatment, and, maintaining a consistent, thorough approach, both during and after treatment, will have a positive impact on the patient's quality of life, and, should be able to enhance the patient's ability to heal and survive the disease.

- **Pre-Treatment Dental Care - Child Patients**

If possible, a child Cancer patient should obtain a complete oral exam and any needed dental work *before* their Cancer treatment begins. Dental care is important during treatment, but even checkups should be avoided when White Blood Cell counts are too low. The patient's parent(s), and/or, Caregiver, should always check with the Medical Team physician(s) prior to commencing some dental work. Conversely, the parent(s) should also let the Dentist know their child will be receiving Cancer treatment in the not-too-distant future. The child may be prescribed and administered an antibiotic before any dental work is done to prevent any possible infections. Keeping the child's teeth, mouth and gums as clean as possible to protect against decay is particularly vital. Ensure that the child's teeth are brushed after each meal using a soft toothbrush, and after each use, rinse the brush thoroughly with cold water, shake it well, and permit it to dry. Provide the child with paper cups to rinse his or her mouth. Dental floss may be used if care is taken not to cut or irritate the gums.

In summary, preparation for a young child or teenage Cancer patient's treatment should include a thorough dental checkup, and a follow-up for any identified conditions. Monitoring of dental health during Cancer treatment is an important aspect of maintaining long-term health. Some dental conditions might be Side Effects resulting from Cancer treatments and harsh related medications. Following a few preventive guidelines and adding a few simple remedies to the patient's daily routine should help them avoid many common dental discomforts in children, and, can often circumvent an unexpectedly dangerous health hazard, both during and after their Cancer therapy.

Engage in Physical Activity

Have you ever heard of the proverb, *"A sound body yields a sound mind?"* Or, maybe this one might ring a bell: *"A sound mind yields a sound body."* Chances are if you've heard one, you've also heard the other, because, quite honestly, they both go hand-in-hand. As we all know, and, as science has proven for millennia, the better that one takes care of their body, the better that their body will take care of them. This reality is classically the case in everyday life, but is especially true in extreme survival-type situations, of which living through and surviving a Cancer experience is at the top of the list.

As was evidenced by my own Cancer occurrence, however, a healthy lifestyle, a strong body, and a positive state-of-mind may not necessarily *prevent* a person from developing Cancer. But, once the person contracts the disease, the time and effort that the patient had invested in being healthy, physically fit, and optimistic *prior* to their diagnosis, may end up paying them large dividends *in the aftermath* of their diagnosis, during their Treatment, Recovery, and Aftercare. A strong mind and body will help the patient better cope with, and overcome, many of the physical, mental, and emotional Side Effects resulting from their treatment. This, in-turn, will beneficially impact their overall outcome, and, their quality of life, after, as a survivor.

Any form of physical activity—even less strenuous kinds—can provide several health benefits to the patient's body and mind. Exercise helps individuals maintain muscle mass, muscular strength, stamina, and bone strength, and can also help to decrease any stress, depression, anxiety, and constipation, in those patients so-affected. Likewise, physical activities could contribute to more relaxing sleep habits (sufficient deep sleep is something that the body and the brain *must* have to be healthy), greater self-confidence, and a higher level of self-esteem. A healthier lifestyle, which incorporates both a stable physical fitness regimen, *and* a reasonable nutritional program, are a winning combination that can not only help to make one's body less prone to minor sicknesses such as Colds and the Flu, but, also will cause it to be less susceptible to more serious medical maladies such as Heart Disease, Diabetes, and Cancer. And, of course, the benefits of a complementary exercise and nutrition plan will also contribute to the losing of unhealthy weight, and the release of Endorphins and Dopamine – those hormones produced by the body that make us feel good, and that give us more energy, vitality, and optimism.

If the Cancer patient isn't involved in an exercise program, some form of physical activity may be just what the doctor ordered for them – literally and figuratively. Patients awaiting their Cancer treatment(s) should talk with their Medical Team physician(s) about the possibility of including lighter or moderate physical activity into their treatment regimen. Of course, the judgment to participate in an exercise plan may be dependent upon the patient's physical state and capabilities, and their age, Cancer severity, treatment schedule, and other circumstances. But, if the doctor does approve of the patient's participation in a fitness plan, the patient should attempt to perform at least 30 minutes or more of moderate activity, such as walking or brisker walking, five or more days of the week, if the patient is able. In all cases, one should err on the side of safety and moderation.

If structured physical activity is new to the patient, they may want to start at a level comfortable to them (perhaps 5 to 10 minutes each day), and, as they are able, work up to the target of 30 minutes. Yoga, biking, swimming, resistance training (with weights or rubber exercise bands), and other aerobic (for the heart and lungs) and non-aerobic (for strength) activities are also wonderful forms of exercise. However, please do keep in mind that some, or all, of these activities may require specialized equipment, and/or, professional instruction, to ensure proper technique, safe use, and optimal results.

Share Pre-Treatment Special Time with Special Ones

Prior to the start of Cancer treatment(s), the patient and their loved one, and/or, family, may want to set aside some quality time together for a brief mini-vacation out of town, or, for a special night out at a fancy restaurant where they've always wanted to go. Or, the patient might desire to schedule time, either alone, or with someone special, in spiritual reflection, or, at a peaceful Yoga Retreat or Spa. Receiving a Cancer diagnosis and making treatment judgments can be very stressful – so, if time and circumstances will permit, before the treatment starts, is the perfect time to take a mental, physical and emotional holiday from all of these many concerns. The decision to go forth, of course, will be contingent upon the patient's health and age, their family and work circumstances, their upcoming treatment schedule, and their Medical Team physicians' concurrence.

If applicable members of the Medical Team will allow, such exciting escapes are highly recommended as they provide the perfect opportunities for the patient and their loved one, and/or, family, to decompress from the stress and to get away—if only for a few hours or a couple of days—to share fun and romantic experiences together before their treatment takes center stage. Possibly just as important, though, is that these well-deserved breaks offer a vital, much-needed distraction from the responsibilities of Cancer planning, meetings, and tests, and the almost inevitable 24x7 immersion in the patient's Cancer situation after they receive their diagnosis.

Once a patient's Cancer treatment begins, the patient's time, and that of their family and Caregiver, will be devoted to a stringent schedule of appointments and a variety of responsibilities for at least a few months—or several—depending upon the patient's variety of Cancer, their treatment protocols, and the patient's response to their treatment(s). Specifically, their non-stop schedule may require them to submit to one, two, or more surgical procedures, and/or, recurring Chemotherapy, and/or, Radiation Therapy sessions; participate in periodic medical tests and examinations; be present at consultations with Medical Team physicians; and, of course, relax, heal, and cope with any Side Effects that may evolve during treatment. Depending upon any Cancer treatment-related Side Effects that the patient may experience, it may take several weeks, or, in some instances, even a quite a few months following the termination of treatment(s), for the patient to feel that they have their "normal" life back again and are physically and mentally able to *go out <u>on</u> the town*, much less *travel out <u>of</u> town*. This may be all the more motivation for the patient and special ones in their life to take full advantage of the "lull before the storm," if possible, and to treat themselves to a very special time!

Plan Ahead for Possible Hair Loss

If a Cancer patient is due to receive Chemotherapy, they may already be well aware that one of the Side Effects of Chemo drugs is the possible, temporary loss of hair from the top of the head. During my own Cancer experience, I was administered an extremely potent "Chemo Cocktail" of two medications that I was told by my Medical Team would probably wipe out all of my hair. Not to be swayed by this presumption, however, I bet my Caregiver and Oncology Nurses that I wouldn't lose any, or very much, of my head hair as a result of my Chemotherapy treatments. They, of course, bet that I would. As it turns out, I didn't lose the golden locks on my head, but, thanks to the Chemo drugs, *I did temporarily say "goodbye" to my eyelashes and most of my eyebrows* – for awhile. In retrospect, all of us won the bet, but while my eyelashes and eyebrows did eventually return, they never grew back as heavy as they were prior to my treatment. I guess that's why they invented *"manscara,"* but, I digress…

With most Cancer treatments, there is no means of knowing how each patient will respond, or, whether the patient will incur any Side Effects as a reaction. But, patients receiving Chemotherapy can be prepared to deal with any temporary baldness should it occur, and they can begin making arrangements prior to the commencement of their therapies. In some cases, both male and female Cancer patients who have *gone bald* as a result of Chemotherapy wear their Cancer-caused hair loss proudly for the entire world to see – almost as if it were a symbol of defiance or a *Badge of Courage*. Others may want to hide or disguise their shortage of head hair, and for these patients, there are a few simple remedy options, depending upon the patient's situation, comfort level, style, budget, and personal preferences.

If the patient plans to purchase wigs, hats, or scarves, they should do so before their first infusion of Chemotherapy medication. Hair may take as long as three weeks to start thinning after the start of Chemotherapy, but, if and when it does occur, the patient will be ready to cover up. If there is a local shop that helps Chemo patients, the patient should take a family member, friend, or Caregiver with them to try on the different styles. Head coverings are also available online. Moreover, the patient should think about whether or not they would choose to go *naturally bald* while their hair takes a Chemo-induced hiatus, or, if they would like to *shave it off* in advance of the eminent "falling out" – the idea behind this being to beat the Chemo medicine to the punch, as it were. Making these decisions ahead of treatment gives the patient some time in which they can process any emotions they may have about their anticipated hair loss, and to take the actions that they feel are the most appropriate, should it occur.

Purchase and Wear Comfortable Clothing

Attending recurring Cancer Chemotherapy, and/or, Radiation Therapy treatments can be somewhat uncomfortable from a mental and emotional perspective, so there is no sense in contributing to the apprehensions from a physical perspective. The name of the game in attending Cancer treatments is comfort, comfort, comfort. It is both impractical and unnecessary (not to say, expensive) for an individual to show up for their Cancer treatment sessions as if they are dressed for the fashion runway or for a night out on the town.

Of course, the Cancer patient is free to wear any clothes that help them feel at-ease, especially if they will be going to, or coming from, work, school, or another public location, either before or after their Cancer treatments. But, if at all possible, the patient's *clothes-of-choice* should give them the non-binding freedom to move, sit, lie down, and to make their body more accessible for "medical things" during their many appointments, as circumstances may dictate. One means of ensuring that the patient is comfortable during their Cancer treatments is for them to buy and wear some loose, soft clothing. In this regard, the good-ole' stand-by—comfortable, cotton sweat suits or athletic wear—may be just what the doctor ordered – literally.

When choosing and wearing the clothes for each prospective Cancer treatment appointment, the patient should take into account that their physicians or nurses may need to gain access to their arms, chest, or various areas of their body to utilize a PIC line or Mediport through which blood can be drawn, and medications delivered. The patient should also remember that they may need to undress partially or completely for treatments (to be replaced with the beloved gown), so they should choose *quick-escape* clothing with a zipper or button front that will not dislodge their wig (if they are wearing one) while undressing. If the patient is going to have Radiation Therapy to the breast, they may prefer to wear soft layers of light fabrics instead of a confining bra that could put pressure on an already sensitive area. Regarding bras, patients may want to look into front-closing bras, in the event that fatigue or Neuropathy makes reaching behind the back a difficult chore. Patients might also want to wear comfortable shoes (with or without socks depending on one's personal preference) with a wide toe (for better circulation) and a good tread. Patients should not have to be worried about being overly cold in the Chemotherapy or Radiation Therapy clinics, as the nurses will be happy to provide the patient with heated blankets and other necessities upon request.

Understand and Verify Insurance Coverage

Prior to a Cancer patient having Surgery, Radiation Therapy, Chemo, or any other treatments relating to their Cancer occurrence (and if they have not already done so), they, and/or, their Caregiver, should contact their insurance company or health care provider and inform them of their Cancer diagnosis and impending treatments, to ensure that the treatments will be covered by their policy. Likewise, the patient, and Caregiver should confirm that their interactions with Physicians, Anesthesiologists, therapists, medical labs, hospitals and medications will also be covered. The patient should also be sure to understand any Deductible or Co-pay requirements, and they should find out what the procedures are for filing a Claim (if applicable), so that they can be quickly reimbursed by their insurance provider.

If the Cancer patient does not have any health insurance, or, if they can't afford to pay for the appointment Co-pays, Deductibles, or treatments and medications due to financial hardship, the afflicted individual must not give in on their attempts to receive the necessary medical assistance they may need to save their lives. It is imperative that Cancer victims try to obtain help and treatments – ***but they must inquire and request to get that help***. Patients with financial hardship conditions *can get monetary assistance,* but they will have to speak with financial personnel at their clinic. These individuals and offices could be able to grant assistance directly, or may refer the individual to other health care organizations which are chartered and funded to accommodate the health care needs of those not having conventional insurance coverage, including for the treatment of Cancer.

Assign Someone to Communicate Status / Progress

There is a good chance that the Cancer patient might wish to keep reports of their Cancer situation and status private among their loved ones and close family members, or maybe, even close friends. This definitely is to be anticipated considering the possible physical, and/or, emotional changes that the patient may undergo during their roller-coaster Cancer journey. But, there also is a possibility that the patient might want to share updates on their progress along the way, because, frankly, their friends, co-workers, school-mates, neighbors, and other individuals close to the patient might like to know how the person is doing – not in a "nosey" way, but purely out of caring and concern. In situations where the patient would feel more contented having a "spokesperson" to communicate the health status to others, the Cancer patient may want to assign a person whom they trust and who is also a good communicator, to be their "press secretary." The patient and their representative will concur beforehand on how much detail will be disseminated, and to whom, and how the news will be broadcast, such as with periodic email messages. The benefit of such an arrangement is that the patient doesn't have to repeatedly tell the same story to others, and can put their focus on beating their Cancer.

Try to Relax and Think Positive As Much as Possible!

You may be familiar with the saying, *"When you're up to your ass in alligators, it's difficult to remember that your original intention was to drain the swamp."* Unfortunately, Cancer patients don't normally have a choice when it comes to landing in the *swamp* that is Cancer. But, as outlined in this Chapter, there are quite a few things that they—and their support network—can do in an effort to avoid many of the *alligators.* Of significant importance is that the patient tries to treat their body like the temple it is, and to attempt to relax both their body and mind as much as possible, before, during, and after their treatment(s). And, along these same lines, it is crucial that the patient do all they can—in spite of the chips they believe are stacked against them—to keep a positive frame-of-mind throughout. Believe me, I know that this is easier said than done, because, for several months, I lived the continuous hell of not knowing what my future held. But, remember this: *No matter how deep the swamp or numerous the alligators, never give up hope on trying to drain it.*

Chapter Five

The Cancer Journey Explained – *Step 7 on the Journey:*

The Cancer Patient's Nutritional Plan

"Nutritious food and water are to a Cancer patient, what air and rest are to a Cancer patient – essential."

- Butch Sickler

Someone was once quoted as alleging, *"You are what you eat,"* a proclamation to which I can most definitely relate, because, admittedly, I *do* consume lots of nuts! But, all joking aside, there is some truth to that sentiment, because—for better or for worse—each of us is a product of our own decisions, environments, and, of life's circumstances, including all of those that can arise in the *Tasty Food Department.* Yes, as one might expect, and as is made perfectly and repeatedly clear on a 24 x 7 x 365 basis in magazines, books, DVDs, and, on television "reality" shows, infomercials, and, in other media, right at the basic essence of who we are as individuals—health-wise, appearance-wise, longevity-wise, and otherwise—is based, honestly, on the quality and quantity of food and beverages that we consume.

➢ *Creation of the Cancer Patient's Nutritional Plan – Step 7 on the Journey*

I would dare say that out of a good-sized group of complete strangers, it wouldn't be all *that* difficult to deduce who in the bunch is eating and drinking healthful, natural, wholesome, and nutritious foods and liquids, and which folks are consuming meals, snacks, and drinks that are loaded with sugar, fat, salt, alcohol, and God-knows-what-else. America has "fast food," and slow learning, to thank for this apparent distinction. But, the material within this Chapter is not about what individuals can do to lose their superfluous body weight. We will leave that up to all the "authorities" in the infomercials and internet blogs pertaining to those subjects. Rather, the information in this Chapter is regarding the vital importance of a patient consuming the necessary quantities of high-quality nutrition and liquids during their Cancer journey. The prescribed Treatments may get rid of the patient's Cancer, but, the patient must have the strength, energy, and endurance to withstand the physical and emotional challenges of the Treatments and the rigors of possible Side Effects. This is exactly where a sound Nutritional Plan can help to save the day.

A Cancer Patient and Good Nutrition Go Together

Generally speaking, as most of us are aware, healthful eating yields healthful living. There are exceptions, of course, (such as *my own incidence of Cancer* in spite of my ultra-healthy nutritional and exercise habits), but, for the most part, if a person takes good care of their body, their body will take good care of them. And, so this also applies to Cancer patients. But, the significance of consuming safe, healthful foods is paramount for *all* Cancer patients, no matter their age or gender, the form and Stage of their Cancer, or, the type(s) of treatment that will be used to, hopefully, rid the patient's body of the disease. And, even if the Cancer patient has been adhering to a well-designed, regimented, and nutrient-rich eating regimen on their own *prior to* their Cancer diagnosis, there might still be a need to re-think and "tweak" their nutritional ingestion in some minor ways to better accommodate the specifics of their unique Cancer-fighting program.

"Gassing Up" for the Cancer Journey

Most individuals *(the sensible ones, at least)* would not think twice about heading off on a several-day cross-country road-trip, or a several-week-long camping jaunt into the wilderness, *without first* planning and preparing to ensure that every known, probable need is considered and taken well-care-of far in advance. These "survivors" will make sure that their vehicle has good tires, and is all gassed up and in perfect working order, and that there is sufficient food, water, and other sustenance to safely see the travelers through the duration of their journey. These adventurous—but prudent—individuals may also even throw in a little extra of the critical things like food, water, and gas to prepare for the worst – should it ever come down to that.

These crucial, spare components, as one would expect, are to ensure that the individuals (and their vehicle) have sufficient fuel to give them the energy and strength to keep them functioning at their best. Without these essentials, people would be leaving it solely up to chance and luck to survive their journeys and reach their intended destinations – which some individuals do, and then, after "missing" for several days, are rescued, write a book about their "heroics," and become rich off of their carelessness. *But, I digress.* While a Cancer patient's journey from diagnosis to hopeful survivorship absolutely does not compare to taking an exciting multi-State drive on historic Route 66 or a lengthy exploration through the Rocky Mountains, the crucial preparations to gear-up for the Cancer journey—nutritionally and otherwise—can be just as important to a successful outcome.

Not unlike a long and winding road-trip from the East Coast of the U.S. to the West, the patient's travels through "Cancer-land" can also be quite prolonged, with many curves, multiple uphills and downhills, and, maybe even a few unforeseen detours along the way. The prospective length of the patient's Cancer journey, coupled with the possible physical and emotional requirements that will be placed upon the patient by a seemingly non-stop, wearisome schedule; the repetitious Cancer-removal therapies; the possible Side Effects; and, the potential deficit of good-quality sleep, could all contribute to the patient potentially "running out of gas" somewhere along the way.

To prevent the dangerous possibility that the Cancer patient might dehydrate or suffer from malnutrition, it is very important that the Cancer patient, and their family member or Caregiver, meet with the Registered Dietician on the patient's Medical Team, and take the recommended steps to keep the patient "gassed up" with nutritious foods and beverages throughout their complete Cancer journey. The Registered Dietician will work with the patient's doctor(s), and the patient, and their loved one, family, and Caregiver, to personalize a healthy, nutritional, and non-allergenic meal plan that is based upon the specific needs of the patient, prior to, during, and after treatment.

The Basics of Healthful Cancer Nutrition

Healthful nutrition is enormously significant for all people—Cancer patients and non-Cancer patients, equally—but, for any who have received a diagnosis of Cancer, consuming sufficient quantities of nutrient-rich foods, protein, and water and other beverages, could, honestly, mean the difference between the patient having a healthful and successful Cancer treatment conclusion, or not. Consuming the foods and liquids that are recommended to them by their Registered Dietician before, during, and after treatment(s), may help the patient feel better, physically and mentally, and, can help the patient remain stronger and more energetic as they progress through what can be a very uncomfortable, stressful, and energy-sapping Cancer journey.

- ### Healthful Cancer Nutrition is a Conscious Effort

"Healthful Nutrition" doesn't just happen with most people. Eating and drinking nutritiously requires that the person *consciously think about* the quality and quantities of the foods and beverages that they are putting into their bodies – or not – and how frequently.

This intuitive, down-to-earth, and mindful process advocates that the average Cancer patient would have:

- A basic understanding about which foods and drinks are healthy, and which ones are not
- An awareness of the quantity of ***healthy*** calories that their body requires to function optimally, both physically and mentally
- The craving and willpower to consume primarily those nutrients and calories that will benefit their body and mind
- The discipline (i.e., power over temptation), when food shopping or dining in or out, to purchase and ingest primarily those food and drink items that are of healthy nutritive and caloric value
- The self-control to not "binge-eat" large quantities of any foods, healthy or not. There truly is good science behind *moderation*

Very simply stated, healthful nutrition is a conscious process that furnishes the Cancer patient's body with the important nutrients, calories, and liquids that it requires, in an effort to enable all organs and bodily systems to function at their tip-top best. Unfortunately, a person's body is at the mercy of their mind, so, if a person does not knowingly make the sensible, healthful, and well-founded decisions on what they put (or don't put) into their body, the wellbeing of their body and mind may end up suffering the consequences.

• Basic Steps to Healthful Cancer Nutrition

The basic steps to healthful Cancer nutrition include:

- A person eats or drinks food and beverages which are comprised of a balanced multitude of healthy nutrients
- The person's bodily systems digest and assimilate the individual nutrients contained in the food and liquids
- The various nutrients travel throughout the person's bloodstream via organs and systems to different parts of the body where they are used (and sometimes stored) as fuel for physical energy and mental processing, for blood circulation, and, as building blocks (such as Amino Acids) for repair and healing of tissues, and for many other purposes, as needed by the body
- Those nutrients that are not utilized by the body or stored for use at a later time, are excreted from the body as waste products

• The Benefits of Healthful Cancer Nutrition

It goes without saying that healthful nutrition is good for our bodies. The unfortunate news for our bodies, however, is that many foods and beverages that are available today at the grocery store and prepared in restaurants (especially those establishments of the "fast food" variety) are anything but healthy, and our bodies tend to suffer the consequences of decisions made by our minds to consume them.

The bona fide "problem" with some foods is that many of the unhealthier nutritional selections are *designed* to be tantalizing to the taste buds and nostrils, and, it is only human-nature to want to chew and drink those things that offer us pleasure, such as ice cream, fried chicken, pizza, and beer. Despite the higher fat, sugar, salt, and other non-nutritious content found in many foods and drinks, Americans, and individuals in many countries in the world, consume billions of dollars-worth of this unhealthy stuff each year. And, while the great taste of these delectable, but potentially deadly, morsels may be only temporary, the longer-term health issues that are associated with the consumption of these unhealthy food renditions are astronomical, as are the healthcare costs ***($150 billion per year!)*** to treat obesity and related health conditions, to which these foods and drinks contribute.

Eating well, on the other hand, means consuming a variety of foods that will provide the Cancer patient with the nutrients that they need—protein, fats, carbohydrates, healthy liquids, and vitamins and minerals—to help protect their health while fighting, and, hopefully, surviving, their Cancer. If a person has been diagnosed with Cancer, it is extremely crucial that the patient, and their loved one, family, or Caregiver, put important emphasis on familiarizing themselves with, and following, the healthy nutritional plan that is developed by the Registered Dietician on the patient's Medical Team. The benefits of healthful, sound nutrition cannot be understated. All Cancer patients, regardless of their ages or genders, and, irrespective of the forms or Stage of Cancer with which they have been diagnosed or its locality, should be ever-mindful of the continued importance of consuming satisfactory quantities of healthful nutrients, calories, and water and other liquids, as they continue throughout their Cancer journey.

The occurrence of Cancer, as well as its treatments and Side Effects, can have a profound impact on the patient's appetite – and, not always in a beneficial way. Additionally, Cancer and associated treatments may impact the patient's body's ability to tolerate, chew, swallow, digest, and eliminate some foods. The nutritional needs of people with Cancer vary from person to person. And, because each Cancer patient is different, as are their forms of Cancer, the resulting treatments, and their own responses to those treatments, the patient's physicians, nurses, and Registered Dietician will help to pinpoint the patient's nutritional goals, and will arrange means to help the patient meet them. These individuals will also help plan meals and develop a grocery shopping list, and should guide the patient in making food and drink choices to help the patient better cope with any treatment-related Side Effects, such as constipation, diarrhea, pain, or nausea.

Following are several of the elemental benefits to the Cancer patient of consistently consuming healthy food, water, and other liquids:

- Feel better – physically, mentally, and emotionally
- Retain strength and energy to face challenging treatments
- Maintain body weight and the storage of nutrients
- Better tolerate treatment-related Side Effects
- Lower risk of infection – 80% of a person's Immune System is within in their digestive tract, so, it stands to reason that a healthy digestive tract will yield a healthier Immune System
- Helps bodily organs and systems function properly, and heal and recover faster from treatment-related Side Effects

Meeting with the Registered Dietician

Eating nutritiously *prior to* the start of Cancer treatment, and continuing to consume sufficient quantities of healthful foods *during* and *after* treatment, is vital to the patient, as it may serve to increase their physical energy, strength, and stamina, and, could also help to improve their mental and emotional state and sleeping patterns. All of these are significant components of successful treatment, healthy recovery, and a favorable, overall Cancer therapy outcome. To help ensure that the patient is consuming the proper amounts and calories of nutritious food through their Cancer journey, a customized eating plan will generally be developed prior to the commencement of the patient's treatment(s). The individual who will assist the patient, and their loved one, family, or Caregiver, in designing and following the patient's plan, will be another vital member of the patient's Medical Team: a Registered Dietician (RD), or a Nutritionist.

The Registered Dietician that will be assigned to the Cancer patient's case will, in general, be one of the patient's best sources of information regarding the customized diet plan that the patient will use, before, during, and after treatment. This health care professional has special training in food, nutrition, biochemistry, and physiology, and will use this knowledge to promote health, and to avoid disease, through counseling and education. Those Registered Dieticians that assist patients, families, and Caregivers in a Cancer setting have the responsibility of making sure that the treating physicians' nutritional requirements for the patient are incorporated into the personal plan. Likewise, they make sure that the patient's nutritional plan not only adequately addresses the patient's critical nutrient, caloric, and other nutritional needs throughout the entire program, but, that it also is compatible with the patient's age and ability to tolerate certain foods and drinks, including allergy considerations. All Cancer patients are distinct, as are their Cancers and resulting treatments, so, all of these important considerations will be brought to light and discussed when the Registered Dietician meets with the patient, and their family or Caregiver, to develop the patient's customized nutritional plan.

Development of the Cancer Patient's Nutritional Plan

Because the Registered Dietician is trained in Cancer-related nutrition, they are very knowledgeable in counseling Cancer patients and developing dietary plans best suited for each patient's individual needs. In so doing, they will work with the patient, and their family or Caregiver, as well as many other members of the patient's Cancer Treatment Medical Team, including the main, treating physicians, to design the most appropriate nutritional regimen for the patient's own circumstances. And, while the "final" developed plan will be based on several different factors, including the patient's treatment(s) and their responses to the therapies, the nutrition plan is also "dynamic," meaning that it can be modified at any given time by the Registered Dietician or others on the Medical Team, as the need evolves.

After the Registered Dietician has employed their knowledge and expertise to develop the patient's primary dietary plan, they will meet again with the patient, family, and/or, Caregiver to go over the final regimen to make sure that the patient, and family or Caregiver, understand it fully. The RD will also take this opportunity to address any worries, and to respond to any questions that the patient, or their family, or Caregiver, might have. Prior to meeting with a Registered Dietician, the patient, family members or Caregiver should jot down any questions they might have prior to the meeting so that they don't forget anything. The patient, family member or Caregiver should be sure to ask the Registered Dietician to repeat or clarify anything that is not clear, especially if the Cancer patient happens to be a young or teenage child, or an elderly individual. These patients may not be fully capable of comprehending, so any help will be beneficial.

Cancer Treatment-Related Side Effects That Can Impact Eating and Drinking

There was an aphorism that was making the rounds in fitness clubs and exercise circles a few years ago, and, which one may still occasionally hear conjectured in exercise-related and other contexts. That memorable phrase, *"No pain – no gain,"* is intended to imply, loosely, that a person will normally have to experience some level of discomfort or inconvenience *(pain),* to be able to reap the benefits of their efforts *(gain)*. There are exceptions to this mode of thinking, of course, such as a person winning the lottery, or an individual being genetically gifted in some respect, but, for the most part, a majority of people normally have to pay, in one form or another, for anything worth having. And wouldn't you know it, the opportunity to survive a Cancer threat also doesn't come without a hefty cost of its own.

As you doubtless are aware, the price that one has to pay for the reward of reclaiming their life comes in the form of unwelcome Cancer treatment-related Side Effects, all of which are inconvenient, and many of which are uncomfortable. In this regard, life irrefutably isn't fair, but, thankfully, not all Cancer Side Effects are terrible, and several can be minimized or eliminated by the Medical Team, with the help of the patient, their loved one, family, and/or Caregiver. An especially critical and continuous consideration in a patient's Cancer journey is the requirement that all Side Effects negatively impacting the patient's ability to eat food and to drink liquids *must* be managed and minimized *as quickly as possible* to ensure that the patient does not have to suffer the harmful effects of malnutrition or dehydration. Either one of these potential, risky conditions—were they to remain unaddressed for more than a few days—would harshly debilitate the patient's health, and could encumber their ability to safely continue with their Cancer treatment(s). Obviously, this is not a prospect that the patient, the Caregiver, or, the Medical Team would want to face.

It is for these reasons that appropriate actions are undertaken by the patient's physicians and Registered Dietician to be sure that the patient's nutritional plan provides for appropriate food and fluids that not only meet the patient's individual nutritional needs, but, that are as comforting, non-irritating, non-allergenic, and, as palatable as possible. Additionally, the patient and all applicable members of the patient's Medical Team will take essential steps to reduce or remove any associated pain to the patient's mouth and throat regions thru the safe use of medications, and/or, other therapeutic methods. Patients, and their loved ones, family members, or Caregiver, should consult with relevant members of the Medical Team, including the Patient's Registered Dietician, if they have any questions or concerns.

Included in the following Table, in no particular order, are the most universal, potential Cancer treatment-related Side Effects that could negatively impact the patient's capacity to consume, and eliminate, food and drink. Also included, are *non-medicinal* recommendations that may be able to help the patient reduce the discomfort of the Side Effects, as well as some nutritional suggestions for easing pain while ingesting. The material below, which is for informational purposes solely, was drawn from my own journaling notes, materials provided to me by members of my Medical Team, and, from online resources of the Government National Cancer Institute (www.cancer.gov):

Side Effect	Recommendation
Loss of Appetite	• Plan and fix a daily menu in advance to make eating easier • Eat small, frequent meals, high in protein and calories to avoid weight loss • Seek foods that smell and taste good • Be creative and experiment with different foods • Consume good-tasting liquids high in protein and calories
Nausea/Vomiting	• Eat dry foods, such as crackers and toast, throughout the day to help absorb liquids and settle the stomach • Sit up for one hour after eating • Eat bland foods • Avoid offensive odors, or anything causing one to "gag" • Suck on candies such as mints, or chew sweet gum

	• Rinse mouth before and after eating • Consume clear liquids with high nutritional value
Diarrhea	• Drink plenty of fluids (room temperature) to avoid dehydration • Try liquids that have electrolytes (Sodium, Potassium) • Limit dairy and gas-forming foods • Limit foods made with Sorbitol (sugar-free foods)
Constipation	• Eat more fiber-containing foods (bran, fruits, vegetables, oatmeal, breads) • Drink 8 to 10 cups of liquid daily • Take walks and perform exercise, as permitted
Taste Alteration	• Eat small, frequent meals and snacks • Use plastic utensils (if foods taste metallic) • Add spices and sauces • Eat meat with something sweet (cranberry sauce, applesauce) to help "awaken" the taste buds • Avoid acidic and spicy foods that can irritate the mouth
Xerostomia (Dry Mouth)	• Use a straw instead of drinking directly from a glass • Increase oral hygiene • Keep liquids handy at all times • Avoid mouthwash that contains alcohol • Consume sweet beverages high in nutritional value

Stomatitis (Sore Mouth)	• Eat soft foods that are easy to chew and swallow • Avoid acidic, spicy, hard foods that may irritate the mouth • Cut food into small, bite size pieces • Use a straw instead of drinking directly from a glass • Practice good mouth care (Dentist will suggest products) • Consume room temperature liquids high in nutritional value

Nutritional Support Options for Cancer Patients Who Cannot Eat "Normally"

As is probably the situation with most people, many Cancer patients might also have an inclination to take different parts of their bodies for granted and to not give them a second thought – that is, as long as "all systems are go," and everything is working as it should be. But, when something bad has happened to the person's body that prevents it—or specific parts of it—from functioning as it should, it can really take a person out of their comfort zone, and can definitely *throw a wrench in the works.* Let's face it, all of us are creatures of habit. Just think of the last time that you injured your dominant arm or hand, and you had to "instruct" your opposite appendage to do the same things that had come naturally to the one you normally use. It completely made things a little awkward, didn't it, at least until you managed to synchronize your brain to direct the *back-up* arm's and hand's movements to complete what needed to be done? The same can be said for injuring an ankle, leg, or foot, as well as one's back, hip, knee, or any other body part that is depended upon to perform a specific function (which, pretty much, encompasses the entire body).

Eating and Drinking is Fun – Unless You Can't

While an individual can certainly educate their non-dominant hand and arm to brush their teeth, or, a person can depend upon their *good* leg and crutches or a cane to help them stay mobile while their broken leg mends, what does a person do when they have, suddenly, and completely, or partially, lost their ability to eat and drink via the normal, oral method of chewing and swallowing with their mouth, tongue, and esophagus? As I alluded to earlier in this Section, these body parts and these functions, are, most likely, taken for granted by most people every time they lift a fork, spoon, chopsticks, or glass to their mouth. Eating and drinking are second-nature to most people, unless we painfully bite our tongues or inner cheeks while chewing, or, should we suffer the consequences of ingesting too much red-hot chili that leads to an upset stomach or a *"Flaming A."* But, usually, the only thoughts that we might give the process of consuming food and beverages will be our appreciation (or non-appreciation) of their flavors, the contentment of "feeling full" at the end of the meal, and, the gratification that may accompany the act of eating and drinking with family and friends in a pleasurable environment. However, take away a person's ability to chomp and swallow food and drink in the normal manner—even for a brief period of time—and we're talking about an entirely different, and disconcerting, set of circumstances.

The reality of this predicament is that some people, including patients suffering Side Effects of their Cancer treatments *(i.e., Head and Neck Cancer patients)*, will forgo—partially, or completely, for either a temporary or an undetermined point in time—their ability to consume food and beverages via the normal method of chewing and swallowing. This may be due to the added adverse affects of Cancer Surgery, in which sections of the Esophagus, Stomach, or Colon are partially or entirely removed along with the Cancer tumor(s). Or, it could be because of excruciating pain in the mouth, tongue, or throat area as the outcome of the patient receiving Chemotherapy, and/or, Radiation Therapy, to the head and neck area. *I can vouch for that!*

No matter the individual or the reason, if the Cancer patient cannot consume life-sustaining foods and liquids, *naturally,* through their mouth, it is vital that essential nutrients and water are delivered into the patient's body by way of the most pertinent means possible. Forget about the patient ingesting food or beverage because it tastes delicious, or because it "crunches" or "fizzes," or, is a cool thing to do on a Friday night at a restaurant with friends. In a perfect world, those are some of the gastronomical pleasures to which most people can relate. But, for some Cancer patients, they are only fantasies.

For Cancer patients who have partially or completely lost the means of consuming foods normally (orally) through their mouth, however, what we're talking about is *good nutrition and survival*, plain and simple. In such extreme situations, changes must be made to the patient's normal ingestion protocol to ensure that the Cancer patient or survivor is receiving the critical nutrients, water, and other liquids that they require to remain strong, energized, and physically capable of withstanding what might often be a very challenging and wearisome treatment regimen. If the Cancer patient has the strength, endurance, bodyweight, and test results to safely continue with their treatment(s), the primary focus can remain on completely and safely removing Cancer from the patient's body – right where it belongs. And, once the treatments have concluded, if the patient still cannot masticate and swallow normally, it is necessary that they continue to consume nutrients, calories, and liquids through alternative methods to help support the critical recovery and healing processes.

Enteral and Parenteral Nutrition – Alternative Means of Delivering Nutrients into the Body

While common eating and drinking through one's mouth and esophagus are always the preferred manner of providing nutrients to the patient's body, should it transpire that the patient is not able to consume sufficient nutrients and calories normally (by chewing and swallowing) due to pain or other reasons, appropriate Medical Team members will present the patient, and their family or Caregiver, with alternative processes for delivering nutrients into the patient's body. Per the National Cancer Institute (www.cancer.gov), in general, the methods that will be recommended will call for the usage of ***Enteral Nutrition*** (a feeding tube introduced from outside the patient's body directly into their stomach or their intestines through the nose or the abdomen), and ***Parenteral Nutrition*** (a thin tube or catheter inserted from outside the patient's body directly into their bloodstream).

In alternative feeding, nutrients delivered in liquid formulas via Enteral or Parenteral tubes are made up of water, carbohydrates, fats, proteins, associated calories, and, vitamins and minerals, which have been specially formulated to ensure that the patient receives the healthful nutrition they require to maintain body weight, and to keep their organs and the bodily systems functioning optimally. If Enteral Nutrition is to be part of the patient's care after leaving the hospital, the patient, and their famly or Caregiver, will be trained to carry out the nutritional support care at home. Enteral or Parenteral Nutrition support can greatly improve a patient's quality of life during Cancer treatment—and also can help to facilitate them continuing to receive their Cancer-killing treatment(s)—but, there are valid, possible risks (such as infection and dependence) with both modes, that should be considered before making the decision to employ them. The Medical Team will discuss the potential benefits and risks of each variety of nutritional support with the patient, their family, or Caregiver.

If a patient has had Surgery to excise a malignant tumor and marginal tissue that entailed the surgical removal of all, or a part of, essential organs associated with their nutritional intake, digestion, or elimination, applicable members of the patient's Medical Team will meet with the patient, and their family or Caregiver, in advance of the surgical procedure(s), to explain how nutrients and water will be safely delivered to the patient after the Surgery has been effectively completed. Similarly, if the patient will be receiving Chemotherapy treatment for their Cancer, and/or, Radiation Therapy, to their head, and/or, their neck area, the Medical Team physicians and Registered Dietician, will, prior to the treatment(s), describe to the patient, and their family, and/or, Caregiver, the likely negative Side Effects they may encounter that could potentially affect their food and beverage consumption. At this time, the Team will also recommend a variety of eating strategies and foods in the patient's Nutritional Plan that may help the patient better cope with any discomfort accompanying their treatment(s). In all such cases, the risks and benefits of Enteral and Parenteral Nutrition are alternatives that the physician(s) on the patient's Medical Team may examine with the patient, the family, or the Caregiver. Physicians should also explain the use of medications that might help to encourage the patient's appetite, and/or, that could assist in reducing or eliminating pain in the affected body areas.

☛***Author's Note:*** The following explanations of Enteral and Parenteral Nutrition are provided to the reader for informational and educational purposes only. A majority of the information below was drawn from my journal notes and materials provided by my Medical

Team, and, via online resources of the Government National Cancer Institute (www.cancer.gov). This information is reliable; however, the patient, and their loved one, family, or Caregiver, should consult with applicable members of the Medical Team for guidance, and to receive answers for any questions they may have, regarding Enteral or Parenteral Nutrition, or, other alternatives for delivering nutrients to the Cancer patient if they are having difficulty eating normally.

The explanations below are provided for the Enteral and Parenteral methods of delivering necessary nutrition to the Cancer patient who cannot receive all essential nutrients through normal, oral, means:

- **Enteral Nutrition**

Enteral Nutrition is frequently referred to as "tubefeeding." Enteral Nutrition is a form of nutrition that is delivered to a person's digestive system in the form of a liquified formula. The ingestion of nutritional beverages or formulas, and tubefeeding, are all forms of Enteral Nutrition. Cancer patients who are not able to complete their complete nutritional needs with normally-consumed whole food and beverages, and, who don't have any vomiting issues or irrepressible diarrhea, may be prescribed tubefeedings to ensure that their bodies are receiving the required quantities of nutrients, calories, and water.

Tubefeedings can be used to supplement, or to add additional nutrients and calories to what a Cancer patient is naturally capable of consuming. Or, tubefeeding of liquid nutrient formulas can be the patient's only source of nutrition, depending on their circumstances. The type of nutient formula used in Enteral Nutrition is based upon the particular dietary needs of the patient. There are special formulas for those patients who have specific health issues, such as Diabetes and Cancer, and, for severely emaciated, and/or, dehydrated patients who require a significant increase in caloric and liquid intake.

With Enteral Nutrition, liquid formula might be delivered to the patient through the feeding tube as a constant drip (referred to as "continuous feeding"), or one to two cups of formula can be given to the patient from three to six times a day (known as "bolus feeding"). Contingent upon the length of time that the Enteral Nutrition will be employed in each patient's case, a small feeding tube may be placed through the patient's nose and down the throat into the stomach or to the small intestine. With both of these types of nasal enteral feeding, the nutrient bag is hung on an IV-type stand, and the feeding tube is fed through a "pump" mounted on the stand that is programmed by the nurse to literally "push" the prescribed quantity of liquid formula into the patient, who is typically lying in bed at the time of delivery.

If the Cancer patient is not able to use the nasal feeding tube, the tube may be surgically placed into the stomach or the intestinal tract through an incision on the outside of the patient's abdomen. In such cases, the tube will have a "shut-off" valve to prevent infection, to which a sizeable, removable syringe-type plastic bottle containing the liquid food can be attached. By using this pump-like device, the liquified formula is physically squeezed through the feeding tube by the patient, their family, or Caregiver. This type of tubefeeding may occur while the individual is seated, standing, or lying down.

Following, are the different types of feeding tubes that may be used with Enteral Nutrition, and the typical durations in which each may be ordered by the responsible health care professional:

- **Nasogastric Tube** – This tube is inserted through the patient's nose and fed down the throat into the stomach or small intestine. This sort of feeding tube is used when Enteral Nutrition is only needed for a few weeks

- **Gastrostomy Tube** – (also known as a Stomach Tube, or Percutaneous Endoscopic Gastrostomy (PEG) tube). This tube is inserted through a surgical incision made on the outside of the patient's abdomen and then in the stomach. This form of feeding tube is usually used for long-term enteral feeding (several weeks, months, or years), or for patients who cannot use a tube in the nose and throat

- **Jejunostomy Tube** – This tube is surgically inserted into the patient's small intestine through an incision in their abdomen. This kind of tube is usually used for long-term enteral feeding (several weeks, months, or years), or, for patients who cannot use a tube in the nose and throat

- **Parenteral Nutrition**

Parenteral Nutrition, also labeled Total Parenteral Nutrition (or TPN), is a method for delivering water and nutrients directly into the patient's blood stream via a catheter (thin tube) that is surgically inserted into a vein in their chest or arm. Parenteral Nutrition *does not* use the digestive system (stomach or intestines), as does Enteral Nutrition (whereby a feeding tube is placed into the Cancer patient's stomach or intestine through their nose or abdominal area). Parental Nutrition may be administered to patients who are not able to absorb nutrients through their intestinal tract because of vomiting that won't die down, or, due to severe diarrhea, or intestinal disease. Parenteral Nutrition may also be prescribed for those patients undergoing high-dose Chemotherapy, Bone Marrow Transplantation, and Radiation Therapy. Due to the potentially excruciating Side Effects from those treatments that can result in pain in the mouth and throat areas, some Side Effects can prevent the normal intake of food and liquids. *Yep!*

Parenteral Nutrition makes it possible to administer all of the water, carbohydrates, proteins, fats, calories, vitamins, and minerals that a Cancer patient needs. Parenteral Nutrition is utilized when the patient cannot consume food by mouth or by Enteral feeding, and is typically used only in patients who need nutritional support for five days or more. The patient is checked often for infection or bleeding at the place where the catheter enters their body. Parenteral Nutrition support may continue even after the patient departs the hospital. If Parenteral Nutrition is to be maintained for the Cancer patient after leaving the hospital, the patient and their family or Caregiver will be trained to administer the nutritional support care at home. When the need for Parenteral Nutrition no longer exists, the discontinuance of Parenteral Nutrition support must be accomplished gradually, and under the supervision of the patient's Medical Team. The Parenteral feedings are decreased steadily over time until they can be stopped, or, as the patient is changed over to Enteral or normal feeding.

Following are the locations on the body where catheters (thin tubes) may be placed with Parenteral Nutrition, and the typical durations of use, during which each form of Parenteral feeding might be ordered by the responsible health care professional:

- **Central Venous Catheter** - This form of tube is placed beneath the patient's skin into a large vein in the upper chest during a surgical procedure. This type of catheter is usually used for longer-term Parenteral Nutrition

- **Peripheral Venous Catheter** – This catheter is placed into a vein in the arm by trained medical staff, including nurses. This type of feeding catheter is typically utilized for Parenteral feeding of patients who need shorter-term nutitional support

Obese Nations / Starving Nations / Untrained Doctors

There is probably nothing more basic, more important, more disregarded, or more misunderstood by a bulk of the people than the foods and drinks that they consume. And, for most Americans, and for tons of other people in developed countries that have seemingly unlimited supplies of food and water, there is also probably nothing that is as taken-for-granted as the vital sustenance that helps to keep them alive. Moreover, I'd bet most people don't give the nutritional composition of their food or drink—good or bad—a second thought, as evidenced by the inordinate numbers of overweight and morbidly obese children and adults in America. These individuals can be very concerned about the food's flavor, receiving monster portions, and, possibly, the cost of the food that they eat, but in many cases, these folks completely ignore how destructive many of these sugar-, fat-, and salt-laden foods can be to their bodies, health, and lives.

It's a very different story, however, for those inhabitants who subsist in food-starved and drought-stricken underdeveloped nations that must depend on external humanitarian assistance to feed, and to provide life-sustaining liquids to their millions of hungry and thirsty mouths. These people are simply happy to get whatever they can to stay alive. In all cultures around the globe, however, no matter the surplus or lack of available, nutritious food and water, it is vital that *all people* receive the nutrients and liquids that their bodies need to be as healthy as possible. And certainly, in a very wide world that suffers over six million Cancer diagnoses each year in men, women, and children, it is of greater significance that these individuals have access to the nutrients and water that they need to survive both there Cancers, *and* life. That's a double-edge sword if there ever was one.

Sadly, however, despite the apparent importance of nutrition to people's health and in the prevention of disease, future doctors in the U.S. only receive about 2-3 hours of instruction on the subject of *Nutrition* in Medical School. Medical practice in the U.S.—at least in comparison to medicine in East Asia and other nations—is more *reactive,* and less *proactive.* Meaning, more emphasis is placed on U.S. doctors and Health Care "fixing" the body after it is "broken," rather than on preventing it from "breaking" in the first place.

Nutrition 101 - A Quick Look at Basic Nutritional Information for Cancer Patients

Any way that you slice, dice, shred, puree, sauté, or fillet it, *"Nutrition"* is big business, and the volumes of information on the topic can be mind-boggling, especially to people who have little, or no knowledge of the vast subject. Absolutely, many self-proclaimed "experts" have recognized this money-making opportunity, and have entered the marketplace to sell their "latest and greatest" ideas about nutrition and related topics that they have to offer. And, thankfully, many educated, qualified, and certified nutritional experts have also joined this mix and have presented their scholarly knowledge and experiences to those disposed to read and listen to their work. But, at the very epicenter of all of this information—regardless by whom it is gathered and transmitted, or why—are the elementary discussions about 6 essential nutrients – Fats, Protein, Carbohydrates, Vitamins, Minerals, and Water. And, it is these six basic components of our available food and drink choices that I will describe in detail below.

☛***Author's Note:*** The following information regarding universal nutrients, which are necessary to human life and proper functioning of all organs and bodily systems, can be found in school textbooks, encyclopedia references, and other topical books and internet sites pertaining to the subject of *Healthy Nutrition.* Because this basic information on nutrients is general and common knowledge that is regularly available in the public domain (*and in my brain),* none of this data is copyrightable, and, therefore, is available to all who wish to use it for their educational and health improvement purposes.

Following are brief explanations about six basic nutritional components that are vital for human life and survival, and that are of even greater importance to Cancer patients. Many Cancer patients require additional strength, energy, bodyweight, calories, hydration, and Immune System integrity to carefully and effectively finish their Cancer treatment(s), and, so they can better cope with any negative Side Effects that may arise during, and after, their treatment(s):

- **Proteins**
    - Proteins are one of the three vital major nutrients that supply calories to the body (the other critical nutrients are Fats and Carbohydrates)
    - The Protein we eat may be broken into smaller units, referred to as "Amino Acids," and are used by the body to develop or repair muscle, bones, skin, blood, and other body tissues
    - The energy produced by Proteins is ~4 calories per gram. (There are about 28 grams in an ounce, so a gram is a very small amount)
    - Proteins are needed for growth, to repair body tissue, and to keep the Immune System healthy. When a person doesn't get enough Protein, it takes longer to recover from illness, and they have a lower resistance to infection. People with Cancer often need more Protein than non-patients. During and after Surgery, Chemotherapy, or Radiation Therapy, extra Protein is usually needed to heal tissues and to help fight infection, especially in Cancer patients coping with harsh Side Effects
    - Good sources of Protein include leaner meats, fish, poultry, dairy products, nuts, dried beans, peas and lentils, soy foods, and also in supplement powders, capsules, pills, etc.

- **Carbohydrates**
    - Carbohydrates, otherwise known as "Carbs," are one of the three crucial major nutrients that supply calories to the body (the other critical nutrients are Fats and Proteins)

- Carbohydrates are the body's primary source of short-term energy. A gram of Carbohydrates produces ~4 calories
- Carbohydrates provide the fuels that are required by the body for physical activity and proper organ function
- The healthiest sources of Carbohydrates are Complex Carbs. Whole grains, vegetables, and fruits, supply needed Fiber, Vitamins, Minerals, and Phytonutrients. Here are specifics:

  - **Whole grains** – Foods made from whole grains contain all the essential components and naturally occurring nutrients of the entire grain seed. If the grain has been processed (for example, cracked, steel cut, crushed, rolled, extruded, lightly pearled, and/or, cooked), the food product should provide about the same rich balance of nutrients that are found in the original unprocessed grain seed. Whole-grain types include wheat, oats, corn, and rye along with lesser-known grains like barley, flaxseed, groats, wheat berries, millet, and spelt. Whole grains are found in some cereals, breads, flours, and crackers, and some whole grains can be used as side dishes or part of an entree. A person can find whole grains at the grocer by looking on the package label for the words "whole," or "whole-grain." Terms such as "stoned wheat," "wheat flour," and "cracked wheat," don't guarantee the presence of whole grains in the product.

  - **Fiber** – The part of edible plant foods that the body cannot digest. Because it is indigestible by humans, fiber helps to move food waste through the body quickly, which is very important for Cancer patients taking Opiate medications

  - **Phytonutrients** – Plant compounds such as Carotenoids, Limonoids, and Phytosterols, which have been proven to have certain health-protecting qualities

- Additional sources of Complex Carbohydrates include bread, potatoes, rice, spaghetti, pasta, some cereals, dried beans, corn, peas, and beans. "Sweets" (desserts, candy, and drinks with sugar) can supply Carbohydrates, but provide very little in the way of Vitamins, Minerals, or Phytonutrients. These "simple sugars" or "simple Carbohydrates" add to a calorie count but normally don't provide other nutrients. Typically, simple sugars are not good for one's health (or teeth!)

- **Fats**

    - Fats are one of the three vital nutrients that supply calories to the body (the other nutrients are Proteins and Carbohydrates)
    - Fats are the body's primary source of long-term energy. The energy produced by Fat is ~9 calories per gram
    - Fats play a very important role in nutrition. Fats and oils are made of Fatty Acids and serve as a rich source of energy for the body. The body breaks down Fats and uses them to store energy, insulate body tissues, and transport some types of Vitamins through the blood. Fats also play an important role in food preparation by enhancing food flavor, making baked products tender, and conducting heat during cooking
    - Some Fats are much healthier for one's overall health than others. When considering the effects of Fats on a person's heart, bodyweight, cholesterol level, and their overall health, *Unsaturated Fats should always be selected* over Saturated Fats or Trans Fatty Acids (also known as "Trans Fats")

        - **Monounsaturated Fats** are found mainly in vegetable oils such as canola, olive, and peanut oils. They are liquid at room temperature. These are considered to be healthy Fats

        - **Polyunsaturated Fats** are found mainly in vegetable oils as safflower, sunflower, corn, flaxseed, and canola. They are also the main fats found in seafood. They are liquid or soft at room temperature. These oils have healthy Fats

        - **Polyunsaturated Fatty Acids**, such as Linoleic Acid and Alpha-Linolenic Acid, are called Essential Fatty Acids, or EFAs, because the body cannot make them. Essential Fatty Acids must come from the foods we eat. These Fats are healthy, and are needed to build cells and make hormones

        - **Saturated Fats (or Saturated Fatty Acids)** are primarily found in animal sources like meats and poultry, whole or reduced-fat milk, and butter. Some vegetable oils such as sunflower and coconut oil, palm kernel oil, and palm oil are made up of Saturated Fats. Saturated Fats are normally solid at room temperature. Fats from these oils are some of the least healthy, and *should be avoided* if at all possible

- **Trans Fatty Acids (or Trans Fats)** are produced when vegetable oils are processed into margarine or shortening. Sources of Trans Fats include those snack foods and baked goods that are made with partially hydrogenated vegetable oil or vegetable shortening. Trans Fats are found naturally in some animal products, like dairy products. Just as with Saturated Fats, *Trans Fats are some of the least healthy fats there are, and should be avoided if at all possible*

- ## Water

  - Clean water and liquids or fluids are vital to a person's good health. All body cells, organs, and systems require water and fluids to function. *If you don't believe me, just ask a fish!*
  - If a person does not consume adequate fluids, or if they lose fluids due to severe vomiting or diarrhea, they may become constipated or dehydrated, which is an unsafe condition
  - The fluids, minerals, and electrolytes (those minerals such as sodium and potassium that are found in a very popular sports recovery drink) that help keep the body functioning properly and hydrated, can become dangerously out of balance if not continuously maintained during activities – especially on hot days or during periods of strenuous, physical activity
  - A person will absorb some water from the foods they eat, but a person should drink about eight 8-ounce glasses of liquid each day to be sure that the cells get all the fluids they need

- ## Vitamins and Minerals

  - Vitamins are key nutrients, like Vitamins A, C, and E, which the body needs in small amounts to grow, function, and stay strong. Most Vitamins can be found naturally in foods. They are also sold as supplements in pill and liquid form

- Minerals are nutrients that are required in small amounts by the body to help the brain, muscles, heart, nerves, and other organs and body systems function properly. Good examples are Calcium, Iron, Magnesium, Potassium, and Sodium
- Vitamins and minerals are required for normal growth and development. They also allow the body to better utilize and assimilate the energy (calories) found in nutritious foods
- A person who eats a balanced diet with enough calories and protein usually gets plenty of Vitamins and Minerals. But it can be difficult to eat a balanced diet when a person is being treated for Cancer, especially if there are treatment-related Side Effects that last for a long time or prevent the ingestion of sufficient food and beverages. In such cases, the patient's physician(s) or Registered Dietician may suggest the patient take a daily multivitamin and mineral supplement
- If a Cancer patient is thinking about taking vitamin, mineral, or other supplements, they should first discuss this with their doctor or Registered Dietician. Some patients with Cancer take Vitamins, Minerals, and other nutritional supplements to try and boost their Immune Systems or even destroy Cancer cells. But, unfortunately, some of these "healthy" substances can be harmful, especially when taken in large doses. In fact, larger doses of some Vitamins and Minerals could actually make Chemo and Radiation Therapy less effective because of their actions to help *mend the damaged Cancer cells*
- During one's Cancer treatment, the patient's Medical Team physician(s) may recommend a Vitamin/Mineral supplement with no more than the Daily Recommended Value (DRV) for all nutrients, either with or without Iron. Again, the patient, or their family members or Caregiver should discuss with the applicable members of their Medical Team whether Vitamin and Mineral supplementation should be considered

- **Nutrient Summary**

Without question (and sometimes, surprisingly), all doctors, nutritional experts, scientists, and dieticians will actually agree as to the importance of *all* people—but especially persons diagnosed with Cancer—obtaining life-sustaining nutrients from their foods, liquids, and, the nutritional supplements that they might consume. Proteins, Carbohydrates, Fats, interrelated Calories, Vitamins, Minerals, and water, are, in most circumstances, naturally-occurring nutrients that contribute to one's physical and mental well-being, and their quality of life. Honestly, if one or more of the essential nutrients is absent from the patient's "nutritional equation" for a great length of time, the resulting health and wellness outcome will be deeply skewed.

One need only look at Prisoners of War, who had all of their Protein rations eliminated from their meals, and, who were forced to consume miniscule quantities of stale bread and water. Their captors were particularly well aware of the importance of protein-rich foods in building strength and maintaining both mental acuity and physical functionality. As such, the enemy deprived them of this significant nutrient so that the prisoners would pose less of a threat and be more controllable. With Cancer patients, however, it is important that this same type of malnutrition or dehydration malfeasance is not allowed to take place. It is essential that these courageous men, women, and children are continually provided with the nutrients and water they require so that they will have the strength and energy to successfully battle and defeat *their* captor—Cancer—and get on with their lives.

Other Nutritional Considerations for Cancer Patients

In addition to the six nutrients previously discussed, there are also some other components found in nature that can sometimes be factored into the patient's nutritional intake, including the following:

- **Antioxidants**
  - Free Radicals are the highly reactive oxygen-free compounds created as by-products of the body's normal processes (think of the exhaust produced by the operation of a lawn mower)
  - Free Radicals can cause significant damage to important cell proteins and enzymes, and, in doing so, can elicit mutations to cellular DNA that can result in the occurrence of Cancer
  - Antioxidants include substances like Vitamins A, C, and E, Selenium, Bioflavonoids, and some enzymes that absorb and attach to Free Radicals, thus preventing them from attacking normal (non-cancerous) cells

- If a Cancer patient is advised to consume more Antioxidants, nutritional experts recommend eating a variety of fruits and vegetables, many of which are good sources of Antioxidants
- Taking large doses of Antioxidant supplements is usually not recommended for Cancer patients getting Chemotherapy and Radiation Therapy
- The Cancer patient, or their loved one, family, or Caregiver, should consult with the patient's Medical Team physician(s) or their Registered Dietician to verify the suitability and the benefits and risks of taking Antioxidant supplements

- **Herbs and Mushrooms**

  - Herbs and Mushrooms have been utilized to treat disease for hundreds of years; however, results have been mixed
  - Today, Herbs and Mushrooms are found in many products, such as pills, liquid extracts, teas, and ointments
  - Many of the commercially available Mushroom products are harmless and safe to use, but others can prompt severe Side Effects of their own – something the patient does not need!
  - Some Herbs and Mushrooms can negatively undermine the Cancer-killing effects of Radiation Therapy, Chemotherapy, and recovery from Surgery. Therefore, taking large doses of Mushroom supplements is generally not suggested while the patient is undergoing these forms of Cancer treatment
  - The patient, their loved one, family members or Caregiver should consult with the patient's Medical Team physician(s) or Registered Dietician to ascertain the tolerability of taking Herb and Mushroom supplements during Cancer treatment

Nutritional Supplement Safety Considerations for Cancer Patients

Many folks think that if they come across a pill, a drink, or a nutritional supplement in stores or on the internet, that it will be safe to use, and, that it will also do what the company says that it will do. *Surprise, surprise!!* Sorry to say this, but that is not always the case. In an effort to help consumers (and keep nutritional and supplement companies truthful), the U.S. Food and Drug Administration (FDA) put out new policies in 2007 to help ensure that supplements contain what their labels claim they do. However, the FDA guidelines do not address the supplement's safety, or, the product's possible effects on the body. Additionally, the FDA does not require manufacturers of these products to print possible negative Side Effects on their labels. Further, the FDA cannot pull a dietary supplement or herbal product from the market unless it can prove that the product is unsafe.

If the Cancer patient is consuming various herbal products or nutritional supplements *prior to* beginning their Cancer treatment(s), or, if the patient is thinking about using these products *during* their Cancer treatment(s), the patient, or their family or Caregiver, should initially inform the physician(s), or the Registered Dietician on their Medical Team of their intent, and to request their guidance. If at all possible, the patient should take the bottle(s) of the supplements to their doctor(s) to discuss the product, and dosage to be used (if any), and to be sure that the supplement ingredients do not interfere with, nor negatively impact, the patient's health or Cancer treatments.

Following are some additional cautionary hints for the benefit of the patient, family members, or a Caregiver, if the patient is considering taking any herbal or dietary supplements during Cancer treatment:

- If the patient is taking herbal or dietary supplements *prior to* beginning Cancer treatment, or, if the patient wants to take such supplements *during* their Cancer treatment, first ask the physician, or Registered Dietician for reliable information on dietary supplements as it relates to Cancer therapies
- Check the supplement labels to determine the quantity and concentration of active ingredients contained in each product
- Stop taking the product and call the physician immediately if the patient experiences any Side Effects such as wheezing, itching, numbness, tingling in their limbs, or other symptoms

Nutritional Considerations AFTER Cancer Treatment

When a Cancer patient finishes their treatment regimen, they hopefully will not throw their personalized nutritional plan, or their conscientious, healthy eating habits, out the window. Long after the last drop of Chemotherapy, or the final dose of Radiation Therapy is directed towards the patient's Cancer, the regular intake of essential nutrients, sufficient healthy calories, and lots of water, will continue to play extremely significant functions in the patient's recovery and healing processes. One of the saving graces of Cancer treatments is that after they are completed, thankfully, most adverse Side Effects associated with the taxing treatments will also disappear. That said, depending on several factors, such as the patient's form, Stage, and location of their Cancer, the patient's either favorable or unfavorable response to the therapies and associated Side Effects, and, the types of treatment that they had to remove Cancer from their body, some resulting Side Effects might persist for a longer period of time than others following the cessation of treatment. And, some Side Effects, regrettably, will never go away, and will impact the patient for life. And, as luck would have it, all of the above holds true for some of the Cancer-related Side Effects that can impact a patient's ability to consume food and drink, normally, through their mouth and throat.

After the cessation of Cancer treatment, many eating troubles experienced during the treatment(s), and soon thereafter, should get better with time. However, some problems, such as any weight loss and changes in taste or smell, may take longer than others to restore. But, as the patient continues to strengthen their body with nutritious, and (hopefully) healthy high-caloric, good-tasting and nice-smelling food and liquids, the lean bodyweight should start coming back on, and the senses of smell and taste should, likewise, return. This might take awhile to normalize in some patients, but, it will – trust me!

However, if the patient has had severely invasive Surgery for some forms of Head and Neck Cancer, or, if parts of their stomach or intestines were removed during Cancer Surgery, eating problems may, forever, be an adverse part of the patient's life. Such cases are enormously unfortunate, but, thankfully, alternative nutrient delivery systems are offered thru the use of Enteral and Parenteral Nutrition, as explained previously within this Chapter. And, while healthy and regular eating and drinking, by themselves, probably cannot prevent Cancer from recurring in a patient, after the patient completes their treatment(s), the proper consumption of nutrients and water *can* help the patient to regain strength, recuperate and heal tissue, and greatly improve their quality of life—both physically and emotionally.

Following are some beneficial suggestions for continuing to provide the Cancer patient with sufficient healthy nutrients, calories, water and other liquids *after the patient's Treatment Phase ends:*

- Prepare simple meals that the person likes and are easy to make
- Buy sufficient ingredients to cook three or four meals at a time. Freeze, defrost, and eat the extras when there's no time to cook
- Gradually experiment with meals, let the Cancer patient sample, and gradually reintroduce foods into the patient's diet that were "off-limits" for one reason or another during their treatment(s)
- Drink lots, and lots, and lots of water and other healthy fluids
- If wanting to put on good-quality bodyweight to make up for the pounds lost during treatment, eat or drink low-fat milk products, and high-caloric, but healthy, foods and protein shakes
- Make cooking easy, by buying vegetables already cut-up
- Eat foods that are low in acidity (dairy products and meats), and that add healthy alkalinity to the diet (raw veggies and fruits)
- Eat and drink many different kinds of foods. No single food has all of the proteins, carbohydrates, fat, calories, and vitamins and minerals that a person—much less a Cancer patient—needs
- Consume lots of fruits and vegetables. This includes eating raw and cooked vegetables, fruits, and drinking fruit juices. These all have essential vitamins, minerals, fiber, and healthy calories
- Eat whole wheat breads, oats, brown rice, or other whole grains and cereals. These grains have healthful complex carbohydrates, vitamins, minerals, and fiber
- Add beans, peas, and lentils to the diet and eat them often
- Go easy on, or avoid altogether, "bad" fats, salt, simple sugars, and spicy, acidic, smoked, processed, or pickled foods
- Eat small portions (about 6 to 7 ounces each day) of lean meats, including fish and poultry, without skin
- Use low-fat cooking methods, such as broiling, grilling, roasting, baking, and steaming

Information on Cancer Nutrition Abounds – Take it in Small, Digestible Bites

Concerning the large topic of "Nutrition" (including "Cancer Nutrition"), it is extremely safe to say that there is more than enough information to go around…and around...and around. In these days of unhealthful "fast food," sky-high obesity rates, and a multi-billion dollar "weight-loss" industry, there are an entire host of resources—including books, DVDs, TV infomercials, mail order diet and fitness plans, weight-loss consultants, nutritional supplement corporations, and zillions of Internet sites, to name just a few—that all attempt to offer nutritional insight, plans, and suggestions, recipes (healthy and unhealthy), and other nutritional and fitness-related information for people who would wish to improve their health, reduce their weight, and firm their bodies – all for a price, and often, a *very hefty* price.

Without a question, there definitely is a large market for such weight loss information and products, at least here in America. And, the purveyors of "educational" materials associated with the subject of Nutrition are not shy about addressing that need. In fact, a quick search in mid-2013 on amazon.com on the topic of *Nutrition-related* books will yield over 54,300 results, of which 4,194 of those works will relate to the topic of *Nutrition and Cancer*. A similar search on google.com in July 2013 comes back with 425,000,000 (that's 425 million!) responses on the word *"Nutrition."* On the term, *"Cancer Nutrition,"* the search returned 107,000,000 different results.

Just think – all of these millions of pieces of information and billions of dollars centering around seven basic nutrients that we put into our bodies: Proteins, Fats, Carbohydrates, Calories, Vitamins, Minerals, and water. Obviously, the consumption of these important, nutritional essentials, the intake of water, and sticking to an exercise program, are all very important elements to consider – not only for those with Cancer, but for every living Human Being. The problem is, that many people do not take the time (or care) to invest in food, drink and fitness activities that will potentially pay them—and their bodies—dividends in terms of better health and longer lives. We all have a choice, but knowing the options makes it easier to choose.

Don't Play "Russian Roulette" With Your Health – Know What You Are Eating and Drinking

While all individuals know that they must consume food and liquids to survive, it's probably a very safe bet that very few of these individuals actually have much of an understanding (or care) about *what exactly* it is that they are putting into their bodies. It definitely is not essential for the everyday person to know what "protein" is, or, in what foods this key nutrient can be found. And, it absolutely is not a requirement for people to know which foods contain healthy fats or carbohydrates, or which foods have the highest percentage of vitamins and minerals, and which foods do not. Still, not unlike the potentially fatal game of *"Russian Roulette,"* in which one chamber of a pistol is loaded with a bullet that is aimed at one's head and the players gamble that the next click of the trigger will not *"make their day,"* some foods and fluids can deliver—albeit not as quickly as a big chunk of lead—the same, potentially deadly outcome if they are not consumed in moderation, or eliminated altogether.

When speaking about the consumption of unhealthful foods and drinks, the bad news is that the damaging "bullet" can come in the form of Heart Disease, Cancer, Obesity, Circulatory issues, High Blood Pressure, Diabetes, or several other health conditions, not to mention the avoidable expenditure of billions of dollars each year to treat health problems caused by poor nutrition. But, the good news is that with some basic knowledge and understanding about healthy nutrients—and the even more significant desire and discipline to put this nutritional knowledge to beneficial use—a person can, in effect, disarm the pistol, and discard the bullet, before it has an opportunity to do them damage. This is especially true for many Cancer patients, whose final outcome of their Cancer-fighting program could depend heavily upon the decisions that they make, either good or bad.

Finally, no discussion about enhancing one's health through responsible nutritional and water intake would be complete without also addressing the significance of the second crucial component of good fitness: ***Exercise.*** Without question, and I know this to be true in my own life and because it has been proven in one Medical Study after another, well-planned and consistently executed nutritional and exercise efforts will pay big dividends in a person's life. This is true just to live a "normal" life, but, it is especially essential if and when life throws one a "curve ball," such as Cancer. There are numerous things in our lives that we cannot control, but, if at all possible, each of us should make a concerted effort to control what we put into our mouths, and what we do to keep our bodies physically fit.

Chapter Six

The Cancer Journey Explained – *Step 8 on the Journey:*

The Cancer Treatments

"Human survival is innate, but not automatic. All individuals, including Cancer patients, must want to survive."

- Butch Sickler

Sometime just after the start of the 19th Century, Thomas Jefferson, the third President of the United States, professed his own views on the subject of War when he stated, ***"It is our duty still to endeavor to avoid war; but if it shall actually take place, no matter by whom brought on, we must defend ourselves. If our house be on fire, without inquiring whether it was fired from within or without, we must try to extinguish it."*** In this poignant, succinct, and judicious proclamation, President Jefferson—the, consummate Statesman, Inventor, Farmer, Architect, Educator, and, the primary Author of the U.S. Declaration of Independence—summarized his patriotic judgment about defending the then, youthful, United States of America, from all enemies, both foreign and domestic.

➢ *Receive Conventional Cancer Treatments – Step 8 on the Journey*

President Jefferson's words and wisdom regarding homeland defense have reverberated throughout U.S. history, and, even to this day, have manifested themselves in the U.S. rejoinders to the rare, but nonetheless costly, foreign attacks on American soil. I believe it to be fitting, then, that the patriotic rationale advocated by President Thomas Jefferson to warrant the security of our Nation via military means, can also be judiciously applied to the extremely grueling and unrelenting war that is being contested on personal fronts each year by over 1.7 million Americans today: ***The War on Cancer***.

World War "C"

Just as with an armed military conflict, in which some lives are injured, some are lost, and some are unharmed, the Cancer Wars can exact just as damaging a toll on its courageous warriors, be their sacrifices physical, emotional, or, the ultimate price to pay – mortal. And, just as with current, conventional U.S. military warfare, which employs state-of-the-art weaponry, very knowledgeable and skilled personnel, and innovative research and investigative techniques, so, too, does the battle campaign against Cancer necessitate the medical equivalents of each of these necessary components. Likewise, it is critical, in both military combat, and in the treatment of Cancer, that proper parties will convene in advance of battle to devise a strategic plan-of-attack that is aimed at successfully annihilating the enemy, while simultaneously protecting and conserving their own. Whether the iniquitous menace is moving about on the battlefield, or lurking inside one's body, President Jefferson's viewpoint on these matters does remain perfectly clear: ***". . . no matter by whom brought on . . . we must try to extinguish it."*** Therein lie both the overarching objective and motive of early and rapid Cancer detection, diagnosis, and treatment: *Neutralize and destroy the enemy before it does you.*

Currently, just a tad under fourteen million Americans alive today—one in every thirty people—are either presently undergoing therapy for Cancer, or, have gone through it in their past. It is these confident fighters, past, present, and future, for which the definitive conventional Cancer fighting weapons—Surgery, Immunotherapy, Chemotherapy, Bone Marrow Transplants, and Radiation Therapy–have been designed, and are deployed, as applicable, to assist each individual in their own personal battles with this menacing disease. When the time does come for the Cancer patient and their Caregiver to "go to war," they will be very well-equipped and extremely well-backed-up by their physicians, their respective staffs, and the other health professionals assembled on their Cancer Treatment Medical Team. *Prevailing* in this war is the only option that a Cancer patient has. There is no coming in "second best" in *this* contest.

A Fight to the Finish

There are numerous opinions about what may constitute the concept of "War," and, there may be just as many definitions for the word, "War," in the dictionary. But, at its bare-bones core, Merriam-Webster's Dictionary defines, *"War,"* simply, as, *"A struggle or a competition between opposing forces to achieve a particular end."* Certainly, the *War on Cancer* will fall into this descriptive category: First, there are the treatments used to destroy the disease in an effort to keep it from growing and metastasizing within the patient's body. And, conversely, there is the lack of genetic "controls" in the mutant cancerous cells that abnormally allows them to continue multiplying and spreading throughout the bodily systems—rather than dying—as would most normal cells. These contradictory objectives will always constitute a competition for "territorial superiority" in the patient's body, and, will invariably result in a fight to the finish. In the end, sometimes the Cancer will "win" the struggle, but, much more often than not, the Cancer treatment(s) will *"achieve a particular end"* by completely eliminating the Cancer from the patient's body. This, of course, is the victory which all Cancer patients strive to attain.

When speaking of developing a strategy to fight the war with Cancer, this might translate into the patient, and/or, their Caregiver: preparing and learning what they can about their Cancer and the best way(s) to eliminate it; convening with the patient's Medical Team to develop, evaluate, and decide upon the final Treatment plan; taking preventive steps to both reduce and eliminate harmful Side Effects; participating in pre-treatment screening tests; obtaining the Cancer-killing treatment(s); recovering and receiving aftercare following the battle; and, ultimately—hopefully—surviving the Cancer war. This positive outcome is not only possible, but is probable for most forms of Cancer, based on Cancer survivability statistics maintained by the National Cancer Institute (www.cancer.gov). In their most up-to-date statistical Study outcomes, the Institute has estimated that there are in the region of 13.7 million Cancer Survivors—men, women, and children—alive in the United States today. Some of these survivors' wars with Cancer were brief and not too injurious, while others were lengthy and possibly quite harmful. But, in the end, all were won.

<u>The Best and Only Option</u>

Taking the concept of "war" one step further as it applies to Cancer, the planning, preparation, and implementation of an anti-Cancer battle strategy by the patient and their family, Caregiver and Medical Team, is not all that different than the many arrangements, tactics, and provisioning processes that Generals and Admirals must discuss, develop, and deploy when they enter a military battle with *their* adversaries. In both instances, all parties must learn everything they can about their enemy in an effort to determine its location and where its strengths and weaknesses lie *(the Cancer Diagnosis);* they must utilize any information and "intelligence" they can obtain from reliable sources to help estimate where and how soon the enemy will advance *(Cancer Staging);* they must evaluate, acquire, and employ materials and the appropriate weapons to the utmost of their abilities *(the patient's Treatment Plan);* and, perhaps, most importantly, they must use all of the data and resources at their disposal to formulate a sound battle strategy aimed at delivering a clear-cut and deadly blow to their opponent *(the patient's Cancer),* while attempting to reduce any "collateral damage" to innocent by-standers, including their own troops in harm's way *(the patient's Normal, Healthy Tissue).*

Whether planning and entering into an armed struggle with destructive cancerous cells, or, with malevolent human rivals, war is not always an exact science—with nature and human nature being as chaotic and unpredictable as they are—and most battles will usually make a mess out of things during the process of attempting to yield some good. But, sometimes, fighting and war are the best and only choices that we may have when our lives, and our health and well-being, have been threatened in an unprovoked assault by something, or someone, that wishes to do us harm. There is no question about it – war, in *any* context, sucks big-time! But, it indisputably beats the alternative, which is what can happen when an individual or a nation gives in and capitulates to the attacking antagonist. Failing to act to protect what rightfully belongs to a person, or to a State or a Nation, should <u>*never*</u> be an option. And, for all Cancer warriors, it never is.

A "Personal" War - With Lots of Persons

Even though the patient's encounter with Cancer is a private matter, and a very personal one aimed at protecting themselves and saving their own life, they absolutely will not be left on their own to fight what could turn out to be a protracted series of physically and emotionally challenging battles with their conniving attacker. To be precise, not only will the Cancer patient have the 24 x 7 back-up of their support network—their loved ones, family members, friends, Caregiver, and others—but, the courageous Cancer patient will also be continually reinforced by the expertise and skilled efforts of the health professionals on their Medical Team. This whole partnership of loving, caring individuals will provide a protective sanctuary and security for the patient. As such, all these people will be there for the important "high-fives," pep-talks, hugs, and emotional and physical support that the patient will need while in the midst of their fight.

As courageous and confident as various Cancer warriors may be, not a one of them—male or female or young or old—will be able to fight and conquer Cancer with their own "bare hands," or, without the involvement and support from those closest to them, personally, or, from those doctors responsible for their health, medically. As the English Poet, John Donne, once stated, "*No man is an island,*" and, with all due respect to Womankind, neither are they. Survivability statistics do show that those Cancer victims that seek and receive the help of others during their time-of-need fare far better—both during and after their Cancer ordeal—than those who do not plead to others for support. Regardless of the type of Cancer that a person has, or its severity, and, no matter whether the patient is a man, woman, child, teenager, or elderly, it is imperative for them to enlist, and trust, the assistance of others in helping them fight their personal scuffle with the disease. Yes, there will usually come a time in each individual's Cancer journey, *either at commencement, or a few miles down the road*, when the patient will need to *hitch a ride* with someone else.

Cancer is a Relative Thing

A Cancer occurrence, like so many goings-on in our lives, is a relative phenomenon, meaning, that Cancer, by its essential nature, is prone to develop in all "sizes, shapes, and colors," as do the very people that it "selects" to serve as its hosts. On the one hand, some Cancer warriors-turned-survivors simply "roll with the punches," do what they have to do to get ahead of their Cancer diagnosis, Cancer treatments, and any Side Effects, and then move on with their lives, typically stronger, wiser, and warier as a result. With many of these individuals, it is almost as if nothing potentially deadly to them had just taken place – *"Que sera, que sera."* On the other hand, several Cancer patients affected by this nasty disease will fall hard and long, and may have quite a difficult time ever getting back on their feet—figuratively and literally—and repossessing their pre-Cancer life that they once knew. And, regrettably, as we all know, some individuals eventually succumb to their nasty Cancers, despite their hard-fought, courageous battles to defeat their Cancers and save their own lives.

There are a good many variables that can come in to play as they pertain to the long and often arduous journeys that each Cancer patient will take to beat their Cancer and to reclaim their lives. But, in spite of the inherent differences in each Cancer patient and their respective Cancers, and, despite the relative ease or complexity with which each patient might get through their Cancer experience, most patients share the common spirit to battle and conquer their Cancers, and, to survive in the best possible condition. When given the option between the two alternatives, *who wouldn't* choose to live a longer, healthier life? Thankfully, most Cancer patients do make the rational choice, and they opt to confront their Cancer straight on in battle, vs. retreat, and turn their backs on their lives and their potential futures. Cancer survivability statistics are definitely in these patients' favor. Patients, families, and Caregivers should know that the medical and health care communities will do all that they can to help maximize a triumphant outcome for the patient, while doing everything possible in an effort to minimize pain, suffering, and an adverse result.

Only One Acceptable Outcome and Support to Get There

There will be many positive days during the patient's Cancer treatment process, and, no doubt, there will also be some bad days in which the patient may question just how in the world they ever got themselves into this freaking mess (which *THEY* did not!). But, it is precisely during these types of moments—the hurtful, stressful, and dreary ones, and those that are pleasant, sunny, and joyful—that the patient's personal support network and their Medical Team will step in and provide the appropriate form and level of help. In such cases, these helpful people will either come to the patient's rescue in their time-of-need, or, will celebrate, along with the patient, their periodic achievements during the journey, and, their hopeful, overall success. Certainly, the goal is to achieve more instances of the latter than the former, but, everyone concerned will be prepared to offer the patient whatever assistance is necessary should things begin heading in the "wrong" direction. We've all heard the famous last words, *"Well, it looked good on paper,"* and, all of us know that things don't always transpire according to plan. Nature, as we're very well aware, can be both predictable (change of seasons), and chaotic (appalling weather events), and Cancer is no different. This is exactly why the patient's support network is always ready to step in and help where they can.

The reality of all Cancer treatment programs—regardless of the patient, their gender or age, or the form of their Cancer—is that some battles will be lost during the Cancer treatment campaign, and that some will be won. But, as with any important altercation, what *really matters more than the outcomes of the daily skirmishes is the end-result.* And, of course, the *"end-result"* in the fight-to-the-finish with Cancer can mean solely one thing: Survivorship, and a ***Cancer-Free*** or ***Cancer-in-Remission*** outcome. The true bottom line is that those responsible for the patient's care will do everything possible to ensure that the patient's needs are being met. This is fundamental so that their patient-warrior will feel comfortable, safe, and strong, and, so that the patient will feel as self-assured and as secure as possible throughout their ongoing, courageous efforts to defeat their disease.

The Patient's Cancer Treatment Arsenal

The patient's individual support network and Medical Team are unquestionably crucial in providing a safe haven for their Cancer warrior should they need to retreat temporarily from battle to receive any assistance and relief. But, equally as important in ensuring that the patient has the best possible opportunity to fight, eliminate, and survive their Cancer, is to provide them with the safest and the most efficient weapons for doing so. Thankfully, there is tried-and-tested weaponry in the Cancer patient's arsenal, all of which that has been medically designed, and scientifically analyzed and tested for safety, and for their ease of administration and effectiveness in eradicating Cancer. And, each of these available, appropriate treatment options will be thoroughly evaluated and discussed by the Medical Team, the patient, their loved one, family, and Caregiver, for their potential and safe use in the patient's customized treatment plan.

During the important Cancer treatment preparatory meetings, the patient, their family or Caregiver, and some of the Medical Team physicians will identify, assess, and talk about conventional Cancer Treatment protocols that might be best-suited for the Cancer patient, including the five most common weapons: Surgery, Chemotherapy, Radiation Therapy, Immunotherapy, a Blood Marrow Transplant, or a combination of two or more. In some cases, for children and other patients having Leukemia and Cancers of the Blood, Bone Marrow Transplantation treatment will typically be considered. In any event, the patient's treating Oncologist, Radiation Oncologist, Surgeon, or other health professionals on the Medical Team, will usually discuss with the patient, family, and Caregiver, the upcoming procedure(s), their benefits and risks, and the potential Side Effects that the patient may experience for each type of treatment. In addition, the patient and their family or Caregiver will want to discuss non-conventional and Alternative / Integrative therapies with the Medical Team, in the event that their Cancer doesn't respond as expected to the prescribed conventional form(s) of treatment. All options are on the table.

The standard process of doctors evaluating Cancer treatment options will consider many factors, including: The patient's form of Cancer; the Stage of the Cancer (its level of severity and progression within the body); the location(s) of the Cancer in the bodily systems; and, the age, gender, and overall health status of the patient. Because all Cancer patients differ from one another, as do the forms, Stages, and locations of their Cancers, so too will the treatment options vary in each patient's unique case. The patients' responses to the Cancer treatments can also differ somewhat from one person to the next. As such, there is not a "one-size-fits-all" Cancer treatment approach for every patient, but, rather, each patient's plan is custom-designed to deliver the most destruction to their respective Cancer, while safely causing the least destruction to the patient, themselves. The patient's treatment plan is very personal and their fight is very personal. But ultimately—hopefully—the patient will defeat their horrible Cancer. Although their victory will be individual, it will be celebrated by all involved – especially their loved one, family, and Caregiver.

Choosing the Best Cancer Treatment Weapons

Holding all of the obligatory information in-hand, along with any diagnostic images and data and pre-treatment screening results, the responsible physicians on the patient's Medical Team will make proposals to the patient, their loved one, family and Caregiver, as to a treatment plan that they believe would produce the best Cancer-killing capabilities, while minimizing the detrimental Side Effects to the patient. The patient and their Caregiver are active participants in developing the Cancer treatment plan with their Medical Team, and, as such, it will usually be the patient's preferences (with input from the patient's family or Caregiver) that will drive the plan from start to conclusion. In some cases, however, patients and Caregivers must comprehend that circumstances with the patient's Cancer, including its form, Stage, location, and/or, other factors having to do with the patient's health status and age, could dictate the form(s) of treatment that will ultimately be prescribed and carried out. In such situations, the patient, and their family and Caregiver will have to accede to the professionals for available options, and, may have little or no choice in helping to settle on the Cancer treatment weapons to be utilized.

In any case, whether the patient and their family members or Caregiver will "have much say" or not about the prescribed Cancer treatment protocol, it is imperative that the patient, and their family or Caregiver, are entirely well aware of the recommendations for the comprehensive treatment plan that have been proposed and planned by the physicians. Likewise, it is just as crucial that the patient, and their family or Caregiver, fully comprehend the potential Risks and Benefits of each treatment protocol, as well as any prospective Side Effects that may arise, and how those will be treated, if, and when, they evolve. It will be the responsibility of each health professional on the patient's Medical Team, along with their staffs, to properly and safely administer the respective treatments, address any physical and emotional concerns, and guide the Cancer patient throughout the course(s) of treatment to their successful conclusions. Ultimately, at the conclusion of the meeting and discussion process, the applicable

Medical Team members, and the patient, and their loved one, family or Caregiver, will determine the Cancer treatment weapons that will be used to, hopefully and completely, defeat the warrior's Cancer.

Consenting to Cancer Treatment

In due course at the initiation of the Cancer journey and after considering the Medical Team's treatment recommendations, it will normally be the patient's decision (with participation of the family, and/or, Caregiver/Guardian, especially if the patient is a young child or teen), as to which form(s) of therapy will be incorporated into the comprehensive Cancer treatment plans and eventually implemented going forward. When the patient, and/or, their family or Caregiver, totally comprehend what is to be expected during Cancer Treatment, and, if they feel comfortable in proceeding with the treatment(s), the patient (or their parent(s)) will be required to sign a form to consent to each type of procedure to be conducted, be it Radiation Therapy, Chemotherapy, Surgery, Immunotherapy, or a combination of two or more of these. Bone Marrow Transplantation might also be given by doctors on the Medical Team in the patient's treatment regimen, contingent upon the type of Cancer to be treated, and other factors.

The Cancer Patient's Private "Declaration of War"

The *Big Stage* is finally set – The patient has been tested and examined; the medical data has been gathered and analyzed; and, all the plans have been developed, agreed upon, and implemented based on that information. Also, during the last few weeks, the patient and their family, and/or, their Caregiver, and applicable members of the patient's Cancer Treatment Medical Team, have each done their due diligence in a team effort to get prepared for what could be the most noteworthy segment of the patient's Cancer journey: the Treatment Phase. With all systems, *"Go,"* the patient has the Team's *"thumbs-up"* to move forward and commence their Treatment(s). Finally, the individual's personal scuffle with Cancer has begun – and there's no turning back. There comes a time in every Cancer patient's journey when they will have to *put it all on the line* – a point when all of the research and education about Cancer; when all of the appointments with members of the patient's Medical Team; and, when each of the pre-treatment exams and other preparations, will all eventually come together in one momentous place and time for an extremely special occasion: *The Inauguration of the Cancer patient's Treatment(s).*

After the patient (or their parent(s) or Guardian in the case of child patients) has read, understands, and signed all of the applicable Treatment Consent Forms, the Cancer treatments will typically start per a prearranged schedule, assuming that there aren't any reasons for the therapy to be delayed, rescheduled, or, in extremely unusual situations, cancelled completely. After the patient, their parent(s), or Caregiver / Guardian provide their approval of the Cancer Treatment strategy, which was developed by the Medical Team in conjunction with the patient, parents, and Caregiver, it is the medical equivalent of patient declaring their own personal "Declaration of War" against the enemy – their Cancer. It is at this juncture in a Cancer patient's program that this new Warrior—whether they are normally passive, assertive, or somewhere in between—should be ready-and-willing to roll up their sleeves, hunker far down in the trenches, and give their evil Cancer the fight of their lives. Combating Cancer is the medical equivalent of entering a war, so the patient must be emotionally and physically prepared to do so. To be perfectly up-front, their survival and their life will be counting on it. I can assure you that the day that the patient, and their family, or Caregiver commit to commence the Cancer treatment(s), will be just as memorable, if not more so, than the fateful day they received the diagnosis that started this big mess.

Cancer Treatment – Converting Obstacles into Opportunities

Mr. Thomas Carlyle, a Scottish writer, historian and teacher during early 19th-century Victorian times, was quoted as saying, *"A block of granite, which is an obstacle in the pathway of the weak, becomes a stepping stone in the pathway of the strong."* The spot-on wisdom of Mr. Carlyle on the topics of fortitude and perseverance is very similar to the insight of Mr. Friedrich Nietzsche, a 19th-century German philosopher, poet, and composer. Mr. Nietzsche famously expressed his thoughts on human robustness and resilience when he stated, *"That which does not kill us makes us stronger."* Over time, in all walks of life, people have confirmed these axioms to be true.

The profound views that both of these distinguished scholars professed on the topics of encountering challenges and overcoming obstacles remain popular even to this day, and, are still actually very germane in most individual's lives – whether they realize it or not. With that being said, though, I am sure that neither of the gentlemen thought at the time when they each uttered their prophetic thoughts about life in general, that their sentiments would also come to serve, more specifically, as anthems for the successful treatment of Cancer.

From the instant that a person is provided a medically sound diagnosis of Cancer, they commence what can be several long days, weeks, or longer, of preparations for the momentous occasion when their treatment—and thus their war with Cancer—will begin. All of the several actions and activities leading up to the commencement of one's Cancer treatments are extremely significant to be sure that the treatments, themselves, go according to plan. But, it is the launch of one's treatment that is actually the "moment of truth." At this point, there is no second-guessing, no giving up, and no turning back. Mr. Nietzsche has it right: Cancer therapy *will* make the patient stronger.

The Transformation from "Hope-less" to "Hope-ful"

As has been established time and time again, and by Cancer survivor after survivor *(13.7 million of whom are currently living in the U.S.!),* the treatments to kill Cancer, while at times challenging unto themselves, will, more often than not, prove to be the force that explodes that "granite block" referenced previously by Mr. Carlyle. These successful therapies may, then, figuratively speaking, convert the obstacle posed by Cancer into a series of "stepping stones" that the patient may utilize on the way to hopefully reclaiming their life. And, equally as significant, the powerful Cancer treatment weapons may very well become the catalysts that will help to transform, what could be a frightened, discouraged, and *hopeless* Cancer victim, into a much stronger, very confident, and more *hopeful* Cancer *Survivor.*

While the actual daily battles with Cancer may seem at times to the patient-warrior to be the equivalent of down-and-dirty "trench warfare" (and for good reason), Cancer treatment weapons, in all of their many forms, have been scientifically designed and tested, and medically verified and utilized for one reason, and one reason only:

To completely remove Cancer while resulting in as little harm to the patient as possible. From this moment on, it is all about killing and eradicating the Cancer, and completing the battle in the best possible physical and emotional condition. Actually, to be more precise, it is all about *Healthy Survival.* The conflict strategy has been evaluated, the decisions have been rendered, and the Cancer treatment weapons have been selected, staged, primed, and loaded. The Cancer warrior will soon be entering into their personal war with the assistance of many, and, the backing of the most state-of-the-art Cancer treatment weapon(s) available. All that remains to do now is for the patient to march off to war, use the knowledge and weapons they have, remain strong and hopeful, eradicate their Cancer, and become a Survivor.

Turning a "Defensive" Reaction into an "Offensive" Response

Someone has to fire the first shot, drop the first bomb, throw the first punch, or inflict the first wound. In any personal squabble, military conflict, political encounter, religious quarrel, or, territorial dispute, one nation, one person, one group, or one animal, must play the role of the attacker, the antagonist, or the provoker. Or, as many of us heard when we were young kids, the person who, *"Started it." (How many times I heard* ***that*** *as a child!).* When this happens, what will usually occur next—again, to use the example of the childhood squabble—the victim retaliates against the aggressor, and before you know it, both parties are "going at it" with all the fists a-flyin'. In a worst-case scenario, the bullets and missiles start trading places.

People, animals, and other opponents (i.e., Cancer) that wish to do harm to another will assume a "proactive" approach, and will strike the first blow in a deceitful effort to accomplish their agenda, including the use of surprise attacks. Think of how effective was the sneaky Japanese assault at Pearl Harbor that brought the U.S. into World War II – but, which, ultimately, led to Japan's undoing. Of course, the clear-cut advantage of an ambush-style attack is that the aggressor will catch the sufferer completely off-guard, and typically will do so with the intention of confusing, harming, paralyzing, and overwhelming them in the process. When this happens, and if those on the "receiving end" of the aggression are in any position to do so, they are left with no choice but to pursue a "reactive" response in an effort to defend what is rightfully theirs, including their lives.

Without a doubt, the surprise attack brought on by Cancer to a man's, woman's, or child's body, certainly meets the criteria of an unprovoked assault, and, its sole mission is to multiply and destroy that which is not its to invade nor overwhelm. Thus, the overarching objective of Cancer Treatment is this: To attack the attacker, and *to transform a reactive, defensive posture, into a proactive, offensive response.* In other words, the ultimate goal of all Cancer treatments is to "fight fire with fire," and, to deliver every strike to the Cancer with such force, with such precision, and with such resolve, that it is not possible for any cancerous cells to *get away* alive. Of course, as with most things in life, there, are, likewise, no solid guarantees with Cancer treatments. Thankfully, however, most Cancer patients do have the statistics in their corner when combating their disease. Per the National Cancer Institute website (www.cancer.gov), the average survival rate for the most widespread adult and childhood Cancers, combined, is just under 80%. *That's* a number worth fighting for!

Cancer Treatment - A Means-to-an-End

Cancer treatment does a pretty darn good job of "leveling the battlefield" to help make for a fair fight between the patient and their disease. Unfortunately, though, some Cancer treatments have a nasty reputation, typically because of the, oftentimes, very distressing and uncomfortable Side Effects associated with some modes of therapy. Chief among the offenders are the most powerful of the anti-Cancer weapons: Chemotherapy and Radiation Therapy. However, despite any potential "collateral damage" that there may be to the patient in terms of wicked Side Effects—which are commonly only temporary in nature—the potent weapons that are engaged to kill Cancer yield far more benefits to the Cancer warrior than they do potential risks.

Admittedly, the possibility of facing and overcoming Cancer treatment-related Side Effects can admittedly seem quite worrisome, especially when one considers the intermittent physical, mental, and emotionally painful, distressful, and inconvenient symptoms that can arise. But, the truth of the matter is that any debilitating Side Effects are a *necessary evil* that come "part-and-parcel" with the favorable,

Cancer-killing benefits that such treatments can provide. Looking at it another way, the Cancer patient can view the all-important Cancer therapies, and any Side Effects, as necessary means-to-an-end.

Reclaiming One's Life – The Ultimate Goal

The benefits of the Cancer therapies can manifest themselves during the thick of the battle, but, they will also expose their positive outcomes *after* all the treatments are finished, when the fighting has stopped, the "dust has cleared," and the patient's cancerous nemesis has, hopefully, been completely exterminated from their body. It is during the patient's Recovery and Aftercare Phases of their journey that they can take the occasion to recuperate from the war, nurse any wounds back to health, and to reflect back upon the fight—that is, if they choose to do so. But, most significantly, hopefully, the Cancer-patient-turned-warrior-turned-Survivor will continue to look forward to their future. A future made possible because of the toughness, the will, and the hope of the patient; the use of highly advanced medical techniques, equipment, and medications; and, the love, skill, caring, and encouragement of many who have supported them during their struggle. Coping with, and surviving, Cancer treatment-related Side Effects can be equated to—albeit it humorously—the saying, *"I like hitting myself over the head with a hammer because it feels so great when I stop."* While in some demented way that may be true, in all seriousness, the hopeful and ultimate outcome of Cancer therapy—eliminating the Cancer and reclaiming one's life—will far outweigh any, typically, temporary inconveniences, pain, challenges, distress, and discomfort that one may experience during the process.

Overcoming Fears about Cancer Treatment

Do you recall that occasionally scary, *"Here goes nothing!"* feeling you sometimes get when you attempt to perform, explore, or experiment with, something new and unfamiliar to you for the very first time? Perhaps it was the trepidation of starting a new job, the apprehensions of asking out a first love, or the fear of going to war – all quite frightening in their own right. And, on the opposite end of those concerns, do you remember how empowered and satisfied you felt after you took (and lived through!) that probably petrifying, but, nonetheless, all-important "Leap of Faith?" It felt good, didn't it? You told yourself you could do it, and...*you actually believed it!*

After you took that courageous, vital jump, if you ended up accomplishing precisely what you had hoped to gain (assuming that what you achieved was constructive, lawful, moral, and beneficial), you not only faced and overcame your worries, but, you also gained a heap of self-confidence in the process. There's no doubt about it, it definitely is a wonderful, relieving feeling when we overcome our apprehensions about attempting something novel or scary. But, it is even more rewarding when we successfully complete that which we set out to do. All of us have experienced the "fear of the unknown," but, that is a built-in survival mechanism designed to make us *"look before we leap."* This same philosophy can also aptly apply to one's attitude and courage when facing the prospect of Cancer treatment.

Taking The Critical "Leap of Faith"

For those first-time Cancer patients who might be leery of, or frightened by, the thought of beginning their treatments and dealing with any dreaded Side Effects stemming from those treatments, the patient will likely have a cloudy combination of fearful, yet hopeful, feelings swirling about in their head. As one might suppose, having indecisive thoughts about unknown situations is absolutely ordinary, and is just as much of a constituent of the human survival process as are adapting to, protecting one from, and countering, any threats to one's well-being. And, knowing that this is how many patients react when confronted by the actuality of undergoing Cancer treatment, is precisely why members of the patient's Medical Team will dedicate as much time as is needed prior to the beginning of the treatment(s) to thoroughly explain all they can regarding the ensuing treatment(s) and Side Effects to the patient, their family, and/or, their Caregiver.

Patient disquietude is also why the Medical Team will ensure that the patient, family, and Caregiver are involved in the decision-making processes, leading up to, during, and after the treatment(s). The Medical Team members will want to make sure that they have addressed all questions or doubts on the part of the patient before the treatments begin. This is so that the patient will feel self-confident and comfortable about taking that courageous "Leap of Faith" when the moment finally arrives to commence their Cancer therapy.

"Ready, Aim, Fire!" - The Patient Calls the Shots

There could be a significant, acceptable rationale why a first-time Cancer patient and their family may be reluctant and afraid for their Cancer treatment(s) to begin. But, the terrific news is that once the initial Surgery to remove the Cancer tumor has been successfully accomplished; once the patient has watched that first critical drop of Chemotherapy medicine travel its way from the IV bag, through the tube, and into their body; once the patient has laid motionless on the Radiation Therapy table for several minutes so that the ultra-forceful beams can precisely hit their mark; or, after the patient has received the necessary Immunotherapy infusion or the momentous matching Bone Marrow Transplantation, the Cancer patient will, finally, after much preparation, introspection, and determination, experience the long-awaited sensation of knowing that ***they*** are in command of the situation; that ***THEY***, not their Cancer, now have the upper hand.

Most importantly, when the patient conveys the equivalent of the military order, *"Ready, Aim, Fire!,"* for their Cancer treatments to commence, they will know that their awaited combat with Cancer has begun, and that the various Cancer treatment weapons they have at their disposal—not to mention their own faith and will to survive; their family and friend support network; and, their Medical Team—will do everything possible to completely and safely get rid of their Cancer. And, hopefully, when this goal has been accomplished, the patient will become a Survivor, and their eventual goal will finally be realized: a ***Cancer-Free, or Cancer-in-Remission*** conclusion!

The Five Common, Conventional, Cancer Treatments – One-by-One ***(Seek Other Resources for Alternative Therapies)***

After the form and location of the patient's Cancer have been confirmed, and, simultaneous with the medical determination of the Cancer's relative severity or Stage, the patient, and their Caregiver and the Medical Team, will begin meeting to discuss any number of topics related to the patient's Cancer. Foremost among these, as one would expect, will be conversations regarding the type, or types, of treatment to be utilized that will provide the optimal Cancer removal and killing experience, while subjecting the patient to minimal Side Effects, and as little "collateral damage," as possible.

The Cancer treatments that will be discussed by the patient and their Medical Team will, presumably, be the five most common conventional tools to fight the disease: Surgery, Radiation Therapy Immunotherapy, Chemotherapy, and, Bone Marrow Transplantation. Most children with Cancer in the U.S. are treated at a center that is a member of the Children's Oncology Group (COG), all of which are associated with a university or children's hospital. As more has been learned about treating childhood Cancers, it has become even more important that therapies be executed by specialists who are not only skilled in addressing these unique Cancers in children and teens, but in best supporting the needs of the patient *and* their families.

☛ ***Authors Note:*** Before the Cancer patient decides to have any medical procedure(s) done, it is important that the patient (and their family, and/or, Caregiver/Guardian) understand the risks involved. Different procedures will have assorted types of benefits, risks, Side Effects, and expected or plausible outcomes. I cannot list all of the possible problems (complications) of every form of Cancer therapy within the pages of this Book. Nor, is that the intention of this work. The material provided in this Book regarding Cancer treatments and their potential Side Effects and other concerns, has been developed from very reliable sources, but, it is made available to the Reader for informational and educational purposes solely. All Cancer patients must discuss the details of their individual cases with the applicable members of their Medical Team. These health care specialists will furnish the patient, their loved one, family, and/or, Caregiver, with information regarding the benefits and risks of each Cancer therapy, as well as the potential outcomes of each. Such information will aid the patient, their loved one, and their family or Caregiver, in making the best possible decisions regarding their treatments and care.

Before beginning Cancer Surgery, Chemotherapy, Radiation Therapy, Immunotherapy, or Bone Marrow Transplantation, some pertinent members on the patient's Cancer Treatment Medical Team and other health professionals, will speak with the patient, and their family members, and/or, Caregiver or Guardian, about the upcoming procedure(s), its (their) benefits and risks, the potential Side Effects the patient may experience, the potential outcomes of the treatments, and the patient's general prognosis. When the patient, and/or, their family or Caregiver, understand totally what is to be expected during and following the prescribed Cancer treatment(s), and, if they feel comfortable with proceeding with the treatment(s), the patient will be asked to sign a form to consent for each therapy procedure. The patient's Cancer treatment(s) will then begin per plan, assuming that there are no reasons for it (them) to be postponed or rescheduled.

Based upon my journaling notes, materials provided to me by my Medical Team, and, on information drawn from the National Cancer Institute online site (www.cancer.gov), following are descriptions of the five most well-known, conventional modes of Cancer treatment. ***Note: Treatment Side Effects are covered in the following Chapter***

• Chemotherapy – Cancer Treatment

Chemotherapy, or "Chemo" as it is sometimes called, is the use of very potent medicines to treat and eliminate rapidly-dividing cancerous cells in the body. Chemo was first used to treat Cancer in the 1950s. This happened, ironically, as a spin-off of "Mustard Gas" Chemical Warfare used by the Germans in WWII. Studying soldiers exposed to the gas, scientists found that Mustard Gas killed quickly-dividing normal cells in the body such as those found in the hair and mucous membranes – similar types of rapidly dividing cells that are characteristic of most Cancers. Since those original applications, the treatment has helped many patients overcome their Cancers entirely, and to continue to live very full, healthy, and productive lives.

The Chemotherapy medications that will be administered by applicable members of the patient's Medical Team have been totally researched, thoroughly tested, and successfully used, to treat Cancer patients in immeasurable instances. A Cancer patient may undergo numerous courses or sessions of Chemotherapy because not every cancerous cell multiplies at the same rate. By irregularly interrupting the division of the cells, it prevents the growth and resulting spread of the disease in the body. Chemotherapy is often used concurrently with Radiation Therapy in an effort to make sure that any cancerous cells are destroyed, including any residual cancerous cells that may be located in the patient's body following Cancer Surgery to remove the tumor and margins (potentially cancerous tissue near the tumor).

Chemotherapy medicines are administered to Cancer patients ***Intravenously*** (through a *Vein*), or ***Orally*** (by *Mouth*). Some forms of Chemo can also be delivered ***Intrathecally***, (via the *Spinal Fluid*), or ***Topically*** (on the *Skin*). When the Chemo enters the bloodstream, the drugs circulate throughout the patient's bodily tissues and wreak mayhem on the cancerous cells. All Chemo drugs function by killing rapidly-dividing cancerous cells, thereby interrupting their ability to divide, multiply, and spread within the body. Regarding Chemo and Childhood Cancers, they all tend to respond well to Chemotherapy, because most Cancers in children tend to be those that are comprised of cells that divide very quickly. And, interestingly enough, research has revealed that children appear to be able to deal with the negative Side Effects of Chemotherapy better than do adults. Good for them!

The point of *Surgery* and *Radiation Therapy* is to get rid of, kill, or damage cancerous tumors and cells in a *localized area in the body*. But, because Chemotherapy medicines are typically delivered via the patient's bloodstream, they can annihilate Cancer *throughout the patient's entire body*. As such, Chemo can "hunt down" Cancer cells that have metastasized or located to parts of the body far away from the Primary (original) Tumor. For these reasons, some Cancer patients are treated with two or three different therapies at the same time, such as Radiation Therapy, Chemotherapy, and Surgery.

By using this treatment protocol, the Medical Team gives the patient's Cancer the "One-Two-Three-punch" by not only physically removing the localized tumor (as applicable) with Surgery, but also by precisely targeting the Primary Tumor site with Radiation to kill any remaining cancerous cells at that location, and then following up with a whole-body Cancer "flush" with Chemotherapy medications. The duration of the patient's Chemotherapy treatment, and the type and number of different Chemo medications used will depend on the form of the patient's Cancer and their response to the drugs – either favorable or not. Every patient's treatment differs, so a patient may receive daily, weekly, or tri-weekly Chemotherapy treatments. The physician may also recommend other cycles of treatment, which will allow the body to rest and recover between periods of Chemo.

At last count, there are more than 300 Chemotherapy drugs currently used to treat most forms of Cancer. A solitary Chemo drug can be utilized by itself, or, it can be used in conjunction with other Chemotherapy medications. For the most part, the drugs work better when used in specified combinations, because each Chemotherapy medication has its own unique characteristics for killing the Cancer cells, as well as its respective, potential Side Effects. Research and the outcomes of actual Cancer treatments have shown that by using "Combination Chemotherapy" with two or more drugs at the same time, it has greatly improved success by interrupting growth of the rapidly-dividing Cancer cells at different intervals. *Sianara Baby!*

Often referred to in slang terms as a *"Chemo Cocktail,"* the combination of multiple drugs with different-but-related actions can work better together to kill more Cancer cells than any singular drug can on its own. The "Cocktail" can also reduce the chances that the Cancer may become resistant to any single Chemo medication. The patient's family member or Caregiver and the applicable member(s) of the Medical Team will decide what Chemotherapy medication, or combination of medications, the patient will receive, and the doctor will discuss the risks and benefits of each. The physician(s) will also prescribe the doses, how the drugs will be administered, and in what frequencies, and for what duration. Each of these stipulations will be dependent upon the patient's form of Cancer, as well as the Cancer's location and Stage, and, how the medication(s) impacts the patient's normal bodily functions and overall health, Side Effect-wise.

• Radiation Therapy – Cancer Treatment

The human body is comprised of *trillions* of normal, healthy cells. Cancer evolves when some factor, or a combination of factors, alters the normal cell and causes it to become a cancerous cell. Left unaddressed, cancerous cells will thrive and multiply out-of-control, typically, until a Primary Tumor is formed. This Primary Tumor can then develop and cause problems all on its own, and, if not detected and treated hurriedly, cancerous cells can then break free and spread from the Primary Tumor thru the Circulatory (blood) or Lymphatic Systems and metastasize in other regions of the patient's body. For obvious reasons, it is of great benefit to remove the Primary Tumor and any cancerous marginal tissues surrounding the tumor as rapidly as possible before the rogue cells have time to multiply and spread. This is where both Radiation Therapy and Surgery come in.

Members of the Cancer patient's Medical Team may suggest Radiation Therapy to suitably treat the patient's disease. Sometimes, the goal is to slow the growth of the Cancer, and at other times, the objective might be to minimize problems caused by growing tumors to *palliate,* or help the patient feel better. As applicable, physicians on the Medical Team will discuss the use of Radiation Therapy for treatment of the patient's Cancer with them and their Caregiver, and will provide them with the information they will need, including any potential risks and benefits and possible outcomes, to assist them in deciding if they wish to proceed with this form of treatment.

Radiation Therapy, which was first used for the treatment of Cancer back in the 1890s, utilizes very sophisticated, scientifically developed and tested equipment that produces high-energy particles or waves to annihilate or damage the cancerous cells. Also known as Radiotherapy and Radiation Oncology, Radiation Therapy directs safe radiation beams to target and kill rapidly dividing Cancer cells. In that sense, it is similar to Chemotherapy, but, Radiation Therapy is delivered to the patient's body thru multiple methods, depending on the form of Cancer being treated and its location in the body, as well as other determining factors. As an illustration, in one radiation delivery method, precisely aimed powerful, high-energy waves from extremely large machines are safely directed from outside the body to the specific tumor or cancerous site within the body. This method literally "fries" the cancerous cells in their boots. And, by the way, it also fries the boots. I am living proof of this method of delivering Radiation Therapy, and how effective it can be in killing Cancer.

Radioactive material can also be safely transported into the Cancer patient's body thru the Circulatory (blood) System—as are Chemotherapy medicines—in an effort to kill the disease wherever it is located in the body. And, additionally, radioactive material may be introduced into one's body in the shape of a radioactive "seed" or a "pellet" that is physically placed near the tumor or cancerous cells inside the body. The strategy behind this safe and innovative method being that the radioactive energy literally "radiates" from the device to the cancerous area, and over time, "cooks" and kills the cancerous cells. Radiation Therapy is also often used with Chemotherapy and Surgery in an effort to ensure the best possible Cancer-killing result

Whereas Chemotherapy medicines are typically administered via the patient's bloodstream and are designed to kill cancerous cells throughout their complete body, Radiation Therapy is delivered thru radiation beams aimed precisely at the tumor and adjacent tissues in one area of the body. In that sense, Radiation Therapy is a localized treatment that only affects that region of the body being addressed. Radiation Therapy is one of the most common treatments for certain childhood and adult Cancers, and it can be employed either by itself, or, depending on the type, location, and Stage (severity and spread) of the patient's Cancer, can be safely delivered in concurrence with Chemotherapy, Surgery, or other forms of treatment. In addressing both childhood and adult Cancers, this amalgamation of treatments has been proven to be an extremely effective and feasible method of completely ridding Cancer cells from the patients' bodies. Radiation Therapy can cause *collateral damage* to normal, healthy cells near the tumor being treated, but, after treatment is completed, the normal cells will usually repair themselves, while the Cancer cells will not.

- ## **Surgery – Cancer Treatment**

Surgery is the earliest-used form of Cancer treatment, having first been employed by a physician in 1600 BC, for the removal of a cancerous tumor in a patient. By the 1890s, Surgery was a common tool for the treatment of some Cancers. Thankfully, both Surgery in particular, and Cancer treatments in general, have come a long way since then. Surgery, or more specifically, *Invasive Surgery,* will be typically performed in the treatment of childhood and adult Cancer patients to physically excise, or cut out, the Primary Tumor and any other tumors or potentially cancerous marginal or surrounding tissue from the tumor site. That is, if the Surgery is deemed safe, and if it presents extremely low risk to perform, depending upon the type and location of the Cancer, and the patient's general state of health.

Cancer Surgery also plays a vital role early-on in the Cancer diagnostic process through the excision of Biopsy tissue samples to determine malignancies, including if Cancer has metastasized from the Primary Tumor to other regions within the body, and its severity. Surgical treatment of Cancer in a child or adult provides the greatest chance for cure for many forms of the disease, especially with those localized, lower-Staged Cancers that have not yet advanced to other locations in the body. Most patients with Cancer will typically have some mode of Surgery, even if it is solely to confirm the presence or absence of the disease. During the last few years, many advances in surgical procedures have permitted Cancer Surgeons to operate on a growing number of Cancer patients with very positive outcomes. In fact, today, many surgical operations to get rid of cancerous tumors involve far less cutting and *collateral damage* to nearby organs and tissues (as with less invasive Robotic-type surgeries), which, in-turn, spares and protects as much normal tissue and function as possible.

For childhood and adult patients with Leukemia (i.e., Cancer of the Circulatory System) or Lymphoma (Cancer of the Lymphatic System), Surgery, normally, will play a minor role. This is because Leukemias and Lymphomas involve two "flowing" bodily Systems that are located throughout the body, which makes it difficult to treat by operating on one specific area, as a Surgeon would do to remove a tumor, for example, from a woman's breast. In patients with solid localized, low-Stage tumors that haven't spread to other parts of the body, however, Surgery can often effectively eliminate Cancer from the patient's body when utilized in combination with Chemotherapy, and/or, Radiation Therapy. Applicable professionals on the patient's Medical Team will discuss with the parent(s) or Caregiver the likely use of Surgery in the patient's Cancer treatment plan, including risks and benefits and Side Effects, prior to a determination being made.

• Immunotherapy – Cancer Treatment

Immunotherapy is a form of *Biologic Therapy* or *Biotherapy* that was first utilized in the early 1900s for the treatment of Cancer. Immunotherapy is a treatment that utilizes certain components of the Cancer patient's own Immune System to locate, identify, and kill the disease. Think of it as the patient's body "deputizing" "good" cells to hunt down the "evil" ones. This is accomplished in two ways:

- By administering synthetic, man-made Immune System proteins to the Cancer patient. These proteins will assist the patient's own Immune System in distinguishing between "friendly," healthy cells in the patient's body, and "unfriendly" Cancer cells. These *deputized* and fortified healthy cells then respond to the threat to the body and destroy the dangerous cancerous cells

- By stimulating the patient's own Immune System to work harder and "smarter" in its identification of rogue, cancerous cells

Although Immunotherapy is sometimes utilized as a singular treatment for Cancer, it is most often performed at the same time as, or sequentially with (i.e., during or after) Chemotherapy, Radiation Therapy, or Surgery, to boost its effectiveness. There is evidence to support the theory that a child's or adult's healthy Immune System can help protect against a Cancer incidence, just as the White Blood Cells typically will patrol, identify, attack, and usually destroy, most internal or external threats to a human's bodily systems.

These Immune System Cell "*Search and Destroy*" missions normally target and kill some viruses, flues, and bacterial infections. But, as we've all realized when we get the Flu, our Immune Systems are not bullet-proof. Some body invaders—external, like viruses, or internal like Cancer—can, and do, manage to attack and overrun our sometimes vulnerable body fortresses. In fact, medical research has confirmed that people with *weakened* Immune Systems are more likely to come down with certain Cancers than are their counterparts whose Immune Systems are functioning at optimal levels. *Really?*

Yes, as highly efficient as our Immune Systems can be, they sometimes cannot perceive the enemy—Cancer—when it is "staring them in the eye." As a majority of us have learned via news reports regarding military urban "street" warfare as it is currently practiced, it is difficult, if not unrealistic, for well-informed and well-equipped, highly-trained soldiers to differentiate between "friend" or "foe," as the identical-appearing individuals intermingle with one another on a dusty street in some far-away town overseas. Dressed in identical local garb, not military uniforms, these people can all appear almost indistinguishable from one another. That is, until the wily offenders physically disclose themselves and their intentions by revealing their visible objectives. Such is also the case with some Cancer cells.

Many Cancer cells "blend in" and will appear to the patient's Immune System to be very similar to normal, healthy cells, when, in fact, these deceitful, abnormal Cancer cells are actually "dressed to kill." When a Cancer patient's White Blood Cells do not recognize these cancerous cells for the hazard they pose to the patient's body, they don't move to annihilate them. When this occurs—just as with their human terroristic counterparts—it gives the Cancer freedom to multiply and to roam freely, undetected. In the case of Cancer, this means that the "terrorists" can scatter throughout the patient's bodily systems and organs without any interruption or resistance. Always hungry to "take new territory," these renegade Cancer cells will then continue to wreak havoc until they are located and killed by external or internal "special forces," including, possibly, Immunotherapy.

Whether or not sneaky cancerous cells *purposely* "disguise" themselves to impersonate *friendly,* normal cells is not well known by science. What is acknowledged, however, is that Cancer cells do have *Antigens* (toxins or other foreign substances that can egg on an immune response in the body, and the production of antibodies), that are not all that different from those of normal cells. Think of Cancer cells *driving around* with the same cars and "license plates" as non-cancerous healthy cells, even as the *"Immune System Police Force"* patrols the patient's roadways, all the while keeping their eye out for cancerous violators. Sometimes the *White Blood Cell Cops* may not correctly identify the "license plates" of the Cancer cells driving by, thus allowing them to "get away" and continue with their dastardly ways. During other times, the law-enforcing White Blood Cells may recognize and stop the threatening cells, but the armed response may not be strong enough or long enough to destroy the sneaky Cancer.

To make matters even worse, Cancer cells, themselves, may produce substances that can deviously mislead the patient's Immune System into identifying these cells, too, as "good guys," and as such, do not respond. Immunotherapy comes into play in such occurrences to *trick the tricksters* through the introduction of manmade proteins that are delivered through the patient's bloodstream. Thru assorted scientific and biological processes, these proteins help these Immune System enforcers to better hunt down and identify the "bad guys"—the mutant cancerous cells—which, in-turn, stimulates the patient's "White Blood Cell Police Force" in strengthening its response to the threat, and in enhancing its ability to kill the Cancer. The definitive goal is to put the Cancerous cells away in the "Slammer" for good.

- ## Bone Marrow Transplantation – Cancer Treatment

First attempted by a U.S. physician in 1959, Bone Marrow Transplantation is a treatment that has been used successfully for the treatment of children, teenagers, and adults. Within the bones of the body, Bone Marrow—the spongy, fatty tissue—develops three types of Blood Cells: Red Cells, White Cells, and Platelets. Bone Marrow Transplantation is used to treat Leukemia (a Cancer that starts in the Stem Cells of the Bone Marrow), and Aplastic Anemia (a condition where the Bone Marrow ceases making the normal quantities of Red Blood Cells, Immune System White Blood Cells, and Platelets).

In healthy children, teenagers, and adults, their Bone Marrow "Blood Cell Factories" make enough blood cells to meet the body's continuous needs. However, if the Bone Marrow does not produce sufficient blood cells, or, if it generates none at all, the condition is referred to as *Bone Marrow Failure*. Factors that may provoke Bone Marrow Failure include, but are not limited to: Chemotherapy (this is quite atypical and Bone Marrow cell production usually returns to normal after treatment), Radiation Therapy, Leukemia, Lymphoma (Cancer of the Lymph System), Tumors, and Aplastic Anemia.

If a patient has a form of Cancer that affects the function or the development of healthy blood cells, a Bone Marrow Transplant (along with Chemotherapy to kill the defective cancerous cells) may permit new, healthy cells to flourish. Bone Marrow produces Stem Cells, and these Stem Cells eventually develop into Blood Cells. If there are any problems with the Bone Marrow, a person can become extremely ill or possibly even die. When a Bone Marrow Transplant is prescribed to treat Cancer, the special Stem Cells normally found within the Bone Marrow are drawn from a person (i.e., the patient or someone that is an exceedingly close "match" to the patient), filtered thru a special piece of equipment, and finally, reintroduced back into the patient. To state this process in simple terms, it is "Out with the old, and in with the new," or, more realistically, *"Out with the bad, and in with the good."* Bone Marrow Transplantation can also be utilized to treat Cancers that do not involve Blood Cells. This, thru the utilization of new Blood Marrow (Marrow that is "fully loaded" with strong White Blood Cells, the Immune System's "enforcers,") allows doctors on the patient's Medical Team to use higher doses of Chemo medication than could otherwise be tolerated by the patient.

The primary objective of any Bone Marrow Transplant is to substitute *unhealthy* Stem Cells with *healthy* cells. This replacement is accomplished during the treatment of certain adult and childhood Cancers via the following two types of Bone Marrow Transplants:

- ***Autologous Bone Marrow Transplant*** - The donor is the patient him or herself

- ***Allogeneic Bone Marrow Transplant*** - The donor is a different person whose body tissue is of the same genetic type as the child patient needing the transplant (the "recipient"). Because bodily tissue types are inherited, similar to a person's hair or eye color, it is more likely that the recipient will find a suitable donor in his or her brother or sister, if there happen to be any siblings in the family. The probability of having a sibling with matching Bone Marrow, however, unfortunately, happens only 25 to 30 percent of the time. Not the best of odds, but at least it's a possibility

If it so happens that the Bone Marrow from a member of the patient's family *does not* match the recipient, applicable members of the patient's Medical Team may search the ***National Marrow Donor Program Registry Database*** in an effort to identify an individual not related to the patient whose tissue type is a comparable or identical match. The Medical Team will keep the patient, family members or Caregiver informed of the results of such searches. It is more likely that a Blood Marrow Donor who comes from the same ethnic group as the patient will have the same tissue characteristics. The chances of an individual who is a Minority in the U.S. finding a match in the Bone Marrow Donor Registry are lower than that of a Caucasian.

Bone Marrow Transplants are not for everyone. Transplants can be accompanied by risks of infection, transplant rejection by the recipient's Immune System, and other complications. Historical use of the therapy indicates that the greater the recipient's age, the lower the success rate of the procedure. Complications are exacerbated for people whose health is already seriously threatened, as in late-Stage (Stage III and IV) Cancers. Accordingly, a patient's age or general state of health may prohibit use of Bone Marrow Transplantation for treatment of their Cancer. In general, the cut-off age for a transplant varies from 40 to 55 years; however, a person's current general state of health is usually the more significant factor. Even in the absence of complications, the transplant and associated treatments are rough on the recipient. Bone Marrow Transplants can be incapacitating. A patient's ability to withstand any bad Side Effects of the transplant is a key consideration in deciding whether to use this treatment, or not.

A Final Word About Cancer Treatments

The information in this Chapter regarding Cancer treatments is a lot to take in, especially for individuals who have little first-hand knowledge or experience in preparing for, or undergoing, any of the therapies. But, that is perfectly alright and to be expected. That also is exactly why the patient's Medical Team will be meeting with the patient, and their family or Caregiver, prior to the start of any of the treatments, so that they can explain available treatment options that are the safest and most effective for the patient's type of Cancer. In other words, the patient, their loved one and family, will be in expert hands each step of the way during the patient's Cancer journey.

Just as with numerous expeditions that we pursue in life, the Cancer journey is not always without its share of detours, obstacles, and scary slopes and turns. The reassuring thing, though, is that the Medical Team members will always be alongside the patient to help them maintain control of the wheel and to keep everything on-track. As I stressed previously, it also can be very helpful prior to the start of treatment for the patient, the family members, or the Caregiver, to read and study the "route" that their journey will take them through the Cancer therapy phase. The more they know about their Cancer and the treatments to get rid of it, the more reassured they will feel about embarking on the trip and reaching their intended destination.

"A diagnosis of Cancer can be devastating, as can the Treatments to kill the Cancer, and the Side Effects from the Treatments. But, no matter how painful and distressing these factors may be, they are faint in comparison to what one's Cancer, if left untouched, will accomplish on its own."

- Butch Sickler

Chapter Seven

The Cancer Journey Explained – *Step 9 on the Journey:*

The Cancer Treatment Side Effects

"Cancer patients soon discover that their bodies and their minds have always underestimated themselves."

- Butch Sickler

All of us have seen the over-the-top television commercials that advertise certain prescription medications for the "treatment" of a host of medical problems, from Allergies and Alzheimer's disease, to Elevated Cholesterol and Erectile Dysfunction *(Watch out for the "4-hour erection!")*. Likewise, we have listened to the raconteurs of these fancy ads as they spout off one warning after another about the possible Side Effects that can be caused by the drugs. In most cases, the potential Side Effects of the medications appear to be far nastier *(i.e., Death - WTF?)* than the medical condition for which the drugs are being prescribed! Unfortunately, as many people are well-aware, several high-powered Cancer medications and treatments also come with their own share of "baggage" and distinctive sets of concerns.

➢ *Managing Cancer Treatment Side Effects – Step 9 on the Journey*

The physical and emotional tribulations that can evolve from some Cancer therapies and various Cancer treatment medications are referred to as *"Side Effects."* And, just as with some of the potential health and safety troubles stemming from their over-the-counter and prescription medicine counterparts, Cancer Side Effects can equally carry with them some relatively uncomfortable, upsetting, and even, life-threatening characteristics. When talking about potential Cancer Treatment Side Effects, nevertheless, as physically, emotionally, and mentally problematic several of them may be to some patients, they are, in reality, a small price to pay for being given a second chance at life. And, without question, they certainly beat the alternative!

Paying the Price to Reclaim One's Life

Just about every undertaking in life will come with a certain potentiality of risk. And, to counter-balance any prospective dangers associated with an endeavor, one would hope that the venture would also carry with it an equal, if not greater, amount of benefit. Such is certainly the case with the five most common, conventional methods for treating Cancer – Surgery, Chemotherapy, Radiation Therapy, Immunotherapy, and Bone Marrow Transplantation. Each of these valuable and effective Cancer-killing modalities unquestionably can produce health-enhancing benefits through the successful treatment of most forms of Cancer for a majority of patients. But, like almost every worthwhile thing in life, the use of these precious, life-saving weapons does not come without some outlay. In the case of Cancer treatments, that price tag comes in the form of Side Effects that can impact the patient physically, mentally, or, a combination thereof.

In some instances, the Side Effects realized will be nominal, causing only minimal disruption to, or discomfort of, the patient. In other situations, though, the Side Effects from Cancer treatment can be quite extreme, and can induce an undue amount of physical pain and emotional anguish. These are the Side Effects that get all of the bad press, and are the ones that most people who are facing Cancer treatment fear and want to pass over if at all possible. The types and severity of Cancer treatment-related Side Effects that a patient can experience will be different from person to person, and usually will be determined by a variety of features. Primary among these will be the form and Stage (severity and progression) of one's Cancer; the type(s) of Treatment(s) that the patient will be receiving; the age and physical condition of the patient; and, in the cases of Chemotherapy and Radiation Therapy, the doses, the frequencies, and the durations of the treatments. Surgery, also, has its own share of possible issues.

Typically, prior to the commencement of any of the Cancer treatments, the physicians and other members of the Medical Team will counsel the patient and their Caregiver on the benefits and any risks that may be encountered with the treatment actions, and, of any potential Side Effects that may be experienced both during and after the treatment(s). If and when a Cancer patient does realize any Side Effects related to their treatment(s), the patient's Cancer Treatment Medical Team will work directly with the patient, and their family, and/or, Caregiver, to establish and carry out the best plan for coping with, and minimizing or eliminating, any treatment-related concerns and problems that the patient may have. Comfort is most important.

Cancer Treatment Side Effects – the Necessary Evils

When thinking about the five common, conventional Cancer treatments—Chemotherapy, Radiation Therapy, Immunotherapy, Surgery, and Bone Marrow Transplantation—it might be beneficial for the Cancer patient to deem the therapies to be a means-to-an-end. Very simply, Cancer treatments, with their associated cadre of Side Effects, are *necessary evils* that will have to be tackled in a hopeful attempt to annihilate an "unnecessary evil"—Cancer—in such a way that the patient not only survives their Cancer, but, that they are able to live as healthy, and as normal of a life as possible afterwards. To express it somewhat matter-of-factly, Cancer Treatment is where the "Rubber meets the road," and, it is the eventual hope of the patient that their *road* after treatment is a *very long, safe, and healthy one.*

To arrive at the intended destination on their Cancer journey, the patient must first navigate what can be a precipitous, narrow, and slippery slope, that can often be scattered with a conglomeration of obstacles and potholes – otherwise known as treatment-related Side Effects. If the Cancer patient has prepared for their journey, and, if they are correctly equipped—emotionally and physically—to safely maneuver either through, over, or around, these obstructions, they—with the support of their loved one, family, Caregiver and Medical Team—will have a much better prospect of successfully completing their treatment(s). And, having achieved that, they will, hopefully, find themselves one big step closer to survivorship and a laboratory-confirmed ***"Cancer-Free,"*** or ***"Cancer-in-Remission"*** outcome.

Cancer-treatment-caused Side Effects can be very *physical* in nature and can manifest themselves in the form of discomfort, pain, nausea, swelling, appearance changes, lack of function, exhaustion, dehydration, or malnutrition, just to name a few. *Emotionally,* Side Effects can also exact their toll on a patient by causing mental stress, depression, anxiety, lack of self-confidence, and, in some cases, the inability of the Cancer patient to think optimistically or clearly about themselves – much less about their life or their future.

In some situations, Cancer patients become so overwhelmed by the demands of the Cancer experience, including the exacerbating Side Effects with which they have to contend, that these individuals, exist, almost literally, day-by-day, and appointment-by-appointment, because they have emotionally "shut off," or disabled, their abilities to project any further down the road than that. In other words, these Cancer patients psychologically give up to, "*Paralysis by Analysis,*" perhaps over-thinking their situation and looking only at its negative downsides, rather than reasoning optimistically about their journey and learning to cope with, and adapt to, whatever may come along..

A sad, ominous "*woe is me*"-type of response and behavior towards any Cancer-related Side Effects, is, by the way, a perfectly normal position for one to assume considering the seriousness of the patient's circumstances, and the pain that they may be experiencing. But, if the Cancer patient is not able to break the "stalemate" of the downward emotional spiral on their own after a reasonable amount of time, or, if they are not taking steps to help themselves better deal with any physical discomfort they may be feeling, their Caregiver or another person close to the patient should connect with the patient's Medical Team so that the patient can be given the professional help that they need. This needs to happen sooner, rather than later.

In other instances of Side Effects, some Cancer patients may take both the Cancer treatments, and the follow-on Side Effects, in-stride, and, their brain may be centered on one thing and one thing only: Getting past their Cancer mess, and getting on with their lives, no matter how challenging, or how prolonged, the journey. There is no telling who will respond which way until the time comes during a Cancer patient's treatment(s). But, for any Cancer patients who have had to cope with some adversities in their past, they may be able to leverage any prior dealings with emotional or physical pain to better help them weather any storms during and after their Cancer therapy. Those who have not known adversity will have a much harder time.

Treatment Side Effects - One Size Does Not Fit All

Whether an individual is a Cancer patient, themselves, has a loved one, family member, or friend who has or had Cancer, or, has learned about this despicable disease and its treatment options thru literature, books, television, Cancer fund-raising events, or any other opportunities, almost all adults, and some children, are familiar with the potential, dreaded Side Effects that can ride in on the coattails of many Cancer treatments. *The word is out: Cancer Side Effects suck!*

While most individuals are conscious of several of the more conspicuous Side Effects of Cancer therapy—such as the temporary loss of hair on the head, nausea, and the noticeable loss of a patient's bodyweight—there are additional Cancer Side Effects that can affect patients that may be less perceptible, and considerably less familiar, to those on the outside looking in. This is because most Side Effects resulting from Cancer treatment(s) are internal to the patient's body, concealed under their clothing, or, tucked away in their mind. And, most Cancer patients, being the brave troupers that they are, will do their best to keep their chins up, to put on a brave front, and, to carry on as "normal" of a life as possible while out in public. This, by the way, is accomplished despite the discontent, the discomfort, and the distress that the patient may be feeling beneath that valiant exterior.

As one might assume, not all Cancer treatment Side Effects are created equally. Just as all Cancer patients will vary from person to person, and, not unlike the differences with each patient's form of Cancer, so, too, will any Side Effects experienced during therapy by each patient be dissimilar as to how, when, why, and where they rear their ugly heads. Likewise as diverse will be each patient's response to Cancer treatment-related Side Effects. Despite these many likely differences, however, the occurrence, harshness, and duration of the

Side Effects will generally be determined in every Cancer patient by some universal factors. Common amongst these will be the patient's age and health status; the type and Stage (severity and progression in the body) of the patient's Cancer; the form(s) of Cancer treatment(s) the patient has undergone; the dosages, durations, and frequencies of the treatments (in the cases of Chemo and Radiation Therapy); and, the carefulness of the Medical Team, and the patient, their parent(s), or their Caregiver in designing and executing a plan for reducing the severity of the Side Effects, if not removing them altogether.

In some situations, and for the reasons just mentioned, some patient's Side Effects will be minimal and manageable, while other patients receiving the same, or similar, treatment(s) and medications will experience Side Effects that are more ruthless and troublesome. Again, how a patient responds to their treatments and Side Effects is largely dependent on the person, themselves, and a variety of other factors exclusive to the patient's individual Cancer program. In any event, prior to the launch of the Cancer treatments, and regardless of the treatment(s) the patient is due to receive, appropriate members of the Medical Team will discuss with the patient, and their loved one, family, and/or, Caregiver, the risks and benefits of the procedures, the potential Side Effects to be encountered with each therapy, and, the remedies that will be undertaken, if and when the time comes to counter the negative consequences of the Cancer-killing treatments.

The Good News about Cancer Treatment-related Side Effects ***(Yes, there actually is some!)***

As we all recognize, there is plenty of *bad* news to go around regarding several Cancer treatment-related Side Effects, no thanks to the discomfort, the sickness, the baldness, the anxieties, the weight-loss, and a host of other life-altering "party-crashers" that most of us have come to know all too well. But, despite the negative stuff, there also is some very *good news* concerning the treatment of these same Side Effects that the patient may be able to *"take to the bank."* The favorable information about Cancer-treatment related Side Effects is that *not all* news about Side Effects is *bad.* For one thing, not every patient having treatment for Cancer will experience Side Effects, or, if they do happen to occur, the Side Effects might be relatively slight and non-disruptive. In such cases, patients will only experience mild discomfort from their Cancer treatments, if any at all. And, in other situations, many Side Effects can be effectively treated and relieved, or, in some situations, can be eliminated altogether.

In a majority of cases, however, the additional good news is that most Cancer treatment-related Side Effects are only momentary in nature, and will go away at some juncture after Cancer treatments have been completed. This is not to say that the patient will notice a reversal of the Side Effect symptoms immediately after cessation of treatment—because some nasty Side Effects may take a few weeks, months, or, possibly even years, to finally discontinue—but, in most cases, the changes will be gradual and continuous, until one day, the Side Effects fade away completely, and the patient doesn't pay them notice anymore. In rare instances, though, Side Effects from Cancer treatment may end up lasting several years or becoming permanent, as could be the situation with "Late Effects" experienced by some childhood Cancer patients later in their lives. But, in such instances, the patient and family would have been advised of such a possibility by members of their Medical Team prior to the start of treatment.

The actual bottom line is that while the risks of most Cancer treatments do include Side Effects that can, admittedly, be radically uncomfortable, inconvenient, and distressing (I can speak to each of these, believe me), the unconstructive affects on the patient can be usually quite manageable, and are typically temporary. This must be compared by the patient to the benefits of Cancer treatment, which, when the patient's Cancer is identified, treated, and destroyed early on, can gift the patient with a second chance at life, and, hopefully, a long and healthy one at that. *I, thankfully, can also speak to this one!*

Side Effects of Conventional Cancer Treatments – One-by-One

In the Sections below, I have provided information regarding the Side Effects that are associated with the five conventional forms of Cancer Treatment, which are: Chemotherapy, Radiation Therapy, Surgery, Immunotherapy, and Bone Marrow Transplantation. With the Cancer patient having an elemental understanding of the possible "downsides" of their Cancer treatment(s) in the way of Side Effects, the patient will be prepared for what might lie ahead, and, will know what to possibly anticipate, plan for, and discuss with their Medical Team, prior to, during, and after, their Cancer Treatment phase.

☛ ***Authors Note:*** In the Sections below, brief explanations and listings are provided concerning the potential Side Effects that could transpire from the different types of conventional Cancer treatment. The following descriptions of Side Effects, which are furnished for informational and educational purposes only, are certainly not meant to frighten, discourage, or distress the Reader. The chief intent of the information in this Section is to enlighten the patient as to what they may come to expect during, or following, their Cancer treatment(s). Cancer patients, their families, and Caregivers should talk about this information with members of the patient's Medical Team to acquire additional knowledge, and to ask any questions they may have.

The information about Cancer treatment Side Effects in the Sections below was extracted from my daily journals, and developed from materials provided to me by my Medical Team doctors during my Cancer experience. Additionally, information was adapted from resources of the National Institutes for Health, the National Cancer Institute (www.cancer.gov), and the Centers for Disease Control.

Following are brief descriptions and listings of the Side Effects that are typically associated with the five common, conventional types of Cancer Treatment *(The patient may, or may not, experience these):*

- ## Surgery Side Effects

Cancer Surgery, which is the physical excision and removal of Cancer Tumors, cancerous tissues, and any margins surrounding the cancerous regions, is one of the foremost treatments for Cancer. Cancer Surgery can be utilized as a primary treatment, a preventive procedure for diagnostic objectives or for Staging purposes, or, in an effort to alleviate Cancer-related symptoms or Side Effects. There are risks that accompany any type of medical procedure, and Cancer Surgery certainly is no exception to the rule. A bulk of the risks of surgical Cancer treatment can depend on the specific form of Cancer being treated, and the mode of Surgery being used. Other risks, such as infection, swelling, and bleeding, apply to any Surgery. Further, there is a possible risk that a patient undergoing Cancer Surgery may experience some problems due to the use of General Anesthesia.

The Surgeon that will be performing the Cancer Surgery, as with the hospital operating room staff and the Anesthesiologist, will ensure that all precautions are followed prior to, during, and after the Surgery, to ensure that the patient is not experiencing any problems with the anesthesia, or, with any other components of the procedure. Doctors have been performing surgeries on humans for a very long time. Advances in surgical techniques and a better understanding of how to prevent infections have made modern Cancer Surgery much safer, and less likely to damage healthy tissues than has occurred in the past. Still, there is always an element of risk involved, no matter how large or small the procedure. The success of a patient's Cancer Surgery procedure will typically depend on several different factors, including the type of the patient's Cancer and the Cancer's Stage (its severity and progression within the body); the location of the Cancer in the body; the type of Surgery being accomplished; the experience of the Surgeon (in treating the patient's particular form of Cancer); and, the patient's age and relative physical health status.

All relevant members of the Cancer patient's Medical Team, to include the Cancer Surgeon, the Anesthesiologist, the operating room staff, and others, will maintain a close watch on the patient for symptoms of the following, and other treatment-related Side Effects. The health care professionals will manage with the patient, and their family, and/or Caregiver, an approach to treat the Side Effects in an effort to reduce, or eliminate, their negative impact on the patient.

Side Effects that ***may potentially*** be associated with Cancer Surgery include the following:

- **Pain**
- **Fatigue**
- **Loss of Appetite**
- **Swelling** (Around the Site of the Surgery)
- **Drainage** (From the Site of the Surgery)
- **Discoloration/Bruising** (Around the Site of the Surgery)

- **Bleeding**
- **Infection**
- **Lymphedema** (Swelling / Build-up of Fluid at the Site of the Lymphatic Surgery)
- **Organ Dysfunction**
- **General Anesthesia Negative Reactions**

- ## Chemotherapy Side Effects

Because Cancer cells develop and divide more speedily than most normal cells, anti-Cancer medicines utilized in Chemotherapy have been developed to track down the rapidly-replicating abnormal, cancerous cells. But, just our luck, certain normal, healthy cells also multiply quickly, and the Chemotherapy drugs, unable to distinguish between the two types of cells, can affect their *collateral damage* on these healthy cells as well. While the body will continue to dispose of the destroyed Cancer cells thru its natural processes, the damage to the rapidly-dividing normal cells may, unfortunately, promote the development of Side Effects that can detrimentally affect the patient. The rapidly growing normal cells that are most likely to be impacted by Chemo drugs are blood cells forming in the Bone Marrow (such as White Blood Cells that are so important in fighting off infection), cells in the digestive tract (linings of the mouth, stomach, intestines, and esophagus), cells in the reproductive system (the sexual organs), and, hair follicles on the head and other regions of the body. Some Chemo drugs may also influence the healthy, normal cells of organs, such as the Heart, Kidneys, Bladder, Lungs, and Nervous System.

Cancer patients undergoing Chemotherapy might experience many, or just a few of the common Side Effects associated with the Chemo. Or, if all of the patient's "planets are aligned" just right, the patient may discard everything in the list of Side Effects provided in this Section, and may experience no negative reactions to the Chemo treatment whatsoever. Certainly, this would be every Chemotherapy patient's dream, and, perhaps, in a perfect world it might occur. But, realistically and unfortunately, this usually will not be the case. The types of Side Effects that one may encounter during Chemotherapy treatment, as well as their severity and duration, will depend largely on the form of the patient's Cancer being treated; the types, dosages, and frequencies of the Chemotherapy drugs being administered; and, the patient's age, health status, and other factors. This will determine the patient's individual response to the therapy, be it minor (few to no issues), major (many problems), or in between (a combination).

If the Chemotherapy patient is also being given simultaneous Radiation Therapy treatments, the combination of the two—being a very powerful anti-Cancer *"One-Two punch"*—can also increase the likelihood of the patient experiencing Side Effects and their relative severity. Meaning, that the Side Effect pain caused by the grouping can be greater than if both treatments were performed individually. I can certainly vouch for this, as the "1-2 Punch" kicked my ass! As for how long the Side Effects may draw out, normal cells within the patient's body usually recover after the Chemo sessions have ended.

Stated another way, most Chemotherapy-related Side Effects will gradually disappear over time after treatment ends, and after the healthy cells have had a chance to develop and grow normally again. Because every patient is different, as is each individual's Cancer and their Chemotherapy regimen, every patient's response to treatment, and the period it takes for each person to get over their Side Effects, will also notably differ. Very rarely are Chemotherapy Side Effects ever permanent, but, it can be possible for some Chemo-related Side Effects to persevere, either partially or completely, for a few months or years. (Or, even for the patient's entire life *(my poor eyebrows!))*.

Patients who face a course of Chemotherapy will be asked to submit to a mixture of pre-screening tests, including a blood test to verify the patient's White Blood Cell Count. A lower White Blood Cell count means that the volume of White Blood Cells in the blood is lower than standard, which places the body's Immune System at-risk, and could render it less able to fight off infections, viruses, and disease should that happen. And, unfortunately, Chemo can have an adverse effect on a patient's White Blood Cell count during therapy by lowering it beneath the acceptable level. So, blood count levels will be monitored very closely and continuously before each Chemo session. If the White Blood Cell count drops below the satisfactory level, the treating physician will typically cease the Chemotherapy sessions until the White Blood Cell count has returned to normal, at which time, the Chemotherapy treatments will normally resume.

Some members of the patient's Medical Team, including the Oncologist, Oncology Nurses, and others, will keep a close watch on the patient for any symptoms of the following, and other treatment-related Side Effects. The health care professionals will work with the patient, and their family, and/or, Caregiver, to monitor and treat any uncomfortable Side Effects in an effort to reduce, or eliminate, their negative impact on the patient.

Side Effects that ***may potentially*** be associated with Chemotherapy include the following:

- **Pain**
- **Fatigue**
- **Nausea**
- **Vomiting**
- **Constipation**
- **Diarrhea**
- **Hair Loss**
- **Taste Changes**
- **Swallowing Difficulties**
- **Dry Mouth** (Xerostomia)
- **Throat Pain**
- **Sleeping Difficulties**
- **Anxiety and Emotional Distress**
- **Low White Blood Cell Count** (Affects Immune System)
- **Anemia (Low Red Blood Cell Count)** (Affects Oxygen Levels)
- **Low Blood Platelet Count** (Affects Clotting of Wounds)
- **Infection**
- **Malnutrition**
- **Dehydration**
- **Severe Weight Loss**
- **Mouth, Gum, and Tongue problems** (Mucositis and Thrush)
- **Skin and Nails Effects**
- **Memory Effects** (Commonly referred to as "Chemo Brain")
- **Kidney and Bladder Dysfunction**
- **Flu-Like Symptoms**
- **Sexual Changes**
- **Dry Skin**
- **Fluid Retention**
- **Tingling Sensations on Skin**

• Radiation Therapy Side Effects

Just as with all Chemotherapy treatments, the primary aim of Radiation Therapy in the treatment of Cancer is to attack and abolish rapidly dividing cancerous cells in an effort to interrupt their ability to multiply, grow, spread, and form additional colonies (metastasize) in other locales in the patient's body. Unfortunately, normal, healthy cells that also happen to divide quickly get caught up in this fray and may also end up suffering some *"collateral damage"* in the form of Side Effects. But, unlike Chemotherapy drugs, which, typically, will normally impact *all* rapidly dividing cells in *different regions* of the patient's body—nasty, cancerous cells and healthy, beneficial ones, equally—Radiation Therapy, by design, is more exclusively directed to the *definite, localized areas* of the body where the Primary Tumor or the targeted cancerous cells exist. In so doing, Radiation Therapy will usually cause Side Effects in the precise area being treated, such as in the head and neck region, the chest area, the abdominal area, or the proximity of the patient's genital region, *but not elsewhere in the body.* The exceptions to this would be universal Side Effects, which the patient may feel regardless of the treatment site, such as fatigue, loss of appetite, anxiety, weight loss, and other negative impacts.

The early effects of Radiation Therapy may be realized a few days or weeks after treatments are underway. It is possible, however, for various postponed Side Effects of Radiation Therapy to manifest themselves months, or even years, after treatments have completed. In some instances, the negative impacts of Radiation Therapy can be permanent, but, in most cases, Side Effects from Radiation Therapy treatments will continue for several weeks after sessions have ended, at which time, the effects will slowly diminish and should disappear completely. As would be expected, the Side Effects stemming from Radiation Therapy are dissimilar for each patient, just as the patients vary themselves, as do their forms of Cancer, and the Stages of their respective Cancers and their location(s) within the body. Because of these differences, and the dosages, frequencies, and duration of each patient's own, personalized Radiation Therapy treatment plan, some people may suffer many or severe Side Effects, while other patients may experience fewer or mild Side Effects. And, as luck would have it, still other patients may realize no negative Side Effects at all.

Those Cancer patients who are receiving Radiation Therapy at the same time as their Chemotherapy treatments are more likely to encounter Side Effects, and, the Side Effects experienced during the combined treatments are generally more severe, than if the therapies were being administered on their own. But, while the Chemotherapy and Radiation grouping works wonders in effectively treating many forms of Cancer, it also gives the same, *"One-Two"* punch to some of the healthy, normal cells. This combo, unfortunately, can increase the impact—and thus, the harshness—of the ensuing Side Effects.

Specific members of the patient's Medical Team, including the Radiation Oncologist, Radiation Oncology Nurses, the Medical Dosimetrist, the Radiation Therapist, and others, will sustain a close scrutiny over the patient for symptoms of the following Side Effects and any others that might develop. The health care professionals will continuously work with the patient, their family, and/or, Caregiver, to monitor and treat any Side Effects that arise in an effort to reduce, or eliminate, their negative impacts on the patient.

Side Effects that ***may possibly*** be associated with Radiation Therapy include the following:

If Radiation Therapy is directed to the Head and Neck area:

- **Salivary Gland Damage** *(Can protect with Amifostine®)*
- **Mouth Sores** (Mucositis and Thrush)
- **Mouth, Gum, Tongue, and Throat Problems and Pain**
- **Swallowing Difficulty and Pain**
- **Dry Mouth** (Xerostomia)
- **Vomiting**
- **Taste Changes**
- **Secondary Cancers** *(This is why Aftercare is so critical!)*
- **Dental Problems**
- **Malnutrition**
- **Dehydration**

If Radiation Therapy is directed to the Abdominal area:

- **Diarrhea**
- **Nausea**

- o **Vomiting**
- o **Loss of Appetite**
- o **Urinary and Bladder Changes**

If Radiation Therapy is directed to the <u>Genital</u> area:

- o **Sexual / Reproductive Changes**
- o **Urinary and Bladder Changes**

<u>General</u> Side Effects of Radiation Therapy include:

- o **Hair Loss** (In the Treatment Area)
- o **Swelling** (At the Site of the Treatment Area)
- o **Sleeping Difficulties**
- o **Anxiety and Emotional Distress**
- o **Fatigue**
- o **Loss of Appetite**
- o **Skin Changes** (Skin is Dry, Flaky, Blistering, or Weepy - Fluid that Releases from Blisters on Skin)
- o **Severe Weight Loss**

• Immunotherapy Side Effects

Immunotherapy is an innovative and relatively newer Cancer treatment approach that—for lack of a better term—"deputizes" the patient's Immune System to help eliminate Cancers and a few other debilitating diseases. In the performance of its protective duties, the always-working-never-resting Immune System uses disease-fighting *mercenary* White Blood Cells and proteins to locate, identify, attack, and sometimes wipe out illnesses like the common cold, the flu, and viruses. By nature, however, the Immune System unfortunately isn't properly equipped to selectively screen out and eliminate cancerous cells. However, because of critical strides in research that have been made in recent years, scientists have discovered brilliant methods to locate Cancer destroyers within the Immune System so that they can be enlisted to seek out, identify, and eradicate cancerous tumor cells. Because Immunotherapies exploit the natural killing influence of the patient's own Immune System, these Cancer treatment methods are much less likely to encourage the physically and emotionally painful

Side Effects that are common to the conventional Cancer treatments such as Surgery, Chemotherapy, and Radiation Therapy.

Some Cancer patients are reluctant and fearful of undergoing Immunotherapy because of the prospective Side Effects. However, Immunotherapy Side Effects are relatively minor when compared to the doozies that can manifest themselves either during or after other conventional Cancer treatment methods such as Chemotherapy and Radiation Therapy. In fact, some Cancer patients experience no Side Effects from Immunotherapy, whatsoever. Whether or not a patient will sense any Side Effects during Immunotherapy will depend upon the individual's health status during treatment, as well as the dosage prescribed by the overseeing physician. Applicable members of the Medical Team will test the patient's limitations to the therapies, and will usually change and stagger the dosages to minimize any adverse reactions. Patients will be monitored in a controlled environment for thirty minutes during each Immunotherapy injection to confirm that there are no risky lingering after-effects. Immunotherapy is a viable method of treating Cancer, and the relatively minor potentiality of having serious Immunotherapy Side Effects should not outweigh the benefits received from this Cancer treatment selection, especially if used in conjunction with Chemotherapy, and/or, Radiation Therapy.

Pertinent members of the patient's Medical Team, including the treating physician(s), and others, will ensure a close watch on the patient for symptoms of the following, and other treatment-related Side Effects. The Medical Team health care professionals will work with the patient, and their family, and/or, Caregiver, to monitor and treat the Side Effects in a team effort to minimize, or eliminate, their negative impact on the patient.

Side Effects that ***may potentially*** be associated with Immunotherapy include the following:

- **Swelling** (At the Injection Site)
- **Bruising** (At the Injection Site)
- **Pain**
- **Flu-like Symptoms**
- **Rash** (At the Injection Site)
- **Lowered Blood Pressure**

- **Fatigue**
- **Breathing Difficulties**
- **Swelling** (Of the Throat)
- **Dizziness**
- **Asthma or Hay Fever-type Symptoms** (Such as Wheezing)
- **Itching, Irritation, and a Lump at the Injection Area**

• Bone Marrow Transplantation Side Effects

The Bone Marrow—the sponge-like tissue that is situated in the core of certain bones—contains *Hematopoietic or blood-forming Stem Cells.* Hematopoietic Stem Cells divide to create more blood-forming Stem Cells, or, they mature into one of three types of blood cells: Good ole' White Blood Cells, which help fight infections; Red Blood Cells, which carry oxygen throughout the body; and Platelets, which enable the blood to clot (such as in a wound). (Hematopoietic Stem Cells are different from the Embryonic Stem Cells. Embryonic Stem Cells can *develop into every type of cell in the body*, whereas Hematopoietic Stem Cells can only *form into blood cells*). All blood cells naturally have a limited lifespan and are always being replaced; therefore, a constant supply of healthy Stem Cells is vital for proper bodily function, and for the health of all human beings.

Under normal circumstances, Red Blood Cells carry Oxygen throughout the body and get rid of Carbon Dioxide ($CO2$) from the body's tissues. And, as I stated previously, White Blood Cells form the cornerstone of the body's Immune System and protect it against infection. Platelets restrict bleeding by enabling the blood to clot if a blood vessel is punctured. A Bone Marrow Transplant is utilized to re-establish the biologic capacity of the body to produce these blood cells and to bring their numbers to normal levels. Illnesses that may be treated with Bone Marrow Transplantation include cancerous and noncancerous diseases. A Bone Marrow Transplant for Cancer may or may not specifically involve blood cells. But, some therapies that target rapidly dividing cancerous cells—such as Chemotherapy and Radiation Therapy—can work against the body's ability to produce new blood cells, which also divide rapidly, and can be a serious Side Effect. That being said, Bone Marrow Transplantation may be used with other treatments, such as Chemotherapy and Radiation Therapy for the concomitant treatment of certain Cancers.

A Bone Marrow Transplant is a medical process employed to replace damaged or abnormal Bone Marrow Cells with healthy Bone Marrow Stem Cells from an appropriate matching donor. According to the National Institutes of Health and the National Cancer Institute (www.cancer.gov), the Side Effects from a Bone Marrow Transplant can depend on numerous factors, including the type of Bone Marrow Transplant the patient will be receiving; the patient's age and health status prior to the transplant; how well-matched the donor's Marrow is to the patient's; what form of Cancer the patient has; and, what is the Cancer's Stage, or its relative level of progression in the body.

Side Effects that ***might potentially*** be associated with Bone Marrow Transplantation may include the following:

- **Infection**
- **Bleeding**
- **Anemia**
- **Graft Failure and Graft-Versus-Host Disease** (Transplanted Bone Marrow Cells Fail to Start Producing New Stem Cells)
- **Skin Rash**
- **Diarrhea**
- **Abnormal Liver Function**
- **Fever**
- **Lung Scarring**
- **Abdominal Pain**
- **Mucositis**
- **Cataracts**
- **Early Menopause**
- **Delayed Growth in Children**
- **Respiratory Distress**
- **Kidney Dysfunction**
- **Fatigue**
- **Nausea**
- **Vomiting**
- **Hair Loss**
- **Changes in Skin Pigmentation**
- **Sexual / Reproductive Issues**
- **Infertility**
- **Swallowing and Eating Difficulties**
- **Lack of Appetite**

- **Weight Loss**
- **Jaundice**
- **Shortness of Breath**

Preparing For, and Managing, Treatment Side Effects

By nature, the loved one, family members, and/or, Caregiver of a patient with Cancer will be concerned with, and attentive to, the patient's Cancer care regimen, including not only the treatment(s) to eradicate the disease, but, the potential Side Effects that may arise as a result. As if the patient doesn't have enough to be concerned about in fighting and surviving their Cancer, they also have to do the best they can to tolerate any potential challenging Side Effects that may come along their way. As the saying goes, *"When it rains, it pours."*

The good news is that the patient will have their loved one, family, parent(s), Caregiver, or Guardian with them every step of the journey. And, the terrific news is that the patient and Caregiver will be continually supported by the appropriate members of the Medical Team, as deemed necessary. The most significant element of the aid provided by the health care professionals will be to ensure that every action taken is centered on delivering the safest and most successful Cancer treatment possible to the patient. Just as significant, though, is that the accountable Medical Team members will work hand-in-hand with the patient, and their loved one, their family member(s), or their Caregiver, to reduce, and, if possible, to remove the negative impact of any treatment-related Side Effects. *All for one: the patient.*

Before the patient's Cancer treatment(s) commence, it can be extremely beneficial for the patient, family members, and Caregiver, to research and find out what they can about Cancer, in general, and about the patient's form of Cancer, specifically. Many books (such as this one), online resources such as those of the U.S Government National Institutes for Health (www.nih.gov), National Cancer Institute (www.cancer.gov), the Centers for Disease Control (www.cdc.gov), as well as the American Cancer Society, and materials provided to the patient, parent(s) or Caregiver by the Medical Team, will contain valuable information that will help guide the patient, and the family and Caregiver of a Cancer patient, thru the entire Cancer program.

Key among these Cancer treatment-related materials will be detailed information about the potential Side Effects resulting from treatment(s), and what can be done to remove or reduce their impact on the patient. Armed with such useful information, the parent(s) or Caregiver of a Cancer patient could then be prepared to discuss with applicable members of the Medical Team, any precautions that must be taken, and, any suspicions that they may have, regarding possible Side Effects. Such information might also stimulate the parent(s) or Caregiver to ask any questions that they may have pertaining to Side Effects, and their effective management, before moving forward.

During the Medical Team meetings, whether they are before, during, or following the patient's Cancer treatment(s), the patient, and/or, Caregiver should ask the Medical Team physicians which of the Side Effects will be the most likely to evolve (with *each* form of Cancer treatment, if more than one type has been prescribed); which Side Effects are the least possible to develop; at what point during or after the treatment(s) are possible Side Effects most likely to present themselves (if at all); and, how will the Side Effects be addressed by the patient's health care professionals if they do surface? Also, ***both during and after the course(s) of treatment(s), it is very important that the patient or Caregiver communicate to applicable members of the patient's Medical Team, any new or worsening Side Effects,*** so that the physicians, nurses, and others on the Medical Team can address the issues and take corrective actions as speedily as possible. The Medical Team members will recommend measures the patient can take, and they may also prescribe medication in an effort to help counteract and eliminate as many of the Side Effects as possible.

Along with modern successes in the triumphant treatment of childhood and adult Cancers with Chemotherapy, Immunotherapy, Radiation Therapy, Surgery, and Bone Marrow Transplantation, the healthcare community has also come to realize that the *quality of life* of a Cancer patient needs similar consideration as well, both during and after treatment. Without improvements in the physical support of Cancer patients during the treatment phase of a patient's Cancer program, many new and advanced therapies, themselves, would not have been possible, much less successful. It is always significant to prepare for, and manage, the Side Effects of the nasty disease and its treatments when caring for men, women, and children with Cancer.

As willing partners with the patient's Medical Team, the family or Caregiver will need to share the responsibilities and the intricacies of the patient's care with the patient's physicians, nurses, and other health care professionals. Together, all of these people can ascertain strategies that can help to reduce the potential negative effects of the Cancer experience, while continually focusing on the patient's well-being and comfort, and in delivering a favorable Cancer outcome.

Late Side Effects of Childhood Cancer Treatment

When one speaks specifically about the Cancer treatment of young children and teenagers, to be realistically truthful about it, the phenomenal survival of childhood Cancers does not come without a price. We've all heard the saying, *"No good deed goes unpunished,"* and these words surely apply to Cancer treatment. Yes, as life would have it, a few courageous survivors of some childhood Cancers may realize treatment-related Side Effects that can materialize months—and in some instances, many years—after the cessation of successful Cancer treatment. In fact, Studies have found that two-thirds of the young children and teens who survive their respective Cancers, end up facing at least one persistent health condition later on during their lives. And, additional research reveals that one-quarter of childhood Cancer survivors suffer delayed Side Effects from their treatment(s) that can be medically categorized as "Severe," or "Life-threatening." These delayed health problems of childhood Cancer survivors, when they do occur, are referred to in medical terms as, *"Late Effects."*

• Good News & Not-so-Good News about Late Effects

The good news regarding some Side Effects stemming from Cancer treatments is that most negative issues appear during, or just after treatment, and that they disappear a short time later after being addressed by the Medical Team, or, when the treatment has stopped. The not-so-good news, though, is that some of the Cancer treatment-related issues might not disappear completely, or, that they may not expose themselves as Late Effects until months, or even years, after the completion of the child's or teenager's treatment(s). Thankfully, however, Studies indicate that childhood Cancer survivors are now living longer, healthier lives, following their respective treatment(s).

As a direct result of this fortunate circumstance of increased longevity, much scientific study and medical research has had to be focused on determining how Late Effects have impacted the long-term health and well-being of childhood Cancer survivors, and, how best to care for, and treat, those so-affected. Just as the Treatment of childhood Cancers requires a unique and very specialized approach, so does Cancer Aftercare, and being watchful for the occurrences of Late Effects. Late Effects may encompass more than one region of the body (or more than one Organ System), and can range from mild to extreme. Careful follow-up and monitoring after Cancer treatment allows physicians to recognize and treat the Late Effects as early as possible. Survivors of childhood Cancers should be aware that they will have to to "be on the lookout" their entire lives for any inward or outward signs or symptoms of anything vis-à-vis their bodies that they sense just doesn't appear, feel, or seem right. If persistent or questionable conditions arise, it is important that the individual seek medical attention to be evaluated, tested, and treated, as necessary.

☛***Authors Note*:** The information included in all of the Sections below regarding the Late Effects of childhood Cancers, was adapted from materials integrated on the online U.S. Government resources of the National Institutes for Health, the National Cancer Institute (www.cancer.gov), and the Centers for Disease Control (CDC). The following information is being provided to the reader for educational purposes only. As with all other subjects addressed within this book, the parent(s), Caregiver, or Guardian of childhood Cancer patients must obtain guidance and assistance from applicable members of the child's Medical Team to be sure that their child receives the safest, and most effective therapies possible. Also, so that the Recovery and Aftercare needs of the child are equally and successfully addressed.

• What Causes Childhood Cancer Late Effects?

Aggressive and very powerful Cancer treatment regimens are administered to childhood Cancer patients at their time of life when they have growing bodies and developing brains. As a result, several Late Effects experienced by former child Cancer patients are caused from the Chemotherapy, and/or, or the Radiation Therapy, that they received when they were younger. Major Cancer Surgery might also be linked to the incidence of Late Effects, but this is less common. While Cancer treatments are centered on destroying the unhealthy, cancerous cells, Medical Research has found that Late Effects are caused by the damage that Cancer treatment, likewise, causes to the healthy cells in the body. Cancer treatments, such as Chemotherapy, Radiation Therapy, and Stem Cell (Bone Marrow) transplants kill cells that grow and divide speedily, such as Cancer cells. In a young child and teenager, however, several normal, healthy cells in organs throughout the body are, themselves, also developing, growing, and multiplying rapidly. Cancer treatment can irreversibly damage these "good" cells that get "caught up in the mixture," which can keep the cells from growing and developing in a natural way as they should. The risks and probability of healthy cell damage occurring should be explained to the patient, and the parent(s) or Caregiver, prior to the commencement of treatments that could result in Late Effects.

• What are Potential Childhood Cancer Late Effects?

As more children and teens are treated for different forms of Cancer, and, as larger numbers of these children, thankfully, survive their diseases and are able to reclaim their health and keep moving forward with their lives, it is becoming increasingly apparent—with the occurrence of Late Effects in these individuals—that childhood Cancer *"is for life."* Studies find that the disease process, itself, or devastation caused by the actual treatment of the childhood Cancers, can result in Late Effects at some point in the person's life. Patterns of Late Effects may include disabilities, persistent health conditions, heart damage, lung damage, infertility, growth deficits, hearing loss, cognitive impairment (problems with comprehending mental tasks), and even subsequent encounters with new or recurrent Cancers. For these reasons, it is imperative that all survivors of childhood Cancer receive on-going monitoring and testing, and continued physical and psychosocial care throughout their young and older adult lives.

• Who is at Risk for Childhood Cancer Late Effects?

Every child or teenager receiving Cancer treatment is one-of-a-kind *(just ask Mom or Dad!).* Similarly, the Cancer treatment(s) performed on childhood Cancer patients may be different from child to child and from one form of Cancer to another. Also varied, might be each child's or teen's response to their Cancer treatment(s), and any Side Effects from that treatment. The occurrences and severities of Cancer treatment Late Effects will also differ, and will typically be dependent on the type of treatment(s) administered, as well as the doses, frequencies, and durations prescribed. Other things that may affect a child's risk for Cancer treatment Late Effects include:

- The form of the child's Cancer being treated
- The Stage (Severity or progression within the body) of the Child's Cancer
- The location of the Cancer in the body
- The age of the child when treated
- The child's overall health before and during treatment
- The child's genetic make-up (Inherited risk for certain health problems)

- **Where can a Parent or Caregiver Obtain More Information on Childhood Cancer Late Effects?**

The Children's Oncology Group (COG) has developed long-term follow-up guidelines for the screening and management of Late Effects in survivors of childhood Cancers. For more information on follow-up after the treatment of childhood Cancers, patients, parents, Guardians, and patients' Caregivers can research the COG website, www.survivorshipguidelines.org, which provides useful information and guidelines. However, please understand that these guidelines are written for health professionals, so, the parent(s), and/or, Caregiver will want to discuss the information with the child's Medical Team.

☛***Authors Note*:** It is extremely important that the parent(s), or, the Guardian or Caregiver of a young or teenage childhood Cancer patient strongly emphasize to their boy or girl the significance of the child having their health habitually and continuously monitored for the rest of their life. Because the treatment of childhood Cancer has been proven to carry with it the very likely possibility that the child will experience negative Late Side Effects as a product of their prior treatment(s), it is incumbent on the former Cancer patient to be ever-watchful for the occurrence of any unusual or abnormal Late Effects that may pop-up during their lifetime. Likewise, should the one-time Cancer patient feel or sense that something "just isn't right," health-wise, with their body, they should seek medical attention at the first sign of symptoms. This is important so that physicians can quickly take any corrective measures to properly deal with the condition(s).

Weigh the Risks vs. Benefits of Cancer Treatment Side Effects – There's a Life Hanging in the Balance

With Cancer treatments and their Side Effects, as with most details in life, there are upsides and downsides, plusses and minuses, and positives and negatives. Life, by its very nature, is a continuous balancing act, and we humans will invariably find ourselves literally caught in the middle of situations—sometimes, of our own making, and others, beyond our control—during which we are duty-bound to make decisions – for better or for worse. Every day of our decision-making lives, whether we give it any conscious thought or not, all of us have to make choices between right and wrong, left and right, yes and no, fast and slow, love and hate, good and bad, and possibly, even, life and death. And, while several of these judgments will be second-nature and not require a lot of cognitive thought, others, such as those which a Cancer patient must make about their forthcoming treatment(s), ***will*** require their focus and undivided attention. This is because there are various "good" benefits that will result from their treatment(s). But, there might also be some "bad" risks, in the form of Side Effects, which can really throw a wrench in the works.

Most Cancer patients will surely agree that there are benefits and risks involved with just about everything we do in life. What is important for the Cancer patient to strongly think about, however, is whether or not the expected benefits—such as improved health and a second chance at Life—outweigh the troublesome and potentially painful, wearisome, distressing, and discouraging Side Effects that are associated with Cancer treatments. For most Cancer patients, it would seem that this choice—typically, temporary body discomfort, vs. a reclaimed, prolonged life—would be a "no-brainer." But, for other Cancer patients, it is not that clear-cut, because there is a lot to think about, and, many of the Side Effects *are* downright scary – not to mention the remote possibility of the patient losing their life.

Prescription Pain Medication Use, Dependency, Addiction, and Worse – ***CANCER PATIENTS BEWARE***

I have chosen to conclude this Chapter on Cancer Treatment Side Effects with a very important discussion about a ***Side Effect of Side Effects.*** Not to bewilder the Reader, but I am referring to the honorable attempts by physicians and patients to reduce pain caused by some Cancer treatments through the proper use of very powerful, very effective, and, ***very addictive*** prescription painkillers. If there ever were a double-edged sword, prescription painkillers would be at the top of that list. As the saying goes, *"You live by the sword and you die by the sword,"* and, for better or for worse, many painkillers that are legitimately prescribed by physicians to relieve discomfort in Cancer patients, can be both a blessing *and* a curse. These potent medical marvels can help make a person's life all the more bearable, or, without warning, they can turn the person's life into a living hell. I know, because I experienced both during my own Cancer journey.

- **A Necessary Evil of Cancer Treatment**

When reviewing the preceding lists of possible Side Effects in this Chapter that are associated with the five conventional Cancer treatments, the Reader might have noticed a common theme running throughout – *pain, pain, pain, pain, and, pain.* Yes, as I have stated numerous times within this Book, there is generally a price that one has to "pay" to acquire something worth having. And, because one's life is the most priceless thing that a person can possibly have, when it comes to them battling and defeating Cancer to reclaim their life, that "gift" will probably cost them more than just a few Side Effects. Physical pain and mental discomfort will be very likely contenders.

Prescription Painkillers are medications that physicians will prescribe to patients—including Cancer patients—who are suffering from excessive physical soreness. Per the National Cancer Institute, (www.cancer.gov), drugs in this category are called *Opioids* because they resemble molecules in the *Opium plant*. (The drug, Morphine, is one such substance present in Opium plants). If the Cancer patient or survivor is having discomfort, physicians on the patient's Medical Team will presumably prescribe some form of powerful painkiller to help make their unfortunate situation more manageable. It is crucial that the Cancer patient is always as comfortable, as vigorous, and as rested as possible so that they will have the physical, emotional, and mental endurance to continue with their treatments, and, to aid them in recovering after their treatments have concluded. In this instance, prescription painkillers are "tools" that doctors on the Medical Team may have to use to improve the Cancer patient's quality of life. But, like other tools—such as many found on a carpenter's workbench—prescription drugs, if not used responsibly, can cut deeply and leave painful scars that may take a long time to heal. Cancer patients and survivors need to be very wary of these necessary evils of treatment.

- **Short-term Painkiller Use = Good**

When they are utilized as prescribed by licensed physicians, Opioids and other painkillers manage pain quite efficiently, and they can improve the quality of life for people with chronic pain. In fact, using Opioids for the short-term, and under a doctor's watchful and steady supervision, will rarely lead to drug addiction or dependence. *This is the side of that sword blade by which a person can live.*

- **Long-term Painkiller Use = Not So Good**

When used long-term, Opioids may promote drug abuse with physical dependence or addiction. Opioids, if used indiscreetly, can also be life-threatening. When Opioids are ingested with substances that can depress one's Central Nervous System—including alcohol, barbiturates, or benzodiazepines, such as Xanax or Valium—there is an elevated risk of Respiratory Depression, and even the possibility of death. Regrettably, several deceased musicians and actors come instantly to mind. *This is the edge of that two-sided sword that kills.*

- **A Prescription Painkiller Epidemic**

As researched by the U.S. Drug Enforcement Administration (www.dea.gov), almost 2 million Americans use prescription Opioid painkillers every year. Between 1997 and 2005, the amount of five major Opioid painkillers sold at U.S. retail establishments rose 90 percent. Honestly, more than 200,000 lbs. of assorted commercially produced Opioids were legally purchased at retail pharmacies during 2005, the most recent year represented in the data. That quantity was enough to provide more than 300 milligrams of painkillers to every person in the U.S. ***Good grief!*** To float another comparison, enough prescription painkillers were prescribed in 2010 to medicate every American adult around-the-clock for a month. That, my friend, is an epidemic, and *drug companies are laughing all the way to the bank.*

Most prescription painkillers are prescribed by Primary Care and Internal Medicine Physicians and Dentists, not Specialists. And, of these health care providers, roughly 20% of prescribers prescribe 80% of all prescription painkillers. Although a bulk of these pain medications were, and are, prescribed for a lawful and valid medical purpose, many have ended up in the hands of people who misused or abused them, which has created problems of its own. But, for the Cancer patient who is working with those on their Medical Team to manage and lessen severe discomfort with prescription painkillers—and specifically Opioids—this sincere effort can come with own set of issues – namely, the possibility that the patient will develop some level of *Prescription Painkiller Dependence* or *Addiction.*

• Painkiller Dependence vs. Painkiller Addiction

According to the Centers for Disease Control (www.cdc.gov), the terms, *"Dependence,"* and *"Addiction,"* are often used as if they are interchangeable, as they pertain to prescription painkillers. But, this is not necessarily the truth. For example, science has found that a person can be physically dependent on a painkiller without being addicted to it. And conversely, it is known that a person can become addicted to a painkiller even if they have never developed a physical dependency with the drug. During the last few years, an individual's ***Dependence*** on prescription painkillers has generally been assumed to be a ***Physical*** circumstance, while one's ***Addiction*** to prescription painkillers has been thought of entirely as a ***Psychological*** problem. Currently, however, scientific and medical communities have come to realize that a drug Dependence has more specific criteria, as does a drug Addiction. There – now that that is as clear as mud, the below information, adapted from www.cdc.gov, may help to illuminate the distinctions between *Dependence* and *Addiction* for the Reader:

- **Prescription Painkiller Dependence**

A person who is physiologically *dependent* on a prescription painkiller needs it to alleviate authentic, severe pain so that they can function as "normally" as possible during their lives. However, this same individual may not necessarily be *addicted* to the drug. Some characteristics of ***Painkiller Dependence*** include:

- Developing a "tolerance" to the medication during which the patient requires more medication (i.e., more pills or higher dosages) to achieve the same pain relief over time
- Experiencing withdrawal symptoms if the patient tries to suddenly discontinue the prescription painkiller without gradually tapering off of the medication in a proper way

An example of physiological dependence on a painkiller is someone who takes Opiates for severe, chronic pain caused by their Cancer or as a result of their treatment Side Effects. *Over time, they may need to increase their dosages to mitigate the pain because their body has developed a tolerance to the drug.* However, their sole purpose for taking the drug is to help in relieving pain, not to *"get high."*

- **Prescription Painkiller Addiction**

An *Addiction* to prescription painkillers implies *drug-seeking* behavior, regardless of the medication's planned medical purpose. A person who is addicted to a painkiller may compulsively search for and take the drug inappropriately, even with knowledge of negative outcomes. These include health complications and social problems, such as losing a job and negatively impacting a person's relationship and friendships, etc. And, as with a physiological dependence on a painkiller, as a patient who is legitimately utilizing the medication to resolve actual physical pain, someone who is addicted to a painkiller may also experience symptoms with withdrawal if they cease taking it, *cold turkey*. However, the striking distinction between the two is that the person who is ***addicted** to a painkiller continues to seek out and use the drug in spite of the potentially negative consequences of doing so.* The Cancer patient or survivor who may be ***dependent*** on the prescription painkiller, along with their doctor who prescribes it, *are trying to **make the best of a bad situation**, as was my own case.*

• Treating Painkiller Dependence vs. Painkiller Addiction

Per www.cdc.com, contingent upon some painkiller(s) being prescribed by physicians, physiological *dependence* may be treated by gradually tapering off the substance(s) and transitioning to other non-addictive pain medications, or, by attempting a combination of both. Physiological painkiller dependence may be compulsory, such as for the warranted mitigation of Cancer-related pain. But, if and when the physical pain subsides, there should come a time that the patient or survivor needs to be physically weaned off the prescribed medication(s). If the pain continues, though, the painkillers will too.

The Cancer patient or survivor (or their family or Caregiver) should be able to recognize when the affected individual has become dependent upon their prescribed painkillers. When this occurs, it is extremely crucial that physicians on the patient's Medical Team be notified so that actions can be taken to gradually, and properly, wean the person off of the drugs. An appropriate member of the patient's or survivor's Medical Team (if they're worth their weight in salt as physicians), should be able to guide or support the affected person in making it safely through withdrawal and off of the medications.

Painkiller *addiction*, however, requires a different approach, and the Cancer patient or survivor will need to seek the assistance of competent Pain Medicine Specialists or other health care specialists ***outside of their Cancer Medical Team*** in order to safely destroy the habit. Someone who is addicted to a painkiller may also experience withdrawal symptoms when they cease using it. Painkiller addiction is also often characterized by relapses, so it is vital that those Cancer patients and survivors so-affected seek professional help ASAP.

☛ ***Authors Note:*** If a Cancer patient or survivor thinks that they may have acquired a dependency on, or an addiction to, the Opioid painkillers prescribed by their doctors, they ***should seek help from health care professionals in an effort to properly discontinue their use. Failure to do so may cause harmful consequences, including, in extreme cases, the possibility of death. Please be advised that in 2010, 18 women per day in the U.S. died of Opiate drug overdose.***

- **The Problems with Prescription Painkillers – *A Hypothetical Example and My Actual Experience***

Here is a hypothetical situation that can, undesirably, also be very realistic, based on my own Cancer experience. In this example, a Cancer patient's or a survivor's physician may have prescribed an Opioid painkiller (or several) to help them manage *pain* Side Effects caused by their Cancer Treatment(s). But, weeks or months after the original discomfort has subsided, the person still feels a need to take the drugs, possibly in a higher dosage than previously, because their body has built up a tolerance. The person needs the drugs, not to *get high*, but, just to get out of bed in the morning and to be fruitful. The medication meant to assist the individual now hurts them. When the person tries to stop taking the very potent drugs on their own—even attempting to steadily taper off of them over time—they experience the exceptionally painful and distressing discomfort of *Withdrawal.* This induces them to take more and more of the drugs just to make it thru each day. Their pain has not eased, but, instead, has intensified. The Cancer patient or survivor has become physically dependent on the prescription painkiller through no fault of their own.

This dire situation requires skillful medical intervention in a safe, humane, and effective environment. But, unfortunately, many well-intentioned doctors are often so centered on eliminating pain in their patients that they have a propensity to fail to see the long-term consequences of painkiller dependence. As such, when the Cancer patient or survivor asks for these same or different physicians' aid in overcoming their dependency on the exact drugs that brought them some reprieve from pain, the physicians are oftentimes not prepared, nor, do they have the training or the knowledge to be able to help the person-in-need. This is where things can get interesting, and I will use my own Cancer experience as a perfect example. Here we go:

When my Chemo and Radiation Therapy treatments began in July 2004, I did not originally have any serious Side Effects such as pain, nausea, loss of hair, mouth sores, or any others for which I had prepared after doing all of my pre-treatment research. In fact, I even got so bold as to ask my Oncologist and Radiation Oncologist if we needed to "up my dosages," because I was not experiencing most of the Side Effects that most patients were. My line of thinking at that time was that if the therapies weren't making *me* feel bad, they may not be killing *my Cancer.* And, while my Radiation Oncologist did call me the "Poster Boy for Radiation Oncology," both she, and my Oncologist, told me that at some point, *"the other shoe would fall."*

And fall it did! About half-way thru my treatments, and for several months thereafter, my mouth and throat felt as if they were on fire, and I found it almost impossible to eat or drink anything – even to swallow a small spoonful of water. To help me tolerate this excruciating and constant pain so that I could eat, drink, sleep, and *live, in general,* my physicians prescribed several Opioid painkillers for me. I was on four or five of these at any one time, and we had to gradually up the dosages to limit the pain as my body was becoming tolerant to them. This, in combination with the Chemotherapy drugs, made me extraordinarily nauseous all the time, which induced me to vomit 2 - 3 days a week (I hadn't thrown up since I was 8 years old). This also caused me to have excruciating constipation and the worst nightmares, in which I was typically dying, drowning, or fighting for breath. I woke up from these soaked in sweat and gasping for air.

When my pain *finally* subsided several months later, I tried my best to discontinue all of the prescription painkillers on my own, one-by-one, by incrementally reducing the dosages of each drug. All went well until I tried to get off of the final prescribed painkiller, the Fentanyl Duragesic® patch, which is a very powerful Opiate that can be ***80 times stronger than Morphine!*** Unsuccessful to do so, I went to my Medical Team for help. Unfortunately—and I hate to say this because they were always so magnificent with everything else—my physicians did not have one clue how to assist me with my painkiller dependency. ***I insisted that I get help***, and I was finally referred to a Psychiatrist who was glad to assist me. He told me, *"Doctors try to help patients with pain issues, but, they hand out pills like they are candy, and in so doing, they teach patients how to fly, but not how to land."* Very profound, true, and sad, I thought. He entered me into a hospital detox unit, where I joined street-drug users and alcoholics facing *their own* demons. After that depressing and scary experience and several days of tapering me off with use of Methadone, I went home, where I faced the horrible hell of withdrawal for three more weeks. *Finally, after one month, I beat my painkiller dependency!*

Chapter Eight

The Cancer Journey Explained – *Steps 10 thru 12 on the Journey:*

Recovery; Aftercare; Hopeful Survivorship

"There is no victory as sweet as Surviving Cancer, and no means of getting there as challenging, or, as rewarding."

- Butch Sickler

If the Cancer patient is able to be given and put up with all or most of their Cancer treatments as scheduled – *fantastic!* In the war against Cancer, all weapons that can be appropriately and safely launched against this adversary are essential to the overall success of each patient's Cancer-removal program. However, contingent upon the specific courses of treatment prescribed, as well as the respective durations, dosages, and, frequencies, and, taking into consideration the general health status of the patient, there is a possibility that the patient will still have to cope with several of the after-affects of their therapies for weeks, months, or, even years, after they have finished.

➢ *Post-Cancer Treatment Recovery – Step 10 on the Journey*

Fairly soon after the Cancer treatments have ended, it is time for the Cancer patient, their family, and their Caregiver and friends, to celebrate, give thanks, and hope and pray for Cancer survivorship.

When a Cancer patient eventually completes their hopeful, disease-eradicating Treatments—be they Chemotherapy, Radiation Therapy, Surgery, Immunotherapy, Bone Marrow Transplantation, or, two or more of these treatments—the significance of this accomplishment can be manifest in a variety of ways. Unquestionably, this important milestone in one's Cancer journey is immense reason for relief. But, even more so, it will surely be cause for celebration – in one form or another. This is, after all, one of the most significant steps a Cancer patient will take during their hopeful journey to reclaim their life.

The triumphant feeling that a Cancer patient might enjoy is a combination of them knowing that they have not only successfully passed the, *"Cancer treatment challenge,"* but, that their courageous efforts have hopefully eliminated their Cancer and have earned them the critical time to recover. For this reason, the conclusion of Cancer treatments is a very momentous occasion when the patient ***must*** be allowed the opportunity for their wounds to mend—be they mental, physical, emotional, spiritual, or a combination thereof. With some Cancer patients, this restorative process will be marked by a smooth transition from Treatment, thru Recovery, and into Aftercare, and, a, hopefully, healthy life beyond. But, with other Cancer patients, the process of healing and recovering from treatments could be long and difficult due to the physical and emotional burdens they continue to carry with them well after their treatments have concluded. For these individuals, Cancer Aftercare will, hopefully, be their saving grace.

"High-fives," Hugs, and Humility

The beneficial conclusion of one's Cancer treatment is a very personal and meaningful conquest, no matter how many family and Medical Team members have been involved in helping to bring this very critical portion of the Cancer patient's journey to a successful, cheery finale. And, because the wrapping-up of the patient's Cancer treatment(s) can be quite a private matter, each Cancer warrior may commemorate this momentous occasion in their own, personal way. With some patients, upon termination of their Cancer treatment(s), there could be *"High-fives"* all around the Oncology Clinic after the final drop of Chemotherapy medicine drips from the bag, slithers its way down the long, clear IV tube, and enters the patient's body like a stealth Commando, its final search-and-destroy mission being to locate and exterminate any covert Cancer cells lingering behind.

Another Cancer patient could communicate their jubilation at the conclusion of their Radiation Therapy treatments by giving hugs to all the folks in the room when they step down from the treatment table after their final session. The confidence that they radiate stems from the knowledge that they fearlessly "stayed the course," despite any discomfort they felt, while the precise, powerful radiation beams thoroughly cooked any Cancer cells that were foolish enough to get in their way. Those patients undergoing Cancer Surgery, however, might not be able to "high five" or hug anybody any time soon after their operation for fear of ripping a stitch or two. But, the successful completion of their procedure(s) will be justification enough for the patient and those close to rejoice, and, to be thankful that they have taken very vital actions in removing Cancer from the patient's body. Still other Cancer patients, after their final Immunotherapy or Bone Marrow treatment, may choose to share their success with simply an intimate cluster of family and friends. And, in yet other situations, Cancer patients may wish to exult or meditate quietly and personally while modestly taking stock of their accomplishments in completing their treatment(s), and, in hopefully surviving their Cancers.

In all cases, no matter the individual, their form of Cancer, or the type of treatment(s) that they received, the Cancer patient, upon termination of their treatment(s), will be celebrated with the positive support, love, and well-wishes from their family, Caregiver, friends, and members of their Medical Team. To plow successfully through Cancer treatments—crazy schedule and physical and emotional Side Effects included—is the equivalent of scaling a tall mountain while simultaneously juggling a bunch of burning torches. . .while walking in high heels! *OK, so I hyperbolize a bit.* But, seriously, it is a very challenging thing for one to achieve, and Cancer patients, young and old, male and female, do what they have to do to get it done. These individuals' lives and futures are, after all, hanging in the balance.

Time to Deal and Heal

While the turbulent, non-stop, and demanding pre-Treatment and Treatment phases of the patient's Cancer program may seem to be difficult enough, the Recovery Phase can be just as bumpy for the patient to circumnavigate, both physically and emotionally. This is because of the excessive limits to which both their bodies and minds have been, and, perhaps will continue to be, challenged and stressed. But, the Recovery Phase of one's Cancer-fighting journey can also be the most inspirational, constructive, and encouraging. This is due to the fact that the patient's enhancement should continue to be well-monitored and evaluated by their Medical Team for many months or years to ensure full recovery. Recovery is also when the outpouring of love and support from family, Caregiver, and friends will help the patient to transcend much of the pain, and/or, anguish, that they may be experiencing at the time. The caring and thoughtfulness of loved ones and friends can be just as powerful and significant, and just as therapeutic—as are the Surgery, Chemotherapy, Radiation Therapy, Immunology, and the Bone Marrow Transplantation treatments—in helping the patient to battle, and hopefully defeat, their disease.

For innumerable reasons, the Recovery Phase of the patient's Cancer journey is extremely important, as it gives the patient's body and Immune System an opportunity to recuperate, and should enable them to build on the successes of their treatment(s), and to gradually get stronger as a result. Ultimately, it will be the patient's favorable responses to their treatment(s), as well as the ability of their body to mend physically, emotionally, and psychologically at the conclusion of their treatment(s), that will play a primary role in determining the ultimate success of the Cancer patient's program. Presently, because of the noteworthy strides that have been made by the scientific and medical communities in both the Treatment and Aftercare of Cancer patients, approximately 80% of patients—or generally, 8 out of 10 patients treated for Cancers—will survive at least 5 years following their treatments. Even greater news is that a considerable number of the Cancer patients that do survive the fight will actually be *cured* of their specific disease. All the more reason to get better and enjoy it!

Why Does Life Always Come With "Strings Attached?"

As this life would have it, the positive, inspirational, and life-renewing benefits of Cancer treatments, unfortunately, do not come without their own unique sets of risks. That is, the very life-saving treatments that allow these patients to live, can also create their own short- and long-term health problems as a result, in the form of Side Effects and Late Effects. Yes, there can be strings attached to getting one's life back. Some of the problems realized can be a result of the Cancer incidence, itself, but, most post-Cancer treatment issues arise as a result of the very treatments or procedures used to eradicate this nasty disease from the patient's body. The therapies used in Cancer treatment can be very powerful and invasive, so, during the process of destroying cancerous cells, healthy tissue can also be harmed due to the *"collateral damage"* sustained during the process.

It is during the Treatment phase and post-treatment Recovery phase that any Side-Effects from the treatments and procedures will typically materialize, and/or, continue. In other words, frequently it is during the Recovery phase of the patient's Cancer program—after all the craziness of the last few months has come to a close—that the *"other shoe drops."* Or, to put it another way, this is when the bill collector comes a'knockin' to settle the account. And, because of the potential severity of the post-treatment Side Effects with which the patient often has to contend, the Recovery phase is when the patient, and his or her Caregiver, must devote much of their time and energy to the healing process. Not unlike any other medical condition that a person might have, from a bad head cold to a surgical procedure, we all know how important it is to "lay low" and let our *boo-boos* heal.

How the patient chooses to rest and relax after the cessation of Cancer treatments is an individual choice. But, it is critical to the recuperative process that a concentrated effort is made, despite other temptations and distractions. Simply put, one ***must* rest and relax** – ***period*** – if they want for their body to heal. Just as with many other things in life, with the treatment of Cancer, it is also, *"Darned if you do, darned if you don't."* But, please take it from a 9+-year Cancer survivor: A person diagnosed with Cancer is much more "darned" if they *don't* have their Cancer properly treated, than they are if they *do* undergo Cancer treatments – nasty, painful Side Effects and all.

A Proverbial "Fork in the Road" During Recovery

After the non-stop activity of challenging Cancer treatments has wrapped up, and the frenzied hustle-and-bustle of the many long weeks or months since diagnosis has finally come to a conclusion, it would seem that at some point during the Cancer patient's recovery, their life would begin coming back together again, and that things would slowly start returning to the way they were before the person was blind-sided by Cancer. *Or not...* For some Cancer patients, this could be the reality, or, it may be partially true. But for others, and I dare surmise that for a considerable number of Cancer patients, just the opposite may be the reality. The simple reason for this is that the potentially deadly Cancer has both the reputation, and the ability, to really clutter up, if not terminate, a person's life. As such, a Cancer diagnosis, itself, and the resulting efforts to rid it from the person's body, can be very unsettling and life-changing, to say the very least.

In some instances following Cancer treatment, many patients will arrive at what equates to the equivalent of a "fork in the road" during their post-treatment journey. It is at this significant juncture during the Recovery phase of the process that the forward-progress of the patient could take one path or another, depending on a variety of different factors. But, in most cases, the direction that the Cancer patient progresses with their life after treatment—that is, how they react and recover physically and emotionally after their therapy has ended—will be dictated by multiple factors that apply universally to most Cancer patients. Key amongst these criteria will be the state of the patient's general well-being following therapy, and, the Stage or severity of the Cancer that was treated. This would, in-turn, dictate the type of treatment performed, as well as the dosages, frequencies, and durations prescribed. Then, most of these factors will determine the severity of any harm caused (or still to be caused) to the patient by any nasty treatment-related Side Effects. In a perfect world, the patient's Cancer would be small and localized, the treatments would be short and sweet, and the bad Side Effects would be non-existent. Well, actually, in a perfect world, there would be no Cancer at all.

- **Taking the "Fast Lane" – Out With Cancer and On With Life**

Following Cancer Treatment and during Recovery, probably, a relatively small number of Cancer patients (when compared to the entire population of patients out there), will essentially conclude that their whole Cancer experience might have been simply an annoying, inconvenient "bump" in their "road of life" – nothing more than just another bothersome obstacle with which they had to contend and get over and beyond. For lack of a better analogy, perchance, one could think of these individuals' Cancers as nothing more than a *flat tire.* That is, when Cancer surprisingly entered these individuals' lives—not unlike the sudden surprise of a tire blow-out while driving—they pulled over to side the of the road (met with physicians and attended treatments); removed the wicked tire (the Cancer), replaced it with a new tire (a body free of Cancer); and, finally, they pulled back on to the Highway of Life, came to that fork in the road (the "fast" lane or the "slow" lane), chose a way, and continued on their journeys as if nothing had occurred (reclaimed and resumed their pre-Cancer life).

o Deal and Heal With Zeal

Believe it or not, with some Cancer patients, a laisser-faire or "fast lane" approach is pretty much the means by which they handle their Cancer experience – they acknowledge the problem, they deal successfully with the problem, they heal physically and emotionally, and, they enthusiastically and optimistically move past the problem and get on with their lives. This may be how some people have been conditioned to deal with *all* major problems in their lives. *"Cancer? – what Cancer?"* is the question that these individuals may ask—but not in a boastful, or an "in your face"-type of way. They just simply did what had to be done, put their Cancer behind them, and off they went. There could be a good many reasons why a number of Cancer survivors may approach their lives following Cancer treatment and other such issues in such a happy-go-lucky manner. In several cases, a Cancer survivor's nonchalant reaction to something so potentially serious and noxious could be directly attributable to the individuals, themselves, and to their personal backgrounds and past experiences.

In such instances, the patient's post-treatment attitude could be the manifestation of their otherwise constant and positive outlook on life; their abilities to weather even the most severe of storms (of which Cancer is at the top of the list); and, their burning desire to get on with their lives as quickly as possible, no matter the impediment, the inconvenience, or the potential severity of the situation. It's not that these Cancer victims *don't give a damn* or realize the severity of their plight. Actually, quite to the contrary, they will know that they have *"dodged a bullet,"* but, after they *dodge,* essentially, they don't dwell upon it. And, in all sincerity, such a casual, but, nevertheless, earnest comeback on the part of the survivor following their Cancer treatments may also be due to specific circumstances of the patient's Cancer, itself, and the treatment(s) prescribed to eliminate it.

For example, if the Cancer was detected early, was localized (Stage 1), and was treated in such a manner that the Surgery, and/or, other therapies were not exceedingly invasive and caused few or no detrimental Side Effects, the patient could, conceivably, go on their merry way following treatment with few or no physical or emotional issues still lingering behind. For lack of a better way of putting it, to these individuals, their Cancer may be a simple case of, *Wham-Bam, Thank-you, Ma'am.* As is true of most Cancer patients, the Recovery and Aftercare phases of their Cancer journeys will be an opportunity for these *lucky* patients to permit their bodies and minds heal, and to readjust to life after Cancer. But, unlike most Cancer patients, those individuals fortunate to have few or no unresolved after-effects from their treatment(s) will transit through these two significant phases of the Cancer journeys much more quickly with few residual problems.

- ## Cancer – Best When Nipped in the Bud

As previously suggested, in the case of some of patients who have the ability to move on with their life immediately after Cancer treatment, this may be due to an amalgamation of not only their own personal characteristics, such as a high level of self-confidence and a healthy, "never say die" attitude, but, it also might be because their Cancer was not too advanced (that is, it was caught in Stage I), was easily treatable, and the Cancer-removal therapies caused negligible or no Side Effects to the patient. This would definitely be an ideal situation, and, could very well be the case, were the person's Cancer detected, treated, and removed, extremely early-on in the process.

Such proactive measures can be because of the patient's self-awareness of Cancer signs and symptoms, and, their promptness in seeing a physician as soon as they noticed something "just not right" with their body. Or, early detection and treatment may be the result of Cancer screening examinations such as the PSA test for men, and

Mammograms for women, or, the patient's carefulness in obtaining routine, but vital, medical and dental physical examinations, during which their Cancer was discovered. In any event, no matter how the patient's Cancer is identified and treated, "early and fast" are always ideal. Thankfully, many Cancer patients do find themselves in this category, and, many of them are able to walk away from their battle with Cancer, almost as if nothing life-threatening had just occurred.

If the patient's Cancer presence is smaller and localized with no or little spread to other bodily areas, it may be very treatable with minimum or no negative affect on the patient's body and mind. In such instances, though, the seriousness of these individuals' Cancers cannot be diminished; nor, can it be implied that these patients' lives are not at risk, as are other patients who have been seriously stricken by the disease in its later Stages (III or IV). That is certainly not the case. ***All*** malignant Cancers are both serious and potentially lethal, no matter how localized, "new," or advanced they may be.

As with so many things in life, when problems are identified early-on and "nipped in the bud"—as is the ideal situation with early Cancer detection and treatment—the chances of doing away with the difficulties with few or zero negative consequences are much greater than if the problem is permitted to get worse and extend. If the latter should occur; that is, if the person's Cancer were to go undetected or untreated for any great length of time, the penalties of a significant delay to the person could be extreme. In such instances, the process for resolving the Cancer incidence may become much more complex and intense, and could be potentially more injurious to the patient on the receiving end and may translate into a less favorable prognosis.

- **Taking the "Slow Lane" - Out With Cancer but On With the Troublesome Aftermath**

To a majority of Cancer patients, the onset of Cancer and the subsequent flurry of activity that ensues for several weeks or months following their diagnosis—to include the busy schedule, treatments, and the potential, resultant Side Effects—can be really intimidating, indeed. For these Cancer patients, their disease can be an extremely threatening, overshadowing, and paralyzing threat that can, literally, stop them in their tracks. Some patients become daunted with their Cancer occurrence for some very good reasons. Many patients, and especially teens or young kids, may never have had to deal with any adversity in their lives, which, on the one hand, is fortunate and can be a positive thing. But, on the other hand, if these same "protected" individuals happen to get assaulted some day with the life-or-death reality of Cancer, their lack of *hands-on* experience in dealing with, and getting beyond adversity, can, unfortunately, place these Cancer patients at-risk should the going get tough. However, even though these patients may not necessarily be pre-conditioned to meet life's troubles head-on, all is not forsaken. All Cancer patients are Human Beings, and humans, like all of God's creatures, are "wired" with an inherent will to survive. Even at that, however, these apprehensive patients will require the uninterrupted support of their loved ones, a Caregiver, and their Medical Team to safely see them through. This would be critical not only during the patient's treatment(s), but also following the treatment(s), and during their Recovery and Aftercare.

- ### When Cancer Causes "Static Cling"

If the Cancer patient has "lingering issues" with their Cancer experience following the conclusion of their successful treatment(s), there could conceivably be many valid reasons why. And, it should be pointed out that such tribulations can be experienced by Cancer survivors well after treatment has ended, and *even though they have received the thankful news from their doctor(s) that their cancerous activity has been completely eradicated.* Yes, despite being told that they are, *"Cancer-Free,"* or that their Cancer is, *"in remission"* and that they have survived their Cancer, some individuals will still have some leftover physical and mental concerns that they might need to address and put behind them in order to reclaim their pre-Cancer life as they knew it. And, just as with many things in life, these Cancer-related, follow-on problems can come in many varieties, and, can hit a Cancer survivor out of nowhere, just when they least expect it.

To begin, as I already alluded, the patient-turned-survivor—through no fault of their own—may not be *naturally equipped* with the necessary physical or mental "tools" to rebound quickly from the often troublesome, demanding, and exhausting stresses that a Cancer occurrence can place upon them, and their bodies and minds. In such situations, the entire Cancer process may have so beleaguered and frightened the individual, that it may have left them with very little energy and strength—physical, emotional, or both—on which to fall back after their treatment(s) have concluded. In other words, some Cancer warriors, and especially the younger and older ones, may not be as resilient as Cancer victims in their prime of life, and, as such, their recoveries may be more difficult, and may take longer to come around. Undeniably, with time, and with the proper professional and family help and support, these Cancer survivors may be able to deal with the issues, get beyond them, and get back to living their lives.

- ### Time to Think About What Happened – *Way Too Much* Time!

As a young boy (and, come to think of it, even as an "adult" boy), if I ever had too much time on my hands, that's usually when I found myself getting into some form of mischief (*clean* mischief, of course!). This same may be true with many boys and men, and, with some girls and women. But, the point I'm attempting to make is that, unless the mind is kept busy and focused on something constructive and useful, there is a very real possibility that it will wander where it shouldn't go. And, believe me, this same premise also holds true for a Cancer patient who has just gotten beyond their Treatment Phase.

Yes, there is the genuine and emotionally taxing aftermath of Cancer treatment that can impact numerous Cancer patients after the hectic, seemingly non-stop activity of meetings, treatments, and tests has stopped, and the person finally has a lot of time on their hands to think about all that transpired over the last few weeks or months. I found myself getting surprisingly snared by this trap during my own Cancer experience, and, honestly, it turned out to be one of the most difficult and challenging aspects of my entire journey. The primary issue is one that I read about when I conducted research concerning Cancer after my diagnosis, and is something that was talked about in Support Group meetings I attended, during, and after, my therapies.
.

The Recovery Phase of the crazy Cancer journey is when the Cancer patient and their Caregiver will finally be able to "catch their breath," after several months of attending what seemed like non-stop appointments, consults, tests, examinations, and treatments. But, the suddenness of having only sporadic medical business when most of the pre-Treatment and Treatment activities have decelerated can also play nasty tricks on the patient and on their psyche. This is because this post-Treatment Recovery period is actually the first time—since receiving their shocking Cancer Diagnosis—that the patient has had the opportunity to slow it down, look back, contemplate, and attempt to make sense of the swift whirlwind that blew into their life one day and abruptly swept them off their feet *(and put them on their ass!).*

For several months following receipt of their Diagnosis, the patient had been preoccupied with an extremely busy schedule, and their primary focus had been on making it successfully through the treatments, and getting safely beyond, perhaps, some accompanying Side Effects. Suddenly, then, with all of this hectic hustle-and-bustle behind them, and a relatively *unoccupied* schedule in front of them, the patient will be left with a plethora of time on their hands *to think, and think, and think.* And, as often occurs post-treatment with some Cancer patients, not all thoughts will be optimistic or productive. A Cancer patient's retrospection can often be rather helpful in bringing clarity or closure to the situation. But, it may also lead the patient to start thinking of the various unanswered questions that have built up over the months, many of which that still may not have any answers.

- **Think Positively – Relax the Body and Mind**

Periods of intense self-examination on the part of the Cancer patient after treatment could cause the patient to develop feelings of regret, self-doubts, or guilt about their Cancer occurrence, including blaming themselves for their Diagnosis of Cancer. Even worse, the Cancer patient can begin questioning their chances of survival, and, perhaps, even contemplating their own mortality. In short, all of this "free time" that the patient has on their hands, during what should be a period of physical and mental healing, can also permit the patient sufficient time to develop pessimistic thoughts and feelings that may lead to severe anxiety, emotional despair, and even deep depression. This blatant negativity can then lead to physical difficulties. Should this happen, health professionals on the patient's Medical Team will take every possible step to provide the patient with the resources and medications they may need to help them cope with these symptoms, and to hopefully get beyond them and back to the healing process.

Without a question, some of the most significant and realistic reasons why a Cancer patient might have difficulty "bouncing back" after running the Cancer gauntlet, are because of the long-term fears of the unknown, and residual questions and thoughts the patient may have about their life and their future. Some patients may be so afraid of *"The Cancer Monster"* still lurking behind every corner—at least in their own mind—that they may have a difficult time transitioning to their new life – albeit, a *Cancer-free life.* And, other patients, still, might be fittingly coping with the aftermath of Side Effects and Late Effects (Side Effects from earlier Cancer treatments that appear later in life), so that, through no fault of their own, they just can't seem to put that *damn Cancer* behind them, no matter how hard they try.

In every situation, and with all Cancer patients, successfully completing Cancer treatment is a very big deal. Whether the patient is an adult, or a young child or teenager, and no matter if they are male or female, putting up with the non-stop treatment schedule and multiple tests and exams, and, overcoming the numerous, potential damaging impacts of treatment-related Side Effects, is one heck of a conquest – for the patient, as well as for their loved one, parent(s), family, and Caregiver. Following this jam-packed and often stressful few months during and after treatments, the patient will have to take time to relax, not only their mind, but their body, and to give each an opportunity to mend and return to "normal." In all instances, though, should the Cancer patient have difficulty adjusting to life after their Cancer treatments, or, should they have fears or display any signs of depression in dealing with the after effects of Cancer treatments, it is important that the patient, and their loved one, parent(s), family or Caregiver, seek professional help on behalf of the patient, as quickly as possible. ***Remember: Seeking help is a strength, not a weakness.***

➢ *Post-Cancer Treatment Aftercare and Monitoring – Step 11 on the Journey*

For the Cancer patient, their journey from Diagnosis through Treatment, Recovery, and Aftercare, may often seem like one, two, or even three marathon races, all clipped together in a never-ending procession of medical and personal commitments, each one aimed at helping the patient to safely and successfully complete their travels. But, unlike the end of a typical marathon race, there is no designated "Finish Line" that awaits the Cancer patient at the conclusion of the most important contest of *their* life. No, instead, the Cancer patient's "breaking of the tape" at the triumphant completion of their journey will welcome them in the forms of favorable follow-up exam results, which indicate that their Cancer has, hopefully, been removed. And, while the 10K or marathon runner may mark their prosperous finish with a medal, a personal-best time, or, simply the private satisfaction of knowing that they completed the race, the Cancer-patient-turned-survivor will subtly commemorate *their* meaningful accomplishment and victory with a trophy like no other: ***A Second Chance at Life.***

Reclaiming One's Life – Starting a "New Normal" Life

After the Cancer survivor has reclaimed their life following Cancer, the individual will gradually begin reacquainting themselves with the many people and things that they held near and dear to their heart prior to Cancer suddenly interrupting their life. In this sense, many things from the patient's pre-Cancer life will remain the same, or change very little, after the patient finally completes their lengthy journey. Definitely, the patient's adoration for, and connection with, their family and friends will probably be stronger than ever, and the patient's own craving to pick up where they left off with their work, hobbies, school, and other activities, may increasingly resume in a determined effort to restore some degree of normalcy back into their life. However, both the occurrence of Cancer within an individual, and the survival of the sometimes punishing, painful, and drawn-out process to eradicate it from their body, might change a person—both physically and emotionally—and, will often cause a Cancer survivor to start looking at life (or some facets of it) from an entirely different perspective. This is a common occurrence in Cancer survivors, and it is typically referred to as living life with a, ***"New Normal."***

In one Cancer survivor's "New Normal" way of living their life, the patient's Cancer experience may have prompted the person to develop a more sensitive understanding of just how delicate their health and life are, and just how vulnerable they can be to a surprise attack by a deadly disease. In this sense, many Cancer patients will never be able to relax comfortably again, always concerned that the Cancer that nailed them one time will come back to do it once again. Another Cancer survivor may recognize just how close to mortality they came, and, it may take the opportunity of their winning Cancer journey to encourage them to get involved in the things that they've wanted to do, but which, they've procrastinated over until the "time was just right." These individuals, knowing that they've been given a second chance, vow to live their life to the fullest every day. More often than not, Cancer survivors will sense their Cancer diagnosis as a "wake-up call," and, in several cases, whether or not the survivor comes to realize a "New Normal" afterwards, the Cancer experience usually does elicit changes in the survivor's life for the better.

Aftercare Support and Monitoring – Being Ever-Vigilant

Most Cancer survivors—regardless of their respective sexes, ages, or forms of Cancer—will likely be monitored continuously for the rest of their lives for the purpose of detecting new or secondary cancerous activity, and/or, to confirm the absence of Cancer in the survivor's body. The latter, of course, is the expectant and eventual desire of all Cancer treatments. And, while most responsible Cancer patients and their physicians will always be "on-guard" and watchful for any future, new Cancer disease when the patient's initial Cancer treatments have concluded, there will, typically, be an incredible and very personal sense of achievement that accompanies the occasion.

Thankfully, as one would suppose, members of the patient's Medical Team are cognizant of, familiarized with, and educated and trained to respond to, the needs and concerns of patients (as well as their loved ones and family members) following their treatment(s). This due diligence is accomplished via the incessant aftercare testing and evaluation of the patient, and thru the constant monitoring of the patient's health status by applicable members of the Medical Team, or by their Primary Physician. In other words, just because a Cancer patient's treatments have concluded, does not mean that the patient is sent home and expected to fend for him- or herself for the rest of their life. To the contrary, the observation and evaluation of Cancer patients/survivors are just as significant subsequent to the Treatment Phase, as they were while the treatments were being performed.

As the days, weeks, months and years go by after treatment, the patient will submit to many follow-up tests, examinations, and evaluations to determine if any malignant Cancer may still exist, or, if by all accounts, it has been removed in its entirety. This period in the journey is called the Aftercare Phase, and it is typically when the patient may join Cancer Support Groups to help them cope with any follow-on problems with which they may be struggling, or, purely to establish a network of fellow patients and survivors with whom they can share ideas and advice. The Recovery and Aftercare phases can also be a very exceptional time because it is when the Cancer patient will, hopefully, continue to receive 100 percent favorable follow-up tests results. And, when that occurs, they can finally transition from being a *Cancer "patient,"* to becoming a Cancer *"Survivor."*

The purpose of conducting periodic follow-up Cancer exams and evaluations is essentially two-fold: To begin, the exams are vital to corroborate the existence or the absence (much preferred!) of any former or new cancerous disease in the body. And, secondly, if any disease *is* identified during the screening process, the outcome of the post-treatment testing will supply the Medical Team with the critical information they will need to ascertain which new treatment options (if any) would be appropriate to pursue. Generally, some physicians on the Medical Team will meet with the Cancer survivor on a usual "check-up"-type basis (i.e., each month, or every 2, 6, or 12 months, as applicable) for the patient's life, following the completion of their treatment(s). Certainly, however, those patients (or, their families or Caregivers whose Cancer survivor is) in need of care *between their scheduled exams,* can contact applicable Medical Team members to arrange for a sooner appointment and necessary services, treatments, and/or, medications, to help resolve any new problems as they arise.

The continuous, regular, and rigorous monitoring of Cancer patients following their treatments (regardless of the type of Cancer or treatment received) is truly one of the "silver linings" of what can be a long, arduous, and often painful, process. Aftercare monitoring protocols and scheduling are based on the particular Cancer treated, and will typically consist of periodic evaluation via the utilization of imaging devices such as Scans or X-rays and could entail the testing of blood or urine, or, the utilization of other non-invasive methods. In some situations, especially where a scan, test, or exam could have yielded a questionable outcome, follow-up Cancer monitoring may require the laboratory examination of body tissue samples removed by way of a Surgical Biopsy. These cell samples will be tested at a medical lab, and the Pathology results will be communicated to the treating physician, who will then convey them to the patient.

For countless Cancer survivors—and I will include myself in this bunch—some of the most anxious, frightening times during the Cancer patient's journey can crop up when the patient is waiting for the lab results to be returned from post-Cancer treatment monitoring tests. While one will always try to think confidently about receiving negative (favorable) outcomes, the "not knowing," and the "what if" thinking (that we are all inclined to do when fearing the worst about something), are what can drive a Cancer survivor crazy. Over time, however, when a Cancer patient has a few favorable post-treatment test results under their belt, they will begin to relax more, feel more confident, and start believing that they may actually be *Cancer-free.*

During my own Cancer experience, over the course of three years, I had three of five individual exams during which post-Cancer treatment PET Scans illustrated areas that "lit up," according to my physician. Throughout the five separate tests, utilizing the "PET" or Positron Emission Tomography exam protocol, I was injected with Radioactive Glucose in a very calm, dark, and cool environment (so as to not become too stressed or excited, which could skew the test results). Because Cancer cells do thrive on Glucose—or body blood sugar—to survive, these PET tests reveal, through electronic scans, any *highlighted* areas where it appears that the Radioactive Glucose may be being consumed in large quantities – such as by a colony of cancerous cells. My Cancer physician told me that these highlighted areas on my 3 scans may reflect the existence of possible cancerous activity. On each occasion, this news scared the hell out of me and dredged up some very memorable, frightening feelings that I had not experienced since receiving my initial diagnosis many months prior.

Following the outcome of these three separate PET Scans, in which some of my bodily tissues appeared questionable, my Cancer Surgeon Biopsied the suspect areas and had the tissue confirmed at a Pathology Lab, or ordered a CT Scan. Thankfully, in each of these cases, medical examination confirmed that there was ***NO*** cancerous activity present, which, of course, was an enormous relief to me. In medical parlance, such occurrences are known as *"False Positives,"* a nice term for Cancer patients to hear during the Aftercare Phase of their journey. To this day, there is no sure way of knowing why the Radioactive Glucose indicated "cancerous" cellular activity as it did during my three separate tests. But, my doctor suggested that it may have been due to my healthy cells or scar tissue consuming the sugar to heal. Nevertheless, as happy as I was to hear that I did not have a Cancer recurrence or residual cancerous cells still hanging out in my body, just the thought of that possibility was *exceptionally scary.*

Cancer Support Groups – Safe Havens for Any In-Need

During the Treatment, Recovery, and Aftercare Phases of a patient's Cancer journey, there is a "Silver Lining" of one's Cancer program that can be particularly beneficial to the patient, their loved one, family members, or Caregiver. These saving graces are known as Cancer Support Groups. Cancer Support Groups are some of the best, most helpful ways for patients, families, and Caregivers to both solicit and provide support, and to become more active (to the extent they wish) in their Cancer communities. Cancer Support Groups are typically led by Social Workers, Doctors, Psychologists, and other medical professionals, and are normally held in churches, hospitals, community centers, and other facilities. Although some groups may be based on Cancer support *in general*, many groups have a *Cancer-specific* basis, meaning that the participants (patients and survivors) may all share the identical form of Cancer, such as, Head and Neck, Breast, Prostate, Colorectal, Leukemia, or others. Having *others "in the same boat"* as the patient can be very beneficial and educational. Most Cancer Support Groups meet on a regular basis and are usually free of charge, but some may require a small registration fee or dues.

Cancer Support Groups provide patients, their families, and their Caregivers with a warm and private environment in which they feel safe to share their own stories—both good and bad—with others who are in a similar place as they. But, perhaps the greatest benefit of Support Groups, aside from the camaraderie that these groups can afford, is that participants can benefit from the lessons, pitfalls, and triumphs that the others have experienced along the way. And, all participants may feel free to ask questions and seek advice to obtain valuable information that will assist them during their own journeys. Often, support group facilitators will invite Physicians, Nutritionists, Psychologists, and other professionals who will talk about particular topics critical to Cancer patients and those enlisted in their support.

If a Cancer patient is experiencing Side Effects as a result of their treatment(s), and cannot attend a Support Group in-person, an online community (on the Internet) could be the best, most effective way for the patient to seek the support, information, and advice they may need, during, or following, treatment. Joining an online Cancer Support Group can also be a very useful, and much more convenient means of obtaining critical, "outside" support while contending with Cancer. Online Support Groups also let the Cancer patients maintain their anonymity, which enables lots of patients to be more outspoken about sharing their personal feelings, fears, and frustrations.

No matter which type of Cancer support a person chooses, it should be remembered that emotional support and caring are just as important as physical care when it comes to facing the disease, and hopefully defeating it and putting it behind them. A Cancer patient doesn't have to feel isolated when coping with their Cancer and the physical and emotional baggage that it can demand. Maintaining a positive outlook on life (and *their* life!), gaining self-confidence, and learning survival and coping skills, are the primary goals of Support Groups. Each of these components helps to make the Cancer journey much easier on the patient, their family, and their Caregiver(s).

➢ *Cancer Survival – The Final, Well-Deserved Destination on the Journey – Step 12*

Imagine that you've just successfully conquered the summit of Mount Everest, and, that you've also just won the big Lottery; the NFL Super Bowl®; a Gold Medal in the Olympics; an all-expense paid trip for two to Hawai'i; a Pulitzer Prize®; the Boston Marathon®; the Most Valuable Player Award in the World Series®; a Nobel Peace Prize®; an Academy Award®; a Blue Ribbon at the County Fair for your mouth-watering Apple Pie; and, you've spelled the word, *"flibbertigibbet,"* to win the National Spelling Bee Championship. Lastly, envision you've just been voted the Sexiest Man or Woman alive – *all in one day!*

Okay, now visualize that you are a courageous Cancer patient who has successfully survived your Cancer journey . . . get the idea?

To survive a Cancer attack is to win the ultimate of all contests; to trounce the toughest of all opponents; and, to conquer the highest of all mountains. Cancer survival is, in a word, *miraculous!* If you are a Cancer patient who has recently concluded their Cancer journey, or, if you are the loved one, family member, friend, or Caregiver of someone who has just converted their long and difficult journey after Diagnosis into a ***Cancer-Free***, or a ***Cancer-in-Remission*** outcome, please allow me to present my heartfelt and well-deserved congratulations. You, or they, have certainly earned a coveted place on the mountaintop!

The Journey Taken – Uphill First, Then Back Down

Even the longest travels to the tallest peak begin with a single step, and this is especially the case with a Cancer patient. Whether the patient realized it or not at the time, the beginning of their long, steep, and winding journey actually started the very moment that their doctor delivered to them their unanticipated Cancer Diagnosis. About a split-second after that, the patient responded to this revelation in a variety of ways, but, most likely, they were astonished, frightened, confused, and possibly, even angry. From the instant that their physician expressed to them those fateful and unforgettable words, *"I'm sorry, but you have Cancer,"* the patient knew that there was no turning back. And, since Cancer diagnoses, as yet, do not come with a "Delete" key or a "Back-Arrow" button (although, I'm sure that some Scientist, somewhere, is working on that as I write this!), the patient was left with no choice but to focus his or her attention and actions in a positive, forward direction, and, to courageously meet the Cancer challenge head-on.

A person can only see so far in the rearview mirror, but looking out front, one can see forever. It is this *ever-forward-never-backward* foundational truth upon which a Cancer survivor will typically attempt to resurrect their life-after-Cancer, and with which most survivors will realize that their bodies and their minds are capable of withstanding—physically and mentally—much more than they ever thought possible. But, it is *after* a patient reaches the high-point of the Cancer journey by overcoming their disease that they will have to endure the reality of the downhill trek to the "base of the mountain" in an effort to return to the life that they knew prior to Cancer. For various Cancer survivors, the "return trip" will be a breeze, but, for others, it may be just as rocky, if not more so, than their uphill hike. It is during any irregular downward regions of the journey that the Cancer patient should use all of the tools at their disposal—both personal and professional—to help them safely reach their ultimate destination: *A reclaimed, healthy, happy life.*

Destination Reached: Hopeful Cancer Survivorship

The final stop on any Cancer patient's long, challenging, and uphill journey—from Diagnosis, then through Treatment, Recovery, and Aftercare—is the promising destination of Cancer Survivorship. More specifically, the eventual objective is a ***Cancer-Free*** outcome, otherwise known as *"Cured Cancer."* From the precise moment that the physician or another health care professional provided the fateful account of the Cancer diagnosis to the patient, every thought, every action, and every minute of every day and night has been devoted to effectively and safely removing the disease from the patient's body. This overarching objective took place while simultaneously ensuring that the patient's physical, emotional, and spiritual needs were being adequately monitored, addressed, and skillfully fulfilled. At the very beginning of a patient's Cancer journey, and throughout the ensuing months, the information and countless unknowns can seem daunting and, practically impossible to comprehend for the first-time Cancer patient, and their loved one, family, and friends. But, as the saying goes, *"When the going gets tough, the tough get going,"* and that is typically what happens when families are faced with an adversity in life, and especially one as serious as a diagnosis of Cancer.

Each Cancer survivor differs from other Cancer survivors, so it stands to reason that each individual will respond differently when their own Cancer experience winds down, whether it is in a physical, emotional, mental, and/or, a spiritual sense. Having, hopefully, and fortunately, reached their long-awaited destination of a ***Cancer-Free*** outcome, some survivors will resume their lives, post-Cancer, as if nothing bad at all had happened to their bodies or their lives. Other Cancer survivors, however, may experience difficulties getting their pre-Cancer lives back on-track, while other survivors still, may end up becoming a combination of the two. In several cases, the Cancer survivor will return to their normal pre-Cancer modes of doing and thinking, while some other Cancer survivors' "New Normal" views of things will cause them to live their own lives—or parts thereof—differently than they did before. In all cases, though, no matter who does what, when, how, why, or where, after the Cancer conflicts are over, the most important thing is that these hopeful, courageous, and determined men, women, and children have defeated and survived their disease. Beating Cancer is Job-One in reclaiming their lives.

These patients who *do* beat their Cancers ***are*** Survivors, and as such, they have joined a very select group of individuals who met their respective Cancers head-on, and who declined to back down to the disease. The courageous people who survive Cancer are, indeed, very fortunate, and they, and their families and friends, are certainly justified in celebrating their triumphant victories for having defeated their attackers. But, those who have skirmished in the trenches and ultimately won their clashes with Cancer will never boast about their accomplishment or take it for granted. They will be content, though, and very thankful for having successfully battled and defeated their Cancers, for they are all proud members of the *"13 Million Club!"*

Most Cancer survivors that I know will humbly acknowledge the recognition that things might have turned out *much* differently, and much scarier, had something not gone right with their diagnosis, their treatments, their Side Effects, or any of a gazillion other things that could have "gone off the tracks" at some juncture down the line. Possibly, most importantly, however, these humbled survivors of the world's second deadliest disease will also remember, pay tribute to, and mourn, those many other Cancer warriors—young and old, male and female—who have given their respective Cancers the fights of their lives, but, who, ultimately and unfortunately, lost their personal battles with this disease. Despite the final outcome of each patient's personal mêlée with Cancer, however, all courageous fighters of the disease will serve as an inspiration to those who may follow in their footsteps. I continually depended heavily on my Mom, a thirty-eight year Cancer survivor, herself, to inspire me during my own journey.

An Enlightening Post-Cancer "New Normal" Way of Life

Thankfully, at some point in their journey, the patient's Cancer program *will* luckily, finally wind down, and will—for all intents and purposes—come to a conclusion as the patient reaches their intended destination: A heartening ***"Cancer Free,"*** or ***"Cancer-in-Remission"*** result. When that happens, and when all of the "dust" has settled from the frenzied, non-stop schedule of the prior few months that was filled-to-the-brim with various medical commitments of one form or another, the Cancer patient's life will eventually return to normal. *Or . . . will it?* Chances are pretty good that some things in the patient's life will fall neatly back into place, almost as though the patient never skipped a beat during what may have been either a brief, or a prolonged, Cancer hiatus. Family interactions, re-connections with friends, and activities such as romancing their loved one, exercising, going shopping or out to eat, resuming hobbies, and returning to work or school, will all most likely be included in the patient's attempt to reestablish some normalcy within their life. With most Cancer patients, just as with many things in life—because each person, and each Cancer are distinct—there will be no common standard or customary manner in which Cancer patients will resume their pre-Cancer life, or begin their post-Cancer life.

With that said, there is a very strong possibility that the Cancer patient, after completion of their challenging journey from diagnosis to survivorship, will naturally assume what is often referred to in Cancer survivorship and other survival circles as a *"New Normal"* perspective on life. In essence, what this term means is that many battle-wise and weary Cancer survivors will view life through a different looking glass than they did prior to their Cancer diagnosis and their challenging fight to save their own lives. For some of these individuals, their pre-Cancer *rose-colored glasses* may have become so remarkably clear because of their eye-opening and death-defying Cancer experience, that they may start seeing things in their world much more plainly and distinctly than they ever have before. To these new Cancer survivors, the "black and white" and the "gray" areas that they may recall from their pre-Cancer days, will, all of the sudden, become more brilliant, more colorful, and, perhaps, more enlightening in their New Normal way of life. To put it another way, these Cancer survivors will actually start "seeing" things that they've always looked at, but seldom ever noticed.

A Distressing Post-Cancer "New Normal" Way of Life

Some Cancer survivors experience a very rough time trying to make sense of the Cancer chaos in which they have found themselves, and their unpleasant, distressing Cancer incidence may have so tainted their outlook on living that the new lenses through which they view the world have become obscure and clouded with anxiety and uncertainty. In such cases, these individuals' New Normal perspective on life may prevent them from being able to look at some things the same way they did prior to their Cancer diagnosis. This very real New Normal way of thinking and approaching life for some Cancer survivors can promote feelings of self-doubt, hopelessness, and a lack of social interaction. It may even involve less-than-positive thoughts about their futures, their lives, their jobs or schooling, or, their family, friends, or relationships.

To make matters lousier, such a Cancer patient's or survivor's emotions could become so "contaminated" by their Cancer experience that they could find themselves living in a mental state so preoccupied with their fear of dying from a recurrence of new Cancer, that—despite their best efforts to the contrary—it may drop them into a never-ending downward spiral of anxiety and depression. *If and when this occurs, it is time for the patient, their loved one, family or Caregiver to promptly seek professional assistance on the patient's behalf.* Depression and Anxiety are a very wicked duo, and no one—and especially a suffering Cancer survivor—should have to subject themselves to the unrelenting depressing feelings that can often accompany the completion of Cancer treatment – even in cases where the survivor has had several successful monitoring tests, and has been declared by doctors to be *Cancer Free.*

I, personally, know very well about post-treatment anxiety and depression. After the conclusion of my Cancer therapies, *"Mr. Happy-Go-Lucky Me"* believed that I had completely, 100%, "Conquered the Beast," and, I was all set to get going with my life. But, I was soon to discover that while I had, in fact, beaten my Cancer, I had no idea that just around the corner from that victory there would be mental despair at such depths, that, after I dropped into it head-first, I thought I would never be able climb out of the darkness and return "to the way I was." Mercifully, I was eventually able to break free of my horrendous, dark depressive state, but it did take many months of Psychotherapy, a huge amount of patience on the part of my girlfriend and other friends at the time, and some real soul-searching on my part, to do it. To this day, I still don't know which I found more disquieting – the atrocious pain in my throat caused by my Cancer and Side Effects, or, the terrible pain in my heart, mind, and soul, caused by the deep depression that ensued.

Fearing the Worst – Hoping for the Best

Having potentially stared death in the face upon receipt of their fateful Cancer diagnosis—because, honestly, all 200+ known forms of Cancer ***can be*** deadly if not promptly and properly addressed—several Cancer patients who have survived the grueling journey will never feel entirely comfortable in their own skin again. For some adult, and some child Cancer survivors, this could be because their Cancer ordeal might have been the first time in their lives that they have ever been coerced into a life-or-death type of situation against their will. Certainly, we all face likely challenges in life every time we walk out of our front doors, or get behind the wheel of a car or hike in the woods. But, we typically are aware of any potential risks "out there," and we (hopefully) will be able to steer clear of them. A Cancer diagnosis, however, represents a different kind of threat to a person than do the *run of the mill, everyday* perils that all of us face throughout our lives. Some Cancer survivors, knowing that they have been ambushed earlier by Cancer, will, for the remainder of their lives, be glancing over their shoulders, bothered that the evil villain will pounce out of nowhere and strike them once again. For this particular Cancer survivor, this will be *their* New Normal.

Other Cancer survivors, however, having effectively run the challenging gauntlet of seemingly ceaseless doctors' appointments, treatments, and Side Effects, will choose to put a more positive spin on their Cancer experience, and will apply both the opportunity and the successful outcome as a springboard-of-sorts to launch them into undertakings that they more-than-likely would have never otherwise pursued. Or, if the Cancer survivor had wanted to carry out certain things or aspire to reach personal objectives, perhaps they, like most people, would have kept putting them off until a "better time," when they "had more money or more time" to chase them. But, when one is fortunate enough to live thru their Cancer, lots of individuals will take advantage of this hopeful blessing—a Second Chance at Life—to reach for their "Bucket List" if they have one, or, if not, to create one, and begin completing things on that list one-by-one. A Cancer diagnosis does an exceptional job of reminding one just how quickly their life can be snatched out from under them. Realizing this, many Cancer survivors reach for their dreams *as if there is no tomorrow.* These Cancer survivors' New Normal way of living is to turn their worst fears into positive and fulfilling thoughts and actions.

The Many Hearts, Hands, and Minds Behind Cancer Survivorship

The fact that just about 80% of Cancer patients survive their disease (depending on the forms and severities of their Cancers, and their general physical states) is a testament, not only to the scientific and medical communities that have developed, tested, and used safe, fast, and effective Cancer-killing drugs, treatments, and state-of-the-art equipment. It's also due to the highly educated and skilled health care professionals that dedicate their own lives to saving the lives of young childhood, teen, and adult Cancer patients. Equally as crucial, however, in obtaining a constructive outcome to a potentially deadly Cancer occurrence, is the support of the patient's loved one, family, Caregiver, and friends, in delivering hope, love, and encouragement to the patient – one smile, one hug, and one positive word at a time.

It goes without saying that the most important consideration, by far, in reaching a successful Cancer outcome, is the strength and determination of the Cancer Warrior, themselves – the valiant boy or girl, the courageous teenager, or the gallant man or woman, that did absolutely nothing to *sign up* for the disease, but who did everything within their power to prevail over it. These courageous patients, who are lying in hospital beds with no hair on their heads, and with tubes coming-and-going in lots of directions from their potentially delicate bodies, are getting a harsh indoctrination to the cruel realities of life. But, having braved all that, and having conquered and survived this occasionally lethal disease, these individuals will be all the stronger, and all the wiser, for what else lies ahead in their lives-to-come.

Cancer Survivorship – An Attainable and Maintainable Objective

Current statistics developed by the National Cancer Institute (www.cancer.gov), specify that there are approximately 13.7 million Cancer Survivors now living in these good ole' United States. This quantity represents an approximate four-fold increase in the last 30+ years, and is expected to continue to climb with time as other valiant fighters conquer their Cancers and join these humbled ranks. These noteworthy increases in the survival rates of Cancer victims are due to many factors, among which are the activities of many to seek and acquire medical intervention at the initial suggestion of questionable symptoms, thus leading to earlier detection and successful treatment of the disease. Also of paramount importance in detecting, locating, and treating Cancer in its earliest Stages have been the concentrated efforts on the parts of both physicians and patients to prescribe and take part in both the Mammogram and the Prostate Specific Antigen (PSA) tests as helpful screening tools. As a result of efforts put forth by many anti-Cancer organizations to inform the masses of—and to encourage their participation in—these Cancer screening techniques, there are within the U.S. today, more than 2.5 million Breast Cancer survivors, and over 2 million survivors of Prostate Cancer. ***Yes!!***

Further responsible for the increase in Cancer survival rates in the U.S. and worldwide are the magnificent strides that have been made in advances in Treatment, and, specifically in the development of medical equipment and technologies, as well as in the enhanced education, skills, and capabilities of the treating doctors and nurses, themselves. And finally, there is no question that the higher survival longevity rates amongst most Cancer Patients have resulted from the continuous testing, monitoring, Aftercare, and support mechanisms that are offered to patients subsequent to their initial Chemotherapy, Surgery, Radiation Therapy, and other medical treatments. Finally, of course, let's be sure not to under-emphasize the importance of the Cancer patients, themselves, and their contributions to the optimistic and reassuring survivorship numbers that are continuing to shoot up over time. It is these unwavering warriors, along with their helpful loved ones, families and friends, who are helping to turn the tide.

Cancer Survivors – Living Better to Live Longer

According to the National Cancer Institute (www.cancer.gov), a review of more than 100 Studies of Cancer survivors indicated that many survivors institute diet, exercise, and other beneficial lifestyle changes following a Cancer diagnosis. In other words, these people used their Cancer occurrence and potential brush with mortality as a *wake-up call* to modify their ways. Many of these constructive and favorable changes in Cancer survivors' habits and lifestyles tend to be beneficial to the individuals who practice them. Cancer survivors are a susceptible population, and as such, are predisposed to a higher risk for new or recurrent Cancers, Osteoporosis, Diabetes, Obesity, Cardiovascular Disease, and other health issues. Any investment in bettering their health should pay them dividends in the long run.

Using Cancer Survivability Databases, researchers from the National Cancer Institute (www.cancer.gov) and two prominent U.S. universities identified and reviewed well over 100 Studies of Cancer survivors since 1996. The Study researchers found that many Cancer survivors adopt healthier behaviors after treatment, as follows:

- 30 to 60% of survivors start consuming healthier diets
- 46 to 96% of survivors with tobacco-related Cancers, such as those of the Lung or Head and Neck, quit smoking
- 47-59% of survivors with Head and Neck Cancers that are closely linked to alcohol use, abstain from drinking alcohol
- 70% of survivors pursue regular physical activity and exercise for 30 minutes a day, at least 5 days a week

As one might expect, according to the Studies, there are also some Cancer survivors—specifically those who are male, older, less educated, and living in rural areas—that are less likely to implement constructive and beneficial alterations to their personal lifestyles and habits after completing Cancer treatments. Additionally, researchers noted that not all Cancer patients went with healthier behaviors post-therapy, with only 25-42% of Cancer survivors consuming adequate quantities of fruits and vegetables, and approximately 70% of Breast and Prostate Cancer survivors remaining overweight, and/or, obese. The analysis also found conflicting data on physical activity as well as smoking status, reporting that although survivors with tobacco- or alcohol-related Cancers were more prone to reduce or do away with these behaviors, 20% of survivors continued to smoke; a figure that is similar to the smoking status of the general population at 24%.

Help Save Others – Help Save Yourself

With billions (with a "B") of dollars, both public and private, being invested in Cancer Research, Treatment, and Aftercare on an annual basis, hopefully, all Cancer survival statistics will continue to improve, right along with the lives of the millions of Survivors that those dollars are benefiting on a very personal basis. Please do keep this in mind the next occasion when you are asked to contribute to a Cancer Cure Cause, to donate money on behalf of Cancer Research and Treatment, or, to help take care of a Cancer patient in-need.

You seriously might want to think twice before not doing so, because your time and your money may assist in not only saving the lives of those who may be very dear to you, but, they ***may also help to save your own life*** some day. Little did I know that the financial contributions to Cancer Research that I've made over many years on behalf of our Mom, Betty—who survived Breast Cancer for over 38 years, herself—would come back to help save ***me*** in my own Cancer experience! *What goes around, comes around...and around...and...*

Learn More – Live More

The data and information provided in this Chapter and in the preceding Chapters about Cancer—and throughout this entire Book for that matter—is a lot to think about, and is a considerable quantity of information about Cancer for one to assimilate, remember, learn, and utilize. But, please don't let the nature of the information, or its volume, frighten or intimidate you. If you have been diagnosed with Cancer, or if a loved one, a family member, or a dear friend has been diagnosed with the disease, it is important that the *patient and their Cancer* come to know each other on a "first name" basis. The best way for this to happen is for the patient, and his or her Caregiver, to take the time to research, study, and to acquire as much knowledge as they can about the disease and their specific form of Cancer.

Being equipped with such information, the brave patient, and perhaps, their loved ones, family, or Caregiver, will become active participants in the plan-of-action to exterminate the Cancer from the patient's body. Each Cancer War is a fight to the finish, and, it is the ultimate manifestation of a person's inborn will to survive. Cancer is an unnecessary evil that must be battled, during which there will be *only two satisfactory outcomes:* First, the *complete and definite annihilation* of the evil Cancer. And, secondly, the *patient's survival* in the best condition possible, physically, mentally, and emotionally. Cancer warriors ***do not*** give up, and, they ***do not*** take prisoners!

"At the conclusion of many travels in life, there is time to rejoice for having succeeded, and there are opportunities to reflect upon one's experiences along the way. So, too, with one's Cancer journey, but, the stakes are much higher, the steps are much steeper, and this triumphant victory is rewarded—not with fame or fortune—but with recovery and renewal."

- Butch Sickler

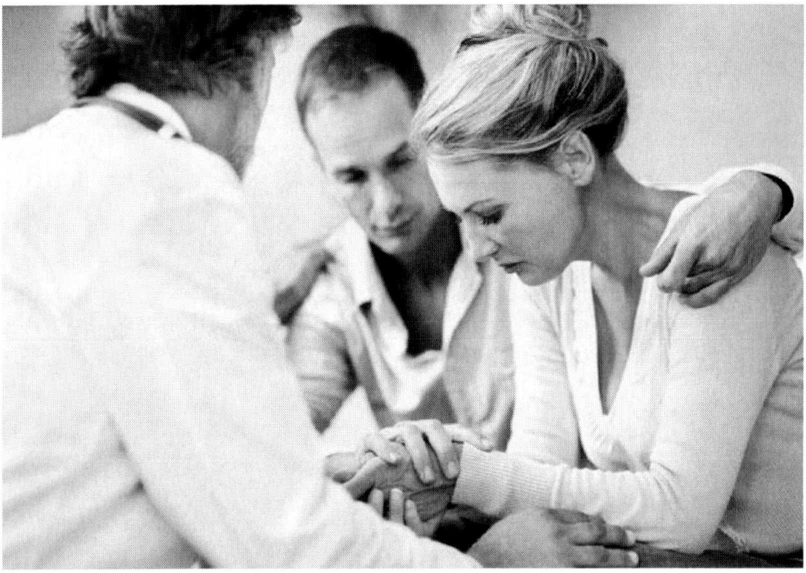

***Cancer. Cancer. Cancer.** Not a pleasant word for doctors to say, or, for individuals to hear. But, regrettably, in scenes much like the one depicted in this stock photo, those words will be delivered by doctors to unsuspecting men, women, and children no fewer than six million times around the world, and one-and-a-half-million times in the U.S. every year. So, the big question is: What will you do if your doctor directs that frightening word towards **YOU** – about **YOU**? Well, the truthful answer is that, initially, you will probably be very terrified, perplexed, saddened, and uncertain. And, if you're anything like me, you'll be pissed off that the Cancer would have the nerve to violate YOUR body, especially if you've taken great care of yours as I have mine. At the same time, you will possibly question, as I did, just how, why, and when you got your Cancer, and, you will wonder whether you will be able to take your Cancer's life before it can take yours. There will be many questions, at least at first, but the answers will be few. However, after the original shock of your diagnosis has had an opportunity to sink in, your fears, anxieties, and feelings of despair should give way to a more hopeful and reassuring outlook. This will usually occur after the new Cancer patient has had time to research and learn about their Cancer; enlist a Caregiver; meet with those on the Medical Team; and, participate in the development of the Cancer Killing Treatment Plan. Finally, when all is said and done, you will hopefully be joining me, and 13.7 million other Americans, who have turned their scary Cancer Diagnosis into Cancer-free Survivorship.*

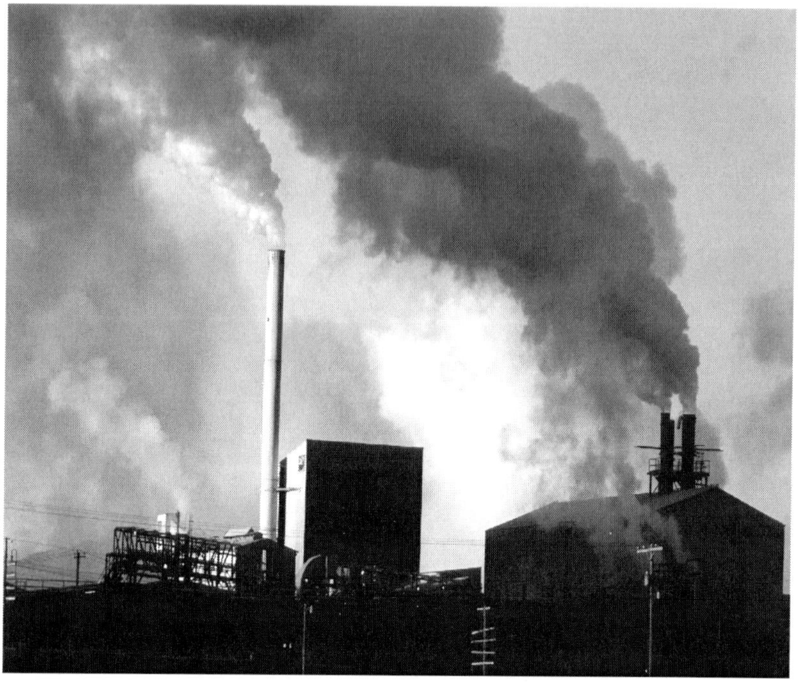

What could possibly go wrong with the noxious waste that is spewing forth from the smokestacks in this stock photo? Well, let's see: Aside from polluting the atmosphere, generating a disgusting eyesore, and negatively affecting the health of all living things that it touches, how about the truths that human exposure to these industrial poisons has been found in several Scientific Studies to be a confirmed risk factor for developing certain forms of Cancer (14,000 Americans die each year from Coal Pollution alone). But, as cancerous as pollution is, it is not alone: Job contacts with harmful chemicals, dusts, and fumes; personal habits such as tobacco and alcohol use; lifestyle behaviors that include exposure to intense sun without protection, or not taking care of one's oral health; transference of a virus during unprotected sex; bacterial infections; and, unhealthy eating and lack of physical exercise, can all contribute to the formation of this dreadful disease. Finally, as if that is not enough, let's add a few more culprits into the mix, such as one's age and gender, and their ethnicity and heredity. There, that ought to do it – right? Not exactly. Even if an individual escapes all of the Cancer-causing threats that life directs their way, there is always that wildest of Wild Cards, Random Chance, that can throw a wrench in the works. But, please, whatever you do, don't let all of this worry you. Studies find that Stress can also cause Cancer.

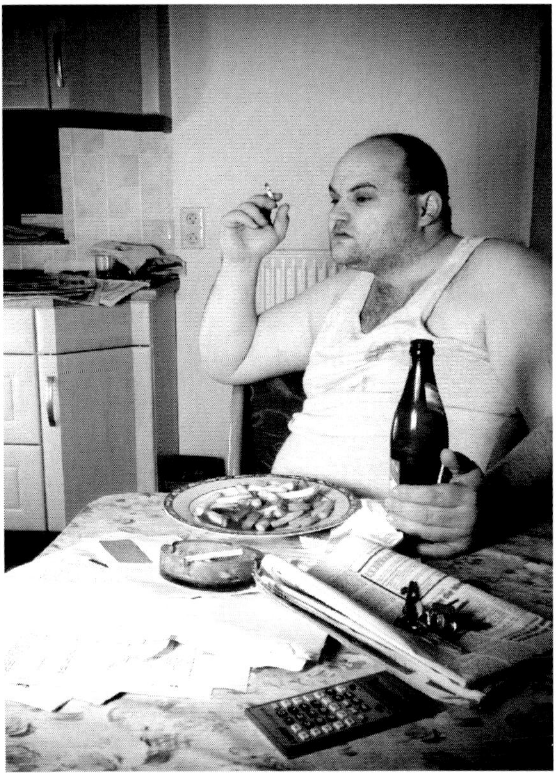

The poor gentleman in this stock photo is a Cancer occurrence (or a Heart Attack) waiting to happen. Or, knowing how wacky life can be at times, he may live to be 100 years old! But, seriously, this person is obese (Strike 1); he is sedentary and doesn't exercise (Strike 2); he drinks alcohol (Strike 3); he smokes cigarettes (Strike 4); and, as evidenced by the French fries on the plate and his portly midsection, he eats fatty, salty, unhealthy foods (Strike 5). You may be thinking to yourself that I personify the exact contradiction to this man, and yet, Cancer still got my number. Yes, that's unfortunately true, but, as I alluded to above, life will sometimes throw us curveballs. There is no telling what caused my Cancer, as I have always taken splendid care of my body. But, ***we are aware,*** *based on Medical Studies, that drinking alcohol, using tobacco, eating harmful foods, being obese, and not exercising, are proven risk factors in both men and women for contracting various forms of Cancer. Several things in life are uncontrollable (thanks again to Random Chance and other factors), but, several activities* ***are*** *within our control, including our personal behaviors. Why, then, roll the dice on these when we don't have to?*

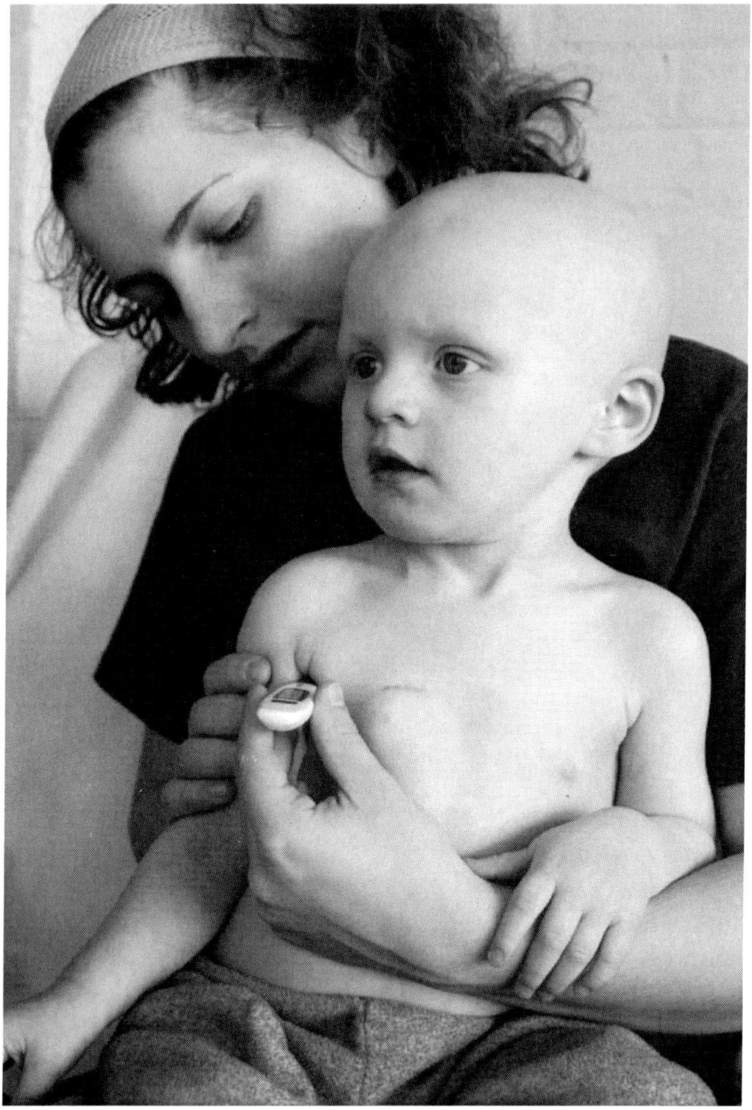

What kind of an evildoer would mess with a child such as the young, innocent patient in this stock photo? Well, Cancer would. Yes, sadly, Studies find that almost 160,000 children, globally, from birth to 19-years old, will be diagnosed each year with some form of Cancer. Of these, about 12,400 will be in the U.S. This equates to approximately one in 300 American boys, and one in 333 American girls, who will get the disease. Thankfully, though, due to major strides in detection and treatment, the overall childhood Cancer survival rate is ~80%! Note the Mediport incision in the right side of this little guy's chest.

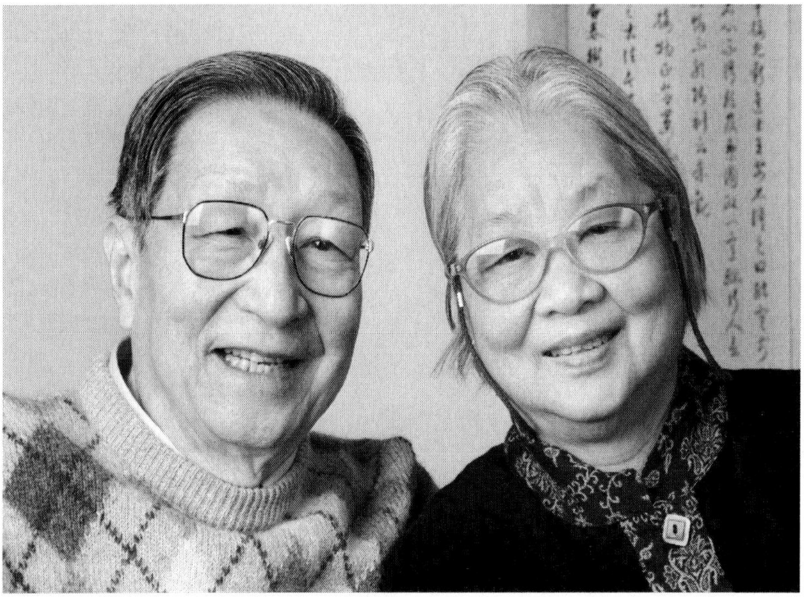

Generally speaking, most Cancer incidence statistics suck big-time. Not to discourage the Reader, but, the truth of the matter (based on Medical Studies), is that one in every three Women may come down with some form of Cancer during their lifetimes. Of course, not to be outdone, Men have strived their damndest to beat the female rate, which they ***have*** *achieved, but, all too successfully: 50% of men (an average of 1 out of 2!) may contract this most despicable disease at some point during* ***their*** *lives. So, yes, I would wholeheartedly agree that this eye-opening information blows. But, wait, there's more... In the rarified coalition of Head and Neck Cancers (the form of Cancer that I had), if you're a White male over 50, you may want to be extra observant for such an offender. That's right, one's age, gender, and race are known risk factors for some Head and Neck Cancers, but, as one might expect, using tobacco and drinking alcohol are the* ***key*** *contributors. And, as peculiar as it may sound, transference of HPV (Humanpapillomavirus) during unprotected sex is also a root of my particular form of Cancer (Cancer at the Base of the Tongue). Since I've always taken superb care of my body, and, because I did not use tobacco or drink alcohol, you be the judge. But, enough negativity. The couple in this stock photo is smiling because they just found out that there is a 75% average combined survival rate for adult Cancer patients, and that there are now 13.7 million Cancer survivors in the U.S.* ***Always remember: The earlier you treat – the easier to beat.***

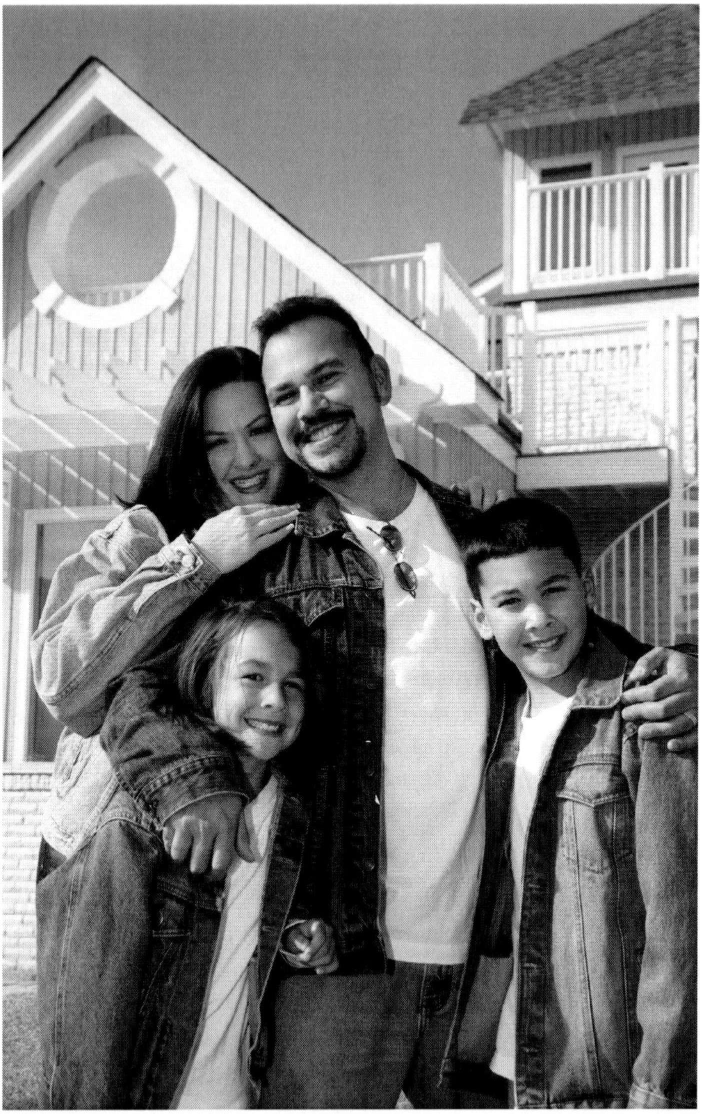

When a man, woman, young child or teenager is diagnosed with Cancer, it is very crucial for the family to maintain an "all-for-one" type of unity to love, encourage, and support their patient-in-need. And, it is also really meaningful—after Diagnosis, but before Treatment, and, if time and doctors will allow—that the family take some time together to enjoy a very special get-away before the hectic, seemingly non-stop activities begin. Once the Treatments and potential Side Effects initiate, there is no telling when the family will be able to do "normal," fun things again.

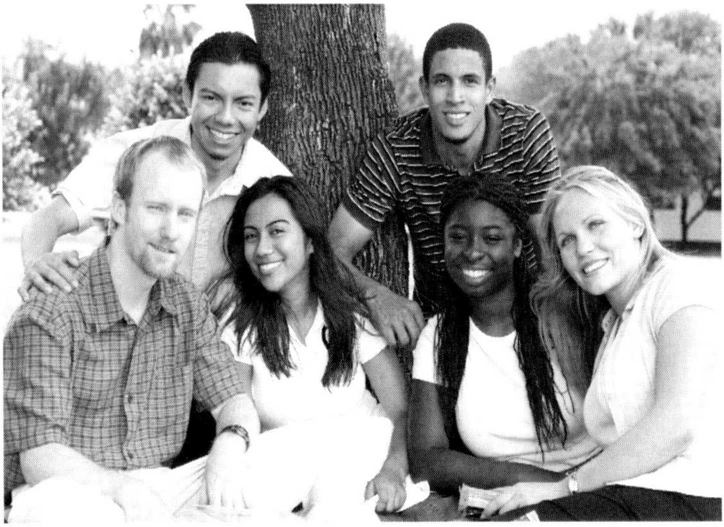

With the possible exception of a Wedding, a Birthday, the Birth of a Baby, or, a Retirement (all fun, happy times), there are few moments in life that will "rally the troops" quite like a family member's or a friend's Diagnosis of Cancer. Definitely, there is nothing to rejoice on such a somber occasion—as one might for the other celebratory events—but, without question, there is strength in numbers, which the Cancer victim will know and sense when their loved ones, family members, and friends all gather around. A Cancer diagnosis is very tough for any person to receive, but, the news of the medical finding can be equally as surprising and scary for those who are close to the individual. Because of this, it can be awkward for some friends, co-workers, school-mates, and, even for some family members, to know exactly what to say or do for the new Cancer patient. That is to be expected, though, as there is no "right" or "wrong" way to express one's sorrow upon hearing the news, while simultaneously trying to communicate their love, prayers, and positive thoughts. The Cancer package comes complete with both good and bad, and happy and sad, and the new patient will soon start to realize that no matter how low the "lows" become, the "highs," provided by their loved ones, family, and friends, will grant them the physical and mental strength to give their Cancer the fight of its life. During my Cancer ordeal, I was very fortunate to have been blessed with loving, thoughtful, and caring family members, friends, and co-workers, who all offered me encouragement and so much else every step of the way. I will always be thankful for their kindness, and for them helping me save my life.

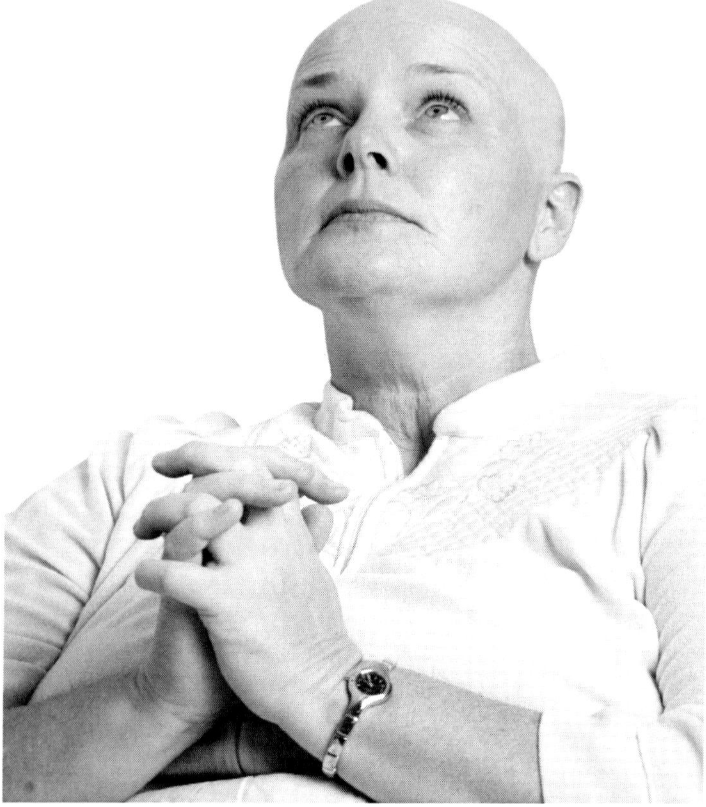

Every Cancer Patient and Survivor, being distinctive, one-of-a-kind individuals, will handle the entire Cancer experience—including the Diagnosis, Treatments, any Side Effects, and their Recovery—unlike any other Cancer Warrior. To some, it may be an inconvenience, but to others, it may seem like a never-ending nightmare. Because all of us are wired differently from birth, and, since all Cancer cases vary from person-to-person, there is no sure way of knowing how we will respond when, and after, we receive the fateful news. But, one thing ***for certain*** *is that each patient will draw upon the faith and strength that is inherent in their heart and soul to survive. It matters not how each patient chooses to will themselves to succeed in their personal war with Cancer. What does matter—at least it did with me—is that we always hope and trust in ourselves and those fighting for our life.*

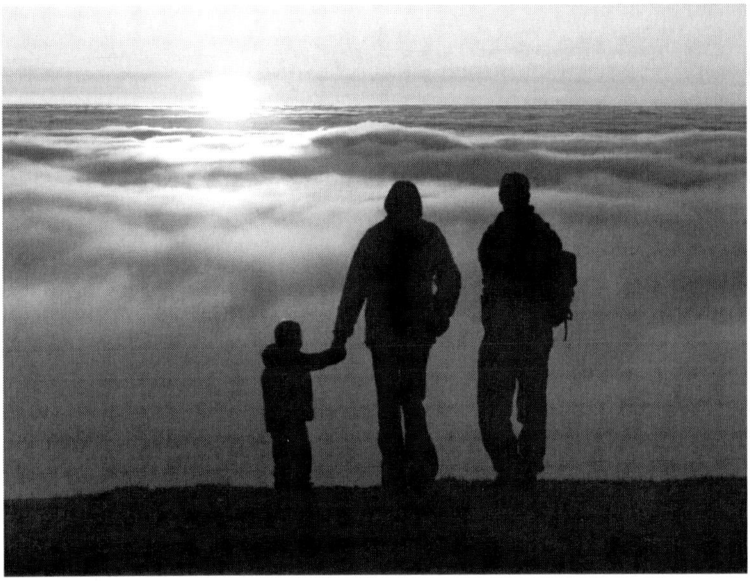

"Every dark cloud has its Silver Lining." These encouraging words were first expressed by John Milton, the 17th Century English Author and Poet. Thankfully, this same sentiment holds true for most brave Cancer patients as they slowly, but surely, navigate their individual Cancer journeys from Diagnosis to hopeful Survivorship. The "dark clouds," when speaking of Cancer, are the shocking and threatening facts that all Cancers are potentially deadly, and, that the patient's sometimes lengthy and difficult Cancer-killing program will often be plagued with unjust feelings of doubt, discomfort, and distress. And, let's also add to that the patient's scary thoughts about an uncertain future, and their worries that even should they survive, their Cancer might return to haunt them someday. All of these concerns are very real and justifiable, and, believe me, I had them all. But, thankfully, this is where the "silver linings" come in to hopefully save the day. To begin, the Cancer patient will be surrounded and encouraged by the love, support, prayers and hope offered by their family members, their loved ones, and their friends. The patient will also be very well taken care of by their skillful Medical Team, who will use the latest and greatest Cancer-killing equipment and medications in an effort to safely remove the Cancer and save the patient's life. And, finally, the greatest "silver lining" is the Cancer patient, themselves. For it is the man, woman, teen, or young child affected by this horrendous disease who has been naturally equipped with the God-given will to survive. It is their strength that will help blow the dark clouds away.

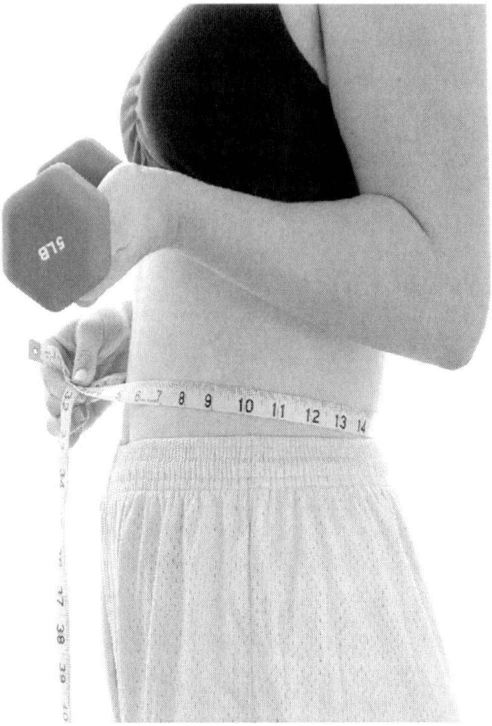

I am living proof that just because a person exercises, eats healthy, isn't overweight, doesn't use tobacco or drink alcohol, and doesn't swim in a pool of toxic waste, it does not render them immune to the possibility of contracting Cancer at some point during their life. But, as Scientific Studies have found, doing all of the "good" things, and avoiding all of the "bad" things, can surely improve one's chances of not instigating a Cancer occurrence. So, with this in mind, it has also been medically proven that an investment in any level of fitness and exercise can offer huge returns in terms of better health, longer life, and, in the important ability to heal and mount a strong "come-back" if ever faced with a big physical or mental challenge, such as Cancer. If a child or adult, male or female, is able to exercise, and, if a health care professional approves, it can be extremely beneficial for them to do something – from walking or jogging, to yoga, biking, weight-lifting, or other healthy activities. For Cancer patients, as in my case, exercising prior to getting Cancer, exercising after Cancer treatments have ended (with approval of doctors), and, continuing to work out as a matter of course, will not only serve to strengthen the body and assist the overall healing process, but, it will also provide the survivor with self-confidence to get their new life back on-track.

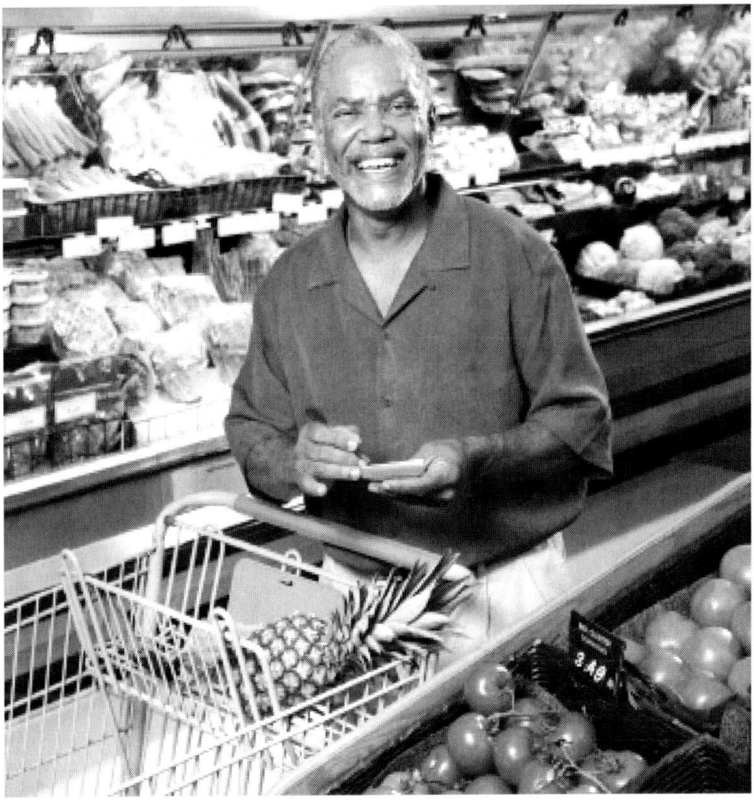

Many people, young and old, give food quite a lot of attention. But, unfortunately, in many cases, the healthful value of that food may be the last thing on their mind. This lack of concern about good quality nutrition might be acceptable for the average person; however, for a Cancer patient, it is vital that they eat and drink healthy foods and fluids that will help them maintain their all-important body-weight, physical strength, and emotional endurance. Cancer Therapies, Side Effects, and a demanding, wearisome schedule can wreak havoc on any Cancer patient, but, especially on younger children and elders. As such, all Cancer patients should repeatedly consume the proper quantity and quality of nutrients to strengthen and fuel their bodies and minds during their tough Cancer journey. I had a heck of a time consuming any nutrients due to constant nausea and the raw pain in my mouth and throat caused by Chemo and Radiation Therapy. As a result, I lost roughly 50 lbs. of hard-earned body-weight. But, after my mind persuaded my body to force down high-calorie, nutritious shakes and foods each day, I was able to remain vigorous enough to continue with my treatments, and, thankfully, to conquer my Cancer.

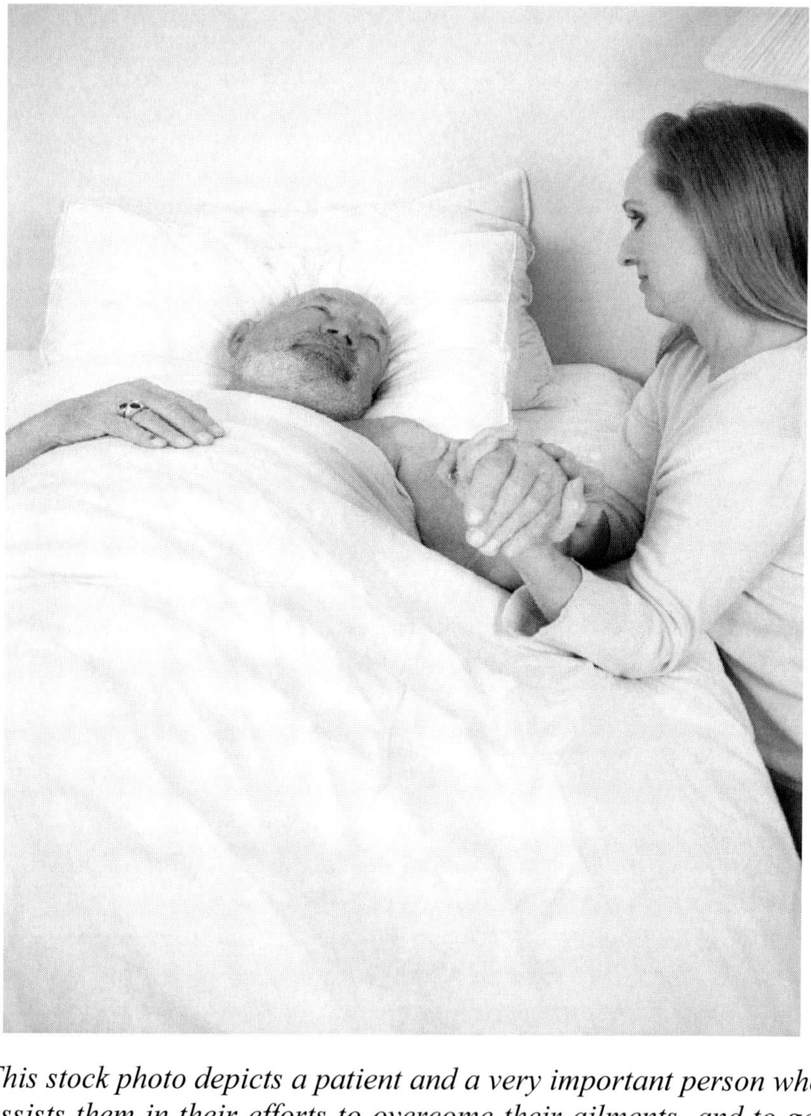

This stock photo depicts a patient and a very important person who assists them in their efforts to overcome their ailments, and to get them back on the road to recovery – their Caregiver. For a Cancer patient, their Caregiver is the voluntary attendant who encourages, assists, and guides them through the entire journey from Diagnosis to hopeful Survivorship. This selfless individual devotes a portion of their own life to help support the patient's, and in so-doing, the Cancer Caregiver not only experiences much of the same pain and challenges as does the patient, but, they also will realize the same successes and victories. The Cancer Caregiver is an unsung hero of the Cancer wars, and they must be appreciated for their efforts.

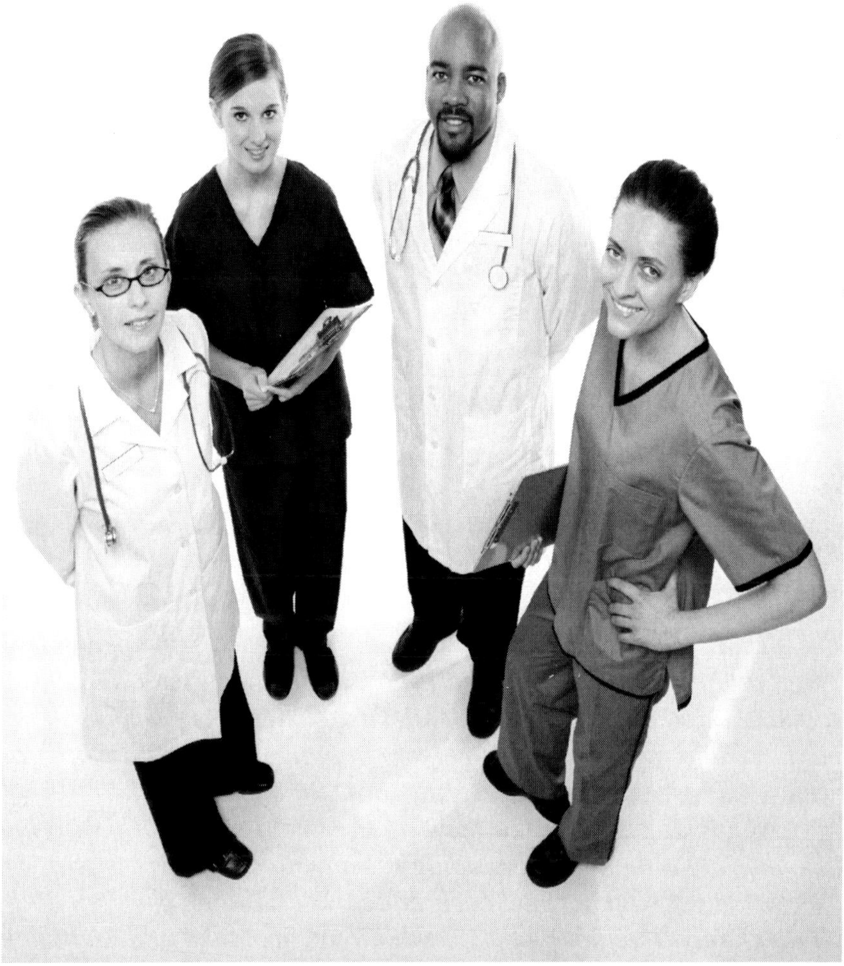

There is no question that the strength, the will, and the faith of the Cancer patient are very significant factors in helping to bring about a favorable Cancer outcome. And, undoubtedly, the loving support of family, friends, and the Caregiver are vital as well to the patient during their battles to conquer the disease. But, equally as crucial in helping to facilitate a successful Cancer result are the use of state-of-the art equipment, powerful medicines, and the knowledge, skill, and compassion of the patient's Medical Team. It is the physicians, nurses, and other specialists, such as those represented in this stock photo, that will do everything within their power to help the patient defeat their Cancer, and do it by the best and safest means possible.

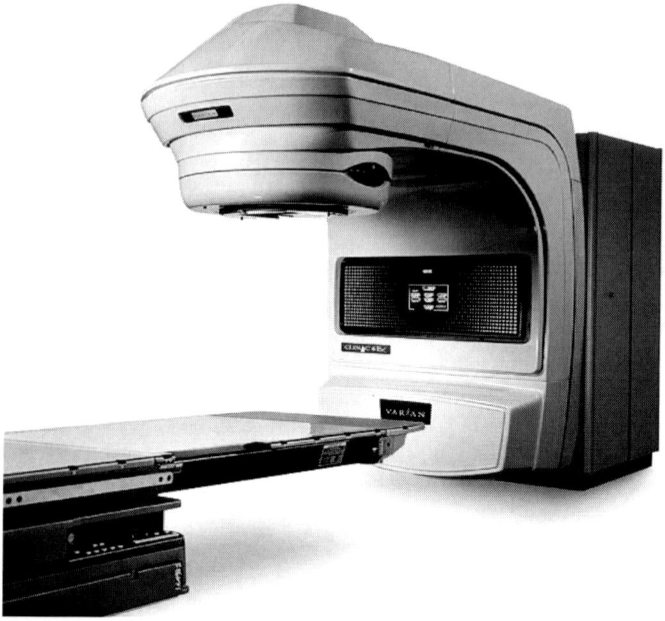

This is an illustration of a massive piece of medical equipment used in Radiation Therapy called the IMRT, which stands for "Intensity Modulated Radiotherapy." This IMRT machine is very similar to the one that I laid beneath for roughly 30 minutes, five days a week, for seven weeks (see accompanying photo of Radiation Therapy Mask). The IMRT is a comparatively new and painless means of delivering Radiotherapy to patients, including those with Cancer. As was the case with my Radiotherapy, each patient's Radiation Therapy Plan is individually developed by the Radiation Oncologist and Radiation Physicist, and the ensuing software instructions are what guides the machine to precisely deliver the radiation from numerous angles in smaller doses to the target – the Cancer Tumor and marginal tissue. The IMRT machine operates much like a filter and shapes the three-dimensional radiation beams to the size and contours of the tumor. These exact beams keep the radiation distribution tightly controlled, avoiding damage to as much healthy tissue as possible. Because of the correctness of the IMRT, it can treat difficult-to-reach Tumors in areas such as the spine, head, neck, prostate, lung, liver, and brain. Dosimetrists and Diagnostic Radiology Technicians ensure that the dosages of radiation are being properly and safely delivered to the Cancer patient to minimize Side Effects and maximize effectiveness.

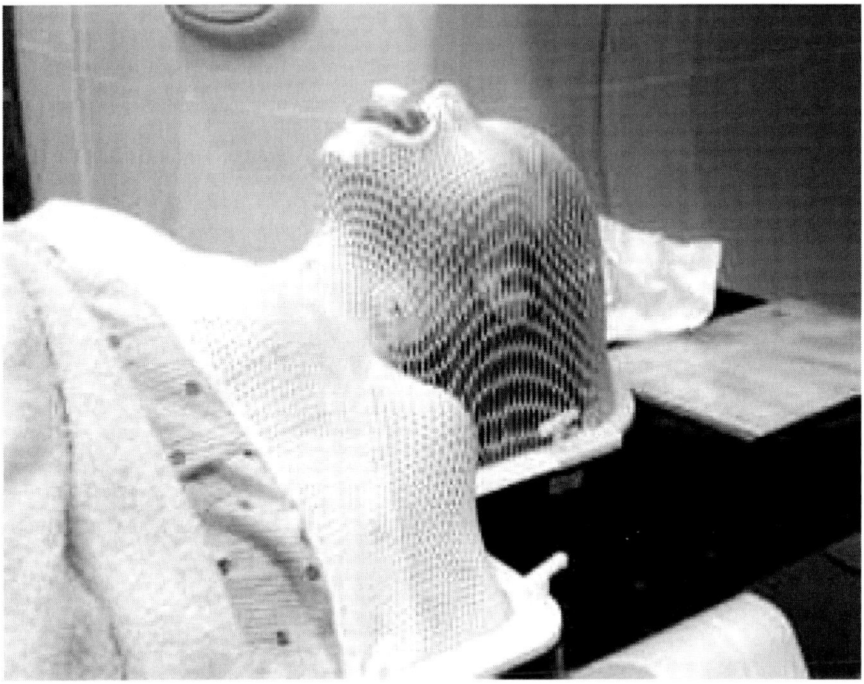

No, this is not a photo from a Frankenstein horror movie. This is a real-life photo of a Cancer patient just about to be given Radiation Therapy treatment to the head or neck area. This is the exact type of mesh mask that I had to "wear" during my ½-hour-long, Mon. thru Fri. Radiation Therapy treatments from July 14, 2004 to September 2, 2004. This mask is made of a substance that is softened in warm water, then molded to the patient's head and neck areas, with extra mesh for the patient's head and shoulders where it is gathered under a clamping mechanism. While the mask is being created, the patient lies motionless for just about 30 minutes, until the plastic cools and becomes stiff. During the patient's ensuing Radiation Treatments, the patient will lie on the treatment table and have their mask (with head, neck, and shoulders inside) snuggly clamped to the table. The principal purpose of the mask is to keep the patient's head and neck completely stationary while the Radiation Therapy apparatus directs the high-powered beams accurately to the desired target area: The Patient's Primary Tumor. Any movement of the patient while this is taking place could dramatically influence the success of the Cancer treatments, and could endanger the patient. The patient is given a plastic "sucker" through the "mouth hole" to help keep their saliva moving. What I found most frustrating were the darned nose itches!

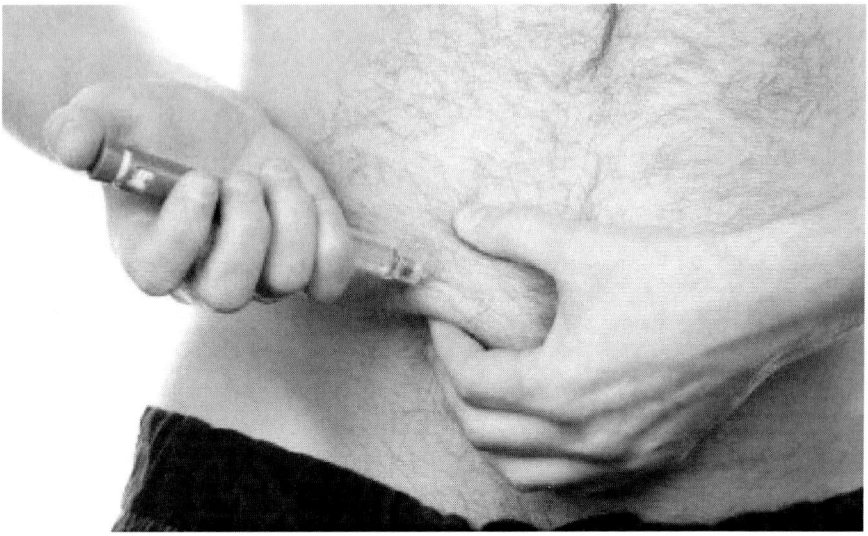

This illustration shows a man injecting himself sub-cutaneously (just beneath the skin in the abdomen) with some form of medication. I similarly self-administered a drug, named Amifostine®, with medical supervision, prior to some of my daily Radiation Therapy sessions. I first found out about Amifostine in 2004, while conducting research on Radiation Therapy prior to my earliest meetings with physicians on my Medical Team. Amifostine is a Protectant Agent that can be used in combination with Chemotherapy and Radiation Therapy. It is approved by the Food and Drug Administration (FDA) to prevent Kidney damage induced by some Chemo drugs in patients who have certain Cancers. It is FDA-approved as well, for patients with Head and Neck Cancer who receive Radiation Therapy after Surgery, just as I did. In this application, Amifostine helps decrease Radiation damage to the Salivary Glands, which could induce a lack of Saliva production and cause Dry Mouth, or Xerostomia. That condition, of course, could lead to possible eating issues and major dental health problems. I listened to the horror stories of people in my Head and Neck Cancer Support Groups who had received Radiation Therapy without protection, and saw that they had to drink water non-stop to keep their mouths wet. After seeing this and learning about the drug, I asked my first Oncologist if I could use it. He told me, "Probably not, because it's very costly." I told him, "If it will save my Salivary Glands, what better reason to approve it?" My insistence paid off, because the drug was authorized for me, and I became the very first Cancer patient at that hospital to use it. Now, I've . . . ***Got Spit!***

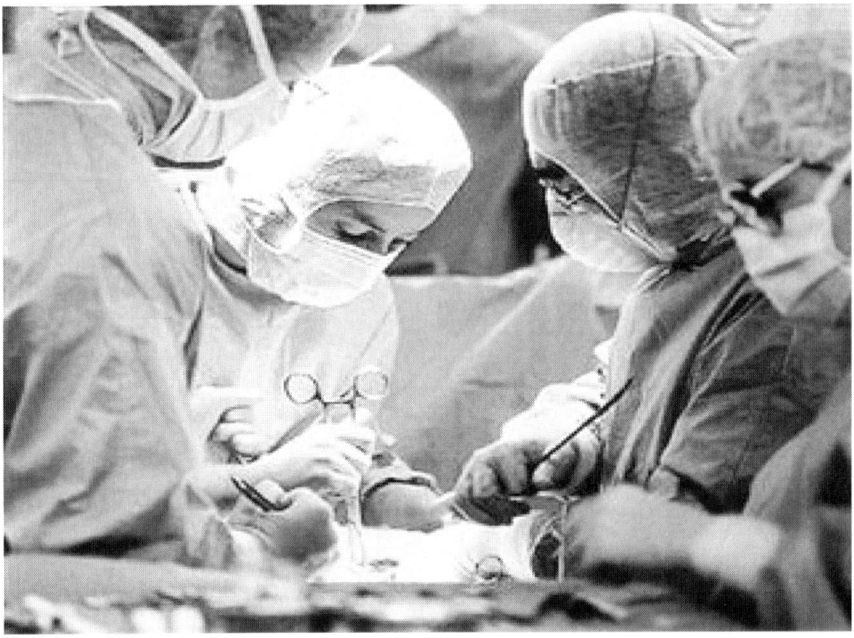

Above is a stock photo of Surgeons doing what they do – repairing things, removing things, restoring things, and assisting patients with all sorts of medical issues to hopefully reclaim their lives. For those patients diagnosed with many forms of Cancer, Surgery is one of the "go-to" Treatments that is used by the patient's Medical Team in an effort to safely and completely remove Cancerous Tumors and cells from the patient's body. In fact, since the late 19th century, Surgery has been regularly carried out for the treatment of several forms of Cancer, and in some cases, it is the ***only*** *form of therapy needed and performed. Generally speaking, Cancer Surgery involves the cutting away and elimination of diseased, unwanted, or sample tissues, but it isn't an option in every case. If the Cancer tumor is still localized (has not spread elsewhere within the body), it may be possible with Surgery to completely take out the tumor and any nearby, potentially affected tissue (i.e., the "margins"), thereby "curing" the patient's Cancer. On the other hand, Surgery might not be a viable option for blood-borne Cancers such as Leukemia, if the Cancer has spread to other areas of the body away from the Primary Site of the tumor, or, if the tumor cannot be safely eradicated without possible damage to vital organs. In addition to me receiving numerous Biopsy Surgeries and a Lymphadenectomy (removal of neck Lymph Nodes), I had a very successful Surgery to remove the residual Tumor on my tongue.*

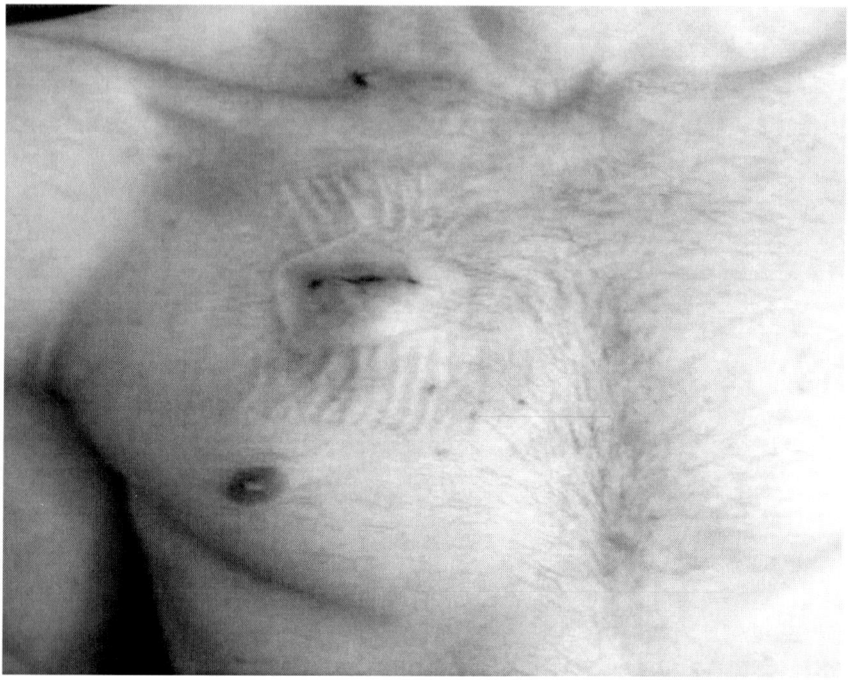

I hope that the above picture does not make the Reader feel "icky," but, this sight is something that most Cancer patients who are given Chemotherapy will become well-acquainted with – male or female, child, teen, or adult. Pictured above is a Mediport that was recently surgically inserted beneath the patient's skin in their chest. A doctor surgically connects the metal/plastic/rubber Mediport to one of the large veins within the chest using a catheter tube. The purpose of the temporary device is to permit the convenient, sterile, and recurrent drawing of blood, and, the infusion of powerful Chemo medications into the port, using a special needle. With the Mediport, the patient doesn't have to continually undergo the possible fear and pain (not to mention, bruises) of being repetitively "stuck" with the standard needle in veins of the arm or hand. To use an analogy, the Mediport could be viewed as a "tap," in which needles are inserted to permit the flow of fluids, both into, and out of, the body. The Mediport is flushed with a blood thinner once a week while it is in use, and once a month when it is not being used. The device will generally stay in place for a considerable time after Chemotherapy has concluded for the drawing of blood samples, and in case additional Chemotherapy is required. My Mediport turned out to be worth its weight in gold, because it was used constantly both during and after my treatments.

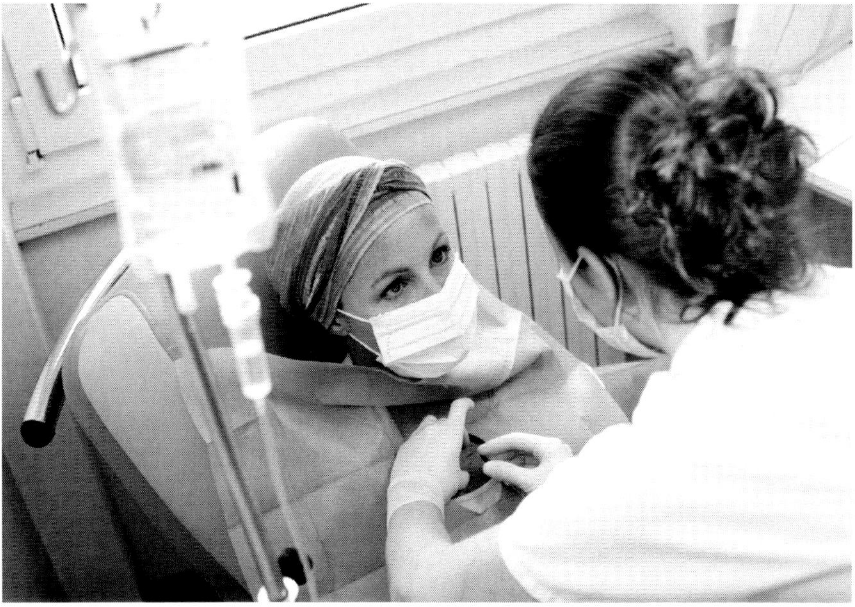

Ah, yes – good ole' Chemotherapy, or, Chemo, as it is often called. Chemotherapy is one of the most powerful weapons in the patient's and Medical Team's arsenal that is used in the, hopeful, life-saving battle against various forms of Cancer. All cells in the human body divide as part of the cell renewal process, but most Cancerous cells divide relatively speedily—and very abnormally—which makes them especially vulnerable to many of the 300+ different types of Chemo medications. Chemotherapy drugs, many of which are derived from natural plant sources, have been developed, tested, and employed by doctors since—believe it or not—the drugs evolved from the use of Mustard Gas by the Germans in World War II. Chemotherapy can be administered through a vein into the bloodstream via a Mediport (as pictured above); injected into a body cavity; delivered orally to the patient in the form of a pill; or, applied topically atop the skin, depending upon which drugs are used. Generally, Chemo treatment does not involve using a singular Cancer medication, but, instead, a combination of medications—"Chemo Cocktails"—that are custom-formulated for particular Cancer-killing purposes for each patient. My "Cocktail" was a mixture of two extremely powerful drugs that I found during my research to be especially effective against my form of Cancer, which, thankfully, it was. While receiving Chemo for 7 weeks, from July 2004 to Aug. 2004, I temporarily lost some of my eyelashes and eyebrows, but I did retain all of the hair on my head!

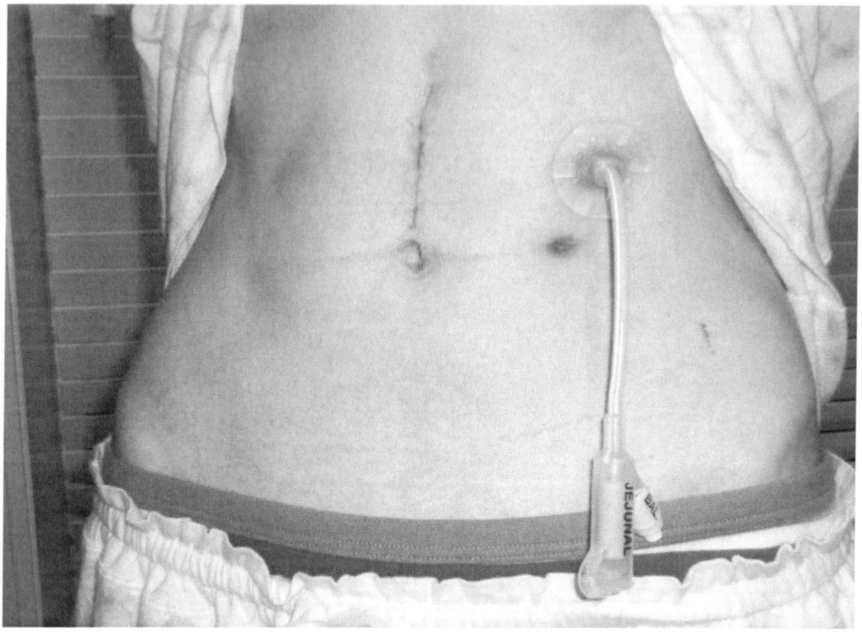

This stock photo shows a woman who has had a ***Jejunostomy*** *Tube inserted into her small intestines via an incision made on the outside of her body. This type of tube is a little different than a* ***Gastrostomy*** *Tube (inserted into the stomach), and is used for long-term Enteral (non-mouth) feeding for several weeks, months, or, even, years. This external means of delivering nutrition to Cancer patients is normally recommended by applicable members of the patient's Medical Team for those who are not able to meet their complete nutritional needs with normally-consumed foods and beverages. If the Cancer patient has had invasive treatments to the neck, throat, and mouth (as do many Head and Neck Cancer patients), or other areas, that prohibit normal injestion of foods due to pain, inflammation, or loss of use, these patients might be prescribed tubefeedings to ensure that their bodies are receiving the obligatory quantities of nutrients, calories, and water to maintain their health, strength, and bodyweight. I did not use a Feeding Tube despite the unfathomable throat and mouth pain I experienced for months while attempting to eat, as a result of my Chemo and Radiation Therapy. My Oncologist chose not to use the Tube with me due to possible infection issues. A fellow Head and Neck Cancer friend of mine* **did use** *the Feeding Tube to assist him through the tough times, but, unfortunately, he was not able to learn how to swallow again. So, he could only "eat" by using the Tube.*

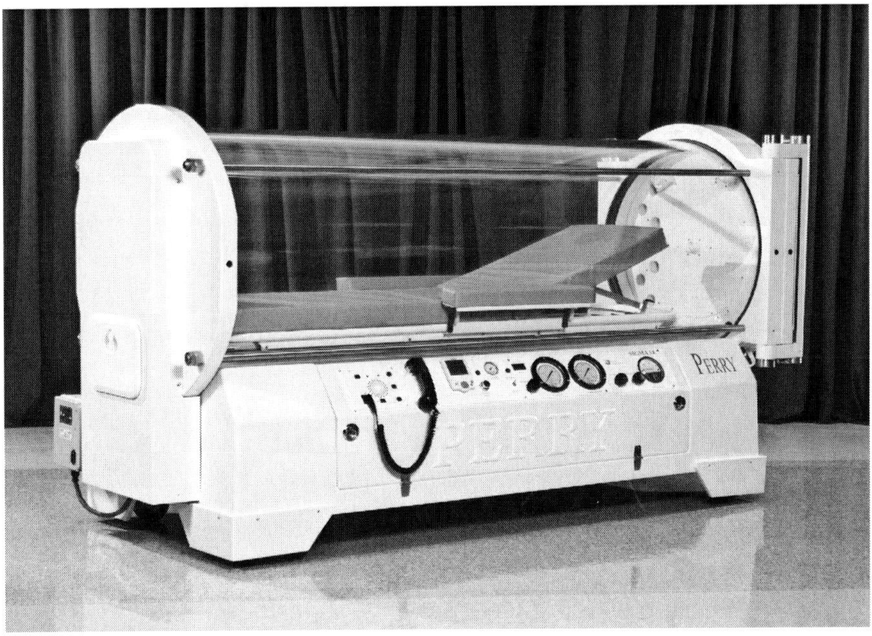

Above is a Hyperbaric Oxygen Chamber, almost identical to the one in which I spent over 2 hours a day for 40 days, from April 27, 2005, to July 13, 2005. A Hyperbaric Oxygen Chamber is a shatterproof pressure chamber (quite similar to those used by Deep Sea Divers to prevent them from experiencing the "bends" when resurfacing) that is designed to force patients to breathe pure Oxygen at higher than normal "Atmospheres." This allows the blood level of Oxygen to be substantially increased, thereby rising tissue Oxygen saturation and promoting healing and helping to eliminate infections. When Head and Neck Cancer patients, such as myself, receive direct Radiation Therapy in the proximity of the Lower Jaw Bone (Mandible), or, to the Upper Jaw Bone (Maxilla), not only do the targeted Cancer cells get destroyed, but any healthy tissue directly in the field of radiation can also become damaged. The very unfortunate Side Effect of this treatment can cause Osteonecrosis of the Jaw (ONJ), which means, "Death of the Jaw Bone." The blood flow restriction and localized bone destruction caused by radiation leads to poorly nourished bone that will typically respond unsatisfactorily to infection, trauma, and wounds, including any tooth extractions and Periodontal Surgery. Therefore, when a Cancer patient receives Radiation Therapy near the jaw bones, they ***MUST*** *receive Hyperbaric Oxygen Treatment to stimulate new blood flow* ***BEFORE*** *they have any dental work done.*

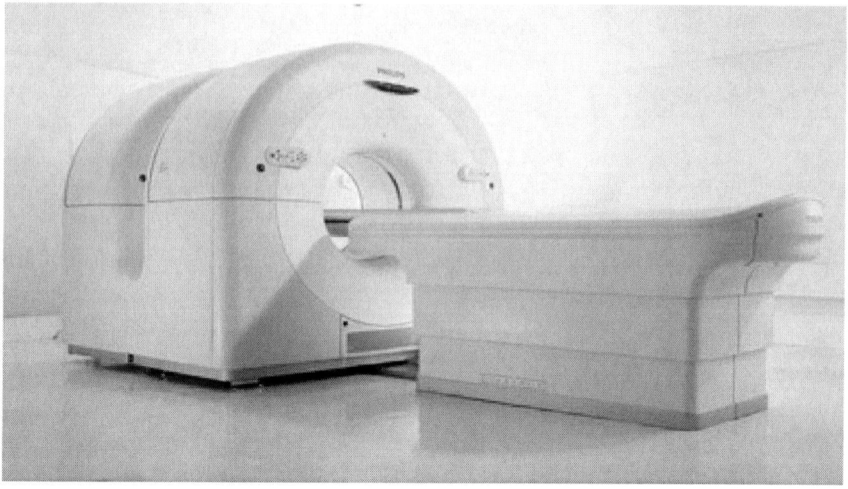

This machine, known as the Positron Emission Tomography (PET) scanner, is not used for Cancer Treatments, but, is utilized for pre- and post-treatment testing in an effort to help determine if there are malignant Cancer cells in the patient's body. It is a very fascinating process: At specialized PET Treatment Centers, the Cancer patient receives an intravenous injection of a Radioactive Glucose (sugar), after which they will rest quietly and comfortably for about an hour. This time period permits the Glucose to travel throughout the body's circulatory system, and allows the patient to calmly relax. After the resting period, the patient is escorted to the scanning room where they will lie down on the scanner table for 15-35 minutes. The table and the patient will pass slowly through the PET scanner, acquiring several sets of images. The procedure is painless and has no Side Effects. The images are interpreted by a qualified Nuclear Medicine Physician or Radiologist, and the results sent to the ordering doctor, who informs the patient. If there is possible malignant Cancer in the body, the Cancer cells will appear much brighter on the images than normal cells, which means that the Cancer cells are consuming the Glucose for energy. I participated in five post-treatment PET Scans, but, unfortunately, in 3 of the 5 Scans, my imagery showed bright "hot-spots," which looked to the Radiologist like cancerous activity. Of course, that terrified me to death, and meant that I had to have Tissue Biopsy Surgery of the suspected areas each time to confirm. Thankfully, all Biopsy results came back negative, which means they were "False Positives" – Scary and good news for a Cancer patient. My doctors attributed my "hot-spots" to the healing of healthy cells.

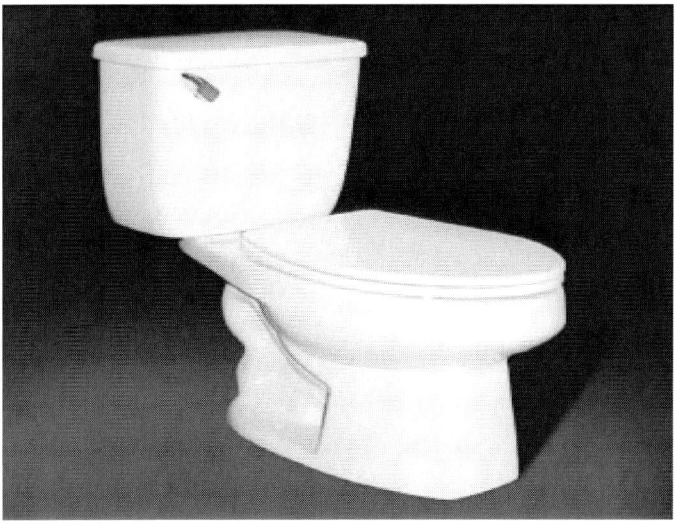

Most Readers should be familiar with this item of technology, known as the Therapeutic Optimized Internal Leftovers Elimination Throne (TOILET). While that terminology is definitely meant to be tongue-in-cheek, one may legitimately ask what a stock photo of a normal, everyday commode is doing in a book vis-à-vis Cancer. Well, please let me explain the method to my madness: If any Cancer patient is to receive Chemotherapy as part of their Treatment Plan, and if that Chemo is coupled with simultaneous Radiation Therapy, there is a high likelihood that the patient will be faced with the accompanying Side Effects of Nausea, Diarrhea, and possible Pain – at least for a period of time. When this occurs, as it did with me during my own Cancer ordeal, the toilet will become a very important appliance in the Cancer patient's life. Because the Chemo drugs affect the fast-dividing healthy cells lining the patient's Gastrointestinal Tract (in the attempt to kill the cancerous cells), the normal cells will become very irritated. This may cause Nausea, which may lead to persistent bouts of diarrhea as well as vomiting. As for the Side Effect of Pain, doctors will prescribe pain killers, as necessary, to help reduce any discomfort. But, any Opiate-based pain killers are a double-edged sword: While Opioids may work wonders in relieving pain, they can also be the ***Mother of all Constipation****. I found that out the "hard" way (pun intended) when I was taking 4-5 different Opioid drugs for my pain, and then tried one day to "give birth" to a "football." As if I wasn't in enough pain, that added insult to injury. I did finally get relief when my doctor prescribed a sugar-based laxative. Phew!*

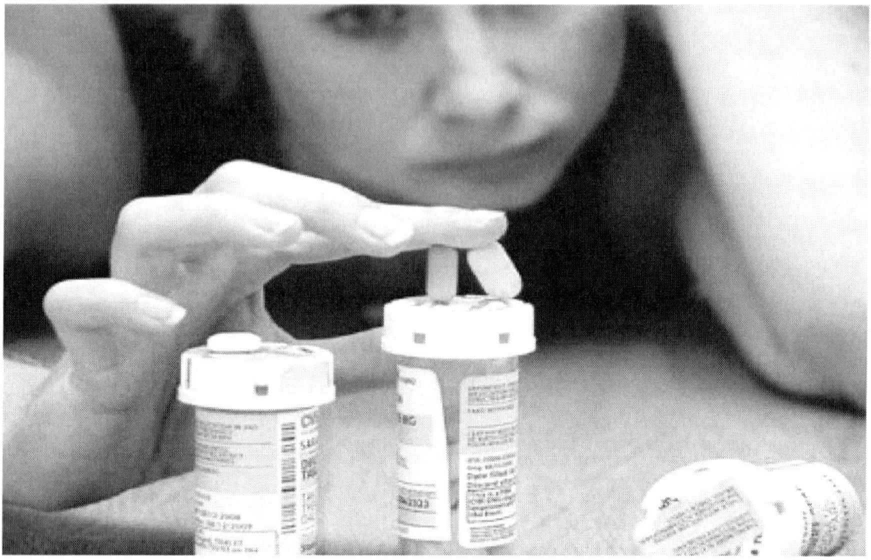

WARNING: Beware of the Prescription Painkiller Monster! *Above is a stock photograph that, regrettably, realistically depicts a major problem experienced by many patients, including Cancer patients – including me. Depending on the form of Cancer a person has and its location, and the form(s) of Treatment they receive and any Side Effects that ensue, the patient's Medical Team may prescribe one or more very powerful—and potentially addictive—Opiate-based drugs to help curb any pain and discomfort. Undeniably, such medications are unavoidable components of a patient's overall Cancer treatment plan if warranted, as they do provide necessary but temporary relief from extreme pain to the patient. God knows I needed all of the pain medications that I was on—typically 4 or 5 at any given time during and after my Treatments—simply to make it through each day. But, unbeknownst to me while I was taking them, my body was becoming dependent on the prescribed medications, which I immediately found out when my agonizing pain subsided and I attempted to discontinue their use. I then found myself in the midst of another type of painful discomfort: The anguish and sting of Opioid Drug Withdrawal. To make matters even worse, my prescribing physicians failed to help me, so I had to request the assistance of a Psychiatrist. He told me, "Doctors try to help, but they hand out pain pills like candy, and in so doing, they teach patients how to fly, but not how to land." The Psychiatrist entered me into a Detox program at a local hospital, and after one* *<u>very</u>* *long and horrible month, I ultimately broke free!*

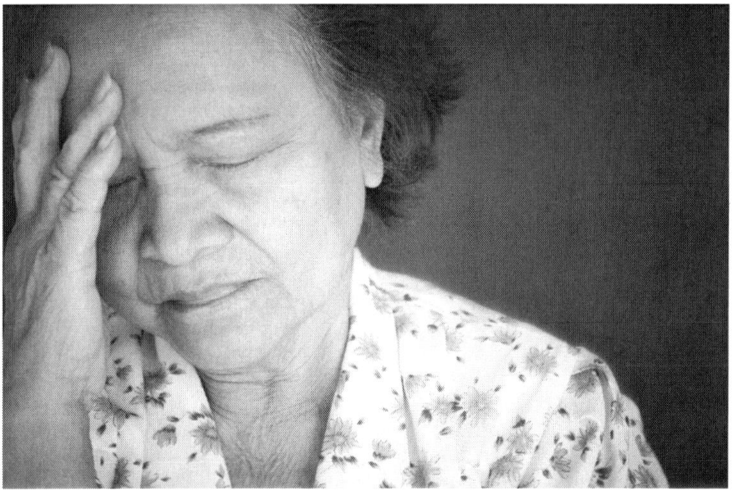

According to Studies, serious Depression impacts approximately 19 million Americans annually, and around 25% of all Cancer patients. Depression not only provokes suffering in those who are depressed, but it can also cause vast difficulties for their family and friends who often do not know how to help. I will personally vouch for all of the above. Immediately after my Cancer Diagnosis, I was very anxious and frightened, but, I don't believe that I was depressed. However, I had read many books, and listened to many of the sad stories told by some of the Cancer survivors in my Cancer Support Group, where it was communicated that serious Anxiety and Depression could often follow the Treatment Phase of an individual's Cancer journey. That is when all of the non-stop activities, appointments, treatments, and other medical commitments have started winding down, and is when the Cancer patient then has plenty of time (too much time!) to think about what had happened, and what their future may hold. It is this continuous speculating about how and why they "got" their Cancer, coupled with the relentless worrying about whether their Cancer is completely gone or if it will return, that can easily drive a Cancer patient into a downward depressive spiral. I know, because, I was sitting at the bottom of that spiral for two long years. I enlisted the services of a Psychotherapist to help me claw my way to the top and out of its clutches, which I did after learning that I was Cancer-free. Because each Cancer patient is different, there is no way of knowing how they will emotionally respond to their ordeal. But, if the going gets tough, they should seek the help of a professional. The physical pain of Cancer sucks; but the mental anguish can be just as ruthless.

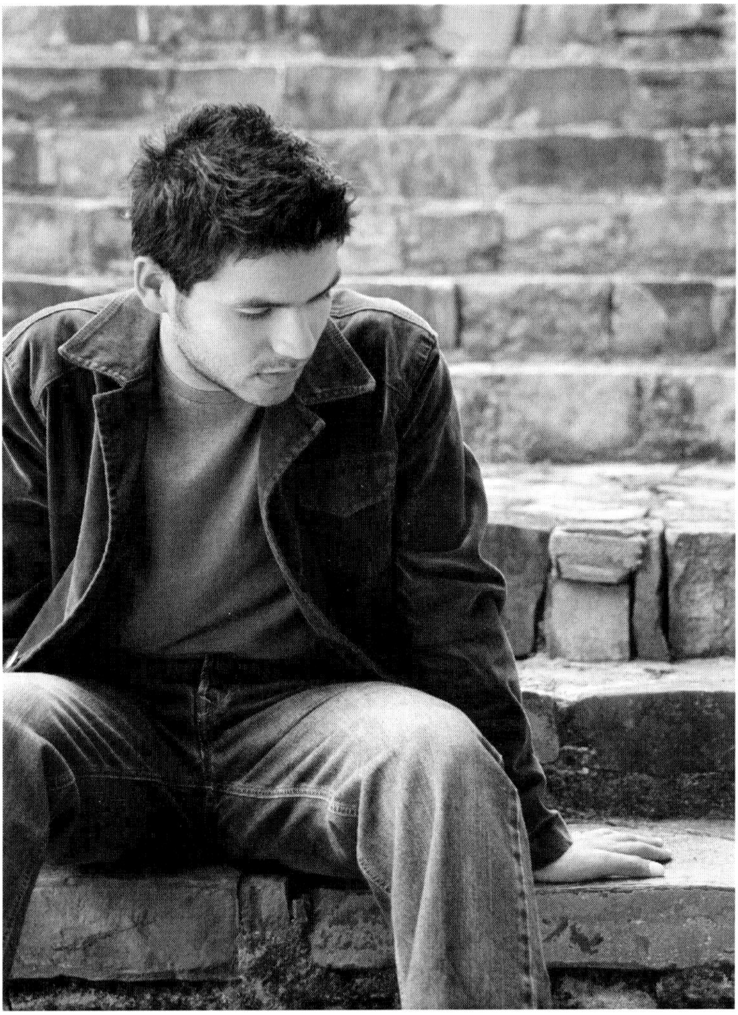

When a person has a loved one, family member, or a friend who has been diagnosed with Cancer, they may have a tendency to withdraw, or attempt to shoulder the burden alone. There will be sadness, to be sure, and many questions, doubts, and fears for what the future may hold. In these situations, whether the distraught individual is older or younger, such as the man in this stock photo, they must know that they are not on their own. There are many counseling services and Support Groups for loved ones and families of Cancer patients that are available through most Cancer Treatment Centers. Cancer can be hard enough on the patient, but, it can also wreak havoc on those who are near and dear to the patient. It is, after all, ***their*** *loved one that Cancer is messing with. They don't have to take it sitting down.*

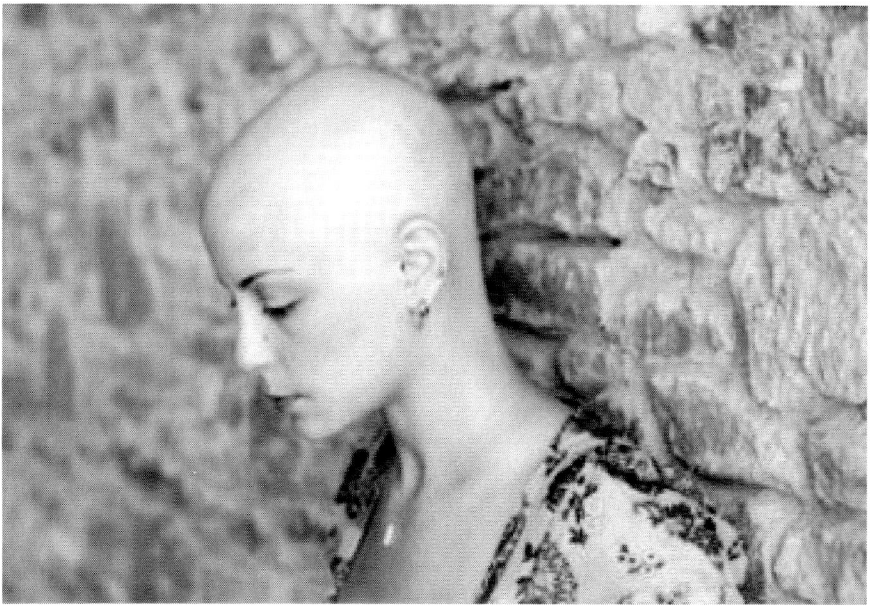

Not unlike a ferocious weather storm that blasts through a town and generates physical harm and emotional distress to many in its wake, Cancer treatment can create its own upsetting versions of a natural disaster to those who would cross in ***its*** *path. These therapy-related physical and mental ordeals, known as* ***Side Effects****, can be slight or severe, and short- or long-term, but, they are always indiscriminate, impacting many Cancer patients in some way – young or old, male or female, and healthy or not. There are no "one-size-fits-all" types of Side Effects, and their harshness—or lack thereof—can depend on a variety of factors, including the patient's overall health status, the form, Stage, and location of the patient's Cancer, the types of procedures used to address the Cancer, and, the actions taken by the Medical Team and patient to minimize or get rid of their negative influences. As strong and physically fit as I was prior to my Cancer treatments, about half-way through and afterwards, I got nailed with several Side Effects that tested my mettle, not the least of which were sickening nausea and extreme mouth and throat pain. I did kick one Side Effect's butt, however: I didn't lose any of my hair despite my super-powerful Chemotherapy drugs! Thankfully, my Side Effects were only temporary, as most are, and I eventually got my life back on-track after they subsided. For lack of a better way of putting it, Side Effects are a "necessary evil" of Cancer treatments, and, as disagreeable as they may be at times, they sure beat the alternative!*

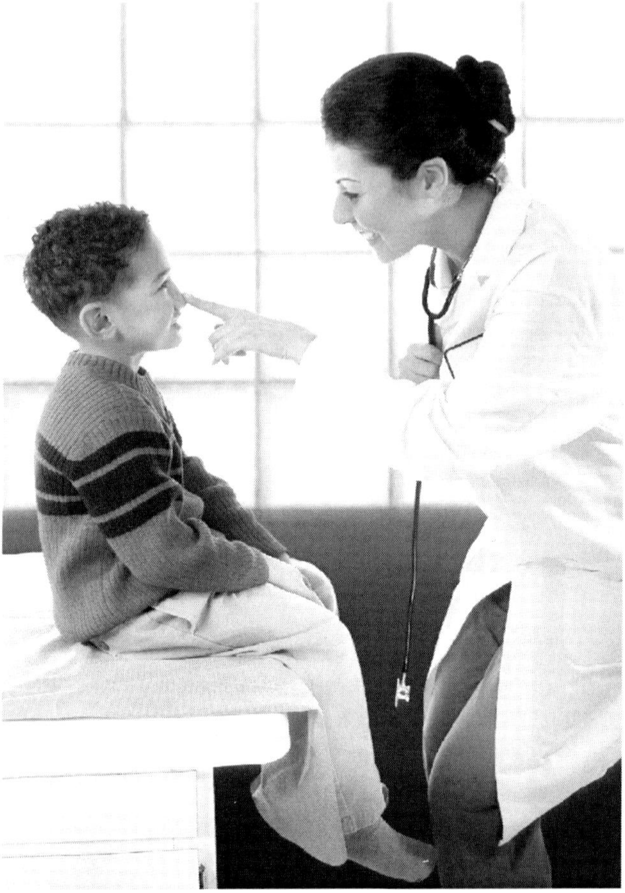

Following the termination of a man's, woman's, teen's, or a child's Cancer Treatments, the patient will typically transition into the next Phases of their Cancer journey: Recovery and Aftercare. Recovery is that all-important period when the patient's healing from any Side Effects will occur, but, unfortunately, is also when many after-effects will get worse before they get better. And, just as Recovery is a time for rest and recuperation, Aftercare is when a Cancer survivor will be regularly tested and monitored to verify that their Cancer is still gone, or, in rare cases, to identify any new or recurrent Cancers so that they can be treated as quickly and safely as possible. Typically, Aftercare monitoring will continue throughout the person's life, with more frequent visits during the first few years of survivorship, and a little less often as time passes by. My follow-up testing started with monthly visits, followed by every two, four, and six months, but now, as a 9+ year Cancer survivor, I have progressed to once each year!

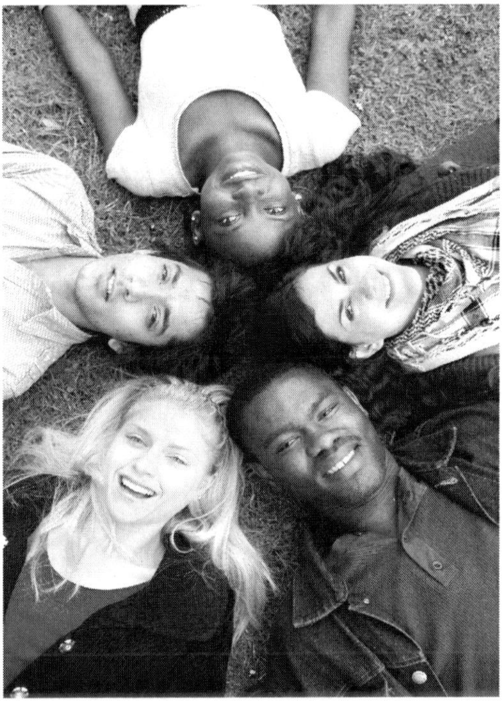

Can you imagine how magnificent this world would be without wars, without criminals, without racists, without bullies, without religious extremists, and, (I'll bite my tongue and exclude politicians) without deadly diseases such as Cancer? Well, regrettably, this is the world in which we now live, and these are the dangers that we all face. As we all know, however, there is strength in numbers in combating all of these threats to humanity, to our rights as human beings, and to our collective lives. When it comes to tackling the bane of Cancer, while it surely is a personal battle fought on a one-to-one basis by over 6 million people, worldwide, each year, Cancer is the common enemy of each of these Warriors. As such, all Cancer Patients and Survivors must know that they are not in this challenge alone. There have been millions who have travelled this way before us, and, there will be many more millions who will make this same journey in our footsteps. But, no matter the potential lethality of this disease, and, despite the numbers of innocent people that it needlessly attacks, at the very heart of this whole Cancer mess is that we all step up and do what we can to help each other survive. Unlike the many radical groups whose aim is to extinguish lives, the sole intent of the entire Cancer community is to save lives. Sometimes, it does take a village.

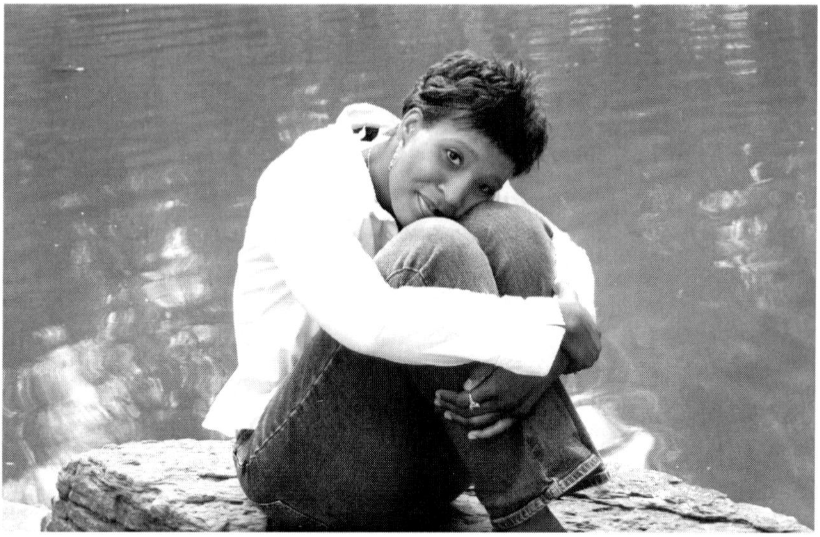

A Diagnosis of Cancer—not to mention the months, or, maybe, even years, of dealing with all of the many ups and downs that come with it—will seriously rock a person's world. And, depending upon many factors, as varied as each patient and their Cancer, the person may or may not come out of their Cancer-killing journey with a different way of looking at life. Some patients will have an optimistic and self-assured sense of contentment, perhaps, like the woman in this stock photo. In many instances, such survivors will go on with their post-Cancer lives almost as though nothing potentially deadly has taken place. Others may realize the significance of the bullet they dodged and will better appreciate life, and, perhaps, fulfill a "Bucket List." Or, the Cancer patients and survivors may realize a "New Normal" way of life in which their capabilities to rebound and return to their pre-Cancer lives may be thwarted by the distress and pain that they experienced before, during, or after their Treatments. These folks' New Normal might have them frightened to look around a corner for fear that the wicked Cancer monster is waiting to pounce upon them once again. Such individuals may never feel at peace or comfortable in their own skin evermore. And then, there will be several Cancer survivors, such as myself, who are a combination of the three – very thankful and content, but, also, fearful and ever-watchful. There is no telling how each Cancer patient will respond after all is said and done with the respective physical and emotional challenges of their personal Cancer experiences. But, one thing every Cancer survivor ***will know*** *is that around every corner, they will find Love and Hope.*

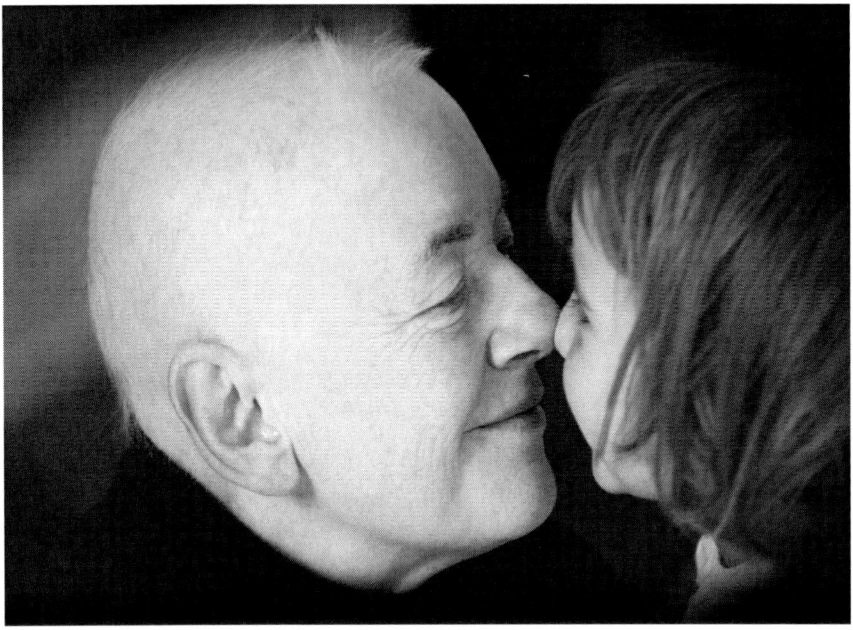

When a Cancer Patient defeats their disease and becomes a Cancer Survivor, there is not a ticker-tape parade to celebrate their success. Nor, is the Cancer Survivor's face featured on a box of Wheaties® or on the cover of Time Magazine®. And, undoubtedly, there will be no brass bands playing the "Victory March" in honor of these valiant men, women, teens, and children who have beaten their Cancers and reclaimed their lives. No, there will be none of that. However, what Cancer Survivors ***will have****—and, I include myself in this bunch—is the inward appreciation and knowledge that they have accomplished something big –* ***really big!*** *In addition to these realizations, though, all Cancer survivors that I have known (again, myself included), will humbly acknowledge the severity of what could have happened, and will be grateful for the miracle that did. All Cancer Survivors, both young and old, have stared death in the face during their individual ordeals. But, through their own strength, and with the support of so many, not a one of them backed down to their disease. Each of these courageous victims gave it their best possible fight – and they won! This, in itself, is an amazing achievement. But, the most significant outcome of these Cancer Survivors' personal plights is that they all got their precious, one-of-a-kind lives back. And, in so doing, they have a much greater appreciation for life, for their life, and for the people in their life. We get one shot at this – we must make it count!*

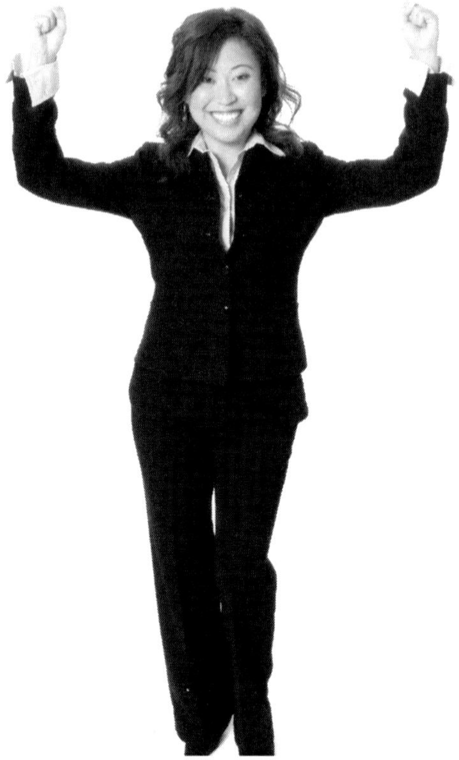

Ahhhh – the reassuring, happy, and hard-earned feelings of victory and success. Some people realize these sensations upon winning a sporting event; others when they conquer a personal challenge; and, still others when they are triumphant in their search for the perfect electronic gadget or pair of shoes. But, let's be serious. What could possibly merit a more significant celebration than that of a Cancer patient who has productively made it through what can be the very long and physically and emotionally challenging Cancer treatment process, coupled with the painful, exasperating, and distressing Side Effects that can ensue? Take it from me, and I had it all—non-stop pain and nausea for months, extreme loss of weight, and follow-on prescription drug dependency and severe Depression—there is only one other thing that can possibly compare to the excitement and joy that a Cancer patient feels upon completing their Treatments: The grateful news from the patient's Medical Team that the Cancer has been completely eliminated, and that the Survivor is "Cancer-free." Nothing like getting one's life back to put a new spin on "winning."

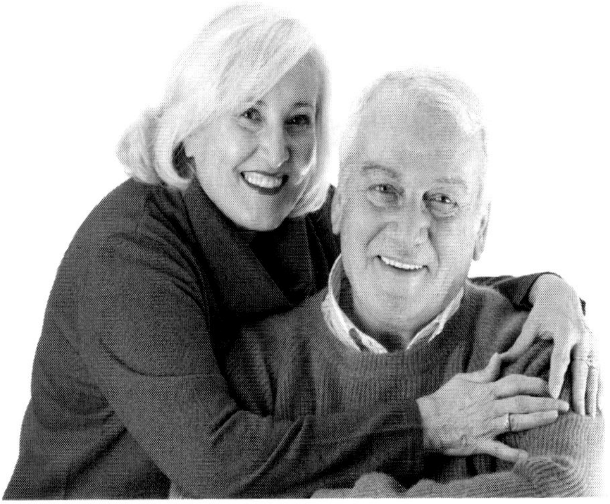

<u>WARNING: White Males Over 50:</u> Head and Neck Cancers Prefer <u>You</u> Over Any Other Ethnicity, Gender, or Age. And, if You Are a User of Tobacco and Drink Alcohol, Head and Neck Cancers Will 'Like You' 6 Times More Than Someone Who Doesn't Use Either.

I certainly don't intend to scare anyone with the above warning, but, sadly, it's all true, and I'm living proof – with the exception that I've never used tobacco and alcohol. There are numerous Cancers that are classified as Cancers of the Head and Neck, and all are found in and around the regions of the throat, tongue, nose, sinuses, mouth, lips, and Salivary Glands. Cancers of the brain, eyes, skull, muscles of the head, and others, have their own specific classifications and are not considered Head and Neck Cancers despite being located in the head. In any case, besides the age, sex, and race of a person and tobacco and alcohol use (that can cause mouth and throat Cancers), Head and Neck Cancer risk factors also include breathing wood and metal dusts and fumes of industrial chemicals (nasal Cancers); poor oral hygiene (mouth Cancers); sun exposure (lip Cancers); transfer of Humanpapillomavirus (HPV) during sex without protection (Base of Tongue Cancers); and, overexposure to radiation (Salivary Gland Cancers). Not a lot of fun, huh? Well, for over 50,000 people in the U.S. (myself included), and over 600,000, globally, each year, who come down with Head and Neck Cancer, it is a reality that must be faced, and a war that must be waged. Ideally, these Cancers would all be prevented, but life usually gets in the way; all the more reason for all adults, but <u>especially White men over 50</u>, to be super-vigilant.

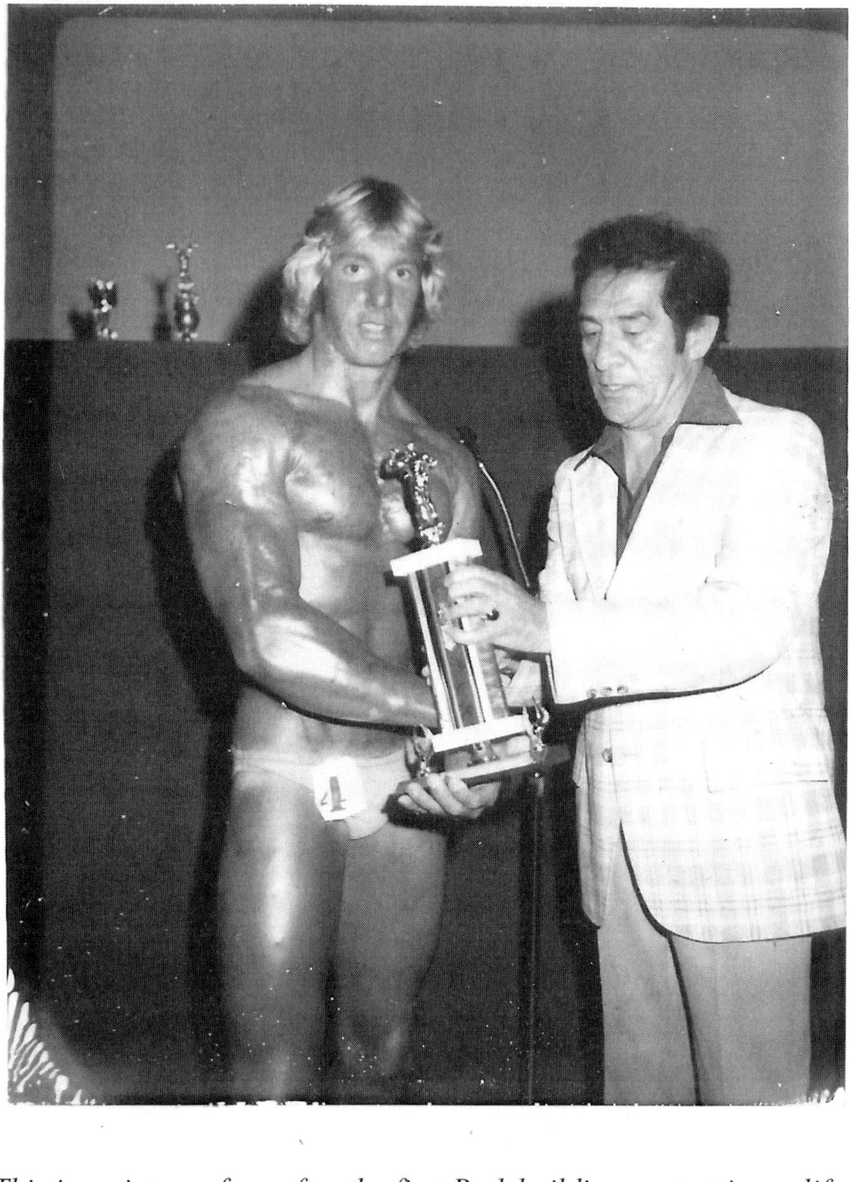

This is a picture of me after the first Bodybuilding contest in my life. My weightlifting buddies at New Mexico State University had talked me into entering the Mr. International Contest in Juarez, Mexico in 1977. In 1977, there were no videos to learn from, and, at that time, Bodybuilding posing routines were not yet set to music. So, I had to "wing it" by learning from magazine photos. Ultimately, it paid off, as I took 3rd Place in the U.S. vs. Mexico contest south of the border. In this photo, the Mayor of Juarez is presenting me with my trophy.

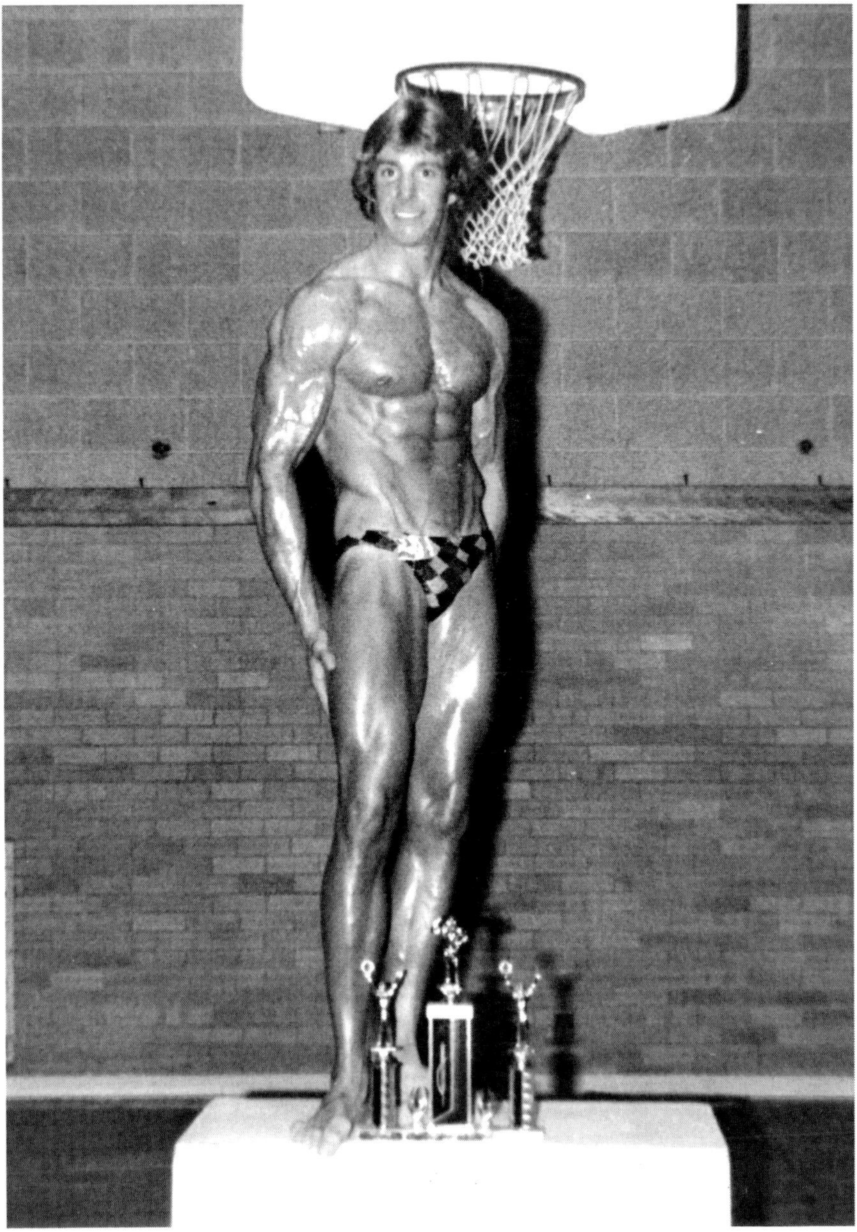

That backboard is just a little distracting, but, this is a picture of me at age 27, in 1978, after my second Bodybuilding Contest, Mr. El Paso, which was held just north of the border from Juarez. I earned 2nd Place in this contest, along with the "Most Muscular" and "Best Chest" awards. Of course, the last thing on my mind at that age and time was that in 26 years, ***my Cancer*** *would be taking center-stage.*

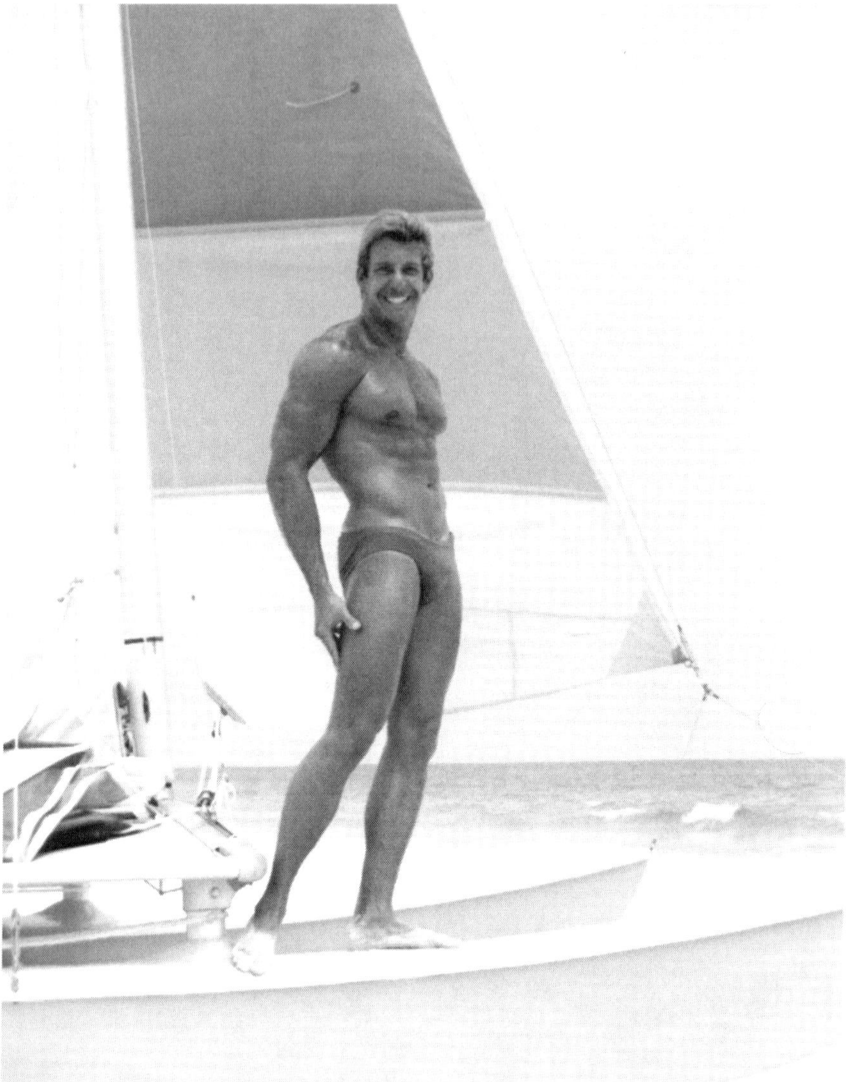

The white sand beaches of Pensacola, FL; now, that's the life! Well, at least it was for a short time after I graduated from Naval Aviation Officers' Candidate School (AOCS) as an Ensign in the U.S. Navy. When this photo of me was taken in 1980, I had been Bodybuilding for about four years, and competing in contests for almost as long. Even throughout my 16 weeks of AOCS, my hard-assed U.S. Marine Corps Drill Instructors gave me special permission and time to work out. They called me "The Hulk," and would always have me "Drop and give 'em 50!" in front of new classes – a scare tactic, I assume.

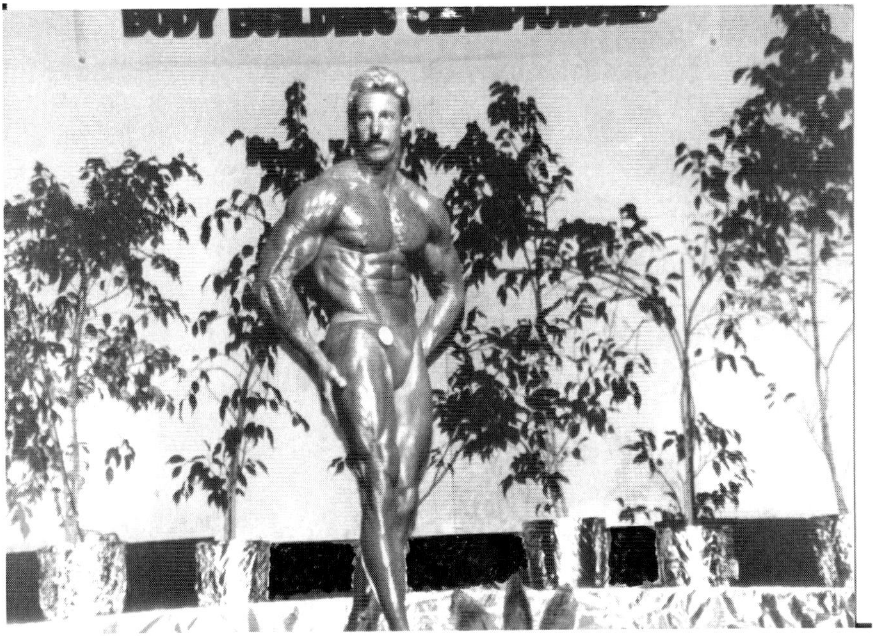

The only Photoshopped thing in this picture is my moustache. Just joking, but this is a photo taken of me in 1984, at age 33, when I was probably in the best Bodybuilding shape of my life. This particular show was the Armed Forces Hawaii Bodybuilding Championship, in which Servicemen throughout the Hawaiian Islands came together to strut their stuff and to compete for top honors. I did not win the competition—I actually placed Third—but, for this contest, as with all the other Bodybuilding shows that I entered from the late-1970s until the mid-1980s, the preparation process was awfully physically exhausting, extremely time-consuming, and mentally demanding. In the interest of becoming strong, muscular, and "ripped," I and other Bodybuilding competitors would train for a minimum of two hours a day (sometimes twice a day!) all year; eat an extremely regimented diet consisting of only the healthiest food and beverage; consume a litany of expensive nutritional supplements (no drugs!) in hopes of gaining and retaining quality, lean muscle mass; choreograph and practice a posing routine to music; work; sleep; and, try to maintain as normal of a life as possible – and all of this for about 45 minutes on stage! Call it loony, but, the mental discipline, physical strength, and never-say-die attitude that I assimilated while preparing for my Bodybuilding contests became invaluable life-savers when I had to gut it out and do battle with the ultimate of competitors – Cancer.

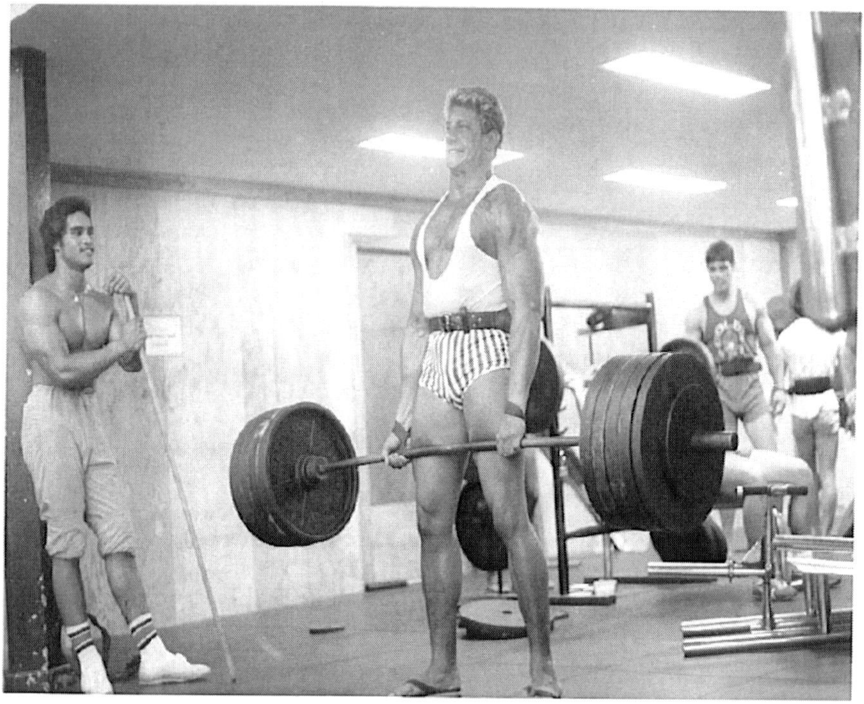

This is a photo of me defying gravity with 545 lbs of iron and steel. This exercise is what is known as a Deadlift, and is one of the three forms of lifts that are performed in Power Lifting competitions, with the Bench Press and the Squat being the other events. The physical training, mental preparation, and discipline that are required to lift heavy weights are not unlike the same qualities that are necessary to be successful in almost everything in life. When this photograph of me training in Hawaii was taken in 1985, I was 34, and I probably weighed roughly 225 lbs., at a height of 6'1". Notwithstanding the striped "shorty-shorts" (which, in my defense, were forgivably worn by well-intentioned manly-men back then), that period in my life was when I was the strongest and heaviest that I had ever been, or would ever become. Unbeknownst to me at that time, however, in a matter of nineteen years, I would be confronted with a physical and mental challenge so unfathomable that it would make that 545 lbs. look like child's play. It was then that I would discover that the body I had worked so hard for so many years to strengthen and protect, would fall victim to the ravaging scourge of Cancer. But, while my body was temporarily devastated by the Cancer, thankfully, everything I had done to keep it fit did help me in the end to defeat my disease.

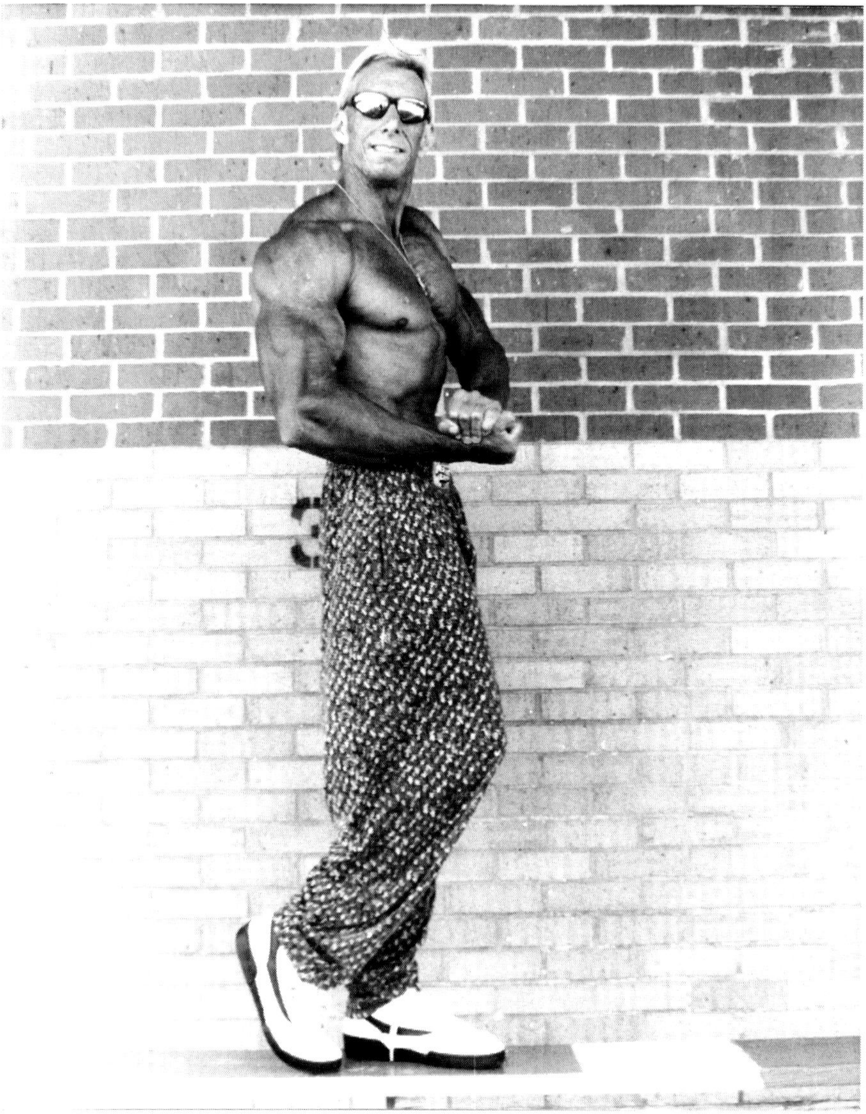

I believe that this was the last posed Bodybuilding photo taken of me before I received my Cancer diagnosis. This photo was taken in VA in 2002 at age 51, and I was diagnosed with Cancer 2 years later, in 2004. This image was one of the many "proofs" taken of me for a calendar photo shoot that we did in the freezing month of February, outdoors, no less. The calendar was being sponsored by a Nutrition and Health Food business with which I was affiliated, and featured male and female fitness athletes from the Northern Virginia area. I was "Mr. November," but only because that's the month I was born.

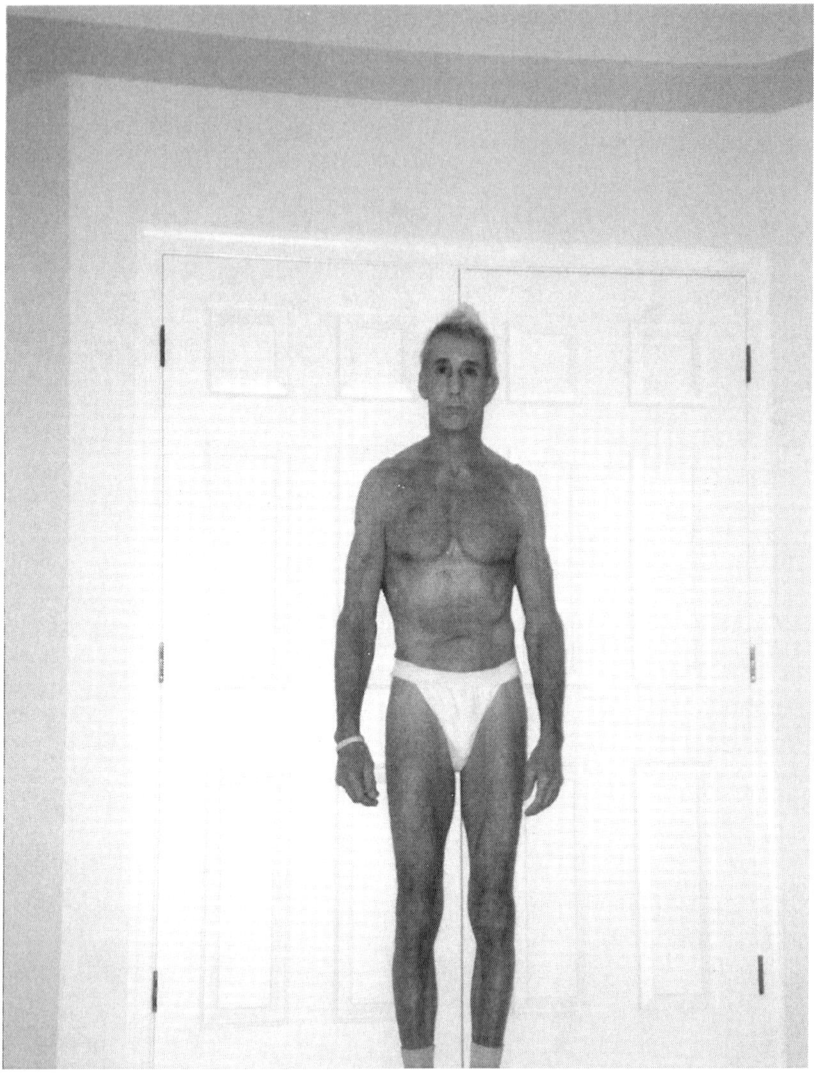

Okay, so I didn't win the "Sexiest Man Alive" contest in 2004, even with my Mohawk-style hairdo. But, at least, thank God, I was alive. And, amazingly, I did keep all my hair during my Chemo treatments. All joking aside, this photo of me was taken in November of 2004, about 2 months after concluding my Chemo and Radiation Therapy treatments. At this point, because I had had such difficulties eating and drinking ***anything*** *due to excruciating throat and mouth pain, I had lost almost 50 lbs. of bodyweight – dropping from 198 to 151 in 5 months! It would be October of 2005 before I would gain all of it back again, thanks to weightlifting workouts and high-quality food.*

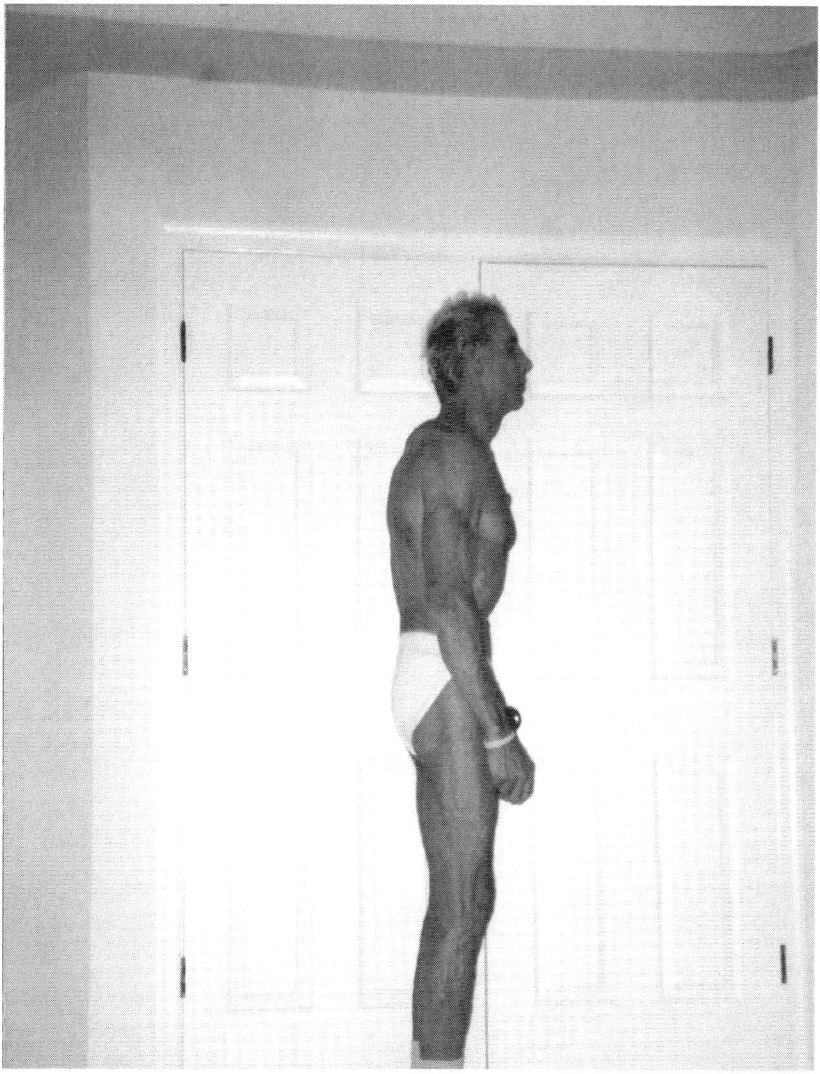

A side view of my less-than-normal-self, taken in November of 2004, at age 53. Not that I expect any sympathy, but, I have the opposite problem of many individuals in that I have a very hard time gaining and holding on to bodyweight – but, I can lose it just like that! This is due to my higher metabolism, thanks to years of working out and eating nutritious foods. The combination of my fast metabolism and limited intake of calories due to pain caused by my treatments, made my body lose any stored fat I had, as well as lots of muscle mass – in just 5 months. By the way, that bump on my Pec is not a misplaced nipple, but my Mediport, used for Chemotherapy and blood draws.

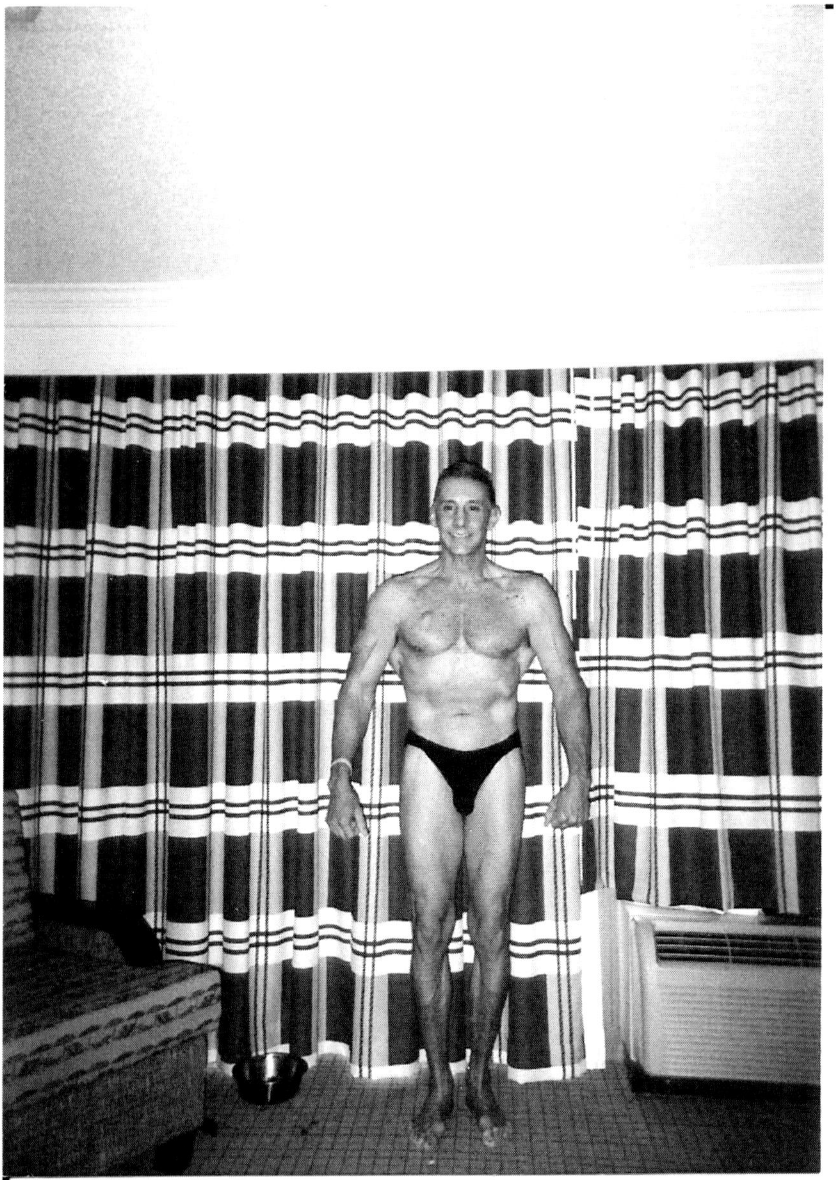

Back on the road to recovery – at least physically. This photo of me was taken in the late-Spring 2005, almost one year after my Cancer diagnosis. After my treatments concluded in September 2004, I was "chomping at the bit" to get back to my workouts. With my Medical Team's approval, on December 20, 2004, I was able to resume my muscle-building regimen. In this photo I weighed 175, which was a gain of 24 lbs. from my low in November, but, 25 lbs. from my goal.

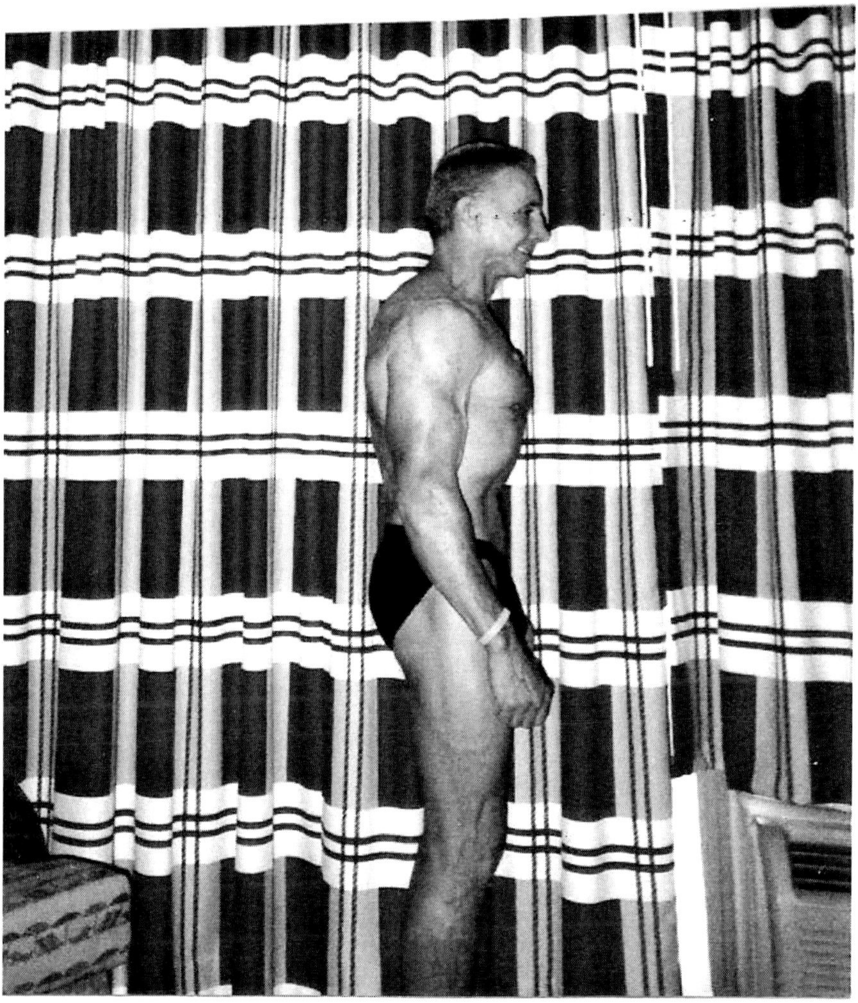

Now, that's a very big smile – and rightfully so. When this photo of me was taken in 2005, I was 54, and I had, thankfully, completed my Cancer treatments; begun working out again and gaining back my bodyweight and strength; successfully made it through a month-long prescription painkiller detox and withdrawal process; received some very encouraging exam results indicating no Cancer presence; and, was half-way thru almost three months of daily 3-hour Hyperbaric Oxygen Chamber treatments. Essentially, I was beginning to get my "new normal" life back on-track. Still to come, however, was a very long struggle with Depression that I eventually also overcame. See that Mediport in/on my chest? It remained there until August 2006.

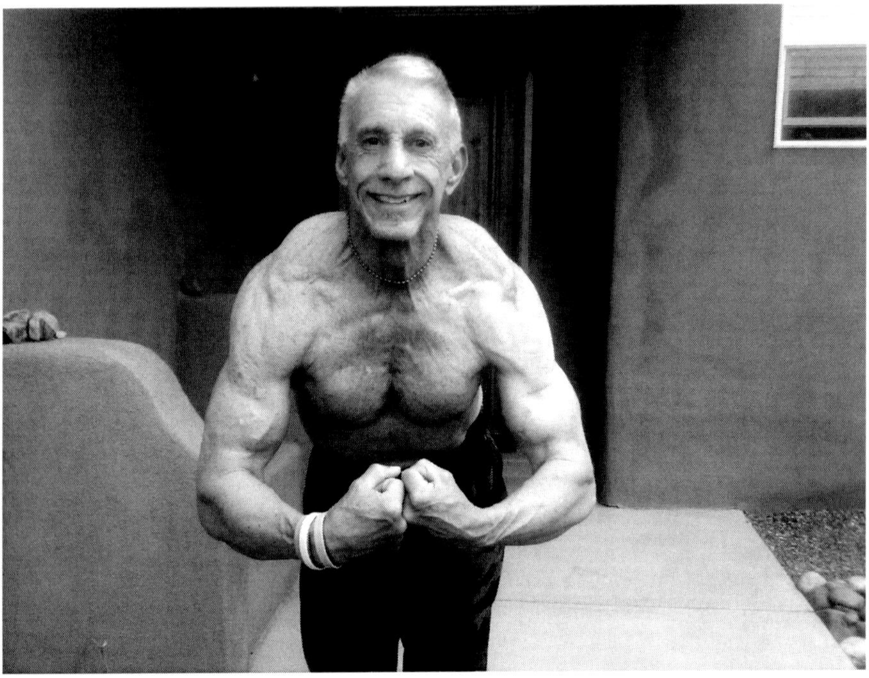

Isn't this just about the wackiest picture you've ever seen? Well, if ***you*** *think that it's a bit awkward, just imagine how I must feel! But, seriously, this pose is, in reality, one of the mandatory Bodybuilding poses that competitors in contests must exhibit for the judges when being compared to other Bodybuilders on stage. The pose is referred to as the "Most Muscular" or "Crab" (it does look a little crab-ish, I must admit), and, its primary purpose is to give the Bodybuilding Contest judges a good look at the overall upper body musculature of the competitors, including their chest, shoulders, and arms. Jayni took this photo of me at 61 ½ years of age in July 2013 at our home. I included this photo in this book to exhibit that no matter what age a person is, they can always make a dork of themselves. All joking aside, though, I actually incorporated this picture to show that I am very much alive over nine years since my Cancer diagnosis, and that I am still taking care of the body that's taken such great care of me.*

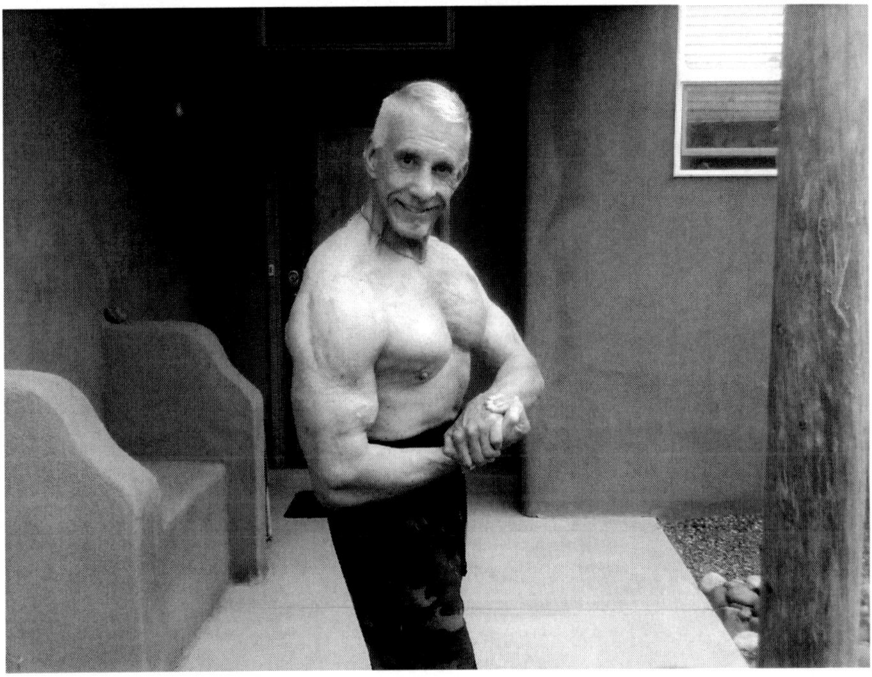

This photo, taken of me in July 2013 at 61 ½ years, demonstrates the ever-popular "Side-Chest" pose that has been displayed by "Muscle Men" throughout the ages to exhibit their physical prowess. Women competing in Bodybuilding contests these days also are asked to use this specific pose to reveal their feminine strength and physique. In any case, I posed for this shot, taken by my wife, Jayni, to exemplify that, nine years after Cancer unceremoniously attacked my healthy and fit body, I remain victorious, and my body is still healthy and fit. I'm not bragging or being boastful, but, I am simply overjoyed and grateful that my body and mind were able to kick my Cancer's butt.

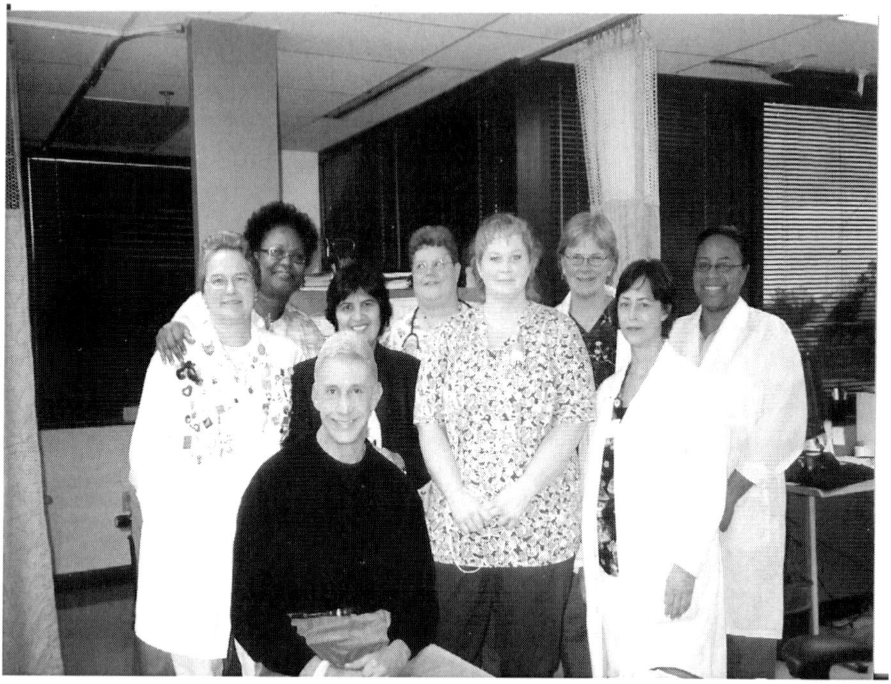

My Oncology Team, above, from L to R, are: Diana, Brenda, Dr. Ahuja – my Oncologist, Tina, Heather, Becky Jill, and Renee.

This photo, taken in the Summer of 2005, is of a ***very*** *happy Cancer Survivor, along with my Oncologist and Oncology Nurses — who I referred to as my "Angels in Disguise." It was these compassionate, skilled, knowledgeable, and encouraging women in the Northern Virginia clinic where I received my Chemotherapy treatments who dedicated their lives to help save the lives of Cancer patients – mine included. And, when the going got really tough for me, it was their kindness, thoughtfulness, caring, and constant smiles that helped me make it through. It is a dreadful thing for a man, woman, teenager, or child to come down with Cancer. But, if it is in the cards and is to be, the patient will want to know that they have the latest Cancer-fighting weapons and the greatest health care professionals in their corner. And, this, thankfully, is exactly what I had – not only with my Chemotherapy treatments, but also with the Radiation Therapy I received, and my many Cancer Surgeries that were performed. I will always be thankful for everything that this wonderful bunch—and all that the other members of my Medical Team—did for me. I mean, after all, here I am 9 years later, writing about it! Thank you, Lord!*

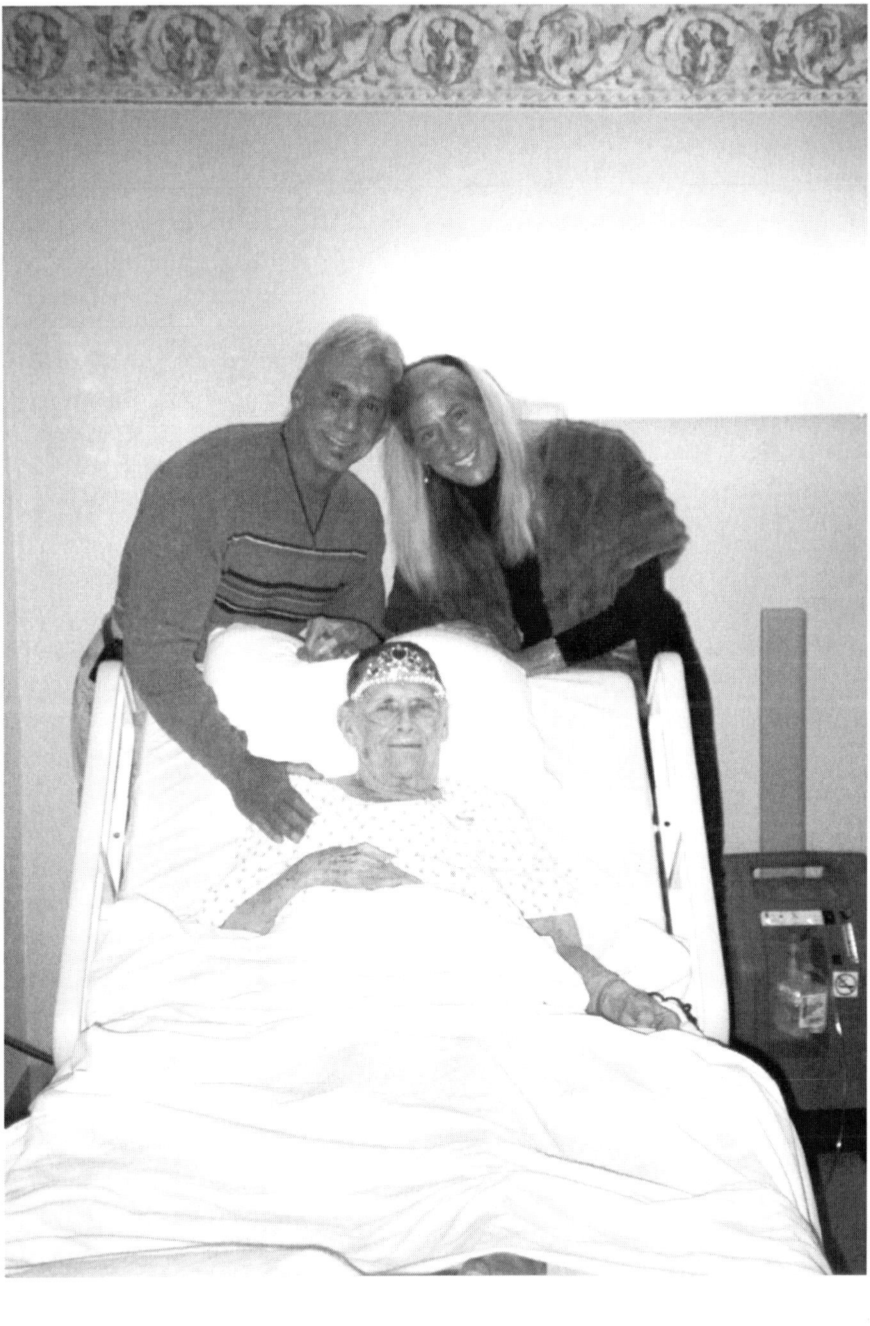

This is a photo taken in December 2010 of me with two very lovely women in my life: My fantastic wife, Jayni, and, my incredible Mom, Betty Lee, who was so beautiful, inside and out. Here, Mom wears a tiara (begrudgingly, I may add), the wonderful Queen that she was.

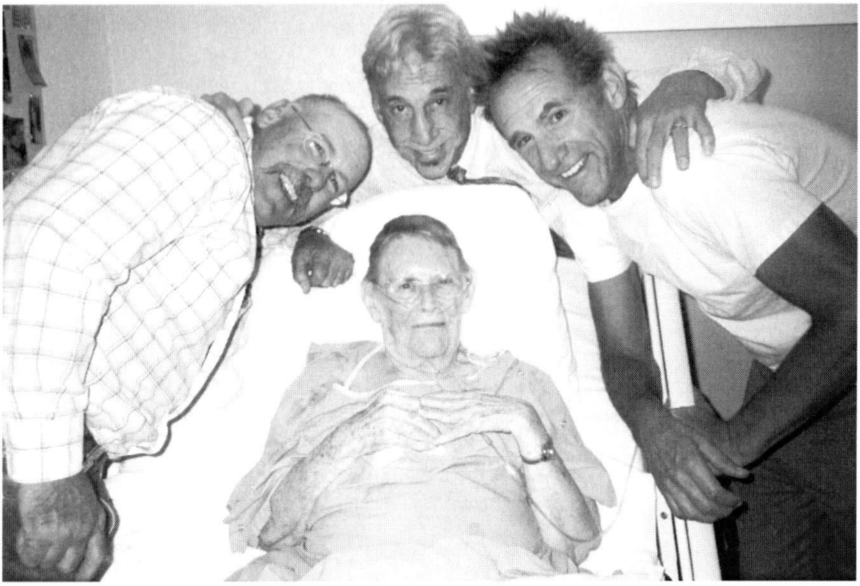

My Brothers, Buz (left), and Rich (right) and I, would constantly tell our Mom, Betty, that we were her fault: that she, and she alone, was responsible for all of our foolishness, and for the stinkers (literally and figuratively) that the three of us had become. Mom, however, as much as she loved every one of us, would have none of that, and would invariably plead innocent to all charges. This photo, taken in Mom's Nursing Home Room in June 2011, gives a pretty good idea of why Mom had her hands full whenever the three of us would end up in her midst. But, despite Mom, rightfully, not taking any blame for any of her Sons' craziness, she would do just about anything else to honor our names, wishes, and lives. Our Mom, unfortunately, was dealt a very tough blow with her first Breast Cancer diagnosis in the early 1970s, and then a second a few years later. And, along with those diagnoses and two Mastectomies would later come more than her fair-share of physical health issues that would eventually take away Mom's mobility, and a good part of her independence. For many people, that would be a death knell, or, at the very least, a beginning of the end. But, for Mom—as strong, positive, and happy as she was—it only seemed to motivate her even more to do as many things as she could; to meet and make as many friends as possible; and, to love, smile, and enjoy every minute of it. Mom was a selfless woman and always put others first, including each of her children – even if she was the chosen recipient of her "angelic" Sons' pranks!

The Following Chapters of This Book Are Devoted to:

- A Detailed Discussion about Head and Neck Cancers Drawn from My Journal Notes, Materials from My Medical Team, and from cancer.gov

- The Story of My 3+-Year Head and Neck Cancer Journey, Including My Journal Notes, from June 2004, to December 2007 (Me "Cancer-Free")

- Musings and Happenings in My "New Normal" Life as a Head and Neck Cancer Survivor, from 2008 to 2013

"Cancer will do many things, none of them good, but, it will humble a person, and, it may cause them to reconsider their life and its place in the grander scheme. But, perhaps, most importantly, Cancer—as lethal as it can be—will prompt us to recognize just how precious and fragile our lives truly are."

- Butch Sickler

Chapter Nine

Head and Neck Cancers – Part 1 – *Getting to Know This Uncommon Foe*

"Some people who take excellent care of their bodies will "get" Cancer, while others, who abuse themselves, will never be affected by the nasty disease. There is no making any sense of it, but, once Cancer occurs, no matter the person or the reason, all efforts must be focused on quickly and completely removing it from their body."

- Butch Sickler

If one were to think of Cancers—generally speaking—as a giant iceberg floating somewhere in the vast ocean, Head and Neck Cancers would, respectively, constitute the very top of the tip. That is definitely not because Head and Neck Cancers are more special or more noteworthy than the over 200 other identified forms of Cancer. It also is not because these types of Cancer are the most well-known. Actually, it's quite to the contrary – Head and Neck Cancers account for only around 3 percent of all malignancies in the U.S. each year.

Rare Cancers but Nonetheless Nasty

The "Big 4" Cancers—Breast, Prostate, Colorectal and Lung—get a volume of the press and attention because these adult forms of the disease are some of the most omnipresent, impacting the lives of over 750,000 men and women in the U.S. who are diagnosed with Cancer every year. By comparison, roughly 55,000 adult American men and women are diagnosed with Head and Neck Cancers on an annual basis, with men being the primary targets, and of those, these forms of Cancer seem to prefer males over 50 years old. ***BINGO!! – that would be me!*** In all seriousness, however, please don't let these relatively small numbers, or the perceptible rarity of this form of the disease fool you – Head and Neck Cancers, being located…well…in a person's head and neck, can be *extraordinarily wicked*, indeed.

☛ ***Author's Disclaimer:*** A bulk of the information that I have incorporated within Chapters 9 through 13 regarding Head and Neck Cancers, has been legitimately acquired and adapted from the U.S. National Cancer Institute website (www.cancer.gov), and accurately included within this Book. Applicable material has been included in accordance with "Web Policies for the National Cancer Institute."

Below, for the Reader's perusal, are the "NCI Web Policies," which I have taken directly from the NCI website, (www.cancer.gov):

"Copyright and Reuse of Graphics and Text

You May Reuse Information from the National Cancer Institute (NCI) Web Site

Most of the information on the National Cancer Institute (NCI) Web site, Cancer.gov, is in the public domain and is not subject to copyright restrictions. No special permission is required to use or reproduce public domain material. NCI's public domain information includes health professional and patient information in NCI's Physician Data Query (PDQ®) cancer information database and patient education brochures, booklets, and fact sheets. However, any reproduced material should acknowledge NCI as the originator and the NCI Web site, www.cancer.gov, as the source. The source can be cited as: the National Cancer Institute (www.cancer.gov)

You Do Not Need Permission to Use text from NCI information products in your own materials.

However, you cannot use the registered trademark logos for NCI, National Institutes for Health (NIH), or PDQ in your materials because NCI has not reviewed or approved your product."

There, now that we have all that legal mumbo-jumbo out of the way, let's get to know these uncommon, but still risky, forms of Cancer – one of which I got to know, ***way-up-too-close-and-personal!***

What the Heck is "Head and Neck?"

According to the National Cancer Institute (www.cancer.gov), ***"Head and Neck"*** is general terminology that is used to collectively describe a family of Cancers that can evolve within the head or neck regions of typically adult men and women (i.e., usually not children or teenagers) in their Nasal Cavity, Sinuses, Lips, Mouth, Salivary Glands, Throat, Larynx (Voice Box), and, the Tongue (front 2/3 and Base, the site of my Primary Cancer Tumor). To be more scientific, Cancers that are known as Head and Neck Cancers usually begin in the thin Squamous Cells that line the moist, mucosal surfaces inside the head and neck. These Squamous Cell Cancers are often referred to as Squamous Cell Carcinomas (SCC) of the Head and Neck.

Head and Neck Cancers can also start in the Salivary Glands, but Salivary Gland Cancers are, in reality, relatively rare. Salivary Glands are made up of many different types of cells that can become cancerous, so there are numerous forms of Salivary Gland Cancer. Cancers of the Head and Neck are further categorized by the areas of the head, and/or, neck, where they occur. In contrast, are Cancers of the Brain, the Eye, the Esophagus, and the Thyroid Gland, as well as Cancers of the Scalp, Skin, Muscles, and the Bones of the head and neck. *These are not normally identified as Head and Neck Cancers,* as each of these Cancers have their own classifications.

Per www.cancer.gov, Head and Neck Cancers are recognized by the area of the body where the Primary Tumor first forms, as follows:

- **Oral Cavity**

The Oral Cavity includes the lips, the front two-thirds of the Tongue, the Gingiva (Gums), the Buccal Mucosa (lining within the cheeks and lips), the floor (bottom) of the mouth beneath the Tongue, the Hard Palate (bony top of the mouth), and the small area behind the Wisdom Teeth in the rear of the mouth.

- **Salivary Glands**

The Salivary Glands produce Saliva, the fluid that keeps mucosal surfaces in the mouth and throat moist. There are many Salivary Glands, with the major ones being in the floor of the mouth, and near the jawbone.

- **Paranasal Sinuses and Nasal Cavity**

The Paranasal Sinuses are small hollow spaces within the bones of the head that surround the nose. The Nasal Cavity is the hollow space that is located inside the nose.

- **Pharynx**

The Pharynx is a hollow tube about five inches long that commences behind the nose, and that leads to the Esophagus (the tube that goes to the stomach), and the Trachea (the tube that leads to the Lungs). The Pharynx has three parts, as follows:

  - **Nasopharynx -** The Nasopharynx, which is the upper part of the Pharynx, is located behind the nose
  - **Oropharynx -**The Oropharynx is located in the middle of the Pharynx. The Oropharynx includes the Soft Palate (the back of the mouth), the Base of the Tongue (***Mine)*** and the Tonsils.
  - **Hypopharynx -** The Hypopharynx is the lowermost part of the Pharynx

- **Larynx**

The Larynx, which is also called the Voice Box, is a little passageway formed by cartilage just below the Pharynx in the neck. The Larynx contains the Vocal Cords. The Larynx also has a small piece of tissue (i.e., a flap), named the Epiglottis, which moves to cover the Larynx, and aids in preventing food from entering the air passages.

- **Lymph Nodes in the Upper Part of the Neck**

Sometimes, Squamous Cancer cells are found in the Lymph Nodes of the upper neck when there is no observed evidence of Cancer in other parts of the head, and/or, neck. When this occurs, the Cancer is called *"Metastatic Squamous Neck Cancer with Unknown (Occult) Primary.* In such diagnoses, follow-up exams, tests, and lab work are ordered in an effort to pinpoint the location of the Primary Tumor and any other metastases in the patient's body, so that they can be properly treated.

Figure 1, below, which was derived from information provided to me in handout materials by a member of my Medical Team, illustrates the multiple areas in which Head and Neck Cancers can occur:

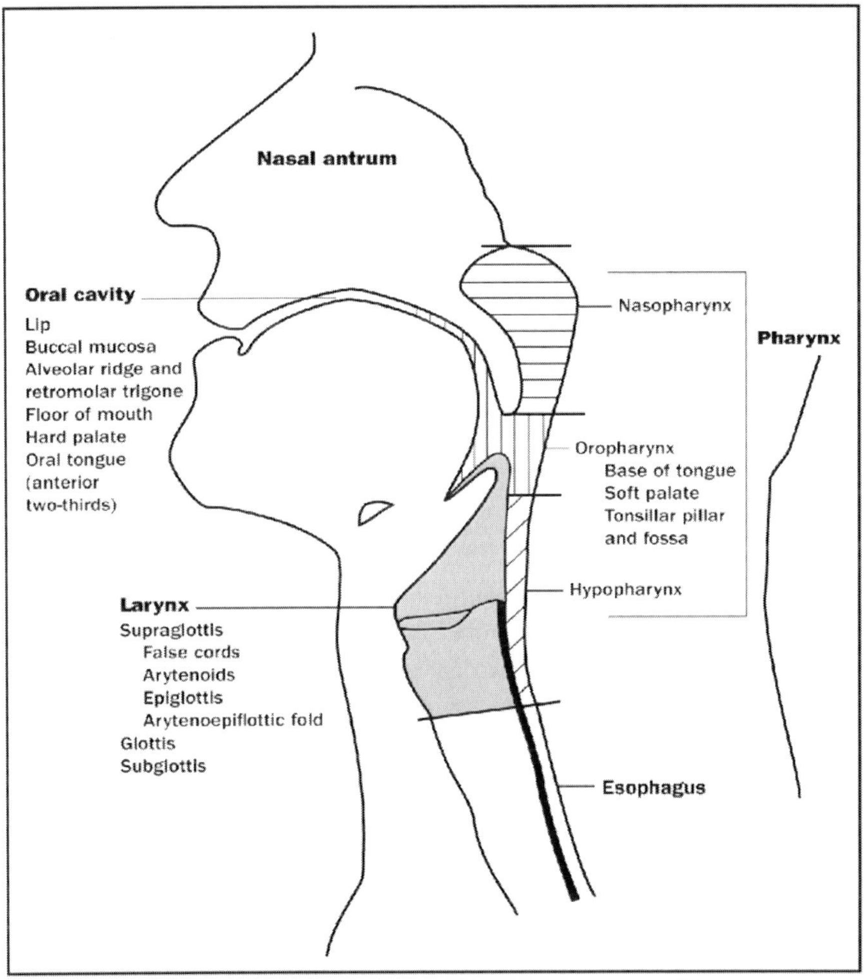

FIGURE 1: Anatomic sites and subsites of the head and neck. The approximate distribution of head and neck cancer is oral cavity, 44%; larynx, 31%; and pharynx, 25%.

How Common are Head and Neck Cancers?

As mentioned elsewhere in this Chapter and in this Book, the many different varieties of the disease that constitute Head and Neck Cancers account for only approximately 3 percent of all Cancers in the U.S. These types of Cancer are nearly twice as common among men as they are between women, and, are also diagnosed more often in individuals over 50 years old than they are within younger people. More than 55,000 men and women in this country are expected to be diagnosed with Head and Neck Cancers in 2013. Per Studies done by the National Cancer Institute (www.cancer.gov), here are details:

The Dreaded Numbers

In 2011, approximately 39,400 men and women (27,710 men and 11,690 women) in the U.S. were diagnosed with Cancers of the Oral Cavity and Pharynx. Of these diagnoses, an estimated total of 7,900 men and women unfortunately succumbed to their respective diseases. Moreover, an anticipated total of 12,740 men and women (10,160 men and 2,580 women) in the U.S. were diagnosed in 2011 with Laryngeal Cancer. Sadly, more than 3,560 of these courageous individuals gave it their best, but perished from their malignancies.

Most patients with Head and Neck Cancers have Metastatic Disease at the time of their diagnosis, meaning that their Cancer had spread from their Primary Tumor to their Lymph Nodes (as did my Cancer), or to other locations in the body, such as the Lungs. In this regard, Studies find that Regional Nodal Involvement was present in 43% of the Head and Neck Cancer diagnoses, and distant Metastases were noted in 10% of cases studied. Further, it has been found that patients with a Primary Head and Neck Cancer often form a Second Primary Tumor later in life. Speaking positively, however, there are now over 500,000 Head and Neck Cancer survivors in the U.S.

Geography and Race

All Head and Neck Cancers, combined, equal the sixth most frequently occurring Cancer, worldwide, and these Cancers account for roughly 3% of all Cancer deaths annually. *Globally, there are an estimated 600,000 new cases of Head and Neck Cancer diagnosed each year,* which represents *about* 5% to 6% of all newly diagnosed malignant Cancers. About two-thirds of these new cases come about in developing or *Third World* countries. Within the European Union, over 100,000 individuals are diagnosed with Head and Neck Cancer every year, and about 40,000 die from the disease. Rates are higher in men than in women, in Western, Southern, and in Eastern Europe. The occurrence of Laryngeal Cancer is greater in African Americans when compared to the Caucasian, Asian, and Hispanic populations. Consequentially, in African Americans, Head and Neck Cancers are associated with lower survival rates for similar Tumor Stages, when compared with other ethnicities. The overall average 5-year survival rate is 60% in Caucasians, and 40% in African Americans.

Gender

Head and Neck Cancers are more common in men, with 66% to 95% of cases occurring in males. ***Lucky us!*** In fact, the disease is more common in men than in women in most countries, including in the United States. With that said, the frequency of Cancer by gender differs with anatomical location of the Cancer in the head and neck. Also, occurrence rates have been changing as the number of female smokers has increased the last few years. The male-to-female ratio is presently 3:1 for Pharyngeal Cancers and for Oral Cavity Cancers. However, in patients with Plummer-Vinson Syndrome, the ratio is reversed, with 80% of Head and Neck Cancers occurring in women.

Age

The risk of an individual developing Head and Neck Cancer increases with age, with the majority of cases happening in patients, 50 years of age and older. And though most patients are between 50 and 70 years old, younger patients can also develop Head and Neck Cancers. It should be mentioned that in contrast to typical Head and Neck Cancer diagnoses, there are more *women and fewer smokers in the younger patient groupings.* Patients with Humanpapillomavirus (HPV)-associated Head and Neck Cancers tend to be younger, and may even be in their 30s or 40s when diagnosed with the disease. In some places of the developing world, Oral Head and Neck Cancer is relatively common in younger people. Rising trends of Oral Cancer in younger and middle-aged men and women have been reported in the UK, other European countries, and in the U.S. So, the moral of the story here, is: ***Males and females of all ages beware; but, men over 50 be especially watchful for any symptoms of these wicked forms of Cancer. At the first signs of any abnormal or persistent health issues, seek medical attention and possibly save your life!***

What May Cause Head and Neck Cancers?

One would not have to be a Cancer doctor, scientist, or other health care professional to figure out that specific things we put into our mouths and noses may not be all too healthy or beneficial for us. And, I'm not just referring to the junk that one can buy at a *fast food* restaurant. No, there are many other *goodies* that we consume, such as tobacco and alcohol, that do a really fantastic job of poisoning our body systems and tissues all on their own. Then, who would assume that breathing wood or metal dust, being a male over 50, or having sex might contribute to the development of Head and Neck Cancers? Well, sorry to break it to you, but these factors, random chance, and others, can all play a role in the formation of the disease.

Adapted from www.cancer.gov, following are some of the verified, prevalent risk factors for Cancers of the Head and Neck:

Head and Neck Cancer Risk Factors - Tobacco and Alcohol Use

As one might think, the most important risk factors that may stimulate the formation of Head and Neck Cancers are ***alcohol and tobacco use*** (including use of smokeless tobacco, sometimes called "chewing tobacco" or "snuff"). ***Smokers, please take notice:*** Head and Neck Cancer tumors occur *six times more often among cigarette smokers than nonsmokers*. Additionally, the threat of mortality from Laryngeal Cancer appears to go up with increased cigarette smoking as a person's age increases. For the heaviest cigarette smokers, death from Laryngeal Cancer is *20 times more likely* than for nonsmokers. Furthermore, *active smoking by Head and Neck Cancer patients or Cancer survivors* is associated with noteworthy increases in the rates of Second Primary Tumor development (when compared with those smokers who have terminated tobacco use, or, those who have never smoked). The use of unfiltered cigarettes, or dark, air-cured tobacco, is associated with further increases in Head and Neck Cancer risk.

The smoking of *cigars*, while often misperceived as posing a smaller health risk than cigarette smoking, has been noted in Studies to cause a change in the incidence of some Head and Neck Cancers. Although the occurrence of several Cancers traditionally associated with cigarette smoking (i.e., Larynx Cancers and Lung Cancers) is decreased in cigar smokers, the occurrence of Cancer is, in actuality, higher at other head and neck sites that are not commonly associated with cigarette smoking. These are usually in the Oropharynx and the Esophagus where the cigar-caused pooling of saliva tends to occur.

Use of *smokeless tobacco (i.e., "snuff," "chaw," or chewing tobacco)* is also associated with an increased incidence of Head and Neck Cancers, especially in the Oral Cavity (mouth). Some users of smokeless tobacco frequently develop premalignant lesions, such as Oral Leukoplakia, at the place where the tobacco quid (i.e., *"chaw"*) rests in the cheek, or just between the lip and gums. Over time, these lesions may form into invasive, malignant carcinomas, meaning that they progress from the less-threatening *minor leagues,* and up to the potentially lethal *major leagues.* The habitual use of snuff has been associated with an increase in Cancers of the Gum and Oral Mucosa.

The risk factors from tobacco use are particularly implicated in Cancers of the Oral Cavity, Oropharynx (throat), Hypopharynx, and Larynx (Voice Box). And, alcohol consumption, by itself, is a known risk factor for the development of Laryngeal and Pharyngeal Cancer tumors. But, even though alcohol is a less potent carcinogen than is tobacco, it should come as no revelation that a majority of all Head and Neck Cancers ***(75%-wow!), are caused by the use of <u>both</u> tobacco and alcohol***. What this means, realistically, is that if at-risk individuals would say "bye" to one, or both, of these unhealthy (and costly!) lifestyle habits, the numbers of Neck and Cancer diagnoses would drop dramatically. Likewise, reduced numbers of Head and Neck Cancer risk factors would, no doubt, lead to lowered numbers of *Lung Cancer* diagnoses for those smokers who quit the habit, and, would most likely contribute to lesser incidences of Heart Attacks!

Maybe in a perfect world people would not smoke and drink, but, not here on Planet Earth – people love to party, and party, and party! And, what soiree, ball game, picnic, or *Happy Hour* would be complete without alcohol and a host of people smoking cigarettes or cigars? In any event, Scientific Studies have found that people who use *both tobacco and alcohol* are at greater risk of developing these Cancers than any who use *either tobacco or alcohol separately*. On the bright side (I guess), the use of tobacco and alcohol are not risk factors for Salivary Gland Cancers, but that's hardly any consolation when use of tobacco (in all its forms) and alcohol can cause Cancers of other areas of the head and neck. *So, put that in your pipe and...*

Head and Neck Cancer Risk Factors - Human Papillomavirus (HPV) – Transference During Sex

Another verified cause or risk factor for some forms of Head and Neck Cancer is an infection with *Humanpapillomavirus (HPV).* HPV is particularly linked to occurrences of Oropharyngeal Cancer that involves the Tonsils, or on the Base of the Tongue. *Hello! That rings some bells, as that was **MY** form of Cancer.* In the U.S., the incidence of Oropharyngeal Cancers caused by HPV-16 infection is increasing, while the incidences of Oropharyngeal Cancers related to other causes appear to be falling. Research has found that practicing *unprotected sex* can amplify an individual's risk of developing HPV. HPV is usually passed between people through unprotected vaginal intercourse and unprotected oral sex (I'm not quite sure how couples "protect" themselves during oral sex short of both wearing a "cone" about their necks - *I digress*), even if the infected partner exhibits no signs or symptoms. The optimistic flip-side of these findings is that many women who contract a higher risk of HPV infection, actually never develop Cervical Cancer, or any other form of the disease.

One recent scientific Study concluded that HPV does sharply increase the possibility of contracting certain types of Throat Cancer among those who become infected while experiencing oral sex with their partner. The Study found that Throat Cancer patients infected with HPV-16 were 32 times more likely to develop one form of Oral Cancer than non-Cancer patients not having the virus. These results could help explain why rates of Oral Cancer have been increasing in recent years, particularly among many younger people who are not smokers or heavy drinkers. *So, kids, just what's going on here?*

In my case, I have never smoked or used any type of tobacco in my life, and, if I drink any alcohol, it may be one or two smallish sips of wine a year, if that. That rules out those risk factors, and only leaves unprotected sex or oral sex as the possible culprit that caused my Head and Neck Cancer. Or, it could have been random chance, or any number of other risk factors I've faced during my life. I will say, though, that if having sex *did* contribute to the formation of *my* Cancer, that is one risk factor that I'm going to have a very difficult time avoiding! *A person's gotta do what a person's gotta do!*

The role of HPV being a genuine risk factor in the incidence of Opharyngeal Cancer is supported by a growing body of evidence. Specifically, per the National Cancer Institute (www.cancer.gov), a case-control *Study of 100 patients with Squamous Cell Cancer of the Oropharynx reported that* ***HPV-16 DNA was located in 72%*** of the tumor specimens. On a favorable note, Studies show that most Head and Neck Cancer patients diagnosed with HPV-caused tumors have been found to have better outcomes after any Surgery, Radiotherapy, and Chemotherapy. Additionally, Head and Neck Cancer *patients with known HPV-induced Cancers have lower incidences of second Cancer occurrences* (thus producing a much improved prognosis for survivorship), and a lower risk of death compared to tobacco-related illnesses (i.e., heart and lung disease). This is all optimistic news for those so-affected. But, as was said previously, Medical Studies have found an astounding, but conclusive, link between the occurrence of Oropharyngeal Cancer and high-risk sexual behaviors, including: an elevated lifetime number of sexual partners; engagement in oral sex; casual sexual relations; and infrequent condom use. As difficult as it may be for lovers of all ages to think about the relationship between HPV and Cancer—especially while in the throes of passion—it is a stark reminder of how serious and prolific this problem has become.

There are over 30 types of HPV that will affect an estimated 75% to 80% of males and females during their lifetimes. For most people, HPV clears on its own, but per www.cdc.gov, for 30 women a day in the U.S. (or about 12,000 women a year), specific types of HPV strains have been determined to cause Cervical Cancer (around

100%), Vaginal Cancers (65%), Vulva Cancers (50%), and, Anal Cancers (95%). Medical Studies have found that HPV may also lead to the development of Non-Melanoma Skin Cancers in some people. Tests are now provided by many health care providers to determine if a person has contracted HPV, and if so, to identify the strain of the HPV. HPV vaccinations are now obtainable which can help protect against some types of HPV. It is hoped that these vaccinations will help to reduce incidences of Oropharyngeal and other Cancers in the future. Individuals concerned with HPV potentially being a Cancer risk factor for them, should consult with their Medical Team.

Head and Neck Cancer Risk Factors – Potential Others

While the most prevalent risk factors for many types of Head and Neck Cancer are tobacco and alcohol use, and, while HPV has been found to promote Cancers of the Head and Neck, there are also other known risk factors responsible for causing many incidences of Head and Neck Cancer in men and women each year. Specifically, exposure to UV light (bright sunlight) without the use of correct sun protectant is a risk factor for development of Cancer of the Lips. At least 33% of patients with Lip Cancer work in outdoor occupations. From a nutritional perspective, studies suggest that dietary intake of vitamin A, β-Carotene, and α-Tocopherol via *fruits and veggies may reduce the likelihood of developing some Head and Neck Cancers.* Smoking Marijuana has been "associated" with the development of certain Head and Neck Cancers, but the level of risk is not known.

From an occupational hazard standpoint, Studies have found that a small group of Head and Neck Cancers may be attributable to on-the-job exposures to specific verified risk factors. For example, Nasal Cancer has been associated with wood dust exposure, such as that experienced by carpenters, sawmill workers, furniture makers, or others within similarly-related construction jobs. Medical Studies indicate that Squamous Cell Cancer of the Maxillary Sinus has been linked to inhaling specific metal dusts (again, related to construction and manufacturing), and, that continuous direct exposure to multiple Petroleum products may be associated with Pharyngeal Cancers. It has also been found that exposure to certain levels of Radiation is a risk factor for the development of Thyroid Cancer, and, has likewise been associated with Cancer of the Salivary Glands. *Good grief!*

What are the Signs and Symptoms of Head and Neck Cancers?

There are quite a few signs and symptoms of Head and Neck Cancers, but, as life would have it, several are comparable signs and symptoms that one could encounter with a bad Cold, Tonsillitis, the Flu, or other conditions. The real trick—and this is why doctors get paid the big bucks—is them being able to distinguish the differences between the occasional, normal illnesses such as Bronchitis or a sore throat caused by a Cold or Flu, and, signs of a more extreme medical condition, such as Cancer, that can display quite similar indications. In medical slang, a Cancer occurrence and symptoms masquerading as another condition is usually referred to as a, *"Red Herring."* The principal and most precarious problem with Cancer *Red Herrings* is that these *false identities* can cause the doctor and patient to devote a lot of time and effort to diagnose and care for a health condition that does not exist, while at the same time, haphazardly disregarding the true cause of the problems – Cancer. In other words, the physicians may start marching down the incorrect path with the patient in-tow, while the patient's Cancer is safe-and-sound and enjoying the ride.

During the outset of my crazy Cancer experience, four of my initial physicians—which includes two Ear, Nose, and Throat (ENT) doctors who are super educated to diagnose and treat Head and Neck Cancers *(which made my occurrence all the sadder and all the more unbelievable)*—started irresponsibly travelling me down the slippery *Red Herring* path. This, they did, by offering their opinions that my multi-month-old sore throat pain was due to Bronchitis. I knew they were mistaken, because I know my body *very* well, and I also knew that no matter what I did to treat my sore throat—which was located ***only on the left side of my neck***—all the over-the-counter remedies didn't work. I was personally very mindful that my throat issue was very different from the "garden variety" Bronchitis. But, despite my attempts to convince them that things were worse than they thought, they stayed with their opinions, because they are ***DOCTORS.*** *And, everybody knows that physicians don't ever commit any mistakes!* (*I say, tongue-in-cheek, but, I digress*). It was only after I passionately asserted myself and insisted that the Primary Doctor order an image of my throat and neck—which then prompted biopsies of my Lymph

Nodes and throat tissue—that we were finally able identify the cause of my constant pain. Yes, you guessed it – ***Head and Neck Cancer at the Base of the Tongue.*** I shudder to think what might have sadly happened to me had I taken these physicians' opinions at their word, and had not taken responsibility for my own health – and *my life!*

The signs and symptoms of several Head and Neck Cancers might include swelling or a sore that does not heal, a sore throat that won't go away, difficulty or pain while swallowing, and a change or hoarseness in one's voice (*I had all of these signs).* These symptoms may also be elicited by other, less serious conditions. It is important for a person to see a doctor or dentist if they experience any of these symptoms. Additionally—and this is a huge one—the Lymph Nodes located beneath the ears and right below the jaw lines on the sides of one's neck, may appear swollen and abnormal. In my own case, it was my enlarged Lymph Nodes, as well as my relentless sore throat pain, that told me something very serious was wrong. It was these two symptoms that, thankfully, caused me to seek medical attention.

Symptoms and Risk Factors of Head and Neck Cancers – By Cancer Type

Adapted from online resources of the U.S. National Cancer Institute (www.cancer.gov), following is information concerning the assorted risk factors and common symptoms for the multiple Cancers that are typically classified as Cancers of the Head and Neck:

Head and Neck Cancers Symptoms and Risk Factors (By Type)		
Type / Locations	**Symptoms**	**Risk Factors**
<u>**Oral Cavity Cancer**</u> The Oral (Mouth) Cavity includes the: • Lips • Front two-thirds of	• A white or red patch on the gums, the tongue, or the lining of the mouth • Swelling of the jaw that causes dentures to fit	• Alcohol or tobacco use, including cigarettes, snuff, chewing, cigars, pipes, etc. • Poor oral hygiene, such as not brushing

the Tongue • Gums • Lining inside the cheeks and lips • Floor (bottom) of the mouth under the tongue • Hard palate (bony top of the mouth) • Small area of the gum behind the wisdom teeth	poorly or become uncomfortable • Unusual bleeding or pain in the mouth	or flossing. Missing teeth may be risk factors for Cancers of the oral cavity • Use of mouthwash that has a high alcohol content is a possible, but not proven, risk factor • Immigrants from Southeast Asia who use paan (betel quid) in the mouth should be aware that this habit has been strongly associated with an increased risk of Oral Cancer • Consumption of mate, a tea-like beverage habitually consumed by South Americans, has been associated with an increased risk of Cancers of the Mouth, the Throat, the Esophagus, and the Larynx
<u>Pharyngeal Cancer</u> The Pharynx is a hollow tube about 5 inches long that starts behind the Nose and leads to the Esophagus The Pharynx has three parts: • Nasopharynx: The	• Trouble breathing or speaking • Pain when swallowing • ***<u>Pain in the neck or the throat that does not go away (My symptom)</u>*** • Frequent headaches • Pain or ringing in the ears • Trouble hearing	• Alcohol or tobacco use, including cigarettes, snuff, chewing, cigars, pipes, etc. • Asian ancestry particularly Chinese, is a risk factor for Nasopharyngeal Cancer, along with Epstein-Barr Virus Infection

upper part of the Pharynx, behind the nose • Oropharynx: The middle part of the Pharynx, including the Soft Palate (the back of the mouth), the ***<u>Base of the Tongue (The location of my tumor),</u>*** and the Tonsils • Hypopharynx: The lower part of the Pharynx		• Occupational exposure to wood dust • Consumption of certain preserved or salted foods during childhood • Humanpapillomavirus (HPV) infection, due to transference during vaginal and oral sexual activity, is also known to cause Oropharyngeal Cancer ***<u>Possibly the cause of my Cancer</u>***
<u>Laryngeal Cancer</u> The Larynx, also called the Voicebox, is a short passageway formed by cartilage just below the Pharynx in the neck. The Larynx contains: • The Vocal Cords • A small piece of tissue, called the Epiglottis, which moves to cover the Larynx to prevent food from entering the air passages	• Pain when swallowing • Ear pain	• Alcohol or tobacco use, including cigarettes, snuff, chewing, cigars, pipes, etc. • Certain industrial exposures, including exposures to asbestos and synthetic fibers, have been associated with Cancer of the Larynx, but the increase in risk remains controversial • People working in certain jobs in the construction, metal, textile, ceramic, logging, and food industries may have an increased risk of Cancer of the Larynx • Consumption of mate, a tea-like beverage habitually

		consumed by South Americans, has been associated with an increased risk of Cancers of the Mouth, Throat, Esophagus, and Larynx
Paranasal Sinus and Nasal Cavity Cancers The Paranasal Sinuses are small hollow spaces in the bones of the head surrounding the nose The Nasal Cavity is the hollow space inside the nose	• Sinuses that are blocked and do not clear • Chronic sinus infections that do not respond to treatment with antibiotics • Bleeding through the nose • Frequent headaches, swelling or other trouble with the eyes • Pain in the upper teeth • Problems with dentures	• Certain industrial exposures, such as wood or nickel dust, or Formaldehyde
Salivary Gland Cancer The major Salivary Glands are in the floor of the mouth and near the jawbone The Salivary Glands produce saliva, which is essential for mouth health and assists with digestion of food	• Swelling under the chin or around the jawbone • Numbness or paralysis of the muscles in the face • Pain in the face, the chin, or the neck that does not go away	• Radiation to the head and neck, for noncancerous conditions or Cancer • Infection with Epstein-Barr Virus

☛ ***Authors Note:*** If a person thinks that they might be at risk for Head and Neck Cancers because of the aforementioned or other risk factors, or, if they have noticed any abnormal, prolonged symptoms or indications with their body ***that just don't seem right,*** they should discuss this concern with their doctor or health care provider. There also are numerous services obtainable through medical facilities and organizations that promote a proactive approach to Cancer detection through regular medical checkups, and the use of Cancer screening tests. **Alert:** ***Early Cancer Detection = Better Cancer Destruction.***

Enlarged Lymph Nodes in the Neck – a Possible Sign of Head and Neck Cancer Presence

Sometimes, cancerous Squamous Cells (the flatter, scale-like Epithelial Cells of the skin or internal tissue linings) can be found in the Lymph Nodes of the upper neck, even if there is no indication of Cancer in other areas of the head and neck, and/or, if the location of the Primary Tumor is unknown. If this should happen, the Cancer is called ***"Metastatic Squamous Neck Cancer with Unknown (Occult) Primary."*** This, actually, is exactly what my Pathology Report said about my Cancerous presence when my physician first delivered my Cancer diagnosis to me. The initial diagnosis of my Cancer resulted from Pathology performed on the Biopsied tissue samples from the Lymph Nodes on the upper left area of my neck, which had become extremely swollen. It was not until supplemental examination—by a doctor outside my HMO that I saw for a Second Opinion—that we were able to discover the Primary Tumor at the *Base of my Tongue.* That is exactly where my sore throat pain had persisted for months.

The cancerous cells had obviously spread from my Tumor on my Tongue via my Lymphatic System, and had metastasized in the Lymph Nodes on the left side of my upper neck. There is no telling how long it took for this process to happen, but, suffice it to say that my Primary Tumor had been growing for quite a long while, and, it took time for the Cancer to spread and for the Lymph Node swelling to take place. This apparent, abnormal swelling, in conjunction with my persistent, non-mitigated sore throat, was what pointed out to me that something unusual with my body was happening. And, it was these "red flags" that caused me to request medical help in an effort to find what, specifically, had been inducing my pain and swelling. Thanks to this, we found and treated my Cancer, and, here I am.

How are Head and Neck Cancers Diagnosed?

To find the cause of the signs or symptoms of a problem in a person's head and neck area, the doctor evaluates a person's medical history, performs a physical examination, and could order diagnostic tests. The exams and tests may vary, however, depending upon the signs and symptoms presented by the patient during the preliminary examination. Biopsy Surgery to physically remove tissue samples from suspect sites in the patient's body, and examination of samples of tissue under a microscope in a Medical Pathology Lab, are always necessary to confirm a diagnosis of no-good, *malignant* Cancer. Not all tumors in or on a person's body are malignancies, as some may be *benign*, and, for all intents-and-purposes, harmless and not lethal.

The Diagnosis of all Head and Neck Cancers will necessitate various medical techniques, technological tools, and a high level of knowledge on the part of the skilled health care professionals. But, of course, for any of the medical exams, technology, and techniques to be of any benefit to the patient, the *person must first seek medical intervention when they become aware of any unusual symptoms or signs with their body.* But, wait, there's more! The second essential component of this very important Head and Neck Cancer Diagnosis process demands that the health care professional whom the patient sees for the exam has the skill, training, and knowledge to recognize potential Cancer symptoms, and to order additional tests to confirm its presence, or lack thereof. There is no room for second-guessing.

Assuming that all actions happen as they should, the patient and their physician(s) will next embark on a medical mission in an effort to identify the cause(s) of the patient's symptoms. During this examination process, an interpretation will be done as to whether the patient has a malignant Head and Neck Cancer that must be treated.

Following, in no particular order, are several of the diagnostic tools that can be used by health care professionals to Diagnose, Stage, and substantiate the presence of malignant Head and Neck Cancer. The explanations of the following medical techniques were adapted from the National Cancer Institute (www.cancer.gov) online resources:

- **Physical Exam of the Throat**

An exam in which the physician palpates the patient's neck with the fingers and feels for swollen Lymph Nodes in the upper neck below the jaw line. The physical exam also includes the physician looking down the throat with a sterilized, long-handled mirror and an intense light to check for areas that appear to be abnormal, swollen, or red.

- **Endoscopy**

A procedure used to view those areas in the throat that can't be seen with a mirror during the physical exam of the throat. An Endoscope (a thin, lighted tube with lubricant) is placed in through the nose or mouth to check the throat for anything that seems unusual. The tube is equipped with a small camera and viewing "monitor" that enables the physician to view the tissue where the Endoscope is directed.

- **Tissue Sample Biopsies**

Although many diagnostic tests can show the presence, location, and size of an abnormal mass in the body, none of the imaging tests can confirm that Cancer is the cause of the growth. Cancer is confirmed by finding cancerous cells during microscopic examination of tissue samples removed from the suspect area(s) through a Surgical Biopsy procedure. The results of Biopsies are ultimately examined under a microscope by a Medical Pathologist, and confirmed in a Pathology Report, which is provided to the ordering physician, and ultimately delivered to the patient – good news or bad. In cases of malignant Cancer, this piece of paper is one of the diagnostic tools the patient's Medical Team will use to help plan the patient's treatment.

- **CT (Computerized Tomography) or "CAT" Scan**

A procedure in which detailed images (i.e., "slices") are captured of areas within the body, taken from different angles. The pictures are loaded into a computer linked with an X-ray machine. A dye may be injected into a vein or swallowed to help the organs or tissues show up more clearly. Whereas an X-ray will generally produce an image of organs and bones and may illustrate any abnormalities in either, a CT Scan will provide the same detail from varying perspectives. CT Scans emit large amounts of radiation, so should be used sparingly.

- **MRI (Magnetic Resonance Imaging)**

Similar to the CT Scan in numerous ways, the MRI, or NMRI, is a procedure that uses magnetic fields, radio waves, and a computer to make a series of detailed pictures of regions within the body.

- **Head, Neck, and Chest X-rays**

An X-ray is a variety of energy beam that can pass through the body and onto special film, thus making a "picture" of regions inside the body. X-rays of the head, neck, and the chest will typically be taken.

- **Barium Esophagogram**

An X-ray of the Esophagus. The patient drinks a liquid that contains Barium, a safe, silver-white metallic compound. The liquid coats the Esophagus and then X-rays are taken, which may reveal "hot spots."

- **Esophagoscopy**

A procedure that enables the physician to look inside the Esophagus to check for regions that appear to be abnormal. Like an Endoscope, an Esophagoscope is a lighted, lubricated tube with a camera that is inserted through the patient's mouth or nose, and down the throat and into their Esophagus. During this exam, Biopsy Surgery tissue samples may be taken of suspect areas for pathological evaluation.

- **Bronchoscopy**

A procedure during which a physician looks inside the Trachea and large airways in the Lungs to see if here are any abnormal areas. Not unlike the Endoscope or Esophagoscope, the Bronchoscope (a thin, lubricated, lighted tube) is inserted through the individual's nose or mouth and into their Trachea and Lungs. Surgical Biopsies of tissue samples may be taken during this procedure of any abnormal areas, so that they can be further evaluated by a Medical Pathology lab.

How are Head and Neck Cancers Staged?

If a diagnosis of malignant Cancer is established by Medical Pathology, the physician will want to learn the Stage (size, degree of spread) of the disease in one's body. Cancer Staging is a careful and scientific means of "grading" a patient's Cancer, which is based on, among other factors, whether or not the Cancer has spread from the Primary Tumor and metastasized in other areas of the body. If one's Cancer has migrated from the Primary Tumor to other body tissues, systems, or organs by way of the patient's Circulatory or Lymphatic Systems, the Stage that is assigned will take into consideration these distant metastases, as well as their degrees of severity at the affected site(s). Knowing the Stage of the Cancer will enable all appropriate members of the patient's Medical Team to plan pertinent treatments to remove the Cancer from the patient's body, while causing as little "collateral damage" as possible to their healthy surrounding tissues.

Per www.cancer.gov, the Stages of Cancer are typically from 0 to IV, with Stage 0 representing possible future cancerous activity; Stage I being a localized Cancer occurrence (Primary Tumor with minimal or no spread); and Stage IV being the most severe due to its size and amount of progression from the Primary Tumor, and/or, its invasiveness in remote areas of the body. Stages II and III indicate varying degrees of Cancer scope and severity between the best- and worst-case scenarios. As one may well envision, the early detection, identification, diagnosis, and treatment of Cancers—at the minimum Stage possible (I or II)—is far more desirable than first locating and addressing one's Cancer when it has had an opportunity to securely entrench itself in one or more locations within the patient's body.

Therapies utilized to address Stage I or Stage II Cancers are, for very good reasons, typically less invasive and problematic, and, usually more successful, than those required to completely eradicate a Stage III or IV Cancer. Stage III and IV Cancers definitely can be effectively treated, but, the methods of doing so, as well as possible negative Side Effects to the patient that may develop as a result, can be rather challenging. So, while a mouse, being the first one to grab the cheese in a mousetrap will potentially lead to a less-than-optimal outcome *(for the mouse!),* a person that takes the initiative to request medical intervention at the earliest indications of questionable health symptoms could be doing themselves a huge favor. In other words, unlike the unlucky, premature mouse that *loses* its life, the proactive, *"early-bird-gets-the-worm"*-Cancer patient could be *saving* theirs.

What are the Stages for Head and Neck Cancers?

As with other forms of Cancer, Head and Neck Cancers are classified into Stages, from 0 to IV, to indicate how relatively severe the cancerous presence is, and, the level of severity if the Cancer has spread to other locations with in the body (i.e., to Lymph Nodes).

Staging Criteria for Forms of Head and Neck Cancer

According to National Cancer Institute (www.cancer.gov) resources, the Stages for different forms of Head and Neck Cancer are:

- **Throat Cancer**
    - **Stage 0**: Abnormal cells that may lead to Cancer are found in the Throat, Voice Box, or Tonsils. This Stage is also called Carcinoma *in situ*
    - **Stage I**: Actual Cancer is found in the Larynx only, which can include the Throat, Voice Box, or Vocal Cords. The Vocal Cords can still move normally
    - **Stage II**: Cancer is still limited to the Larynx only, but the Vocal Cords may not move normally
    - **Stage III**: Cancer may have spread to Lymph Nodes near the neck or to tissues near the neck. If Cancer is confined to the Larynx, the Vocal Cords cannot move
    - **Stage IV**: Cancer has spread to tissues outside the Larynx, such as the Thyroid Cartilage, the Neck, the Esophagus, or the Lymph Nodes, and it may have spread to distant areas of the body, such as the Lungs or the Liver

- ## Oral Cancer

  - **Stage 0**: Abnormal cells are seen in the lining of the Lips or Oral Cavity. These cells may develop into Cancer. This Stage is also called Carcinoma *in situ*
  - **Stage I**: Actual Cancer has formed, but the tumor is small and has not spread to Lymph Nodes
  - **Stage II**: The tumor is larger (between two and four centimeters), but it has not spread to any Lymph Nodes
  - **Stage III**: The tumor can be of any size and has spread to one Lymph Node on the same side of the neck in which the Cancer began, or, the tumor is larger than four centimeters
  - **Stage IV**: The Cancer has spread through the Lip and Oral Cavity to nearby tissues such as the Jaw, the Tongue, the floor of the mouth, the Sinuses in the cheek area next to the nose, or the skin on the chin or the nose

- ## Sinus and Nasal Cavity Cancers

Some Cancers of the Sinus, such as Cancer of the Sphenoid Sinuses (back of the skull), and frontal Sinuses (near the forehead), have no standard Staging system. Other Sinus Cancers are Staged as follows:

o Maxillary Sinuses

Maxillary Sinuses are in the cheek area next to the nose.

- **Stage 0**: Abnormal cells are found in the Inner Lining of the Maxillary Sinus. These cells may develop into Cancer. This Stage is also called Carcinoma *in situ*
- **Stage I**: Actual Cancer has formed in the Mucous Lining of the Maxillary Sinus
- **Stage II**: Cancer has spread to bone around the Maxillary Sinus, which includes the roof of the mouth and the nose. Cancer has not spread to bone at the back of the Maxillary Sinus or the base of the skull
- **Stage III**: Cancer may have spread to bone at the back of the Maxillary Sinus, to the eye socket, to tissues under the skin, to the base of the skull, or to Sinuses in the upper part

of the nose near the eyes (the Ethmoid Sinuses). Cancer may have spread to a Lymph Node on the same side of the neck where the Cancer began

- **Stage IV**: Cancer has spread to one or more Lymph Nodes. It may also have spread to areas far away from where the Cancer started, such as the back of the Eye, Brain, or Lungs

○ Nasal Cavity and Ethmoid Sinuses

These are the Sinuses at the top of the nose near the eyes.

- **Stage 0**: Abnormal cells are found in the inner lining of the Nasal Cavity or the Ethmoid Sinuses. These cells may develop into Cancer. This is also called Carcinoma *in situ*
- **Stage I**: Actual Cancer has developed. It is found in only one area - either the Nasal Cavity or the Sinuses in the upper part of the nose near the eyes. It may have spread into bone
- **Stage II**: Cancer is found in both the areas - the Nasal cavity *and* the Ethmoid Sinus. It may or may not have spread to any bone
- **Stage III**: Cancer may have spread to a Lymph Node on the same side of the neck as the original Cancer. It has also spread to areas adjacent to the Nasal Cavity, such as the Eye Socket, the roof of the mouth, the Maxillary Sinus, or the bone between the eyes
- **Stage IV**: Cancer has spread to one or more Lymph Nodes and has spread to more distant areas, such as the front of the nose and cheeks, base of the skull, back of the eye, or brain

• Metastatic Squamous Neck Cancer With Occult (Unknown) Primary

There is no standard Staging System for Metastatic Squamous Neck Cancer with Occult (Unknown) Primary. As a consequence, tumors are described as being in one of the two following categories:

- **Untreated**: The Cancer has been diagnosed but not treated except to relieve painful or other unconstructive symptoms

- **Recurrent**: The Cancer has returned after treatment. The Cancer may have come back in the neck or in other areas

The "TNM" Cancer Staging System

According to the National Cancer Institute (www.cancer.gov), the *"TNM System"* is one of the most generally used Cancer Staging Systems by both the medical and scientific communities. The TNM System is based on the extent (size) of the *Tumor (T),* the amount of Cancer spread to the *Lymph Nodes (N*), and the presence of distant *Metastasis (M)* (Cancer located in other organs/tissues of the body). A number may be added after each letter (for example, T3, N2, M1) to indicate the magnitude of the Primary Cancer Tumor, the amount of Cancer in the Lymph Nodes, and the level(s) to which the Cancer has spread to (or metastasized in) other areas of the body.

Not all Cancer incidences will have numerical values (1 thru 4) for *N* or *M*, however, as there might be only a Tumor (T) present, in which case the Cancer may not have spread to the Lymph Nodes (N), or Metastasized (M) elsewhere in the body. Thus, the Staging would comprise a numerical value for *T*, but a 0 value for *N* and *M.* Likewise, there could be the existence of Cancer in the Tumor and Nodes, but no Metastasis, in which circumstance, the Staging would reflect numbers for the *T* and *N*, but a 0 for *M. Starting to sink in?* Lastly, in conditions whereby a decidedly advanced Cancer has been detected in all the above – that is, in the Tumor(s), Nodes, and other Metastases located within the body, the Staging data would include numerical values for all three: *T, N,* and *M.* In some Cancers, such as Leukemia, cancerous cells are found in the Circulatory System, so a Tumor may not be present to quantify a Stage. In cases when the *T, N,* or *M* cannot be evaluated, this will be indicated accordingly. ***My own Cancer Stage and TNM rating was: Stage IV T1(2)N2bM0.***

☛ ***Author's Note***: The TNM Staging information below is being provided for informational purposes only. It may assist the patients to have a better understanding of Cancer Staging data if it is given to them by their treating physician(s), or, if they should read it in their own Cancer Pathology Lab Report. The Cancer Staging information featured below is not intended to be used by the patient to attempt to diagnose, assess, Stage, or treat their own, or another's Cancer, or to estimate one's prognosis. These actions are solely the responsibility of qualified medical professionals, whose job it is to advise patients accordingly in these areas. Patients should consult with their doctor.

Following are values and rudimentary criteria of the "Tumor, Node, Metastasis" (TNM) System of Staging Cancer, as extracted from the National Cancer Institute (www.cancer.gov) online resources:

- **Tumor, Node, and Metastasis (TNM) Staging System**

Value	Description
	Primary Tumor (T)
T0	There is no evidence of a tumor
T is	The tumor is *"in situ,"* meaning that it has not spread to nearby tissues
T1	The tumor cannot be viewed without using imaging techniques (X-Ray, CT Scan, PET Scan, etc.)
T2 – 4	The higher numbers indicate the involvement of the Lymph Nodes and the extent of the Primary Tumor
	Nodes (N)
N0	The Cancer has not spread to the Lymph Nodes
N1 - 4	The Cancer has spread to the Lymph Nodes. The higher numbers indicate how many Lymph Nodes are affected and how far away the Cancer has spread
	Metastasis (M)
M0	No distant metastasis, meaning the Cancer has not spread to other organs
M1	Distant metastasis, meaning the Cancer has spread to other organs

How are Head and Neck Cancer Tumors Graded?

To better understand how Cancer Tumors are graded, it may benefit the Reader for them to learn again how Cancer Tumors form. As I have stated previously in this Book, the human body consists of *trillions of millions* of different kinds of cells. Normally, cells will grow and divide to produce new cells that replace older, dead cells, and, they typically will do this in a controlled and regulated manner. Sometimes, however, new, *extra* cells continue to be produced when they are not needed, which can result in a mass of spare tissue called a *Tumor*. This tumor can be ***Benign*** (non-cancerous), or ***Malignant*** (cancerous). The cells in malignant tumors are irregular because of damaged DNA that can be caused by a variety of risk factors. These mutated cancerous cells divide rowdily without any control or order, and can invade and cause harm to adjacent tissues. These destructive cells can also spread to, and metastasize in, other parts of the body.

☛***Author's Note***: The following material regarding the Grading of Cancer Tumors is provided for informational purposes only. The Cancer Tumor Grading information offered below is not intended to be used by the patient to endeavor to diagnose, assess, Stage, or treat their own or another's Cancer, or to estimate one's prognosis. These proceedings are the responsibility of qualified medical professionals, whose job it is to advise patients accordingly in these areas.

The following information regarding the Grading of Cancer Tumors was adapted from the National Cancer Institute (www.cancer.gov):

Cancer Tumor Grading

Cancer Tumor Grading is a system used to categorize Cancer cells in terms of how abnormal they look under a microscope and—based upon scientific evidence of the same forms of cancerous cells observed in multiple Studies—how quickly the tumor cells are likely to develop and multiply within the patient's body. Many factors are considered when determining Tumor Grade, including the structure and growth pattern of the cancerous cells. Also, the specific factors used to determine Tumor Grade vary with each type of Cancer.

The Tumor Grade should not be mistaken for the Stage of a Cancer. Cancer Stage refers to the degree or severity of the Cancer, based on factors including the location of the Primary Tumor, tumor size, magnitude of tumors, and Lymph Node involvement (spread of Cancer cells into the Lymph Nodes), and other metastasis within the body. *Histologic Grade*, also called *Differentiation*, pertains to *how much the tumor cells resemble normal cells of the exact tissue type.* *Nuclear Grade* relates to the sizes and shapes of the Nuclei in tumor cells, and the percentage of tumor cells that are dividing.

Determination of Cancer Tumor Grade

If a tumor is suspected to be *Malignant*, a doctor will remove a sample of applicable localized tissue, the entire tumor, or both, in a Biopsy Surgery procedure. A Pathologist (a physician who identifies diseases by evaluating cells beneath a microscope) will examine the samples in a Medical Lab to determine whether the tumor is Benign (non-cancerous) or Malignant (cancerous). The Pathologist will also verify the Tumor Grade and other characteristics of the tumor cells.

The Lab Pathologist will document the results of the Biopsy exam findings on a Pathology Report, which will be provided to the physician that performed the Biopsy Surgery. It is this Pathology Report—a simple piece of white paper, full of several fancy medical terms—that the physician will deliver and read to the patient during their Biopsy follow-up exam. And, it is this same document that will carry the news of a malignant Cancer diagnosis for about 1.7 million unsuspecting men, women, teenagers and kids in the U.S. each year. The Pathology Report, without question, is one very powerful piece of paper that can change a person's life in a heartbeat - *literally!*

What the Different Malignant Tumor Grades Signify

Based upon the microscopic appearance of Cancer cells, Lab Pathologists commonly describe the Tumor Grades by four levels of severity: Grades 1, 2, 3, and 4 *(hmm, I wonder where they came up with that? Sorry, I digress).* The cells of Grade 1 Tumors resemble normal cells, and tend to grow and multiply slowly and are the least aggressive. The cells of Grade 3 or Grade 4 tumors, however, do not appear like regular cells of the same type. Grade 3 and 4 tumors tend to grow rapidly and spread much faster than lower Grade tumors.

The American Joint Committee on Cancer (AJCC) recommends the following guidelines for grading malignant Cancer Tumors:

Grade	Cancer Tumor Grading Criteria
GX	Grade cannot be assessed (Undetermined grade)
G1	Well-differentiated (Low grade)
G2	Moderately differentiated (Intermediate grade)
G3	Poorly differentiated (High grade)
G4	Undifferentiated (High grade)

Grading Scales Differ Depending on Form of Cancer

Grading Systems are different for each type of Cancer. As an example, Pathologists use the Gleason System to describe the degree of differentiation of Prostate Cancer cells. The Gleason System uses scores ranging from Grade 2 to Grade 10. The lower Gleason scores describe well-differentiated, less aggressive tumors. Higher scores illustrate tumors that are poorly differentiated and more aggressive. Tumor Grading Systems also include the Bloom-Richardson System for Breast Cancer, and the Fuhrman System for Kidney Cancer.

Tumor Grade Affects a Patient's Treatment Options and Prognosis

Doctors use Tumor Grade and many other factors to develop a personalized treatment plan for the Cancer patient and to forecast the patient's prognosis. Generally speaking, a lower Grade indicates a better prognosis (the perceived outcome of the Cancer after efforts to remove it, or the chance of recovery or recurrence). However, the importance of Tumor Grade in planning therapies and estimating a patient's prognosis is greater for particular types of Cancers, such as Soft Tissue Sarcomas, Primary Brain Tumors, Lymphomas, and Breast and Prostate Cancer. Patients who wish to learn more, or who have questions about Tumor Grades, should speak with their doctor about how the Grade relates to their own diagnosis and treatment.

Who are the Health Professionals that Treat Patients with Head and Neck Cancers?

Patients with Head and Neck Cancers are typically treated by a team of specialists that represent numerous health care disciplines. These professional individuals, who encompass the patient's Cancer Treatment Medical Team, are extremely skilled, knowledgeable, and well-trained in the multi-disciplined elements of Cancer Treatment, Recovery and Aftercare. Additionally, because of several of the very distinctive health care concerns and requirements of Head and Neck Cancer patients, all of the professionals on the Medical Team should be well-suited to address any and all needs as they evolve. That said, the health care specialists on the Medical Team may differ at times, depending on several factors, including the patient's variety of Head and Neck Cancer, as well its Stage and its location within the body, and, the age, and general health status of the patient being treated.

While the Medical Team will have a core faction of doctors, nurses, and others who will be treating and looking after the patient from the beginning to a, hopefully, successful outcome, a few of the health care professionals will come and go depending on whether or not their services are needed at the time. In this respect, the Medical Team is a dynamic force whose principal responsibility is to convert a frightening Cancer diagnosis into Cancer survivorship, and to do it as capably and as safely as is possible. Medical Team members may include Dentists; Oral Surgeons; Ear-Nose-and-Throat doctors (also referred to as Otolaryngologists); Pathologists; Medical Oncologists; Radiation Oncologists; Plastic Surgeons; Primary Care Physicians; Registered Dietitians; Social Workers; Nurses; Physical Therapists; Speech-Therapists; and, others that may join the Team, as necessary.

Each of these health care professionals, individually, and all of them working together as one, make up the collection of certified, highly skilled, well-educated, talented, experienced, and (hopefully) compassionate people on whom the Head and Neck Cancer patient, and their family and Caregiver, will depend throughout the patient's entire Cancer journey. From the moment that the unsuspecting man woman, or child is told of their Cancer diagnosis, and, typically, for the remainder of their life, these folks will *have the patient's back.*

"'Cancer Survival' is a multi-step process. First, there is survival of the Diagnosis and resulting worry. Next, will be survival of the Treatment preparations, followed after by the Treatments, themselves, and any uncomfortable Side Effects. Finally, one has to survive any despair that may ensue with the doubt of not knowing if all of their Cancer is gone after treatment, or, whether it will strike once again. The journey to Cancer Survival is not an effortless one, but, with faith, hope, and the support of many, the road can be safely traveled, and the final destination can be reached. That destination is Survivorship."

- Butch Sickler

Chapter Ten

Head and Neck Cancers – Part 2 – *Getting to Know This Uncommon Foe*

"The only way Cancer wins is if we forget what matters most."

- Butch Sickler

Very rarely will most people in the general population ever hear any mention of the description, *"Head and Neck Cancer."* This is because, as I've stated previously, Head and Neck Cancers are not *"household name"* Cancers such as Breast, Prostate, Colorectal, and Lung. Some Readers might recall the actor, Michael Douglas, being diagnosed with Stage IV Cancer in 2010, but, most might not have realized that his Cancer was classified as, *"Cancer at the Base of the Tongue" – the form of Cancer that I had.* And, not unlike *my* Cancer experience, Douglas' Cancer also "revealed" itself with a sore throat that wouldn't heal. In truth, he told a national magazine that he had visited doctors for 9 months to try to figure out why his throat hurt, but none of them could locate the reason. I also visited doctors about my never-ending throat pain who could not identify its source. Then, in Mr. Douglas' situation, as in mine, we steadily forced the doctors to eventually find the problem. Head and Neck Cancers are so rare, I guess that even Hollywood doctors aren't aware that they exist. As with my Cancer, I read that Mr. Douglas is not sure what caused his.

Is There Screening for Head and Neck Cancers?

According to the National Cancer Institute (www.cancer.gov), men and women who believe that they may be at risk for developing

Head and Neck Cancers could be screened as a preventive measure. Cancer screening can also be utilized as a useful tool to help indicate a Cancer existence in its original Stages, when it is less invasive and safer to treat, and is more susceptible to conventional treatment(s).

The Upside of Cancer Screening

Basic Screening for Cancer is the examination (or testing) of people to medically determine if cancerous activity may be present, even though the individual may display no outward or obvious signs or symptoms. Scientists and doctors have studied patterns of Cancer in the population to learn which people are more likely to get certain types of Cancer, including of the Head and Neck variety. They have also researched the potential environmental inducers of Cancer. This information sometimes helps physicians recommend who should be screened for specific forms of Cancer, what types of screening tests individuals should have, and how often these tests should be done.

The Potential Downside of Cancer Screening

It has been realized during medically-controlled Studies that not all Cancer screening tests are beneficial, and that various follow-on actions could carry some risk, such as bleeding and infection, if Biopsy Surgery tissue samples must be taken to confirm Cancer due to an abnormal Screening exam, or a test indicating "false positives" (i.e. looks and acts like Cancer, but isn't). For these reasons, medical scientists from the U.S. National Cancer Institute (www.cancer.gov) are researching Cancer Screening tests to determine how useful they are, and, to ascertain their relative benefits and risks. If a patient's doctor suggests certain Cancer Screening tests as part of their health care plan, *this does not mean they think that the person has Cancer.*

To Screen or Not to Screen? – That is the Question

Screening tests are typically performed when an individual is exhibiting no Cancer symptoms. Since decisions about whether or not to receive a screening can be difficult to make, the patient will want to discuss the topic with their physician. The individual should ask their physician questions about the potential benefits and risks of

Screening tests, and, whether the tests have been proven to decrease the risk of Cancer mortality. If a person's doctor suspects that they could have Cancer, he or she will order specific diagnostic tests such as Image Scans, and/or, Biopsy Surgery, to pathologically determine if Cancer is present. *These exams are used for diagnostic purposes, but are not suitable for screening people who have no symptoms.*

How Can a Person Reduce Their Risk of Developing Head and Neck Cancers?

As is elucidated in the lists of Cancer causes and risk factors back in Chapter 9, and ahead in Chapter 11, medical authorities have a pretty good handle on the identified and suspected risk factors for every type of Head and Neck Cancer. Therefore, the logical way for a person to lessen their chances of developing any form of Head and Neck Cancer is to abstain from exposing oneself to any of the listed prospective causes. I know – easier said than done, especially when it comes to age, gender, race, and, yep, you guessed it, sex and HPV.

Age? Sex? Gender? Vices? – What's a Person to Do?

As mentioned a few times previously, a person's age is a risk factor for Cancer, unto itself, as one gets older. And, as we all know, there is not a whole lot that a person can do about that, short of them climbing into a Time Machine (if you can locate one, *please* let me know!). Then, just our luck, there's that gender thing. As was stated earlier in this Chapter, Head and Neck Cancers are two times more prevalent in men, than in women, which means that being a Male is yet one more risk factor to pile onto the seemingly never-ending list. However, if there are any 50-year-old men thinking of having a sex-change operation in a desperate attempt to outsmart a possible Head and Neck Cancer occurrence, that *is* a very nice try. But, they might want to hold off on buying any lingerie *for themselves* just yet!

All joking aside, as stressed by the National Cancer Institute (www.cancer.gov), men and women who believe that they may be at high risk of developing some form of Head and Neck Cancer—and particularly those who use or abuse tobacco and/or, alcohol—should speak with their doctor about ways that they may be able to diminish their risks. And, knowing what we now know about HPV-16 and its relationship to unprotected sex and certain Cancers, those who think that they could be at risk for Head and Neck Cancer because of these circumstances should ask their doctor whether or not they should be tested for HPV, and, how often they should have medical physicals.

"Preventive Medicine" – Regular Exams and Vaccines

Regular patient examinations are highly recommended by all physicians as they serve as a very useful tool to help determine if the "coast is clear," or, if further actions should be taken in an effort to test, detect, identify, and tackle any abnormal physical conditions—including Cancer—that may have stoked the physician's curiosity or seemed "suspect" during the exam. In addition to the patient and the physician doing their due-diligence through periodic medical check-ups, Cancer Researchers and Food and Drug Administration (FDA) Scientists have partnered with each other in ongoing Clinical Trials.

The intention of the Clinical Trials is to test the effectiveness of assorted medications and vaccines that have been developed in a hopeful effort to prevent the incidence of Head and Neck Cancers in persons who have a high likelihood of developing these forms of the disease. In particular, the FDA has recently authorized two vaccines to prevent HPV infection, and both vaccines have been found during tests to be extremely effective in preventing infections. Researchers are also studying the effects of a HPV vaccination to see if it reduces the incidence of the forms of HPV infections in the Oral Cavity that can lead to the formation of Oropharyngeal Head and Neck Cancers – the type of Head and Neck Cancer with which I was diagnosed.

Can Patients with Head and Neck Cancers Take Part in Medical Clinical Trials?

Medical Clinical Trials are Research Studies conducted with those patients who volunteer to take part. As stated by the National Cancer Institute (www.cancer.gov), for many patients with Head and Neck Cancers, participation in Clinical Trials may be an option that they may want to consider. Clinical Treatment Trials with Head and Neck Cancer patients are designed to develop more effective Cancer

Treatments and better ways to use current Treatments. Members of the patient's Medical Team should be able to provide information to the patient, their family or Caregiver, that explains Head and Neck Cancer Clinical trials, and their overall, potential risks and benefits.

Clinical Trials for Individuals to Hopefully Benefit Many

While the outcomes of Clinical Trial Studies are essential to Cancer research and are aimed at finding newer and improved ways to effectively treat Cancers—in general—the primary purpose of the Clinical Trials is to distinctively treat ***all participating patients*** *with one, and only one, objective: To eradicate the patient's disease as completely and safely as possible.* In other words, while the patient volunteers are told by doctors—and they completely comprehend—that their involvement in the Study is aiding Cancer research efforts, overall, that definitely doesn't mean that these courageous souls are "guinea pigs," or that they will be receiving inferior care, placeboes, or other procedures that will position them in harm's way during the treatment of their particular Cancers. Much to the contrary, many of these patients will be on the receiving-end of cutting-edge medicine, techniques, and technologies in an effort to rid them of their Cancers and to save their special lives. Whether involved in a Clinical Trial, or receiving "normal" Cancer treatment at a local hospital or Cancer Clinic, ***all Cancer patients*** are treated with a complete cure in mind. That is, if the patient's overall health status and age, and their form of Cancer, and its Stage, location, and other factors, will permit.

Clinical Trials - The Ultimate "Science Fair Projects"

In some Head and Neck Cancer Clinical Trials, all patients in the Study receive the "new" treatment being tested. In other Cancer Trials, physicians compare the effectiveness of different therapies on different Head and Neck Cancers by giving the new treatment to one group of patients and standard therapy to another group. Doctors are also continually studying new methods and schedules for delivering Radiation Therapy; new anti-Cancer drugs; new drug combinations (for the *"Chemo Cocktails"* prescribed for some patients); and, new means of combining treatments (i.e., adjuvant use of Chemotherapy and Radiation Therapy, etc.). Scientists are also researching ways to treat Head and Neck Cancers using Biological Therapy (i.e., a type of treatment that stimulates the patient's personal Immune System to fight Cancer with Cancer Immunotherapy drugs), either by itself, or in amalgamation with other anti-Cancer drugs or Radiation Therapy. Of significant interest to all Head and Neck Cancer patients are the Clinical Trials being conducted by scientists to find better means to resolve the often painful, nauseating, and distressing Side Effects of Chemotherapy and Radiation Therapy. These critical Clinical Trials, called *Supportive Care Trials,* explore ways to improve the comfort and quality of life of Cancer patients and Cancer survivors.

Guidance for Participating in a Clinical Trial

Head and Neck Cancer patients who are interested in taking part in a Clinical Trial should discuss this possibility with one of the applicable physicians on their Cancer Treatment Medical Team. The physician should be able to provide the patient with information on Clinical Trials, in general, or, possibly, on specific Clinical Trials of which they may be aware. Additional information about Head and Neck Cancer Clinical Trials is available through the National Cancer Institute (www.cancer.gov) booklet entitled, ***Taking Part in Clinical Trials: What Cancer Patients Need to Know.*** The aforementioned booklet describes how research Studies are carried out and explains potential benefits and risks and other considerations. In addition, the U.S. National Cancer Institute online resources at www.cancer.gov offer comprehensive materials about Head and Neck Cancer Clinical Trials, and includes links to *"PDQ,"* a Cancer information database developed by the National Cancer Institute, which provides detailed information regarding specific ongoing Cancer Studies. And, finally, patients can obtain information concerning Head and Neck Cancer Clinical Trials the *good, old-fashioned way,* by using the telephone. Interested patients can phone the National Cancer Institute's Cancer Information Service at 1–800–4–Cancer (1–800–422–6237).

Is There Follow-up Care for Head and Neck Cancer Patients, and What Does it Involve?

According to the National Cancer Institute (www.cancer.gov), the relatively positive news for Head and Neck patients is that if the initial treatment(s) for their Cancer is triumphant—meaning that the patient is cured of their disease—there is a relatively low risk (2% to 3% per year) of the patient developing a new, completely unrelated Head and Neck Cancer. *(**Note:** These percentages are assuming that the Cancer survivor does not aggravate their post-treatment Cancer risks by using tobacco, drinking alcohol, or, experiencing excessive exposure to other would-be Cancer causes).* But, 2%-3% is not 0%, which means that there will forevermore be a slight possibility that a second, new Cancer will rear its irritating head out of nowhere. And, not unlike the hard-to-get critter in the *"Whack-a-Mole"* game at the County Fair, every effort will be taken by the responsible physicians and Pathology specialists to attempt to find and identify the Cancer, and to *whack* it into oblivion as quickly and as safely as possible.

Follow-on Tests – the Medical "3,000 Mile Oil Change"

As I've mentioned a few times previously in this Book, when a Cancer patient completes their scheduled treatments, they do not fall off of the "medical radar screen." In fact, they're watched closer than a spy in Washington, D.C. But truthfully, all Cancer patients—no matter their gender or age, or the form of the disease they had, or the therapies used to treat it—will be closely monitored, examined, and tested for a Cancer recurrence, or any new, unrelated Cancer, on a regular schedule throughout their lives. It is one thing for a person to be completely surprised by deceitful Cancer when it unexpectedly comes knocking the first time. But, once a Cancer patient and their family, Caregiver, and Medical Team have done all the right things and invested their hearts and souls to purge the *original* Cancer from the patient's body, the furthest thing that anyone wants to happen is for another Cancer to rear its horrible head and multiply, undetected, *once again.* So, from a follow-up standpoint, as one might presume, *Head and Neck Cancer survivors* are subject to the precise forms of regular aftercare tests and monitoring as are other Cancer survivors.

Treatment Follow-up Examinations and Frequencies

Subsequent to the achievement of a Head and Neck Cancer patient's Treatment phase of their journey, and during the Recovery and Aftercare phases and beyond, the patient will be asked to submit to many follow-on tests and exams so that all responsible physicians can continue to monitor the health status of the patient, typically, for the remainder of their lives. If, *"An ounce of prevention is worth a pound of cure,"* as the proverb goes, then all post-Cancer treatment follow-up tests and examinations have got to be priceless.

Following are specific reasons cited by the National Cancer Institute (www.cancer.gov), for post-Head and Neck Cancer therapy follow-up examinations for patients and survivors:

- To monitor the acute Side Effects of the Radiation Therapy
- To detect recurrent Cancer (from the initial Primary Cancer Tumor) and possibly try further treatment, such as Surgery, if the Radiation Therapy, and/or, Chemo is unsuccessful
- To detect and treat Late Side Effects (i.e., *Late Effects*) or complications from prior Radiation Therapy, should they manifest themselves after treatment
- To detect and treat unrelated, Secondary Head and Neck Cancers, or other forms of Cancer, that may occur

Following are the *general frequencies* of follow-up examinations to which Head and Neck Cancer survivors will be asked to submit after the conclusion of their treatment(s):

- **First Year:** **Every four to six weeks**
- **Second Year:** **Every two months**
- **Third Year:** **Every three months**
- **Fourth/Fifth Year:** **Every six months**
- **Thereafter:** **Annually (Every 12 months)**

In addition to Head and Neck Cancer patients adhering to the above follow-up exam schedule, they should also get a Chest X-ray once each year to monitor potential Cancer metastasis in that suspect region of the body. Further, Thyroid functions should be confirmed annually to recognize any occurrence of Hypothyroidism (decreased Thyroid function), which may be caused by Radiation Therapy, and can be easily treatable. Sometimes, additional tests are used, such as a CT scan, Positron Emission Tomography (PET) scan, or an MRI. The survivor's physicians will apply all the appropriate tools to help verify absence (good), or presence (bad), of post-treatment Cancer.

After Cancer Treatment – Tests, Tests, and More Tests

As stated in prior Sections of this Chapter, regular follow-up care is very important after treatment for all Head and Neck Cancers to verify whether or not the patient's Cancer has relapsed or recurred (returned), or if a Second Primary Cancer (new and unrelated to the initial Cancer incidence) has developed within the patient's body. It goes without saying that the preferred outcome of all post-treatment follow-up exams will be that no new or remaining cancerous activity will be found throughout the patient's entire body during any of the follow-up exams. Undeniably, every Cancer patient, when provided with the results of their follow-up tests by their doctors, will want to hear the physician utter the phrase, *"The coast is clear," "We see no cancerous activity," "Your tests came back negative for Cancer,"* or, some similar iteration of these thrilling, optimistic words. When all Cancer patients—young or old, male or female—are told by their doctors that there are no new signs of Cancer presence, that is a very celebratory and memorable moment, indeed. Each negative Cancer test and examination propels the Head and Neck Cancer *Patient* just one step closer to becoming a well-deserving Cancer *Survivor.*

Depending upon the patient's type of Head and Neck Cancer and the form of therapy they received, follow-up medical checkups could include exams of the Stoma (a mouth-like incised opening that is kept open for drainage or other purposes), if one has been created, and physical exams of the mouth, neck, and throat. Regular Dental or Oral exams by a qualified Dentist or an Oral Surgeon may also be called for to verify that no new signs of potential Cancer are present, or, to become aware of them, and take necessary action, if there are.

According to the U.S. National Cancer Institute (www.cancer.gov), regular follow-on tests that the doctor may perform could include:

- A physical exam, especially of the Head and Neck region that was treated for Cancer, including the site of the Primary Tumor (if known) and Lymph Nodes *(I receive this exam)*
- Blood tests
- X-rays
- Computed Tomography (CT or CAT) Scan

- Positron Emission Tomography (PET) Scan
- Magnetic Resonance Imaging (MRI) Scan
- Endoscopy *(typically what I get during my follow-on exams)*

The treating physician may also monitor Thyroid Gland and Pituitary Gland function, especially if the Head or Neck areas were treated with Radiation. If the patient is a smoker, the doctor is likely to counsel the patients to cease their smoking. Research has shown that continuous smoking by a Head and Neck Cancer survivor might decrease the effectiveness of treatment(s), and could exacerbate the chance of a Second Primary Cancer forming somewhere in the body.

Discovery and Confirmation of "Possible" New Cancer

What every Cancer patient, including those treated for Head and Neck Cancers, must be aware of, is that occasionally, during the post-Treatment follow-on testing process, the patient's exam results may ***suggest*** the existence of cancerous activity. What this means, is that, according to a physical exam of the tumor site conducted by the physician, or, based upon other tests or the results of imaging scans performed with one or more medical diagnostic machines (CT, PET, X-Ray or MRI), the apparent indications could point to the far-flung *possibility* that live Cancer cells ***may*** be present in the patient's body tissue. *There's a VERY BIG difference between "may" and "are."*

When the surprising and disheartening discovery of possible cancerous activity is made during Cancer follow-up testing (as took place with me during *three of my five* post-treatment PET Scans), I am not lying when I tell you that the news will frighten the patient to no-end. Any remark from the doctor that a follow-up Cancer test or exam has revealed a *potential new Cancer* is all it takes to dredge up the terrified and distressing feelings that the patient experienced the moment their doctor *first* told them of their initial Cancer diagnosis. For lack of a better way of putting it, this type of eye-opener can be a Cancer survivor's worst nightmare. *I can certainly vouch for that!*

If and when any follow-up exams suggest that new Cancer may have formed in the patient, the treating physician will typically want to corroborate the correctness of the test by ordering a Surgical

Tissue Biopsy procedure of the suspect area(s). During the Biopsy procedure, as detailed elsewhere in this Book, the Surgeon will take samples of the patient's tissue that appeared or felt during the exam as if it may be tainted with cancerous cells. The Surgeon will ensure that all tissue samples are properly marked before being sent off to a Pathology Lab for microscopic examination. From the time that the Surgeon performs the Biopsy procedure, until the moment when the patient's treating physician delivers the Biopsy results to the patient, I can assure you that it will seem like an eternity. While the patient is awaiting receipt of the follow-on test results, their heart and mind will most likely be overwhelmed with concern, distress, fear, and—not unlike their original diagnosis—some aspect of doubt about their future. It's one thing to meet and overcome the Cancer monster one time, but, to potentially come face-to-face with it again can be very scary and extremely unsettling to any Cancer patient or survivor.

Positive and "False Positive" Follow-on Test Results

After Biopsy samples have been surgically removed and are analyzed by a Medical Pathologist, sadly, some Cancer patients' and survivors' worst fears will be realized when their treating physician informs them that a new or recurring Cancer has been found in their body. For these individuals—and I've known of quite a few of these gutsy warriors including my Mom, to whom this has happened—the notion of having to "go to the mat" with this evil disease once again is almost too much for them to bear. But, just as they did when they courageously conquered and survived their First Round with Cancer, these valiant Cancer Warriors, along with their families, Caregivers, and Medical Teams, will, once again, do what they can to safely and completely vanquish the nasty disease once again, in Round Two.

Thankfully, not all *"apparent"* Cancer activity that is located during post-treatment follow-up exams, either by a physician or via a diagnostic machine, ends up testing positive for malignant Cancer. In my Cancer experience, I had five Positron Emission Tomography (PET) Scans in the several months following my Cancer treatments for the purpose of looking for any new or residual cancerous activity at the site of my tumor, and within my entire body. During three of the five Scans, my doctor told me that my PET images appeared to be *"lighting up"* in the area of my Primary Tumor at the Base of my

Tongue. *Lighting up* is the best way to depict it, because on the PET scan image, suspect areas appeared much brighter than other tissue.

Each time that the "red flag" of potential Cancer went up the pole, I, of course, freaked out, thinking, as my doctor had led me to believe, that I could still have some cancerous cells wreaking havoc within my body. And, with each round of "possible" Cancer came the need for me to undergo Biopsy Surgery of the suspected areas – with each of those Surgeries carrying with them their own elements of risk. The *"potential of Cancer"* worried me beyond compare on each occasion, and, I found that there was nothing that anyone could say or do to eliminate the angst that I felt while I was waiting for the results of the laboratory tests to come back. Fortunately, in each of the three cases, my physician told me that the tissue samples tested negative for malignant Cancer. As one can well imagine, in the three instances, I was extremely relieved about the false alarms—or as my physician referred to the outcomes, *"False Positives."* However, the circumstances still beg the question, *If it wasn't* ***Cancer*** *on the PET Scans, what was it?* Not knowing on what to "blame" the erroneous PET Scans, my doctor attributed the *lit up* areas on the images to the healing of healthy cells – a reasonable guess, I guess. W*ho says that Medicine isn't an exact science? I often wonder if throwing a dart at a dartboard may actually be a more scientific method!* I digress.

What Rehabilitation and Support Options are Available for Head and Neck Cancer Patients After Treatment?

Rehabilitation after Cancer Treatment is a very critical aspect of the entire program for patients with Head and Neck Cancer. The goals of rehabilitation during the patient's Recovery phase are aimed at providing the patient with the support mechanisms and tools they will need to help bring about the most encouraging Cancer outcome possible. As one might expect, the final Cancer result that is realized will depend on many factors, including: The extent of the disease in the body; the invasiveness of the treatment the patient had received; any ensuing Side Effects with which the patient had to contend; the patient's response—favorable or not—to the treatments and Side Effects; and, lastly, the age and overall health status of the patient.

The Rehab Needs of Head and Neck Cancer Patients

The Head and Neck Cancer patient's Medical Team makes every attempt—with the assistance of the patient's family members and Caregiver, as applicable—to help the patient return to normal, *pre-Cancer* activities as soon as is reasonably possible. The primary purpose of treatments for all Head and Neck Cancers is to safely and thoroughly control and eradicate the disease from the patient's body. However, physicians are, likewise, concerned about maintaining the function of the affected, treated areas as much as they can. Such due diligence is extremely important for Head and Neck Cancer patients, essentially, because of the life-critical locations in the head and neck regions where their Cancers occurred. Many Head and Neck Cancer patients exit their treatment phase bearing not only external physical scars, but deeper, debilitating wounds of an emotional or mental sort as well. Rehabilitative Therapy is a very significant component that aids the patient in confronting and coping with a lot of the *collateral damage* that was incurred both during and after Cancer treatment.

Post-treatment rehabilitation may involve a multitude of therapeutic techniques, facilitated by a disparate group of health care specialists. Per www.cancer.gov, following are three of the more common forms of rehab support that are offered to Head and Neck Cancer patients:

- ### **Physical Therapy After Cancer Surgery**

Following their Cancer treatment, the Head and Neck Cancer patient may notice changes in his or her physical strength, muscular range of motion, equilibrium, endurance, and flexibility. During the Rehabilitation process, Occupational Therapists educate patients and their families and Caregivers about these alterations and how to use adaptive equipment and compensatory procedures to stabilize and to improve patients' independence throughout their daily routines. The Therapists also teach patients methods that will help them complete basic daily activities such as bathing, dressing, and moving around.

Some Head and Neck Cancer patients may realize a decrease in vision after Surgery. Therapists can evaluate and teach the patient techniques to help make up for diminished eyesight. Therapists may also prescribe therapeutic exercise regimens to help affected patients improve their speech and pronunciation, swallowing, posture, range of motion, and, the strength of both their neck and shoulder muscles following treatment. They may also provide therapies to improve the efficiency of breathing and coughing after Surgery, as well as some assistive devices to help patients walk and perform other functions.

Depending upon the type and location of the Head and Neck Cancer in the patient’s body, and the type of treatment(s) the patient received, rehabilitation may also entail training on how to care for a Stoma. A Stoma is an opening into the Windpipe through which the patient breathes after a Laryngectomy, which is a Surgery to remove the Larynx. Sometimes, especially with Cancer of the Oral Cavity, a patient may require Reconstructive and Plastic Surgery to rebuild bones and tissues. However, Reconstructive Surgery may not always be possible because of damage to the remaining tissue caused by the original Surgery to eradicate the Primary Tumor, or from Radiation Therapy. If Reconstructive Surgery is not possible, a Prosthodontist might be able to fashion prosthesis (an artificial dental, and/or, facial part custom-fitted to the patient) to restore satisfactory swallowing, speech, and outward appearance. Therapists will provide Head and Neck Cancer patients with training on how to use the device(s).

- **Swallowing Therapy and Potential Problems**

Eating and drinking may be difficult after treatment for some Head and Neck Cancer patients because of the Side Effects of their treatment(s) they received, be it Chemotherapy, Radiation Therapy, Surgery, or a combination of these. In such cases, some patients may have trouble chewing, drinking, and swallowing food via the normal means through their mouth and Esophagus. In these cases, patients may be ordered to receive nutrients directly into a vein, or through a nasal or stomach feeding tube until they can eat on their own.

A feeding tube is a flexible plastic tube that is passed into the stomach through the nose, or through an incision in the abdomen. In both cases, the liquid “food” is externally pumped into the tube, and subsequently finds its way into the patient’s stomach. This means of “eating,” or consuming foods and fluids obviously does not compare to the life-sustaining benefits and pleasure of eating and drinking in the conventional manner of chewing, tasting, and swallowing. But, if the Cancer patient or Cancer survivor is not able to put away life-essential food, nutrients, and beverages thru normal processes, these alternative methods of consumption could help to save the day – and even the patient's life. (Please see Chapter 5 for detailed information about Enteral (Tube) Feeding, and Parenteral (Vein) Feeding).

As just stated, alternative means of consuming food certainly have their life-saving and beneficial uses. But again, unconventional nutritional consumption can also come with drawbacks, especially if the patient is utilizing the Gastrostomy Tube (otherwise known as a Stomach Tube, or the PEG (Percutaneous Endoscopic Gastrostomy Tube)). If the Head and Neck Cancer patient is not able to consume nutrients and beverages normally through their mouth and throat, a Gastrostomy feeding tube might be ordered by the treating physician on the patient's Medical Team. In such instances, the physician will explain to the patient, and to their family or Caregiver, the rationale for the tube, and its risks and benefits. If the Feeding Tube is agreed upon, it will be surgically put in place into the stomach by way of an incision into the patient's abdomen. The benefits of the Gastrostomy Tube are realistically apparent in that the device does allow for life-sustaining nutrients and beverages to be delivered into the patient, who might not be able to eat and drink foods and fluids via normal methods. The potential issues with the Stomach Tube, however, are very real, and I can speak from personal experience about these.

Specifically, infection at the site of the incision and insertion into the abdomen is a potential hazard. I am aware of two Head and Neck Cancer patients to whom extremely bad infections occurred at the insertion site. An infection can become a genuine problem for a Cancer patient who received (or is receiving) Chemotherapy drugs, because the powerful Chemo treatments, themselves, could have a negative impact on the patient's Immune System by harming White Blood Cells along with Cancer cells. When this occurs, the patient is at higher risk for developing additional health complications, thus compromising their safety and their capability to continue with their Cancer therapies. This is exactly what happened to the two people I am aware of. It is because of this very real threat of infection with a Gastrostomy Tube that my Oncologist did not authorize the Tube for me to use. She did this, despite my plea, and in spite of the truth that I was losing significant bodyweight due to the fact that it was almost impossible for me to eat and drink normally thanks to the unbearable throat pain caused by my Chemotherapy and Radiation Therapy.

An additional threat of Enteral feeding via the PEG Feeding Tube is that the patient may eventually become dependent upon the Tube for ***all*** nutritional consumption – meaning that they will lose their ability to swallow food via their mouth, tongue, and esophagus. Most people do not know that the act of swallowing does not come naturally – it is a learned behavior that babies acquire and grow into after they latch onto Mom’s nipple the very first time for food. Once again, I witnessed first-hand the problems that can be realized when the Gastrostomy Tube is used for *all* food consumption for a lengthy period of time. A fellow Head and Neck Cancer patient that had the exact form of Cancer I did (Cancer at the Base of the Tongue), was prescribed a Gastrostomy Tube because he was completely unable to eat or drink food via his mouth due to pain caused by his Chemo and Radiation Therapy treatments. Unfortunately, after several months of “eating” in this fashion (and his dedicated wife blending a variety of nutritious foods into a liquid that he could pump into his stomach three+ times a day), he had become completely dependent upon the apparatus. Yes, despite several months of Swallowing Therapy, and him even attempting to “eat” melted ice cream by, literally, dripping it on his tongue and unsuccessfully attempting to swallow it, he was never able to swallow food or drink via his mouth and throat again.

Please note that I mention the above real-life risks regarding Gastrostomy Tube feeding for educational reasons only. Appropriate members of the Head and Neck Cancer patient’s Medical Team will advise the patient, and their family or Caregiver, if there is reason to believe that alternative feeding would be appropriate in the patient’s case. These health care professionals will also ensure that all parties are very well-informed of any potential benefits and hazards of such methods. With all of this being said, Head and Neck Cancer patients should be aware that a qualified Speech / Language Pathologist can help patients try to learn how to swallow again after Cancer Surgery, or, after they receive Chemotherapy, and/or, Radiation Therapy. For other assistance on this subject, please note that the National Cancer Institute (www.cancer.gov) booklet, ***Eating Hints: Before, During,***

and After Cancer Treatment, contains many useful suggestions and recipes that may be of benefit to Head and Neck Cancer patients.

- **Speech Therapy After Cancer Surgery**

For many of the same or similar reasons specified in both of the preceding Sections regarding Physical Therapy and Swallowing Therapy Rehabilitation, Head and Neck Cancer patients could also have a need to receive Speech Therapy. If, due to Cancer Surgery or other reasons associated with the patient's Cancer or Side Effects of Cancer treatment, the patient is having difficulty speaking normally, Speech Therapy may be prescribed by the treating doctor to help the patient overcome their vocal problem(s). Often, a Speech/Language Pathologist will accomplish therapy with the patient in the clinic and teach speech exercises or alternative methods of speaking. Speech Therapy usually continues after the patient returns home until such time that the patient feels that he or she has successfully regained control of their ability to communicate normally once again.

Support for Head and Neck Cancer Patients Suffering from Depression

According to the National Cancer Institute (www.cancer.gov), severe Depression occurs in up to 25 percent of all Cancer patients. Along with fears about their appearance and vital bodily functions, Head and Neck Cancer patients could become depressed over many of the same issues that all Cancer patients cope with, such as loss of income, changes in social roles, reshuffling their goals, uncertainties about their futures, and, whether or not they will even have a future. Material below was derived from my journal and my Medical Team:

- **Reasons For Depression**

Head and Neck Cancer can leave patients especially prone to Depression and Suicide because these forms of Cancers—and their resulting Treatments and Side Effects—can directly affect the basic, necessary, and pleasant life-sustaining functions. Several Head and Neck Cancer treatments can be terribly extreme, simply because the therapies can invasively and detrimentally impact the portions of the patient's head and neck areas that are vital to eating, breathing, and communicating. On top of that, if there is associated disfigurement of the patient's head, and/or, neck areas, due to Cancer Surgery, any abnormalities may be apparent for others to see. This, of course, can cause the Cancer patient to be embarrassed and self-conscious about their appearance, thus making them withdraw from important social situations and interactions with others. Although it is very normal to experience sadness and grief in response to a Head and Neck Cancer diagnosis, Depression that is merciless and disabling can occur. In such cases, the patient should quickly seek professional assistance.

• Warning Signs of Depression

If a Head and Neck Cancer patient experiences symptoms of Depression, that doesn't automatically mean that they are Clinically Depressed. As we all know, for a variety of reasons and influences, we all have good days and bad days every now and again. But, if the patient's doldrums are continuous and last for more than two weeks, the patient should ask for help with their depressive condition. And, if the patient does not initiate efforts to seek assistance, the patient's family members or Caregiver should step in and request help on the patient's behalf. Often, Cancer patients can become so preoccupied with the stress and anxieties they are feeling at the moment (or fears that they have for their future), that they may fail to recognize their world closing in around them and shutting them off from others.

According to the National Cancer Institute (www.cancer.gov), the most common symptoms of Depression that Head and Neck Cancer patients and their families or Caregivers should be aware of, include:

- Feeling hopeless or helpless, or unable to enjoy anything
- Being unable to concentrate, or socially withdrawn
- Experiencing changes in sleep or appetite (less of either)
- Having (or demonstrating or voicing) thoughts of suicide

• Asking for Help With Depression

Take it from me, dealing with the misery of relentless mental Depression during and after Cancer therapy can be almost as painful as enduring the physical discomfort and nausea associated with the Side Effects of Cancer treatments. As a matter of fact, *Depression is a common Side Effect of Cancer therapy.* Seven weeks of Radiation Therapy to the patient's fragile head or neck areas, and three months of Chemotherapy can take their toll on anyone, no matter how tough they believe themselves to be. During my own Cancer experience, I literally had to get up the guts to force myself to eat and drink water during the day—as implausibly agonizing as it was—so that I could be strong enough to continue my Cancer treatments. And, just a few months after my Cancer treatments completed, I discovered that it took every ounce of physical and mental strength that I could muster at times just to get out of bed and *do anything* during the day, much less exercise, use my brain, or expend any energy. It was after my Cancer treatments concluded that "the other shoe dropped," and, that is when I first, unexpectedly, fell into a very deep, dark Depression – something that I had never experienced during my entire life.

During my depressive state, I permitted myself to continually question how and why I got Cancer, despite the excellent care I had taken of myself. Because of this, I started worrying that my Cancer would return, and I was continuously anxious about whether I would keep on living, and for just how long. The commonly optimistic and positive person I was prior to my Cancer diagnosis had transformed into an apathetic and pessimistic version of my former self. I didn't want to be with people, watch the News (which is *always* bad), and I always wanted to curl up into a ball in my dark basement. There was nothing my Caregiver could do to assist, so I knew that I had to seek professional assistance, which I did thru my Medical Team. Finally, after working with a Psychotherapist for almost two long years, and, after receiving results of post-treatment tests which found that I was Cancer-free, I was able to clamber out of that horrible hole in which I had lived for so long. In retrospect, I know that had I not obtained professional help to assist me in dealing with my severe Depression, I'm not so sure that I would have ever broken free of it on my own.

Depression is a frequent Side Effect of Cancer treatment and is nothing to be ashamed of. Health care professionals and hospitals and Cancer Clinics are very well aware of its debilitating effects on all Cancer patients—including Head and Neck Cancer patients—and they are fully staffed and prepared to deal with it. Help is available for the asking, and it works. If a Head and Neck Cancer patient is struggling with Depression (or even thinks that they are), they need to speak with a member of their Medical Team about it, and seek a referral to a Mental Health professional. Likewise, family members, Caregivers, or friends of a Head and Neck Cancer patient who might be suffering from Depression should inform the Medical Team if the patient does not. Sometimes, what a Head and Neck Cancer patient needs most of all is a person to talk with that will listen, and a safe place to communicate. Mental Health Therapists are ready to help.

According to the National Cancer Institute (www.cancer.gov), some treatments that have been found to work for Head and Neck Cancer patients who are suffering from Clinical Depression include:

- **Anti-Depressant Medications -** These medications are effective and are given to about 16 percent of Cancer patients. Anti-Depressants may take up to six weeks to work, but most show results sooner. A recent Study, while small in scale, showed that Citalopram (Celexa®) may be helpful as a preventive measure to ward off major depression in patients undergoing treatment for Head and Neck Cancer

- **Psychotherapy -** Talk Therapies are also effective and can be combined with Cancer education as well as relaxation and stress reduction techniques. It is often helpful to include family members in some of these sessions

- **Support Groups -** A Head and Neck Cancer Support Group may be helpful in treating Depression. Cancer Support Groups have been shown to improve participants' moods, coping skills, and quality of life. Cancer Support Groups are available at most treatment centers and online. Participants benefit by listening to, and sharing, their Cancer experiences

One of the greatest self-coping mechanisms that a Head and Neck Cancer patient can practice is to try to remain focused on each day, and to not forecast too far into their future. As I learned during my own Psychotherapy sessions, *"Shoulda, coulda, woulda"*-types of thinking, as well as *"What if"* thinking will only cause the patient more worry and consternation. These should be avoided, as nothing productive will come of it. It took my Psychotherapist many months to convince me that I could once again believe in my body and trust my mind, because, admittedly, I had lost all faith in both when I got Cancer after living such a healthy lifestyle. Head and Neck Cancer patients should do their best to educate themselves about Head and Neck Cancer, and its *modus operandi.* Likewise, they should try to remain as positive as possible and retain their senses of humor. The most noteworthy thing for Head and Neck Cancer patients to know, however, is that ***they can get through and ahead of*** their Head and Neck Cancer obstacles. *But, first, they* ***must believe in themselves.***

Head and Neck Cancer Support Groups

The physical and emotional effects of Cancer are often much more apparent in patients with Head or Neck Cancer than in people who have other forms of this dire disease. Facial deformities, speech impairments, or issues with normal eating and drinking can result in physical, emotional, and social complications that are special to this group of patients. Due to the Cancer Treatments employed, or as an outcome of the Side Effects from those therapies, problems for Head and Neck patients could include disfigurement, painful chewing and swallowing, speech issues, mouth sores, dry mouth and other issues, contingent upon the location of the patient's Cancer. Head and Neck Cancer patients learn that they may have to limit their work through treatments, which might be difficult. Additionally, their expectations about healing and returning to work or becoming involved in social situations can be unrealistic. All of this can lead to Depression.

For every Cancer patient—but especially for Head and Neck Cancer patients—it is significant to be able to gather and speak with others who have *"been there and done that,"* and, to be able to hear, and see, personally, that recovery from their terrible experience with Cancer and its Side Effects, can, and does, take place. And, it is for these important motives that the concept of Cancer Patient Support Groups were first established: To provide existing Cancer patients and survivors, and members of their families and Caregivers with an opportunity, and a safe, comfortable location, to meet and talk about the day-to-day complexities of living with Head and Neck Cancers, and their aftermaths. Numerous hospitals, Cancer Clinics, and other Cancer-treatment health care facilities will provide the space and the professional staffs to plan, schedule, conduct, and facilitate regular *(and free!)* Head and Neck Cancer Support Groups for the benefit of all concerned individuals. Most Support Groups will focus on the multidisciplinary approach with a Social Worker, Dietician, Speech Therapist, Nurse, and, occasionally, a doctor, providing educational information and talking about services available to Cancer patients.

Head and Neck Cancer Support Groups have been proven to be a significant part of patient wellness. In the last 15 years, research has shown that membership in such groups improves overall quality of life, both during and following Cancer. Psychological distress in Cancer patients has also been found to reduce greatly with ongoing participation of patients and their families in these groups. Groups provide an informal and supportive atmosphere in which folks share common treatment experiences, coping strategies, and their feelings. Additionally, facilitators of the groups seek to provide patient-driven education and information about the disease along with a setting for open discussions about Treatments, Side Effects, and the emotional and physical changes that can take place, and how best to cope with those. Quite simply, nobody knows what it is like to have Head and Neck Cancer better than the patients, survivors, and Caregivers who have already been through it. And, there is no better way for these people to meet and share their experiences than in a Support Group.

Attendance by existing Head and Neck Cancer patients and survivors, and, perhaps, their significant others and family members, is encouraged at all Support Group gatherings. Dress is comfortable and casual, and, perhaps, beverages and some food may be served. I participated in several of the Head and Neck Cancer Support Group meetings (both during and after my treatments) at the hospital where I received Radiation Therapy. I personally found the experience to be very helpful and educational, but honestly, also, often a little sad.

One of the most significant benefits of the Support Groups, I think, aside from the generous support components that they offer, is that the other participants remind the patient that they are not alone in this conflict – that there are many others facing the same or worse problems as them, and, that everyone in the room has the exact same goal in mind: To survive their Cancer, and to try to reclaim as much of their pre-Cancer life as possible – as soon and safely as possible.

Support Groups for Head and Neck Cancer patients come in many sizes, shapes, and formats. Following are some of the most common:

- **Face-to-Face Support Groups**

These Head and Neck Cancer Support Groups are probably the most common, and are those I've discussed in the Section above. Most face-to-face-type of Support Groups are typically facilitated by professional staff at Cancer Treatment Centers and Cancer Clinics and are recurrently scheduled and well-publicized meetings that can be attended by active Cancer patients, Cancer survivors, significant others and family members. Those interested in participating should check on the Internet or through their local Cancer Clinic or Cancer Treatment Center for information and guidance.

- **Online Support Groups**

Online (Internet) Head and Neck Cancer Support Groups are facilitated by Oncology social workers, are password-protected, and participants must go through a registration process. After completing the registration process (which can take up to 5 to 7 business days), members can participate 24 hours, 7 days a week. Those interested in participating should check on the Internet or at their local Cancer Clinic or Cancer Treatment Center for information and guidance.

- **Telephone Support Groups**

Telephonic Head and Neck Cancer Support Groups permit Cancer patients to connect on the phone with Head and Neck Cancer patients and health care professionals around the country who share similar concerns. Typically, these "conference call"-style meetings are regularly scheduled, one - two hour sessions. Those interested in participating should check on the Internet or with their local Cancer Clinic or Cancer Treatment Center for information and guidance.

- **Grief Support Groups**

The death of a loved one or a friend deeply affects surviving family members and friends in various ways. The emotional, social, and spiritual reactions can be overwhelming. Grief Support Groups facilitate a supportive environment where experiences and feelings can be shared, and where learning about the mourning process may begin. Group participants are also able to explore their own distinct resources and strengths in dealing with a loss. While these types of forums exist for the benefit of those who are grieving the loss of any family member or friend, special groups that assist with the loss of Cancer patients are also available. Those interested in participating should look on the Internet or consult with their local Cancer Clinic or Cancer Treatment Center for information and guidance.

- **Support for People with Oral and Head and Neck Cancer (SPOHNC)**

Support for People with Oral and Head and Neck Cancer, Inc. (SPOHNC), was organized in 1991. SPOHNC is a not-for-profit 501(c)(3) organization concerned with the development of self-help support programs for Head and Neck Cancer patients, and is a vital component of the healing process for these patients. SPOHNC has had an enormous positive impact on meeting the psychosocial needs of Head and Neck Cancer patients, as well as preserving, restoring, and promoting patient physical and emotional health. Additionally, SPOHNC serves as the foundation for patient and family education and awareness about the topic of Head and Neck Cancer. Head and Neck Cancer Patients, or their loved ones, their family members, or their Caregivers who are interested in the services that SPOHNC has to offer, can access this information at www.spohnc.org.

How Can People Who Have Had Head and Neck Cancers Reduce Their Risk of Developing a Second Primary (New) Cancer?

As I have mentioned elsewhere in this Chapter, if the initial treatment for the patient's Primary Cancer is successful, and, if, after follow-up exams, the patient has been declared *Cured, Cancer Free,* or *in Remission,* there still is a relatively low risk (2 to 3 % per year) that the patient will develop a new and completely unrelated Cancer of the Head, and / or, Neck. This is per the National Cancer Institute (www.cancer.gov), who also states that the risk of developing a new or second Head and Neck Cancer can be exacerbated in those who received Radiation Therapy for treatment of their original Primary Tumor. Yes, as if ***UNO*** Cancer is not enough, several years-worth of scientific research has found that individuals who have been treated for Head and Neck Cancer have an increased chance of developing a new Cancer, usually in the Head, Neck, Esophagus, or Lungs. *WTF?*

Tobacco and Alcohol Users Should Not Tempt Fate

According to the National Cancer Institute (www.cancer.gov), the potentiality of developing a Second Primary Cancer (i.e., not a *recurrence of the First Primary Cancer)* differs, depending upon the patient's original diagnosis. However, research has proven that the chance of developing a new, second Cancer is higher for people who smoke and drink alcohol. ***Patients who do not smoke should never start, and those who smoke should do their best to stop.*** Scientific Studies reveal that Cancer survivors that still smoke or drink alcohol increase their chances of forming a Second Primary Cancer ***for up to 20 years*** after the first Cancer diagnosis. Information about stopping smoking is found in the National Cancer Institute (www.cancer.gov) fact sheet titled, ***Questions and Answers About Smoking Cessation.***

Patients who use tobacco have a greater risk of developing a Second Primary Cancer, so physicians caution these patients to stop. Guidance about quitting smoking is also available from the National Cancer Institute's (www.cancer.gov) Cancer Information Service at 1–800–4–CANCER (1–800–422–6237), and in the fact sheet ***Where To Get Help When You Decide To Quit Smoking.*** The main U.S. government's resource to assist people in stopping using tobacco is the website www.smokefree.gov. The U.S. government also sponsors www.smokefreewomen.gov, a site to help women quit using tobacco. The toll-free number is 1–800–QUIT–NOW (1–800–784–8669).

What are the Rates of Head and Neck Cancer Diagnosis and Survival?

You just knew that I *had* to include a Section in this Chapter on Head and Neck Cancers with some not-so-rosy information about the Diagnosis and Survival rates associated with this vicious disease. Well, as difficult as it is for me to write about these topics *(believe me, I have anguished over **this** Section of this Book more than any other!)*, I know that it might be just as hard for you as the Reader, to view, or to even casually peruse, the information that follows. I can definitely understand if the Reader would choose not to learn of the statistics concerning Head and Neck Cancer incidence and survival. This is, because, quite frankly, when I first became a Head and Neck Cancer patient in 2004, and for numerous years following, I wanted nothing to do with the disheartening, and very impersonal, numbers. ***Therefore, if the Reader would like to disregard the following data, and jump to another point within this Book, please go for it – you have my blessings.*** On the other hand, if the Reader would prefer to know just how Head and Neck Cancers stack up against one another in terms of their relative occurrence rates and extents of survival, the information below may help to shed some light on those curiosities.

All Cancer Mortality Statistics Suck – No Doubt About it

I have decided to include in my presentation regarding Head and Neck Cancers some diagnosis and survivability figures from the resources of the National Cancer Institute (www.cancer.gov). It is my wish that the Reader will utilize this information for educational purposes only. It certainly is not my intent to frighten, discourage, or worry anyone with this material, but, unfortunately, death is a fact of life. Whenever individuals talk about mortality, death, or dying, the subject can't help but be upsetting, sad, morbid, and even, off-limits, for many people. I can say that I will include myself in that group.

In any honest discussion concerning Cancers, however—due to their deadly nature, and the fact that some forms can, thankfully, be cured in some patients—I believe it is quite important to not only talk about the "good" stuff, such as the potential for Cancer survival, but, also to be cognizant of the not-so-good reality that some people will not survive their respective Head and Neck Cancer occurrences. The fact of the matter, as I have stated previously, is that while all Head and Neck Cancers are relatively rare in the Cancer world, they can be some of the most horrible forms of the disease on the planet. As a result of this—the Tasmanian Devils that they are—they can do some serious harm to those on the receiving end of their wickedness.

The National Cancer Institute SEER Study

There have been numerous Studies conducted concerning the diagnosis and survivability of the several different forms of Cancer. When it comes to Head and Neck Cancer Study results, perhaps the most conclusive and comprehensive research has been conducted in conjunction with the ***Surveillance, Epidemiology, and End Results (SEER)*** Program, which is administered, funded, and chronicled by the National Cancer Institute (www.cancer.gov). In my attempts to provide the Reader with the most up to date information available on this topic, I, unfortunately, was only able to acquire records that, as I write this, were over twelve years old. That is, the SEER Study for Head and Neck Cancer Diagnoses and Survivability Data that I will refer to in this Section was evaluated for patients diagnosed between the years 1998 and 2001. And, while this statistical information in the Head and Neck Cancer SEER Study is not current as I write this in 2013, I do believe that it is still very relevant. This is because the eye-opening and stark statistics do paint a very apparent and realistic picture as to the omnipresence of the Head and Neck versions of this menacing disease, and the extremely serious threat to health and life that it continues to pose to over 55,000 adult Americans each year.

- ### Head and Neck Cancer SEER Study: Who/What

This SEER Study—the information for which I have adapted from National Cancer Institute (www.cancer.gov) online resources—provides diagnosis and survival analyses for 40,811 histologically confirmed (verified in a Medical Laboratory) male and female adult cases of Cancers of the Head and Neck. These Study cases included Cancers of the Paranasal Sinus, Oropharynx, Salivary Glands, Oral Cavity, Hypopharynx, Lip, Nasopharynx, and Nose. The National Cancer Institute SEER Program contracts individually with Central Cancer Registries, which are situated in organizations such as State Health Departments and Universities, to solicit facts on all Cancers diagnosed in applicable patients within the Registry's relevant areas. SEER Cancer Registries are selected on the basis of two criteria:

1. The Registry's ability to capture data, and operate, maintain, and report via a population-based Cancer reporting system

2. The epidemiologic significance of their group's population

While some Cancer Registries have continued in the SEER Program since it began, others have left; additional Registries have joined at a later date, or left for a period of time and rejoined the Program later.

- ## Head and Neck Cancer SEER Study: Where/When

The National Cancer Institute SEER Study assessed the data studied from twelve geographic areas in the U.S., which collectively represent approximately 14% of the total U.S. population. Included in the SEER Study was information from the States of Connecticut, Iowa, New Mexico, Utah, and Hawaii, and the metropolitan areas of Detroit, Atlanta, San Francisco, Seattle, San Jose, and Los Angeles, plus ten counties in rural Georgia. Los Angeles contributed data for diagnosis years 1992 to 2001. Data from other geographic regions in the Country was gathered for diagnosis years from 1988 to 2001.

- ## Head and Neck Cancer SEER Study Results: An Upfront Summary

The actual, in-depth results from the Head and Neck Cancer SEER Study are detailed in Tables in the Section following. To help the Reader in interpreting the voluminous amount of data contained in the Tables, I provide this upfront summary: **1)** Overall, the five-year average survival rate for patients with Head and Neck Cancers was 57%: **2)** The average five-year survival rate for Head and Neck Cancers for Whites was 60%; for Blacks was 40%: and, **3)** The five-year average survival rate for males was 45%; for females, 55%. As a function of race and sex, average 5-year survival rates tended to be elevated for White males and females than Black males and females. For the purposes of the SEER Study, when a patient has a five-year relative survival rate of 100%, the patient has the identical chance of living for 5 years as a demographically similar *Cancer-free* person.

- **Ethnicity and Diagnosis**

Racial distribution tends to reflect the collective population from the Study geographic regions (Caucasians 81%, Blacks 11%, and other

Races at 9%), with the exception of Cancer of the Lip, which can be found overwhelmingly in Whites (98%), as are Cancers of the Oral Cavity and Pharynx. Cancers of the Hypopharynx and Oropharynx were elevated in Black patients at 17%, and 15%, respectively.

- **Most Frequent Cancers Diagnosed**

The most commonly occurring Cancers in the Head and Neck group were Tongue (21%) *(Not exactly the type of "No. 1" I'd hoped for!)*, Gums and other mouth sites (15%), and Salivary Glands (10%).

- **Age and Diagnosis**

Most Head and Neck Cancers are diagnosed at older ages, including my form, Base of Tongue. Nasopharynx Cancer is found at younger ages at diagnosis than other Cancers in the Study, with 40% of these cases being diagnosed at ages younger than 50. Cancer of the Lip is diagnosed more often at older ages than are the other Head and Neck Cancers, with almost 70% of cases diagnosed at age 60 or older.

- **Gender and Diagnosis**

While each of the Head and Neck Cancers are diagnosed more often among males, the percentages for males and females are closest for Gum and other Mouth Cancers (54% male), and for Salivary Gland Cancers (56% male). The distribution by gender is most extreme for Cancers of the Lip (81% male), and Hypopharynx (78% male).

• The SEER Study Results: The Cold, Hard Facts of Head and Neck Cancer Diagnoses and Survivability

The Tables below contain the actual SEER Study data pertaining to Head and Neck Cancer Diagnosis and Survivability. Please note that differences in survival rates for each form of Cancer are dependent upon the Stages of the patients' Cancers when treated, as well as the ages, genders, and races of the patients, and, could be affected by the *patients' efforts to avoid risk factors after treatment.* In any event, as I'm sure you will notice below, as far as Head and Neck Cancers are concerned, *it REALLY SUCKS to be a **WHITE MALE OVER 50!!***

National Cancer Institute SEER Head and Neck Cancer Incidence and Survivability Study Results – 1988 to 2001			
Diagnosis / Survival Averages	**Head and Neck Cancer Type**		
	Floor of Mouth	**Gum and Other Mouth**	**Hypopharynx**
% Diag. of All Head & Neck	**8.0**	**14.6**	**8.0**
% Age 20-49	**14.8**	**15.2**	**10.6**
% Age 50-80+	**85.2**	**84.8**	**89.4**
% Male	**68.8**	**53.6**	**78.2**
% Female	**31.2**	**46.4**	**21.8**
% White	**83.4**	**82.3**	**76.6**
% Black	**13.1**	**11.6**	**16.4**
% Other	**3.5**	**6.1**	**7.0**
1 Yr. Surv. %	**82.8**	**82.8**	**67.4**
3 Yr. Surv. %	**61.7**	**65.8**	**38.3**
5 Yr. Surv. %	**52.7**	**59.5**	**29.5**
8 Yr. Surv. %	**43.3**	**59.1**	**22.0**
10 Yr. Surv. %	**37.7**	**48.1**	**18.2**

NCI SEER Diag/Surv Avg 1988 - 2001	**Head and Neck Cancer Type**		
	Lip	**Nasopharynx**	**Nose and Paranasal Sinus**
% Diag. of All Head & Neck	**9.8**	**6.9**	**5.7**
% Age 20-49	**15.2**	**40**	**20.7**
% Age 50-80+	**84.8**	**60**	**79.3**
% Male	**81.2**	**69.6**	**57.8**
% Female	**18.8**	**30.4**	**42.2**
% White	**97.7**	**42.7**	**80/1**
% Black	**1.0**	**8.0**	**9.7**
% Other	**1.3**	**49.3 - Asian**	**10.2**
1 Yr. Surv. %	**99.6**	**84.1**	**79.8**
3 Yr. Surv. %	**96.2**	**65.3**	**61.9**
5 Yr. Surv. %	**93.5**	**56.6**	**54.0**
8 Yr. Surv. %	**90.4**	**48.3**	**50.3**
10 Yr. Surv. %	**88.0**	**44.7**	**46.6**

National Cancer Institute SEER Head and Neck Cancer Incidence and Survivability Study Results – 1988 to 2001			
Diagnosis / Survival Averages	**Head and Neck Cancer Type**		
	Oropharynx and Tonsil	**Other Oral and Pharynx**	**Salivary Gland**
% Diag. of All Head & Neck	**13.4**	**2.5**	**9.9**
% Age 20-49	**22.5**	**10**	**27.2**
% Age 50-80+	**77.5**	**90**	**72.8**
% Male	**74.7**	**69.4**	**56.2**
% Female	**25.3**	**30.6**	**43.8**
% White	**81.0**	**79.7**	**84.1**
% Black	**14.6**	**17.4**	**7.8**
% Other	**4.4**	**2.9**	**8.1**
1 Yr. Surv. %	**79.8**	**63.8**	**90**
3 Yr. Surv. %	**58.8**	**38.9**	**77.7**
5 Yr. Surv. %	**49.8**	**29.8**	**73.9**
8 Yr. Surv. %	**43.5**	**23.6**	**70.7**
10 Yr. Surv. %	**39.3**	**21.5**	**68.5**

NCI SEER Diag/Surv Avg 1988 - 2001	**Head and Neck Cancer Type**		
	Tongue (Total)	**Anterior 2/3 of Tongue**	**Base / Rear 1/3 of Tongue**
% Diag. of All Head & Neck	**21.2**	**56% of all Tongue Cancer**	**44% of all Tongue Cancer**
% Age 20-49	**21.3**	Not Avail.	Not Avail.
% Age 50-80+	**78.7**	Not Avail.	Not Avail.
% Male	**66.7**	Not Avail.	Not Avail.
% Female	**33.3**	Not Avail.	Not Avail.
% White	**82.5**	Not Avail.	Not Avail.
% Black	**10.5**	Not Avail.	Not Avail.
% Other	**7.1**	Not Avail.	Not Avail.
1 Yr. Surv. %	**80.8**	**83.1**	**77.8**
3 Yr. Surv. %	**59.4**	**62.6**	**55.3**
5 Yr. Surv. %	**53.1**	**57.5**	**47.5**
8 Yr. Surv. %	**46.3**	**50.6**	**40.9**
10 Yr. Surv. %	**42.1**	**46.2**	**36.8**

- **SEER Study Results are Scary but Shouldn't Be**

When reading and absorbing Cancer survival rate statistics—including those specified in the above Tables for the SEER Study—one must recognize that not all Head and Neck Cancer survivors will fit perfectly into these obscure "statistical pigeonholes" as if they are just another number on some *cold* Cancer survivability spreadsheet. For obvious reasons, every Cancer patient is different, each patient's Cancer, and its Stage, Treatments, and Side Effects will vary, as will each patient's favorable or unfavorable responses to the Treatments and Side Effects. *And, clearly, one cannot even think about Cancer survivability without also taking into consideration the survivors' or patients' efforts—**post-Treatment**—to either take better care of their bodies by living a healthier lifestyle, free of as many risk factors as possible, or, by perhaps inviting a new Cancer because of their risky behaviors, habits, or exposures.* Each of the aforementioned factors can contribute to either a longer life after an initial Cancer diagnosis and Treatment, or, to a life that is unnecessarily cut much too short. In either case, according to several Cancer Survivability Studies, the handwriting is on the wall: ***Play with fire and you may get burned.***

Conclusions from Additional Head and Neck Cancer Survivability Studies: One Cancer is One Too Many

It should not come as a shock to anyone (especially because I've mentioned it within this book at least a *half-million* times), and, it should be apparent to any person who has not lived their entire life inside a cave or under a rock, that tobacco and alcohol use are major risk factors for many Cancers, including those of the Head and Neck variety. There are other causes of Head and Neck Cancer, of course, such as overexposure to sun; Humanpapillomavirus (HPV); contact with, or breathing of, environmental toxins; one's age and sex; the ubiquitous Random Chance; and, others. But, for very good reason, tobacco and alcohol use and abuse are some of the most prevalent—yet avoidable—causes of Head and Neck Cancers. And, regrettably, they're both also *very good* at eliciting recurring and new Cancers.

Because of the preponderance of evidence pointing directly from tobacco and alcohol use to various Head and Neck Cancers, it would be sensible to assume that if a Head and Neck Cancer patient successfully makes it through and beyond the Cancer Treatment and Side Effect "obstacle course" and has an uneventful and constructive recovery, that the patient would desire to do everything within their power to survive their Cancer for just as long as possible – and, this would include dropping any questionable, risky behaviors that could incite a Cancer recurrence, or the occurrence of a new Cancer. Well, not only is common-sense on the side of this concept, but, so are the conclusions of the following Survivability Studies, which have been adapted from National Cancer Institute (www.cancer.gov) materials:

- **Head and Neck Cancer Survivability Study - 2004**

In this 2004 Study, 50 Cancer survivors that were smokers, and 50 Cancer survivors that were non-smokers, were assembled by their ages and genders; their varieties of Head and Neck Cancer; the Stages and localities of their respective Cancers; and, the modes of Cancer treatment(s) they each received. By matching these factors in each pair of patients, researchers were able to measure the effects of smoking on a patient's longevity. Factors such as alcohol use, other health problems, and Cancer-related symptoms were also analyzed.

This Study indicated that non-smokers with Head and Neck Cancers survived longer after the completion of their treatments, and that they were less likely to have their disease return when compared to the Head and Neck Cancer patients who were actively smoking or who had smoked in their past. As a matter of truth, the Study found that the danger of death or the return of their Cancers was more than ***three times greater for smokers*** than for non-smokers. Researchers did emphasize that these findings indicate that smokers experience a different, and possibly more aggressive, form of the disease than do non-smokers. Scientists also noted that alcohol abuse, other health problems, or more severe Cancer treatment-related Side Effects may contribute to the reduced length of life in smokers with the disease.

- **Head and Neck Cancer Survivability Study - 2009**

Researchers queried 504 Head and Neck Cancer survivors in this 2009 Study about their smoking and their alcohol habits; their nutritional intake (the quality and quantity of foods and liquids that they consumed); their levels of exercise and physical activities; and, how many hours they slept each day or night. The research subjects were then consequently surveyed every three months for two years, and then once per year. Not surprisingly, when the research data was calculated and analyzed, it illustrated that the Cancer survivors with the shortest longevity after Treatment were those who used tobacco. The Study also exposed that drinking excess amounts of alcohol was associated with shorter survival times, as was eating little or no fruit. In fact, although nutritional experts recommend consumption of two servings of fruit per day, 1/3 of the Head and Neck Cancer survivors reported ingesting *fewer than four servings of fruit per month! Their Grandmas would not be happy!* Finally, a lack of exercise was also shown to decrease survival times of Head and Neck Cancer patients.

Complicating the situation even more from a Head and Neck Cancer survival standpoint, is the fact that many of the poor health habits can be inter-related. For example, smokers are also frequently heavy drinkers of alcohol. So, it may not be enough for a doctor to refer a patient for a smoking cessation program when alcohol could also be affecting their general health and Cancer survival. It should come as no surprise to anyone that scientific research has shown that a healthy lifestyle can help prevent Cancer. However, take it from me, that is not always the case. I tried my entire life to maximize all the "right" things and minimize all the "wrong" things to stay fit and healthy to "prevent" Cancer, but I still turned into one of the Cancer *diagnosees* nonetheless. With all that being said, Medical Studies *do* reveal that not smoking, drinking alcohol only in moderation, eating several servings of fruits and vegetables, and exercising, can have a big impact on a person's risk of *not getting Cancer in the first place.* Now, it appears that these exact factors could also impact Head and Neck Cancer survival longevity *after diagnosis and treatment.*

- **Head and Neck Cancer Survivability Study – 2009 – Humanpapillomavirus (HPV) Diagnoses**

The Humanpapillomavirus (HPV) is most commonly passed from person to person during sexual activity. A Study conducted in 2009 found that people with more than *six* lifetime oral sex partners *(not five, not seven, but six!)* have the greatest chance of contracting

Oropharyngeal Cancer. It's not obvious why some people with HPV come down with this form of Cancer while others don't (good ole' Random Chance, perhaps?), but Study findings suggest that decades can pass by between the actual HPV infection, and the appearance of Cancer. So, that crazy night a college kid had in their Twenties may come back to haunt them in their Fifties. Can't a person have some fun without having to look over their shoulder for *damn Cancer?*

Sadly, while the prevalence of HPV-induced Head and Neck Cancer is steadily increasing, Study data suggests that the Cancer is easily addressed, and that patient longevity is much longer for HPV-caused Oropharyngeal Cancers than for those driven by smoking or alcohol use. Particularly, researchers found that people with Stage III or IV Oropharyngeal Cancer (Cancers of the upper throat and the Anterior Tongue and Base of Tongue, such as mine) that have (had) tumors with Humanpapillomavirus (HPV) live longer. For example, Cancer survivors with *HPV-induced Oropharyngeal Cancer have a disease-free survival rate of 85-90 percent over five years*. This is in contrast to the characteristic Cancer patient population of excessive smokers and alcohol users diagnosed with severe (Stage III and IV) disease who have a 5-year survival rate of approximately 25 to 40%.

A Final Word about Head and Neck Cancer Survival Statistics – Take Them with a Grain of Salt

In reviewing and interpreting factual Head and Neck Cancer diagnosis and survival statistics obtained from dependable sources, the Reader should understand that all the statistics simply speak for themselves for a given study group, at a given place (or places), and, during a given timeframe. Therefore, the statistical figures make no claims, assumptions, assertions, or predictions about other Head and Neck Cancer patients or survivors, past, present, or future. Stated another way, based on past history, data suggests that there is a good chance that X number of men and women will come down with one of the several Head and Neck Cancers each year; X number of men and women will survive their individualized Head and Neck Cancers every year; and, X number of men and women will, unfortunately, perish every year due to their Head and Neck Cancers. I definitely don't intend to be insensitive, careless, detached, or irresponsible by offering this, because, please don't forget, I, also, find myself in two of those three "Xs." But, the point I'm trying to make is that while statistical data analyzed from prior Cancer Studies may be relatively precise in documenting *previous diagnoses and survival rates*, that doesn't necessarily indicate that the same Study results will translate into precise predictions of *current or future Head and Neck Cancer diagnoses, prognoses, or survivability.* So, for lack of a better way of putting it, take the stats, but please take them with a grain of salt.

My Personal Opinions about MY Head and Neck Cancer Diagnosis

When I was a youthful lad, I didn't know what a *scapegoat* was, but I had one: *Marney* was his name, and I gave him my blame. Yes, my make-believe Marney "took the fall" for me a lot of times for problems I had caused, but, the *Court of Mom* knew the truth and busted *me,* not Marney. I was then tried and sentenced accordingly. Looking back at my Cancer diagnosis, I know how easy it would be to hold Marney responsible for the whole mess, and to simply move on. But, the *Court of Life* is not quite as fast to rush to judgment.

I've stated a few times in this Book that the Cancer patient or survivor should not blame themselves for their Cancer occurrence – no matter what. Staying truthful to my word, I've never held myself responsible for causing my Cancer. But, I do have to admit that I am still really curious how a very healthy guy like me could get tripped up by this wicked disease. In this regard, I think back to my college years and jobs in which I accidentally deluged myself with gasoline, or breathed in Zinc fumes while cutting galvanized steel with a blow torch. Both made me very ill. Then, there was my job as a Nightclub Bouncer in which I breathed in second-hand cigarette smoke every night, or, the many years that I've laid and worked in the sun with little or no protection. And then there's the stress – the *damn stress.*

Since I've never used tobacco and the only alcohol I've ever drunken was an occasional sip of wine, my Cancer could have been caused by some of those risk factors I stated above, it could be due to random chance, or, perhaps, even HPV with unprotected sex. I'll probably never know, but I'm sure Marney's in there somewhere!

Chapter Eleven

Head and Neck Cancers Explained – *One-by-One*

"Knowledge is a wonderful thing to have, and an even better thing to use."

- Butch Sickler

Even though a few things in life may be rare, that does not necessarily mean that they are precious or priceless. And, that logic definitely applies to many of the uncommon health problems that we Humans try our best to outrun, outfox, and outlive through our lives, including the King and Queen of them all – Cancer. And, converse to many Cancers, those of the Head and Neck ilk are comparatively unusual. But, as the Reader has probably discerned in reading these pages, the various Head and Neck Cancers are anything but coveted, and, in fact, are extremely malicious to have around. It is because of these truths that it may be beneficial to those impacted by Head and Neck Cancers—and individuals interested in, hopefully, preventing the disease—to learn what they can about this *Gang of Ten (or so).*

Head and Neck Cancers Explained – One-by-One

Realizing that I may run a slight risk of presenting redundant material concerning the multiple forms of Head and Neck Cancer, I thought that it still might benefit the Reader to restate prior material, and to include detailed summaries of the many different forms. This is because each type of Head and Neck Cancer is unique, as are their divergent causative factors, their numerous head and neck locations, the assortment of tests used to diagnosis the individual Cancers, and, the treatments employed by the Medical Team to safely eradicate the Cancer – which are based on various factors associated with both the patient *and* their Cancer. Therefore, in this Chapter, I provide a brief review of the different forms of Head and Neck Cancer.

☛ ***Author's Disclaimer:*** Included in the following summaries of each of the forms of Head and Neck Cancers are their locations in the Head or Neck; any potential Risk Factors; the signs or symptoms of each form of Head and Neck Cancer that individuals may identify (and which, hopefully, will prod them to seek medical intervention); the diagnostic tests for each type of Cancer; and, lastly, those factors that may influence the treatment and prognosis of each form of Head and Neck Cancer. The Reader should be cognizant that the materials concerning Head and Neck Cancers in this Chapter are furnished for informational and educational purposes only. In all cases, Head and Neck Cancer patients should consult with applicable members of the patient's Medical Team to obtain relevant information and answers to any questions they may have regarding Cancer, or *their* Cancer.

The following material in this Chapter regarding the particular forms of Head and Neck Cancers has been adapted from the resources of the National Cancer Institute (www.cancer.gov):

❖ *Hypopharyngeal Cancer*

- ### Hypopharyngeal Cancer Location(s)

Hypopharyngeal Cancer is a Head and Neck Cancer in which malignant cancerous cells mature in the tissues of the Hypopharynx. The Hypopharynx is in the bottom part of the Pharynx (throat). The Pharynx is a hollow tube roughly five inches long that starts behind the nose, extends down the neck, and ends at the top of the Trachea (Windpipe), and Esophagus (the tube that goes from the throat to the stomach). Air and food pass through the Pharynx on the way to the Trachea or the Esophagus. Primarily, Hypopharyngeal Cancers form in the Squamous Cells, the thin, flat cells that coat the walls on the inside of the Hypopharynx. The Hypopharynx is comprised of three different areas, and Cancer may be found in one or more of these.

- **Hypopharyngeal Cancer Risk Factors**

  - Smoking tobacco and chewing tobacco
  - Heavy alcohol use
  - Consuming food and drink with insufficient nutritional value
  - Having Plummer-Vinson Syndrome

- **Hypopharyngeal Cancer Symptoms ***

  - A sore throat that does not go away
  - Ear pain
  - A lump in the neck
  - Painful or difficult swallowing
  - A change in voice

* Seek medical attention if any of the above are persistent or unusual, so that exams can be performed to determine cause

- **Hypopharyngeal Cancer Diagnostic Tests**

  - Physical Exam of the throat, and exam of the neck to identify any swollen Neck Lymph Nodes
  - Endoscopy
  - Biopsy Tissue Samples
  - CT (Computed Tomography) Scan (or CAT Scan)
  - MRI (Magnetic Resonance Imaging (also called Nuclear Magnetic Resonance Imaging (NMRI))
  - X-rays of head, neck, and chest
  - Barium Esophagogram
  - Esophagoscopy
  - Bronchoscopy

- **Hypopharyngeal Cancer Treatment Considerations**

  - The Stage of the Cancer
  - The patient's general health status
  - Whether or not the Cancer is a recurrence (second Cancer)
  - The need to retain the patient's ability to talk, eat, and breathe as normally as possible

- **Hypopharyngeal Cancer Prognosis Considerations**

  - The Stage of the Cancer (whether it affects part of the Hypopharynx, involves the whole Hypopharynx, or has spread to other places in the body). Hypopharyngeal Cancer is usually detected in later Stages because early symptoms rarely occur that are noticeable to the affected individual
  - The patient's age, gender, and general health status
  - The location of the Cancer
  - Whether the patient smokes during Radiation Therapy

- **Hypopharyngeal Cancer Recurrence Possibility**

Patients who have been diagnosed with Hypopharyngeal Cancer are at a heightened risk of developing a second Cancer in the head or the neck. ***After treatment for Hypopharyngeal Cancer, frequent and careful medical follow-up is extremely important.***

❖ *Lip and Oral Cavity Cancer*

- **Lip and Oral Cavity Cancer Location(s)**

Lip and Oral Cavity Cancers are Head and Neck Cancers in which malignant cancerous cells form in the lips or in the mouth.

The Oral Cavity includes the following:

- The ***front two-thirds*** of the Tongue **(*NOT* the Base)**
- The Gingiva (Gums)
- The Buccal Mucosa (the lining of the inside of the cheeks)
- The floor (bottom) of the mouth under the tongue
- The hard palate (the roof of the mouth)
- The Retromolar Trigone (the small area behind the Wisdom Teeth)

Most Lip and Oral Cavity Cancers start in Squamous Cells, the thin, flat cells that line the Lips and the Oral Cavity. These are referred to as Squamous Cell Carcinomas. Cancer cells may spread into deeper tissue as the Cancer continues to enlarge. Squamous Cell Carcinoma usually develops in areas of Leukoplakia (white patches of cells that do not rub off) in membranous tissues that line many bodily areas.

- **Lip and Oral Cavity Cancer Risk Factors**

  - Using tobacco products
  - Heavy alcohol use
  - Being exposed to natural sunlight or artificial sunlight (i.e., tanning beds) over long periods of time without protection
  - Being male
  - Being infected with Human Papillomavirus (HPV)

- **Lip and Oral Cavity Cancer Symptoms ***

  - A sore on the lip or in the mouth that does not heal
  - A lump or thickening on the lips or gums or in the mouth
  - A white or red patch on the gums, tongue, tonsils, or lining of the mouth
  - Bleeding, pain, or numbness in the lip or mouth.
  - Change in voice
  - Loose teeth or dentures that no longer fit well
  - Trouble chewing or swallowing or moving the tongue or jaw
  - Swelling of jaw
  - Sore throat or feeling that something is caught in the throat

* Seek medical attention if any of the above are persistent or unusual, so that exams can be performed to determine cause

(***Note:*** Lip and Oral Cavity Cancers may not demonstrate any signs or symptoms that are externally noticeable to the affected individual. Lip and Oral Cavity Cancer is sometimes identified by Dentists and Oral Surgeons during dental exams and other oral procedures)

- **Lip and Oral Cavity Cancer Diagnostic Tests**

  - Physical Exam of the lips and oral cavity (insides of the cheeks and lips; the gums; the roof and floor of the mouth; and, the top, bottom, and sides of the tongue). The doctor will feel the neck for swollen Lymph Nodes

- Endoscopy
- X-rays of the head, neck, and chest
- Biopsy Tissue Samples
- MRI (Magnetic Resonance Imaging (also called Nuclear Magnetic Resonance Imaging (NMRI))
- CT (Computed Tomography) Scan (or CAT scan)
- Exfoliative Cytology (A procedure to collect cells from the lip or oral cavity. A piece of cotton, a brush, or a small wooden stick is used to gently scrape cells from the lips, tongue, mouth, or throat. The cells are viewed under a microscope to find out if they are abnormal and malignant)
- Barium Swallow with X-rays of Esophagus and Stomach
- Positron Emission Tomography (PET) Scan (A procedure used to identify malignant tumor cells in the body. A small amount of Radionuclide Glucose (sugar) is injected into the patient's vein prior to the PET Scan, and the scanner then rotates around the body and takes pictures of where Glucose is being used by cells in the body. Cancer cells are more active than other cells, and therefore utilize more Glucose for energy than the normal cells. When this happens, the PET Scan images "light up" where this Cancer activity occurs)

- **Lip and Oral Cavity Cancer Treatment Considerations**

    - The Stage of the Cancer
    - The size and Grade of the Tumor
    - The location of the Tumor is in the Lip or Oral Cavity
    - Whether the Cancer has spread to Blood Vessels

- **Lip and Oral Cavity Cancer Prognosis Considerations**

    - The Stage of the Cancer
    - The size and Grade of the Tumor
    - The location of the Tumor in the Lip or Oral Cavity
    - The need to retain the patient's ability to talk, eat, and breathe as normally as possible
    - The patient's age and general health status

- ## Lip and Oral Cancer Cavity Recurrence Possibility

For all Lip and Oral Cavity Cancer patients who smoke, the chance of recovery is better if they cease smoking prior to beginning Radiation Therapy. Patients diagnosed with Lip, and/or, Oral Cavity Cancers have an increased risk of developing a second Cancer in the head or neck. Clinical Trials are studying the use of Retinoid Drugs to reduce the risk of a second Head and Neck Cancer. Information about continuing clinical trials is available from the National Cancer Institute (www.cancer.gov) website. ***Following therapy for Lip and Oral Cavity Cancer, frequent and careful follow-up is important.***

❖ *Laryngeal Cancer*

- ## Laryngeal Cancer Location(s)

Laryngeal Cancers are Head and Neck Cancers in which the malignant cancerous cells form within the tissues of the Larynx. The Larynx is a part of the throat, between the base of the tongue and the Trachea. The Larynx has the Vocal Cords, which vibrate and make sound when air is directed against them. This reverberation echoes through the Pharynx, mouth, and nose to make an individual's voice sound and resonate the way it does. Most Laryngeal Cancers form in Squamous Cells, the thin, flat cells lining the inside of the Larynx.

There are three main parts of the Larynx, as follows:

- ***Supraglottis*** **-** The upper area of the Larynx above the Vocal Cords, including the Epiglottis (Flap that covers Windpipe)
- ***Glottis*** **-** The middle portion of the Larynx where the Vocal Cords are located
- ***Subglottis*** **-** The lower part of the Larynx between the Vocal Cords and the Trachea (i.e., Windpipe)

- ## Laryngeal Cancer Risk Factors

- Smoking tobacco and chewing tobacco
- Heavy alcohol use

- **Laryngeal Cancer Symptoms ***

  - A sore throat or cough that does not go away
  - Trouble or pain when swallowing
  - Ear pain
  - A lump in the neck or throat
  - A change or hoarseness in the voice

* Seek medical attention if any of the above are persistent or unusual, so that exams can be performed to determine cause

- **Laryngeal Cancer Diagnostic Tests**

  - Physical Exam of the throat, and exam of neck to identify any swollen Neck Lymph Nodes
  - Laryngoscopy
  - Endoscopy
  - Biopsy Tissue Samples
  - CT (Computed Tomography) Scan (or CAT Scan)
  - MRI (Magnetic Resonance Imaging (also called Nuclear Magnetic Resonance Imaging (NMRI))
  - Barium Swallow with X-rays of Esophagus and Stomach (This procedure is know as an *Upper GI Series*)

- **Laryngeal Cancer Treatment Considerations**

  - The Stage of the Cancer
  - The location, size, and Grade of the Tumor
  - Whether or not the Cancer is a recurrence (second Cancer)
  - The need to retain the patient's ability to talk, eat, and breathe as normally as possible

- **Laryngeal Cancer Prognosis Considerations**

  - The Stage of the Cancer
  - The location and size of the Tumor
  - The Grade of the Tumor
  - The patient's age, gender, and general health status, including whether the patient is Anemic

- **Laryngeal Cancer Recurrence Possibility**

Smoking tobacco and drinking alcoholic beverages decrease the effectiveness of treatments for Laryngeal Cancer. Patients with Laryngeal Cancer who continue to smoke and drink are less likely to be cured and more likely to develop a second tumor. ***After treatment for Laryngeal Cancer, frequent and careful follow-up is critical.***

❖ *Nasopharyngeal Cancer*

- **Nasopharyngeal Cancer Location(s)**

Nasopharyngeal Cancer is a Head and Neck Cancer in which malignant cancerous cells develop in the tissues of the Nasopharynx. The Nasopharynx is the upper portion of the Pharynx (throat) behind the nose. The Pharynx is a hollow tube around five inches long that starts behind the nose and ends at the top of the Trachea (Windpipe) and the Esophagus (the tube through which foods and liquids travel from the throat to the stomach). Air and food and drink pass through the Pharynx on their way to the Trachea, or to the Esophagus. The nostrils connect to the Nasopharynx and an opening on both sides of the Nasopharynx leads into each ear. Most Nasopharyngeal Cancer commonly starts in the Squamous Cells that line the Nasopharynx.

- **Nasopharyngeal Cancer Risk Factors**

  - Chinese or Asian ancestry
  - Exposure to the Epstein-Barr Virus
  - Drinking large amounts of alcohol

- **Nasopharyngeal Cancer Symptoms ***

  - A lump in the nose or neck
  - A sore throat that does not go away
  - Trouble breathing or speaking
  - Nosebleeds
  - Trouble hearing
  - Pain or ringing in the ear

- Headaches (Continuous and out of the ordinary)

* Seek medical attention if any of the above are persistent or unusual, so that exams can be performed to determine cause

- **Nasopharyngeal Cancer Diagnostic Tests**

  - Physical Exam of the throat, and exam of the neck to identify any swollen Lymph Nodes
  - Nasoscopy (A procedure to look inside the nose for abnormal areas. A Nasoscope is inserted through the nose. A Nasoscope is a thin, tube-like instrument with a light and a lens for viewing. It may also have a tool to remove tissue samples, which are checked under a microscope for signs of Cancer)
  - Neurological exam (A series of questions and tests to check the brain, spinal cord, and nerve function. The exam checks a person's mental status, coordination, and ability to walk normally, and how well the muscles, senses, and reflexes work. This may also be called a Neuro Exam)
  - MRI (Magnetic Resonance Imaging (also called Nuclear Magnetic Resonance Imaging (NMRI))
  - CT (Computed Tomography) Scan (or CAT Scan)
  - Positron Emission Tomography (PET) Scan (A procedure used to identify malignant tumor cells in the body. A small amount of Radionuclide Glucose (sugar) is injected into the patient's vein prior to the PET Scan, and the scanner then rotates around the body and takes pictures of where Glucose is being used by cells in the body. Cancer cells are more active than other cells, and therefore utilize more Glucose for energy than the normal cells. When this happens, the PET Scan images "light up" where this Cancer activity occurs)
  - Laboratory Tests (Medical procedures that test samples of tissue, blood, urine, or other substances in the body).
  - Biopsy Tissue Samples

- **Nasopharyngeal Cancer Treatment Considerations**

  - The Stage of the Cancer

- The type of Nasopharyngeal Cancer
- The size and Grade of the Tumor
- The patient's age and general health status

- **Nasopharyngeal Cancer Prognosis Considerations**

  - The Stage of the Cancer
  - The type of Nasopharyngeal Cancer
  - The size and Grade of the Tumor
  - The patient's age and general health status

❖ *Oropharyngeal Cancer* *(My Form of Cancer)*

- **Oropharyngeal Cancer Location(s)**

Oropharyngeal Cancer is a Head and Neck Cancer in which malignant cancerous cells develop in the tissues of the Oropharynx. The Oropharynx is the middle region of the Pharynx (throat) behind the mouth, that includes the rear one-third of the tongue *(or Base of Tongue)* the soft palate, the side and back walls of the throat, and the Tonsils. The Pharynx is a hollow tube roughly five inches long that starts behind the nose and ends at the top of the Trachea (Windpipe) and Esophagus (the tube that connects the throat with the stomach). Air and foods pass through the Pharynx on their way to the Trachea (breathing) or the Esophagus (eating/drinking). Most Oropharyngeal Cancers are Squamous Cell Carcinomas *(as was the case with mine).*

- **Oropharyngeal Cancer Risk Factors**

  - Smoking tobacco and chewing tobacco
  - Heavy alcohol use
  - A diet low in fruits and vegetables
  - Drinking *Maté*, a stimulant drink common in South America
  - Chewing *Betel Quid*, a natural stimulant found in Asia
  - Being infected with Humanpapillomavirus (HPV) ***(This MAY have contributed to my Cancer occurrence)***
  - Being a Caucasian Male
  - Being over 50 years of age

- **Oropharyngeal Cancer Symptoms ***

  - A sore throat that does not go away, sometimes on only one side of the mouth, throat, and/or, neck
  - A dull pain behind the breastbone
  - A non-stop cough
  - Trouble swallowing
  - Weight loss for no known reason
  - Ear pain
  - A lump or swelling on/in the mouth, throat, neck, or tongue
  - A change in voice, such as hoarseness

* Seek medical attention if any of the above are persistent or unusual, so that exams can be performed to determine cause

- **Oropharyngeal Cancer Diagnostic Tests**

  - Physical Exam of the throat, and exam of the neck to identify swollen Lymph Nodes. The doctor does a complete exam of the mouth and neck and looks down the throat with a small, long-handled mirror and bright light to check for abnormal areas. A history of the patient's health habits and past illnesses and treatments will also be gathered and evaluated
  - CT (Computed Tomography) Scan (or CAT Scan)
  - MRI (Magnetic Resonance Imaging (also called Nuclear Magnetic Resonance Imaging (NMRI))
  - X-Rays of the organs and bones
  - Positron Emission Tomography (PET) Scan (A procedure used to identify malignant tumor cells in the body. A small amount of Radionuclide Glucose (sugar) is injected into the patient's vein prior to the PET Scan, and the scanner then rotates around the body and takes pictures of where Glucose is being used by cells in the body. Cancer cells are more active than other cells, and therefore utilize more Glucose for energy than the normal cells. When this happens, the PET Scan images "light up" where this Cancer activity occurs)
  - Endoscopy (A procedure to look at organs and tissues inside the body to check for abnormal areas. An Endoscope is inserted through the patient's nose or mouth to look at areas

in the throat that cannot be seen during a physical exam of the throat. An Endoscope is a thin, tube-like instrument with a light and a lens for viewing)

- Biopsy Tissue Samples

- **Oropharyngeal Cancer Treatment Considerations**

  - The Stage of the Cancer
  - The size, Grade, and location of the Tumor
  - The patient's age and general health status

- **Oropharyngeal Cancer Prognosis Considerations**

  - The Stage of the Cancer
  - The size and Grade of the Tumor
  - The location of the Tumor
  - Whether or not the Tumor is associated with HPV infection

(***Note:*** Researchers have found that individuals with Stage III or IV Oropharyngeal Cancer (Cancer of the Upper Throat and the Base of Tongue) who have tested positive for Humanpapillomavirus (HPV), survive longer than those that test negative for HPV, whose Cancer may have been caused by tobacco use or excessive alcohol use)

➢ ***While on the Topic of Oropharyngeal Cancer...***

- **Squamous Cell Cancer of the Base of Tongue – A Brief Summary**

☛ ***Author's Note: This is the specific form of Cancer I had, and the ultimate location of my Primary Tumor***

Like the Oral Tongue (the Anterior or front 2/3 of the tongue that one sees in the mouth and upper throat), the Base of Tongue (or Posterior 1/3 hidden in the throat) can also be home to several forms of Cancers. The National Cancer Institute (www.cancer.gov) found Squamous Cell Carcinoma (also referred to as *SCC*) to be the most common form of malignant Cancer diagnosed in the Oropharyngeal region. Squamous Cells are thin, flat cells found in tissues that form the surface of the skin and the lining of body cavities such as in the mouth. Per www.cancer.gov, Anterior Tongue Cancers account for 56% of all Tongue Cancers, and Base of Tongue Cancers for 44%.

○ Diagnosis of Base of Tongue Cancers

While *Anterior Tongue SCCs* are generally more apparent to the affected person because of the visibility of the tumor growths on the tongue and any pain they may cause, even in their earlier Stages of development, *Base of Tongue SCCs* are typically larger and more advanced when at first diagnosed. This is because in both the earlier Stages (i.e., 0, I, and II), and also in later Stages (i.e., III and IV), the Primary Tumor cannot be seen by the impacted individual because it is hidden deep down in their throat. Further, detection during earlier stages of Base of Tongue SCC development is very difficult because the tumors may prompt few, if any, noticeable symptoms. In other words, during its infancy, this nasty disease is growing, feeding, and staking its territory in the person's healthy tongue tissue, while he or she has no clue that something very atrocious is taking place within their body. That was definitely what happened in my situation.

It is usually not until the Base of Tongue SCC has advanced in size, Stage, and progression within the body *(as was the case with my Cancer),* that the affected individual first begins noticing signs and symptoms that (hopefully) cause them to question what's going on, and to take steps to seek medical intervention. In Stages III and IV, Base of Tongue Cancer may induce very perceptible symptoms, which include: Unremitting pain on the side of the throat where the Tumor formed *(a symptom I had*); changes in what the voice sounds like; difficulty swallowing in general; some extent of discomfort and pain when swallowing any food and drink *(a symptom I had)*; Neck Lymph Node involvement on same side as pain *(a symptom I had).*

○ Lymph Node Impact of Base of Tongue Cancers

Because a Base of Tongue Cancer diagnosis typically comes later on in the Cancer's formation, a greater number of patients with this calamity of the disease will have already had a Neck Metastasis.

Meaning, that by the time the person notices the abnormal signs and symptoms and makes an appointment to go and visit their doctor for an examination, the Cancer cells have already spread to the Lymph Nodes in the person's upper neck on the side of the Primary Tumor, just below the jaw line. This effect on the Lymph Nodes can also be very apparent to the affected individual because that portion of their neck will become irregularly swollen, and, they can actually feel the enlarged Lymph Nodes just beneath the skin with their fingers. Once again, this was my precise situation, and it was these odd, abnormal, and persistent symptoms that caused me to seek medical assistance.

Even though I had no idea what was going on with my *one-sided* sore throat, hoarseness, swallowing issues, and a swollen neck, the first four physicians I saw, including my Primary Care Physician and *two Ear, Nose, and Throat Specialists who treat Head and Neck Cancer patients all the time,* didn't have the slightest clue what was provoking the problems. How can it be possible that physicians who treat Head and Neck Cancers can fail to see what turned out to be an obvious Cancer diagnosis, especially when I was experiencing all of the trademark symptoms? That is a rhetorical question, I understand, but, had I only known then what I know now, it would have saved me plenty of time and frustration. And—this is the most important part—we may have "caught" my Cancer earlier, such as Stage III vs. Stage IV, which would have been huge! *20/20 hindsight,* you say?

- ## Treatment of Base of Tongue Cancers

From a Cancer Treatment standpoint, after a Cancer tumor at the Base of Tongue has been identified, diagnosed and Staged, and, after the Treatment strategy plan has been developed by the Medical Team and patient, the treatment(s) to eliminate the Cancer at Base of Tongue will commence. According to the National Cancer Institute (www.cancer.gov), Surgery is commonly used to remove some Base of Tongue Cancers, whether they are lower or higher Stage Cancers. However, the Institute also stresses that Base of Tongue SCCs can, and should, also be treated by Radiation Therapy whenever possible. Medical findings show that Base of Tongue tumors are considerably more susceptible to Radiation Therapy treatments than several of the other Cancers, so Radiotherapy is frequently employed in an effort to safely and completely remove the disease from the patient's body.

In elevated Staged (i.e., III and IV) Base of Tongue Cancers, such as my own (Stage IV), the treatment strategy determined by the Medical Team, patient, family, or Caregiver, may not only call for Surgery and Radiation Therapy, but, also, for a complete course of Chemotherapy, to-boot. The concomitant Chemotherapy / Radiation Therapy / Surgery plan has been found to be very successful against many forms of Cancer, as the extremely powerful mixture combines to interrupt the cellular division / growth cycles of the Cancers. This impediment results in Cancer cell obliteration, not only at the site of the Tumor (Radiation Therapy), but, also throughout the rest of the body (Chemotherapy). Absolutely, there are exceptions to this, but these treatments *can* be extremely effective. *I am living proof that!*

Radiation Therapy can also be utilized to control and kill any cancerous cells that have metastasized in the Neck Lymph Nodes, as long as the Cancer is not too advanced. In some cases, massive and advanced cancerous Neck Node disease is surgically removed before Radiation Therapy is commenced. This protocol is typically utilized when the treating physicians on the patient's Medical Team are able to determine that the use of Radiation Therapy, alone, would not be 100% successful in controlling the cancerous disease in the neck.

- ## Prognosis of Base of Tongue Cancer Patients

From a patient prognosis perspective (anticipated outcomes following the completion of treatment), the patient's prospects after treatment of Base of Tongue Cancer will vary from patient to patient as with any other variety of malignant cancerous disease. That being said, however, Studies carried out by the National Cancer Institute (www.cancer.gov), have noted that the cure rate for Base of Tongue Cancers is good…but, not as good as for Anterior Tongue Cancers.

The cure rate disparity between Anterior Tongue and Base of Tongue Cancers, as stated previously, is typically because the more visible Anterior Tongue disease is detected sooner than the Base of Tongue forms, as the latter are hidden, and usually more advanced at their time of diagnosis. With that being said, one must also consider medical Studies which find that Oropharyngeal Cancers known to be incited by Humanpapillomavirus (HPV) have a greater overall cure rate—approximately 90%—and much higher patient longevity, than Oropharyngeal Cancers caused by tobacco use and alcohol intake.

❖ *Salivary Gland Cancer*

• Salivary Gland Cancer Location(s)

Salivary Gland Cancer is quite a rare form of Head and Neck Cancer in which malignant cancerous cells form in the tissues of the Salivary Glands. The Salivary Glands make saliva (otherwise known as *spit),* and release it into the mouth. Saliva has enzymes that help digest food, and it contains antibodies that help engender protection against infections of the mouth and throat. In other words, it's vital.

There are three (3) pairs of Primary Salivary Glands (one Gland on each side of the head in three (3) different locations), as follows:

- **Parotid Glands -** These are the largest Salivary Glands and are located in front of, and just underneath, each ear. Most cancerous Salivary Gland Tumors begin in this Gland
- **Sublingual Glands -** These Glands are positioned below the tongue in the floor of the mouth
- **Submandibular Glands -** These Glands are found below the lower Jaw Bone (Mandible)

In addition to the three pairs of large (Major) Salivary Glands, there are also hundreds of small (Minor) Salivary Glands that line parts of the mouth, nose, and Larynx. These smaller Glands can only be seen beneath a microscope. A majority of Minor Salivary Gland Tumors begin in the Palate (i.e., Roof of the Mouth).

*(**Note:*** On the optimistic side, Medical Studies have found that more than half of all Salivary Gland Tumors are Benign (not cancerous) and do not broaden to other bodily tissues. Nevertheless, individuals that notice anything unusual and persistent occurring with their head or neck should seek medical intervention as early as possible so that Malignant Cancer can either be ruled out (hopefully), or diagnosed, and the cancerous presence can be treated promptly and completely. *Note: All Cancers must be considered lethal until proven otherwise)*

- **Salivary Gland Cancer Risk Factors**

  - Older age
  - Radiation Therapy to the head and neck (for past Cancers)
  - Exposure to noxious industrial chemicals and substances

- **Salivary Gland Cancer Symptoms ***

  - Trouble swallowing or opening the mouth widely
  - A lump (usually painless) in the area of the ear, cheek, jaw, lip, or inside the mouth
  - Fluid draining from the ear
  - Numbness or weakness in the face
  - Pain in the face that does not go away

* Seek medical attention if any of the above are persistent or unusual, so that exams can be performed to determine cause

(***Note:*** Salivary Gland Cancer may not cause any symptoms that are perceptible to the affected person. The disease is sometimes located during a standard dental check-up, an oral exam, or a physical exam. Symptoms caused by Salivary Gland Cancer can present themselves to be the same or similar to symptoms of other health problems. As such, individuals experiencing the above-specified symptoms should not attempt to self-diagnose their condition, but should seek medical intervention to determine the cause of the problem(s))

- **Salivary Gland Cancer Diagnostic Tests**

  - Physical Exam of the body to check general signs of health, including checking for signs of disease, such as lumps or anything else that seems unusual. A history of the patient's health habits and past illnesses and treatments will also be taken and evaluated by the physician
  - Physical exam of the face, and exam of the neck to identify any swollen Lymph Nodes. The doctor does a complete exam of the mouth and neck and looks down the throat with a small, long-handled mirror and bright light to check for abnormal areas, redness, swelling, etc.

- MRI (Magnetic Resonance Imaging (also called Nuclear Magnetic Resonance Imaging (NMRI))
- Positron Emission Tomography (PET) Scan (A procedure used to identify malignant tumor cells in the body. A small amount of Radionuclide Glucose (sugar) is injected into the patient's vein prior to the PET Scan, and the scanner then rotates around the body and takes pictures of where Glucose is being used by cells in the body. Cancer cells are more active than other cells, and therefore utilize more Glucose for energy than the normal cells. When this happens, the PET Scan images "light up" where this Cancer activity occurs)
- Endoscopy (A procedure to look at organs and tissues inside the body to check for abnormal areas. An Endoscope is inserted through the patient's nose or mouth to look at areas in the throat that cannot be seen during a physical exam of the throat. An Endoscope is a thin, tube-like instrument with a light and a lens for viewing. It may also have a tool to remove tissue or Lymph Node samples, which are checked under a microscope for signs of disease)
- CT (Computed Tomography) Scan (or CAT Scan)
- Ultrasound exam (A procedure in which high-energy sound waves (ultrasound) are bounced off internal tissues or organs and make echoes. The echoes form a picture of body tissues called a Sonogram. The picture can be printed for reference)
- Fine Needle Aspiration (FNA) Biopsy (The removal of tissue or fluid using a thin needle. A Pathologist views the tissue or fluid under a microscope to look for Cancer Cells)

(***Note:*** Because Salivary Gland Cancers can be difficult to diagnose, patients should make sure that appropriate members of their Medical Team ***have the Biopsy tissue samples checked by a Pathologist who has knowledge in the diagnosis of Salivary Gland Cancer.*** Due to the rarity of this form of Head and Neck Cancer, it may be difficult for a Pathologist with no experience to accurately diagnose Salivary Gland Cancers and properly identify the disease in the laboratory)

- **Salivary Gland Cancer Treatment Considerations**

  - Stage of the Cancer (especially the size of the tumor)

- Type of Salivary Gland affected by the Cancer
- Type of Cancer cells (Their appearance under a microscope)
- The patient's age and general health status

- **Salivary Gland Cancer Prognosis Considerations**

  - Stage of the Cancer (especially the size of the tumor)
  - Type of Salivary Gland affected by the Cancer
  - Type of Cancer cells (their appearance under a microscope)
  - The patient's age and general health status

❖ *Metastatic Squamous Neck Cancer With Occult (Unknown) Primary*

☛ ***Author's Note: This is the initial Diagnosis that I received from my physician, as the location of my Primary Tumor had not been found at that point***

Metastatic Squamous Neck Cancer with Occult Primary is a disease in which Squamous Cell Cancer spreads to Lymph Nodes in the neck, but it is not known where the Cancer first developed in the body. In other words, it is known, due to Pathology confirmation of tissue sample biopsies of the neck Lymph Nodes, that the patient has Cancer. But, what is not known at the point of diagnosis, is the exact location of the Primary Cancer Tumor. Because the Tumor Site has not yet been identified, the Cancer Tumor is referred to as "Occult," which means *hidden.* Applicable members of the patient's Medical Team will attempt to locate the tumor in follow-on tests and exams.

- **Squamous Cell Description and Locations**

Squamous Cells are thin, flat cells found in tissues that form the surface of the skin and in the linings of body cavities such as the mouth, hollow organs such as the Uterus and Blood Vessels, and the linings of the Respiratory Tract and Digestive Tract. Some organs having Squamous Cells include the Esophagus, Lungs, and Kidneys. Cancer can begin in Squamous Cells anywhere in the body and can spread (or metastasize) throughout the Circulatory System or Lymph

System to other parts of the body, including the Neck Lymph Nodes. It is this migration of Cancer cells from the Primary Tumor to other bodily regions that increases the Stage of the Cancer, and, which can create additional challenges in successfully treating the disease.

• Tests and Exams to Locate the Primary Tumor

When Squamous Cell Cancer spreads to Lymph Nodes in the neck area or around the collarbone, it is called Metastatic Squamous Neck Cancer. In most cases of Occult Cancer, the physicians on the Medical Team will conduct appropriate exams and tests in an effort to find the Primary Tumor (the Cancer that first formed in the body), so that the Cancer can be accurately treated. To use an analogy, just as a hunter will want to be properly geared up for whatever game he or she may encounter in the field, the patient's Cancer Surgeon and Oncologist will also want to know what they will be up against with this big *Cancer Beast.* Please be informed that sometimes, however, despite their finest efforts, doctors cannot find in the patient's body where their Cancer first began to develop. In other words, they can't locate the Primary Tumor from which the cancerous cells spread to the neck or other body parts. If this occurs, applicable members of the patient's Medical Team will inform the patient and all concerned parties, and they will discuss the treatment options that are available.

• Treatment of Metastatic Squamous Neck Cancer

For obvious reasons, it is very important that the members of the patient's Medical Team have as much scientifically substantiated information about the patient's Cancer as is possible. They will use the Pathology Report and the scientific data to work with the patient and their family or Caregiver to design a safe and powerful Cancer-eradication treatment regimen that best takes into account the form of the Cancer, as well as its Stage, its location, and the extent of its metastasis in other parts of the body. The treatment for Metastatic Cancer is the same as treatment that would be applied to the Primary Tumor. For example, if confirmed Lung Cancer spreads to the Neck Lymph Nodes, the Cancer Cells in the Neck are *Lung Cancer Cells* and, they would be treated the same as Cancer in the Lung. In such a case, the Cancer would be referred to as *Metastatic Lung Cancer.*

- **Metastatic Squamous Neck Cancer Symptoms ***

    - A lump or swelling in the upper neck just below the jaw line, and is sometimes coupled with a sore throat on the same side
    - An unusual pain or soreness in the neck or throat

* Seek medical attention if any of the above are persistent or unusual, so that exams can be performed to determine cause

(***Note:*** Symptoms provoked by Metastatic Squamous Neck Cancers might be the same or similar to symptoms of other health conditions. As such, individuals who experience the abovementioned symptoms should not endeavor to self-diagnose, but, should proactively request medical intervention to determine the cause of the problem(s))

- **Metastatic Squamous Neck Cancer Diagnostic Tests**

    - Physical Exam of the body, especially the head and neck, in an effort to locate the Primary Tumor, and to search for any signs of disease, such as lumps, redness, or anything else that seems abnormal in the organs and tissues of the Respiratory Tract, the upper regions of the Digestive Tract, including the lips, mouth, tongue, nose, throat, Vocal Cords, and regions of the Trachea and Esophagus, and the Genitourinary System
    - Endoscopy (A procedure to look at organs and tissues inside the body to identify the Primary Tumor, and to discover any abnormal regions. In this situation, an Endoscope is inserted through an incision (aperture) in the skin or an opening in the body, such as the mouth or the nose. The Endoscope is a thin tube-like instrument having a light and a lens at the end for viewing, and, it could also have a tool for taking out tissue or Lymph Node samples, which are confirmed by a Pathologist beneath a microscope for any signs of disease. Additionally, the Larynx, Pharynx, Trachea, Bronchi and Esophagus will be checked in a attempt to locate the Primary Tumor)

    (Note: It was an Endoscopy, performed by a Cancer doctor outside my HMO whom I saw for a Second Opinion about my diagnosis, which finally located my Primary Tumor)

- Biopsy Tissue Samples (The removal of cells and tissues so they can be viewed under a microscope by a Pathologist and tested in the medical laboratory to check for signs of Cancer)

  Two types of Biopsy may be performed by the Surgeon:

  - **Fine-Needle Aspiration (FNA) Biopsy -** The removal of tissue or fluid using a thin needle
  - **Excisional Biopsy -** The surgical cutting and physical removal of an entire section of tissue

- Sinus X-ray (An X-ray of the Sinuses (hollow spaces in the head)
- Chest X-ray (An X-ray of the organs, such as the Lung, and bones inside the chest)
- Bronchoscopy (A procedure to look inside the Trachea and large airways in the Lung for abnormal areas. A bronchoscope is inserted through the nose or mouth into the trachea and lungs. A Bronchoscope is a thin, tube-like instrument with a light and a lens for viewing. It may also have a tool to remove tissue samples, which are checked under a microscope for signs of Cancer)
- MRI (Magnetic Resonance Imaging - A procedure that uses a magnet, radio waves, and a computer to make a series of detailed pictures of areas inside the body. This procedure is also called nuclear magnetic resonance imaging (NMRI))
- Positron Emission Tomography (PET) Scan (A procedure used to identify malignant tumor cells in the body. A small amount of Radionuclide Glucose (sugar) is injected into the patient's vein prior to the PET Scan, and the scanner then rotates around the body and takes pictures of where Glucose is being used by cells in the body. Cancer cells are more active than other cells, and therefore utilize more Glucose for energy than the normal cells. When this happens, the PET Scan images "light up" where this Cancer activity occurs)
- CT (Computed Tomography) Scan (or CAT Scan)
- Serum Tumor Marker Test (A procedure in which a blood sample is checked to measure the amounts of certain substances released into the blood by organs, tissues, or tumor cells in the body. Certain substances are linked to

specific types of Cancer when found in increased levels in the blood. These are called Tumor Markers)

The test will be done to detect the following Tumor Markers:

- Alpha-fetoprotein (AFP)
- Beta-human Chorionic Gonadotropin (β-hCG)

- **Metastatic Squamous Neck Cancer Treatment Considerations**

  - In which part of the neck the Cancer is located
  - Whether certain Tumor Markers are found

- **Metastatic Squamous Neck Cancer Prognosis Considerations**

  - The numbers and sizes of Lymph Nodes that have Cancer in them, as confirmed by microscopic Laboratory Pathology
  - Whether the initial Cancer has responded to treatment or has recurred (come back). (If the patient's response to treatment was favorable, as verified by regular follow-on testing, and there has been no diagnosis of recurrent Cancer, the patient's prognosis is improved)
  - The amount of difference between normal, healthy cells, and the Cancer cells when viewed under a microscope
  - The patient's age and general health status

❖ *Paranasal Sinus and Nasal Cavity Cancers*

- **Paranasal Sinus and Nasal Cancer Location(s)**

  - **Paranasal Sinuses**

Paranasal Sinus Cancers and Nasal Cavity Cancers are Head and Neck Cancers in which malignant cancerous cells mature in the tissues of the Paranasal Sinuses and Nasal Cavity. *Paranasal* means *near the nose.* The Paranasal Sinuses are hollow, air-filled spaces in bones around the nose. The Sinuses are lined with cells that create mucous, which helps to keep the interior of the nose moist and helps to prevent the nasal passages from drying out during breathing.

The Paranasal Sinuses are named after the bones that surround them. Specifically, the four (4) Sinuses and their locations are as follows:

- **Frontal Sinuses** - Located in the lower forehead, just above the nose
- **Maxillary Sinuses** - Located in the cheekbones on either side of the nose
- **Ethmoid Sinuses** - Located beside the upper nose, between the eyes
- **Sphenoid Sinuses** – Located behind the nose, in the center of the skull

Nasal Cavity

The nose opens into the Nasal Cavity, which divides into two nasal passages. Air moves through these passages during breathing. The Nasal Cavity is positioned above the bone that forms the roof of the mouth and curves down towards the back to join the throat. The region just inside the nostrils is referred to as the Nasal Vestibule. A small area made up of unique cells in the roof of each nasal passage sends sensory signals to the brain, which become the sense of smell. Together, the Paranasal Sinuses and the Nasal Cavity both filter and warm the air we breathe, and they make the air moist before it goes into the Lungs. The movement of air thru the Sinuses and other parts of the respiratory system help to make the sounds that are associated with talking. *Think of all this during your next important speech!*

Varied types of cells in the Paranasal Sinus and Nasal Cavity may become malignant. The most common form of Paranasal Sinus and Nasal Cavity Cancer is Squamous Cell Carcinoma. This type of Cancer forms in the Squamous Cells (thin, flat cells), which line the inside of the Paranasal Sinuses and the Nasal Cavity.

Other types of Paranasal Sinus Cancers and Nasal Cavity Cancers, and their potential locations, include the following:

- **Sarcoma** - Cancer that starts in muscle or connective tissue.
- **Melanoma** - Cancer that forms in cells named Melanocytes, the cells that give skin its natural color
- **Inverting Papilloma** - Benign (non-cancerous) tumors that develop inside the nose. Studies indicate that a small number of these incidences will transform into malignant Cancer
- **Midline Granulomas** - Cancer that forms in tissues in the middle part of the face

- ## Paranasal Sinus and Nasal Cancer Risk Factors

  - Being exposed to certain workplace chemicals or dust, such as those found in the following jobs:

    - Furniture-making and woodworking (carpentry), etc.
    - Sawmill work
    - Outdoor construction in an environment with fine dust
    - Shoemaking
    - Metal-plating, grinding, welding, etc.
    - Flour mill or bakery work
    - Other vocations in which particulate matter is breathed

  - Being infected with Humanpapillomavirus (HPV)
  - Being male and older than 40 years
  - Smoking

- ## Paranasal Sinus and Nasal Cancer Symptoms *

  - Blocked sinuses that do not clear, or sinus pressure
  - Headaches or pain in the sinus areas
  - A continuous runny nose
  - Unexplained nosebleeds
  - A lump or sore inside the nose that does not heal
  - A lump on the face or roof of the mouth
  - Numbness or tingling in the face
  - Swelling or other trouble with the eyes, such as double vision or the eyes pointing in different directions
  - Pain in the upper teeth, loose teeth, or dentures that no longer fit well

- Pain or pressure in the ear

* Seek medical attention if any of the above are persistent or unusual, so that exams can be performed to determine cause

(***Note:*** The above symptoms and others may be caused by Paranasal Sinus and Nasal Cavity Cancers, but, be aware that other conditions may also cause the same or similar symptoms. Medical intervention is necessary to differentiate and identify the cause of the symptoms. Also, there may be no perceptible symptoms in the earlier Stages of Cancer, but may appear and become apparent as the tumor grows)

- **Paranasal Sinus and Nasal Cancer Diagnostic Tests**

  - Physical Exam of the body to check general signs of health, including checking for signs of disease, such as lumps or anything else that seems unusual. A history of the patient's health habits and past illnesses and treatments will also be taken
  - Physical Exam of the nose and face, and exam of the neck to identify any swollen Lymph Nodes. The doctor does a complete exam of the mouth, nose, and neck and looks down the throat with a small, long-handled mirror and bright light to check for abnormal areas
  - X-rays of the head, neck, and chest
  - Nasoscopy (A procedure to look inside the nose for abnormal areas. A Nasoscope is a thin, tube-like instrument with a light and a lens for viewing that is inserted into the nose. It may also have a tool to remove tissue samples, which are checked under a microscope for signs of Cancer)
  - Biopsy Tissue Samples

- **Paranasal Sinus and Nasal Cancer Treatment Considerations**

  - Where the tumor is located in the Paranasal Sinus or Nasal Cavity, and whether it has spread
  - The size of the tumor
  - The specific type of Cancer

- The patient's age and general health status
- Whether the Cancer is a first-time diagnosis, or a recurrence

- **Paranasal Sinus and Nasal Cancer Prognosis Considerations**

    - Where the tumor is in the Paranasal Sinus or Nasal Cavity and whether it has spread
    - The size of the tumor
    - The specific type of Cancer
    - The patient's age and general health status
    - Whether the Cancer is a first-time diagnosis, or a recurrence

(***Note:*** By the time that assorted Paranasal Sinus Cancers and Nasal Cavity Cancers are diagnosed, they have metastasized in other parts of the head or body, and could be difficult to cure completely. After treatment has concluded, *it is critical that the patient frequently and carefully follow-up with doctors **knowledgeable of** Paranasal Sinus Cancers and Nasal Cavity Cancers.* This is because these forms of Head and Neck Cancers come with an increased risk of developing a second type of Cancer in the head or neck area later in life. As such, it is important that it be identified and treated as quickly as possible)

A Final Word about the Many Forms of Head and Neck Cancers

Now tell me, Reader, was this not the most interesting, *keep-you-on-the-edge-of-your-seat* Chapter that you've ever read in your life? Yeah, I know, it sucked. However, for any current or past Head and Neck Cancer patients, or, for anyone who wants to do what they can to ***NOT become a Head and Neck Cancer patient***, the material provided in this Chapter (which has been adapted from the National Cancer Institute (www.cancer.gov)), is a wealth of information and *"to dos,"* and *"not to dos."* Believe me, I know how overwhelming and frightening this information can be, because I've read it, studied it, and employed it—in one way or another—during my own Cancer experience, for several years now. But, it is what it is, and, when one of these Head and Neck Cancers strikes a person, they'd better know all about *it*, because, believe me, it knows all about *them*.

Chapter Twelve

Head and Neck Cancers – *The Common Treatments*

"Life never prepares a person for getting Cancer, but it spends years teaching them how to survive it."

- Butch Sickler

Any person who has been in a scary and nerve-racking, ***Oh crap!***-type of situation has had the possible dread, the worry, and the *"How did I get myself in this predicament and what do I do to get out of it?"* feelings. My first memory of such a terrifying experience was when I was roughly four years old, and my Sister, Vikki, and I thought that we were under attack by "killer cats" owned by the man next door. I can still recall how quickly we both "barely escaped" by putting that 3'-high fence between us and them (not realizing at our young ages that cats can jump over 10 feet, but that's a minor point). The major point, though, is that we both got out of that *harrowing* experience and lived another day. Well, then, welcome to Head and Neck Cancer Treatment, where Cancers are, hopefully, fenced in for good, and patients can come safely out the other side to live again.

How are Head and Neck Cancers Treated?

Generally speaking, the three common forms of treatment for eradicating Head and Neck Cancers are Radiation Therapy, Surgery, and Chemotherapy. However, the primary techniques for treating a bulk of all Head and Neck Cancers are Radiation Therapy, Surgery, or both, combined. Chemotherapy, the utilization of very powerful medications to treat Cancer, is often used in advanced Stage Head and Neck Cancers (Stages III and IV) in conjunction with Radiation Therapy, and/or, Cancer Surgery. This powerful combination gives the patient's Cancer a *"1-2-3 punch,"* which can be very effective.

Cancer Stage + Type + Location = Cancer Treatment

The Cancer treatments that are decided upon for the patient's treatment plan may depend on several factors. But, key among these are the age and overall physical condition of the patient; the form of Head and Neck Cancer the patient has; the head or neck locale of the Cancer; and, the Cancer's Stage, or, its level of progression within the patient's body and metastasis in other tissues and systems.

The following general information regarding Head and Neck Cancer treatments was adapted from www.cancer.gov:

- ### Stage I and II Head and Neck Cancer Therapies

Patients with earlier-Stage Head and Neck Cancers, such as those classified as Stages I or II, and, particularly those localized at the site of the original Primary Tumor – the ***best case*** – are typically treated with one procedure – either Radiation Therapy, to "zap" the Cancer Tumor and the surrounding marginal tissue, or, Surgery, to physically remove the Primary Tumor and any adjacent, potentially cancerous tissue. In Stage III and IV Head and Neck Cancer cases, however, such as my disease, Chemotherapy may also be employed with Surgery and Radiation Therapy as an optimal combination to completely destroy and remove the disease from the patient's body. Chemo is typically used to treat most Stage III and IV Cancers.

- ### Stage III and IV Head and Neck Cancer Therapies

Head and Neck Cancer patients who have more "entrenched" Cancers (meaning, that they are of the higher-Stages, such as III and IV), are often treated with concurrent Chemotherapy and Radiation Therapy. And, in still other incidences of Head and Neck Cancer, dependent upon the patient's situation, the patient may first undergo Surgery to physically remove the tumor, and then might back that up with Chemotherapy, and Radiation Therapy. If the plan of treatment for Head and Neck Cancer calls for Radiation Therapy to target the Primary Cancer Tumor, the surrounding marginal neck area is also treated with Radiation Therapy to annihilate any residual cancerous cells. And, finally, in several instances (such as my own), Stage III and IV Head and Neck Cancers are treated initially with Chemo and Radiation, and later with Surgery to remove any remaining tissue.

Common Treatments for Head and Neck Cancer – One-by-One

Head and Neck Cancers, like many of the other 200+ known forms of Cancer, are distinct unto themselves. However, while they may have their own specific causative factors, locations in the body, and distinctive *modus operandi,* Head and Neck Cancers are similar to many other Cancers in that they *can be* effectively addressed with the conventional Cancer treatments—Surgery, Radiation Therapy, and Chemotherapy—if the Cancers are detected, confirmed, Staged, and aggressively treated, as early in the process as possible.

☛***Authors Note:*** General information about *five* conventional Cancer Treatment options—including for Head and Neck Cancers—is explained in Chapter 6 of this Book, The Cancer Treatments, *Step 8 of the Cancer Journey.* Further, as would be anticipated, supplemental information regarding all of the various conventional and alternative Cancer treatments is available in a multitude of resources regarding Cancer, including the National Cancer Institute at www.cancer.gov, and, in materials provided to the patient by appropriate members of their Medical Team. Following receipt of the Head and Neck Cancer diagnosis, it might be very beneficial for the patient, and their family or Caregiver, to research treatment options for their form of Head and Neck Cancer, and to learn what they can about the treatments' success rates, possible Side Effects, and other pertinent information.

In all Cancer cases, however, the patient, and their family or Caregiver, will consult with appropriate Medical Team members to determine—based on the patient's variety of Head and Neck Cancer, its Stage and location, and, the patient's general state of health—the most appropriate treatment(s) to be utilized to safely and (hopefully) completely remove the patient's Cancer. These individuals should discuss each type of treatment, the risks, benefits, and potential Side Effects, and how each form of the treatment(s) might temporarily or permanently alter the way the patient looks, talks, eats, or breathes.

Adapted from the U.S. National Cancer Institute online resources at www.cancer.gov, my journaling notes, and materials provided to me by my Medical Team, following are brief descriptions of the three most widespread and effective conventional treatment modalities for all Head and Neck Cancers: Chemotherapy, Radiation Therapy, and, Surgery. *Note: Side Effects are addressed in the following Chapter.*

• Surgery – Head and Neck Cancer Treatment

If the patient's Medical Team determines that the Head and Neck Cancer patient must receive Surgery in an effort to physically remove the cancerous tissue, the doctor will discuss with the patient and their loved one, their family members, or Caregiver, the safest and most appropriate mode(s) of surgical operation(s) that should be performed on the patient. This determination will be based on many factors, including the type, size, and location of the Cancer Tumor, the Cancer's Stage (the level of its spread to any other regions of the body), and the patient's age, physical status, and other factors. It's extremely noteworthy for Head and Neck Cancer patients, and their loved one, families, or Caregiver, to have pre-treatment discussions with the physician(s) on the Cancer Surgical Team pertaining to the forthcoming surgical procedure(s). This will permit questions to be answered, and will help all parties to understand exactly what tissue is planned to be removed, and from what location(s) on the patient's body. These meetings will also permit the doctor to fully explain the anticipated benefits and potential risks of the surgical procedure(s), and how the operation(s) may, likely, have an effect on the patient—good and bad—in both the short term, and further down the road.

o Removal of Tumors, Margins, and Lymph Nodes

During Head and Neck Cancer Surgery, the Cancer Surgeon will typically remove the Primary Cancer Tumor, itself. This is Job One. If it is deemed safe and prudent to do so, the Surgeon will also physically extract some of the healthy tissue surrounding the Tumor. These adjacent areas, which might potentially still be cancerous, are known as the *"Margins,"* and they are commonly removed to ensure that no lingering, possibly cancerous cells remain behind to provoke more problems for the patient in the future. Further, removal of any affected Lymph Nodes and marginal tissues in the patient's upper neck may be necessary if laboratory testing of Biopsy tissue samples indicates that the quantity of disease in the Neck Nodes is relatively extensive. In such cases, Neck Dissection Surgery may be essential. Neck Dissection Surgery will also universally be performed if it has been determined by follow-up Biopsy Surgery that the Cancer cells in the Neck Nodes have not been thoroughly gotten rid of following the conclusion of the patient's entire course of Radiation Therapy.

- ## Reconstructive Surgery After Cancer Removal

Unfortunately, as one might suppose, not all Head and Neck Cancers can be removed from the patient's affected regions without there being some degree of "collateral damage" to healthy tissues in adjoining and nearby areas. Regrettably, due to the chancy locations in which some Head and Neck Cancer can invade—and with higher-Staged Cancers, depending upon how entrenched the disease might be—the Cancer Surgeon could be left with no choice but to radically impact other head and neck tissues through the practice of removing the cancerous cells. In severe circumstances some patients may need to have Reconstructive Surgery performed on one or more areas of their face, and/or, neck. The Surgeon will discuss all potential risks and the benefits of Reconstructive Surgery with the Head and Neck Cancer patient, and will do all they can to see to it that post-surgery results are as normal-looking and as normal-functioning as possible.

As adapted from National Cancer Institute (www.cancer.gov) online resources, following are forms of Reconstructive Surgery that may have to be performed on some Head and Neck Cancer patients:

- ### Skin Flap and Bone Graft Surgery

Depending upon the form of Head and Neck Cancer that the patient has, its head or neck location, its Stage, and other factors, the

Cancer Surgeon may need to remove part of the mouth, tongue or throat lining and occasionally, some facial skin. Removed facial skin can be replaced using a piece of skin taken from another part of the body – typically the forearm or chest. When this sort of Surgery is performed, it is known as a ***Skin Flap***. Typically, a successful Skin Graft procedure will do a very decent job of concealing the surgical site, and, after healing, will leave little or no trace of what had been performed beneath the dermis to remove the patient's Cancer. If the Head and Neck Cancer has infiltrated and is affecting some or all of the patient's Jaw bone, the affected bone might have to be surgically separated from the patient's head, along with the cancerous tumor. In this event, part of a bone will typically be surgically taken from elsewhere in the patient's body and will be fitted and inserted in the patient's head to replace the missing jawbone. In a majority of these forms of Surgery, the replacement portion of bone is taken from the patient's leg. When such an operation is performed, it is referred to as a ***Bone Graft***. Many modern surgical techniques usually enable the patient to normally move their jaw again as soon as the operation is finished, and after the surgical site has had an opportunity to heal.

- ## Prosthetic Surgery

Seldom, in order to entirely eradicate the patient's Head and Neck Cancer, the Cancer Surgeon may also need to remove some of the facial bones such as the Cheekbone, or the Palate. Additionally, depending on the form of the Cancer and its location in the head and the severity of its invasiveness into surrounding areas, any impacted soft tissue, such as portions of the patient's lips or nose, may have to also be surgically taken out by the doctor. Depending on the extent of the surgical operation and its affect on functionality and outward appearance, the patient could be offered use of an artificial substitute called a ***Prosthetic*** (false part). The prosthetic is a specially designed soft plastic replacement for the part of the patient's face that had to be removed. The most commonly used Prosthesis is an ***Obturator*** – a denture with an extension that is used to replace the upper jaw.

Modern Prostheses can be designed to suit the needs of Head and Neck Cancer patients. Although, such replacement devices will not feel like normal, live tissue, they still can look very realistic and can work very well. But, most importantly, as with any sort of false or imitation "cover up"—such as cosmetic make-up, wigs, and even Plastic Surgery and padded bras—the main purpose of Prosthetics is to help the person feel "normal" and good about themselves, and to *be acceptable* in public (i.e., in the mind of the person so-affected). Basically, it's all about self-confidence and reclaiming that part of their lives that the patient's Cancer tried to take away from them. If the Head and Neck Cancer patient is likely to need a Prosthetic, the appropriate Medical Team physician will discuss this fully with the patient, and their family or Caregiver, prior to the surgical operation. As a part of this discussion, the doctor will point out the advantages and disadvantages, and any benefits or risks of Prosthetic devices so that there are no questions. If it is then decided that the patient will be using a Prosthesis, the patient will meet and talk to a Prosthetics Technician, who will custom-design and make the Prosthetic. When complete, the patient will learn how to attach and detach the device.

• Chemotherapy – Head and Neck Cancer Treatment

Normally, a person's cells will mature and die in a controlled way. Cancer cells, however, which are the result of mutations within the cells' internal structures, can continue developing, growing, and spreading in a person's body with a lack of controls. Chemotherapy works by stopping or slowing the growth of Cancer cells throughout the body, which, by nature, grow and divide quickly. But, the super-powerful Chemo drugs can also do injury to healthy cells that divide rapidly too, such as cells that line a person's mouth and intestines, or those that cause their hair to grow. Any destruction to healthy cells, including the ever-important White Blood Cells (the body's Immune System "enforcers"), may cause some uncomfortable, inconvenient, and distressing Side Effects. Often, any Chemo-induced Side Effects will get better or go away after the Chemotherapy is completed, but, some may have a longer-lasting impact on the patient and their life.

o Strategies for Treating with Chemotherapy

Chemotherapy has been used for the treatment of Head and Neck Cancers in a diversity of strategies, with each having their own terminology and main objectives. Specifically, per www.cancer.gov,

Chemotherapy is commonly used in the treatment scenarios below:

- **Induction Chemotherapy**

Induction Chemotherapy is a first-line treatment for Cancer in which the patient is administered doses of Chemotherapy ***prior to all other treatment(s).*** Extremely high doses of Chemo medications are often given in Induction Chemotherapy with the *goal of avoiding repeat cycles in the future by attempting to kill all Cancer presence during the first few rounds.* The hope of Induction Chemotherapy is that this intense form of treatment will put the patient's Cancer into remission. In some cases, even though the Induction Chemotherapy will eliminate much of the Cancer, follow-on tests could reveal that Cancer is still present, so additional treatment(s) will be required.

- **Adjuvant Chemotherapy**

Adjuvant Chemotherapy is conducted ***after Cancer Surgery***, to reduce the risk of Cancer returning, and to kill any cancerous cells (which the Surgery did not capture) that might have spread from the Primary Tumor to other locations in the body. Adjuvant Chemo has been used following both Cancer Surgery and Radiation Therapy as *a therapy for patients felt to be at higher risk for Cancer recurrence.* Adjuvant Chemotherapy has also been used as Palliative Therapy in patients with advanced *unresectable* or *metastatic disease.* A tumor could be unresectable (inoperable) because of the size or the location of the tumor; the spread of the cancerous cells to distant areas of the body (metastasis); or, other health issues concerning the patient that could raise any risks with Cancer Surgery. In these cases, Adjuvant Chemotherapy may be employed in a best effort to kill or control the cancerous tumor, and any "rogue" Cancer cells within the body.

- **Neoadjuvant Chemotherapy**

Neoadjuvant Chemotherapy is delivered ***prior to the Cancer Surgery*** procedure, and *its ultimate objective is to attempt to shrink the Cancer Tumor so that the surgical procedure may not need to be as extensive or invasive.* Neoadjuvant Chemo can also be employed prior to Radiation Therapy where organ conservation is the goal, and it has been utilized concurrently with Radiation Therapy in locally advanced tumors (early Stage) where it has been verified to control and minimize the risk of distant Cancer recurrence. The physicians on my Medical Team and I determined that Neoadjuvant Chemo would probably be the most effective in treating my Cancer, so I had both Chemotherapy and Radiation Therapy first, with Surgery after, to excise what was left of my Primary Tumor and any margins.

o Methods for Administering Chemotherapy

Chemotherapy for many Head and Neck Cancer patients can be administered via numerous safe and successful means. Because the powerful and scientifically designed and formulated medications saturate tissues within the body and circulate throughout the body, they can effectively expel cancerous cells that have spread distantly from the Primary Tumor to other organs and bodily systems.

Following are the common methods for administering Chemo drugs to Head and Neck Cancer patients, as adapted from www.cancer.gov:

- **Intravenous (IV)** - Chemotherapy goes directly into a vein
- **Injection** - Chemotherapy that is given by a shot in a muscle in an arm, thigh, or hip, or just under the skin in the fatty part of an arm, leg, or belly
- **Intra-Arterial (IA)** - Chemotherapy that enters straight into the artery that is feeding the Cancer
- **Intraperitoneal (IP)** - Chemotherapy that transports directly into the Peritoneal Cavity—the area of the body that contains the Intestines, Stomach, Liver, and Ovaries
- **Topically** - Chemotherapy in a cream that can be put onto the skin, and which is absorbed into the body thru the skin
- **Orally** - Chemotherapy ingested in pills, capsules, or liquids

o Intravenous (IV) Chemotherapy – The Method Often Used for Head and Neck Cancers

Intravenous (IV) Chemotherapy is usually given to Head and Neck Cancer patients via a thin needle placed in a vein on the hand or the lower arm, or, in the chest, using a Mediport. The nurse will put the needle in at the beginning of each treatment and will remove it when treatment is finished. Patients should tell staff immediately if they feel pain or burning while they are getting IV Chemotherapy.

Head and Neck Cancer patients receive IV Chemo via Catheters or Ports, and often with a Pump. The following is per www.cancer.gov:

- **Catheters:** A Catheter is a soft, thin tube. A Surgeon places one end of the Catheter in a large vein, usually in the patient's chest area. The other end of the Catheter stays outside the body, and may be connected to a Port. Most Catheters stay in place until all the Chemotherapy treatments are done. Catheters can also be used to administer drugs other than Chemo, and to draw blood. Patients must watch for signs of infection around the Catheter

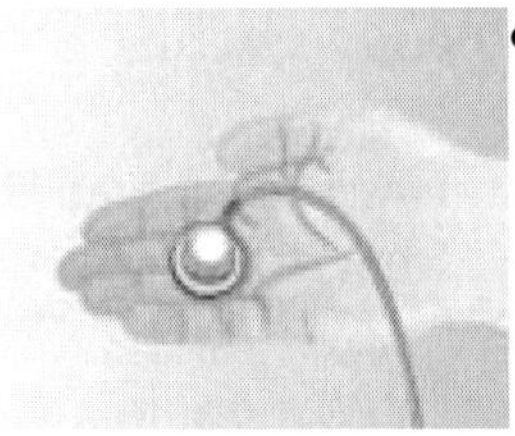

- **Ports:** A Port (often called a *Mediport)* is a small, round disc made of plastic or metal that is surgically placed under the skin. A Catheter connects the Port to a large vein in the chest. The nurse inserts a needle into the Port to deliver Chemo and other medications, or to draw blood. The Mediport is usually left in place for Chemotherapy treatments and for several months after. Patients must watch for signs of infection around the Port

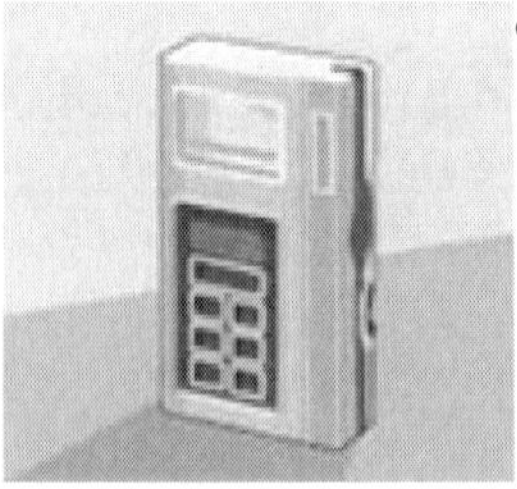

- **Pumps:** Pumps are normally attached to Catheters, or Ports. The electric pumps control how much, and how quickly, the dosage of Chemo drugs enters the body. Pumps can be either inside or outside of the body. Internal Pumps are positioned beneath the skin by a Surgeon. External Pumps remain outside the patient's body and can be mounted on a stand in the Cancer clinic, or, can be carried by the patient

o Frequency of Chemotherapy Administration

Chemo is given to Head and Neck Cancer patients in cycles, alternating between sessions of treatment and the very important rest that patients need to recover from their last Chemotherapy session. In the case of my Cancer treatments, the Oncologist on my Medical Team felt that I could probably withstand larger doses of the Chemo drugs because of my overall strong health status. So, they slammed me with a *giganta*-dose of my *"Chemo Cocktail"* (a combination of two Chemotherapy drugs) on a weekly basis. In between those one-week sessions, I honestly did take every moment I could to rest and recover so that I would have the strength to endure my next round of Chemo. Thankfully, the timing of my Chemotherapy sessions and the prescribed dosages worked extremely well in combination with the Radiation Therapy that I concurrently received…when it came to killing my Cancer. But, I will say that these two therapies, coupled together, definitely kicked my ass in the *Side Effects* department.

Courses of Chemotherapy can last several weeks, or longer, depending upon the patient's form of Cancer, the patient's treatment plan, the health status of the patient, and other factors considered by the Medical Team. While Chemotherapy medications and *"Chemo Cocktails"* (mixtures of two or more Chemo drugs) are developed to kill certain forms of Cancer, some Cancers will respond to particular medications, and some will not. Realizing this, the patient's Medical Team may need to adjust the patient's treatment plan over time in an endeavor to capitalize on the effectiveness of the medications for the particular type of Cancer. As stated previously, Chemo medications have been created to disrupt the cellular division and growth cycles of Cancers. As such, varying delivery strategies in terms of dosages and frequencies of the drugs are used in an attempt to interrupt these processes. In any event, the patient's individualized Chemo plan may call for one of the following protocols (which will be evaluated and possibly tweaked by the Oncologist as circumstances dictate):

- A low daily dose
- A moderately low weekly dose
- A relatively higher dose every three to four weeks

o Common Head and Neck Cancer Chemo Drugs

Per www.cancer.gov, there are more than 300 types of Chemo medications, and all of them have been investigated and tested with their safety and success with treating most Head and Neck Cancers. The Chemotherapy medications found, as of this writing in 2013, to be the most effective in destroying Head and Neck Cancers, include:

- Cisplatinum®
- Carboplatinum®
- Taxanes
- 5-Fluorouracil®
- Methotrexate®
- Ifosphamide®

The Chemo medications listed above have been used on their own, or in combination (there's that *Chemo Cocktail* again) in a multitude of frequency and dosage protocols. Each of the above medications varies in their rate of response and toxicity (i.e., their Cancer-killing capabilities when used singularly, or in combination with others).

☛***Author's Note***: Product or brand names of drugs that appear in the previous listing are for informational intentions only. The U.S. Government, the National Cancer Institute, and the Author do not endorse any specific product or brand. If products or brands are not mentioned, it does not mean or imply that they are not satisfactory.

- ### Common Head and Neck Cancer Chemo Drugs Used Concurrently with Radiation Therapy

According to the National Cancer Institute (www.cancer.gov), (and I can personally attest to the accuracy of these findings) recent Studies indicate that *Chemotherapy given to Head and Neck Cancer patients at the* ***same time*** *as Radiation Therapy is* ***more successful*** *than if Chemo is administered before a course of Radiation Therapy, or, if either treatment protocol is* ***delivered individually.*** Therefore, the treatment plans for several Head and Neck Cancer patients (and especially those with advanced Stage Cancer (Stage III or IV) such as mine), could incorporate simultaneous Radiation Treatment along with the Chemotherapy. This synergistic therapy combo, along with Cancer Surgery (as applicable), gives the Cancer the *"1-2-3 Punch"* that I've mentioned several times within this Book, and, which has proven to be very effective in eradicating Head and Neck Cancers.

There are quite a few Chemo drugs that are most commonly employed in conjunction with Radiation Therapy for Head and Neck Cancers, as listed below in 2013. The Reader should know, though, that this is just a partial list of medications and that physicians on the patient's Medical Team may elect to administer other Chemotherapy agents in the patient's treatment plan, as circumstances dictate:

- Cisplatin® (Platinol®)
- Cetuximab® (Erbitux®)
- Fluorouracil® (5-FU®, Adrucil®)
- Carboplatin® (Paraplatin®)
- Paclitaxel® (Taxol®)

☛***Author's Note***: Product or brand names of drugs that appear in the previous listing are for informational intentions only. The U.S. Government, the National Cancer Institute, and the Author do not endorse any specific product or brand. If products or brands are not mentioned, it does not mean or imply that they are not satisfactory.

- **National Cancer Institute Chemotherapy Book**

Further information about Chemotherapy is available in the National Cancer Institute (www.cancer.gov) (NCI) booklet, ***Chemotherapy and You: Support for People with Cancer***. NCI publications and materials can be obtained by calling the Cancer Information Service (CIS) at 1-800-4-CANCER (1-800-422-6237), or through the NCI Publications Locator at www.cancer.gov/publications.

• Radiation Therapy – Head and Neck Cancer Treatment

Radiation Therapy, also called Radiotherapy, entails the use of high-energy X-rays, and is a standard treatment method for Head and Neck Cancers, in combination with Surgery and, occasionally, with Chemotherapy. Radiation Therapy is also used to kill localized solid tumors like Cancers of the Breast, Skin, Prostate, and Cervix. Radiation Therapy may also be used to treat Lymphoma (Cancer of the Lymphatic System), and Leukemia, which is a Cancer affecting

Bone Marrow and Blood. Radiation Therapy works by disrupting the capacity of cancerous cells to divide, develop, and spread in the body by destroying the DNA structures of the Cancer cells (which are the cells' sets of instructions). Radiation exposure is employed with the hope of eradicating the Cancer and "curing" the disease. While the most significant goal of Radiation Therapy, as expected, is to target the Cancer cells only, there is a possibility that healthy cells adjacent to the Cancer tumor could be caught up "in the line of fire," and could be affected by the Radiation exposure, thus causing damage to those healthy cells. That "collateral damage" could lead to somewhat uncomfortable Side Effects, depending upon the area being treated, as well as the dosages of Radiation being directed to the site. Most of the Side Effects will typically go away over time.

- **Strategies for Treating with Radiation Therapy and Surgery**

In general, if surgical removal of the Head and Neck Cancer Primary Tumor has been directed by the Medical Team, Radiation Therapy might be performed *afterward*, if necessary, in an effort to destroy any lingering, potentially cancerous tissue in the immediate vicinity. Sometimes, though, the cancerous cellular activity at the affected site may be rather widespread, or, it may not be feasible or safe to completely extricate the initial Cancer presence via surgical intervention. In such instances, Radiation Therapy is *administered first* in an attempt to shrink the Tumor, and, then, Cancer Surgery is performed following Radiation Therapy in an effort to remove any remaining cancerous tissue (including any marginal body tissue that may be suspect) from the site of the Cancer occurrence. This is the type of Radiation Therapy and Surgery scenario that was performed in my personal situation: I had Radiation and Chemotherapy first, then Surgery to evict any cancerous cells at the site of my Primary Tumor that were lagging behind. *Take that, you latent SOB cells!*

- **Methods for Administering Radiation Therapy**

Radiation Therapy can be directed to Head and Neck Cancer patients via two methods: *External* or *Internal*. Some patients have both, one after the other, but several patients who receive Radiation

Therapy for Head and Neck Cancer have External Radiation only. External Radiation Therapy is usually given during outpatient visits in a clinic or a Cancer Treatment Center. During External Radiation Therapy, a massive, specially-designed apparatus scientifically and accurately directs the high-power X-rays to the Cancer Tumor, and a sizeable margin of the normal tissue surrounding it. Following are the forms of Radiation Therapy, as adapted from www.cancer.gov:

▪ External Radiation Therapy

The large machines utilized for external Radiation Therapy function in slightly different ways. Some of the machines are better for treating Cancers near the skin surface, while others work better on Cancers that are positioned deeper within the bodily tissues. The most universal type of machine that's used for Radiation Therapy is a *Linear Accelerator.* Some of the radiation machines use a variety of radioactive substances as the source of the high-energy beams.

Following are the two types of External Radiation Therapy that the Medical Team may employ to treat Head and Neck Cancers:

- **External Beam Therapy (EBT)**

  EBT is a method for delivering a beam of high-energy X-rays to the exact location of the Primary Tumor. The beam is generated outside of the patient (usually by a Linear Accelerator machine) and is targeted directly toward the Tumor site. These X-rays can destroy the Cancer cells, and, careful treatment planning allows a significant amount of surrounding normal tissues to be spared. No radioactive sources are placed inside the patient's body

- **Intensity-Modulated Radiation Therapy (IMRT)**

  IMRT is an advanced modality of high-precision Radiotherapy that utilizes computer-controlled X-ray Accelerators to transport precise radiation doses to a malignant Tumor or to specific areas within the Tumor. The prescribed radiation dosage is calculated specifically for each Head and Neck Cancer patient to conform to the three-dimensional shape of their Tumor by modulating, or controlling, the intensity of the radiation beam to focus a higher radiation dose to the tumor while minimizing radiation exposure to healthy cells. The IMRT is a humongous piece of machinery, but has the dexterity and deft movements of a dainty ballerina.

Subsequent to my diagnosis but prior to commencing my Cancer treatments, I "discovered" the IMRT while conducting research to look for the most effective means of treating my form of Head and Neck Cancer. I found during my exploration that the IMRT, when utilized in conjunction with Cancer Surgery, and also with Chemotherapy (for treating advanced Cancer Stages III and IV, such as mine), yielded excellent results on actual patients having Base of Tongue Cancers. When I first consulted my Radiation Oncologist at the Northern Virginia hospital where I was to have my Radiation Therapy, I asked her if they had an IMRT machine that would be used to treat my Cancer. She answered, "*It sounds like you've been doing your homework...and yes, we will use the IMRT to treat your Cancer.*" That news made me ecstatic!

Ultimately, when my Radiation Therapy started, I recall lying on the Radiation table with my head and neck firmly clamped down beneath my mesh mask. Lying motionless, I had no choice but to listen to, and watch, the huge, revolving arm of the equipment as it dutifully followed its human-calculated software commands and safely delivered the prescribed dosage of radiation precisely to its anticipated target: the Tumor on the Base of my Tongue. I recalled thinking to myself, *"All that power, all that size, and all that detailed planning simply to kill cancerous cells that are so miniscule in size, yet so VERY big in the problems they cause."*

- **Internal Radiation Therapy**

When Internal Radiation Therapy is employed, the radiation source is actually placed inside the body. This protocol of radiation treatment is called *Brachytherapy,* or *Implant Therapy.* The source of the radiation (such as Radioactive Iodine, for example), which is sealed in a small holder, is called an Implant. Implants may be thin wires, plastic tubes (catheters), capsules, or "seeds." The Implant could be surgically placed straight into the Tumor, itself, or inserted into a body cavity contiguous to the Tumor site. Sometimes, after a Tumor has been removed by Surgery, the Implant is placed in the "Tumor bed" (the place from which the tumor was removed) to kill any tumor cells that may remain. Another type of Internal Radiation Therapy uses unsealed radioactive materials which may be taken by mouth or injected into the body. If the Cancer patient has this type of treatment, they may need to stay in the hospital for several days.

- ### Radiation Therapy Treatment Preparations

If the Medical Team, patient, family or Caregiver determine that External Radiation Therapy may be employed for treatment of the patient's Head and Neck Cancer, a new set of actions will be set into motion. To begin, the patient, and their family or Caregiver, as applicable, will have a one- to two-hour meeting with the Radiation Oncologist(s) on their Cancer Treatment Medical Team. The initial visit with the Radiation Oncologist is for a consultation, whereby the Radiation Oncologist and patient, their loved one, family member or Caregiver, will meet each other, and begin to talk about the patient's medical history, the details surrounding the patient's Head and Neck Cancer, and the type of Radiation Therapy that may be employed in the patient's specific case, along with its benefits and potential risks.

Additionally the Oncologist will point out to the patient and their family or Caregiver, any potential Side Effects from Radiation Therapy, including strategies for minimizing or removing them, as well as any other factors that should be considered in designing the patient's customized Radiation Therapy plan. Soon after the initial meeting with the Radiation Oncologist, the patient will be scheduled for, and submit to, a physical exam, and will also be tasked to attend imaging tests, which are crucial in planning the patient's care. The Radiation Oncologist will also consult with other physicians on the Head and Neck Cancer Medical Team, such as the Surgeon, Chemo Oncologist, Pathologist, and Dentist. It is very important to have the input of various members of the team who will be taking care of the patient before a treatment plan is decided and treatment begins.

After the recommended Radiation Therapy Treatment Plan and prospective choices are made clear to the patient by the Medical

Team, and, after the patient and their loved one, family or Caregiver decide on a course of treatment in conjunction with doctors on their Medical Team, a date will be set to meet again and begin the actual planning of the patient's custom Radiation Therapy Treatment Plan.

- **Designing the External Radiation Therapy Treatment Plan, and "Simulation" Session**

After the Medical Team physicians and the Head and Neck Cancer patient, and loved one, family, or Caregiver have decided on the form of External Radiation Therapy that the patient will receive, the patient will be scheduled for a treatment planning session called a *Simulation.* The Simulation process typically involves the patient submitting to conventional X-rays or a Computed Tomography (CT) scan. During the Simulation, the patient will be asked to lie very still so that the X-ray or CT images will be extremely high quality. The Radiation Oncologist and Radiation Physicist (or Therapist) will use the imaging data to define the patient's Treatment Area (also called a *Treatment Port* or *Treatment Field*) for planning purposes.

The results of the Radiographic Studies will subsequently be used by the Radiation Oncologist and Radiation Physicist to plan the type and direction of the Radiation Beams that will be used to target the patient's Cancer. The Radiation Therapy planning process is very scientific and extremely technologically sophisticated in nature. This is to be expected, because the protocol is employed to calculate and develop a completely personalized approach for addressing each patient's specific form of Head and Neck Cancer. If the Physicist's calculations are off at all, the consequences could be very damaging.

Following the completion of the patient's Radiation Therapy Treatment Plan, the Simulation Data will be loaded—in the form of software—into the Radiation Therapy machine, which could be the Intensity Modulated Radiotherapy, or IMRT machine. This was the type of machine that we utilized for treatment of my Head and Neck Cancer. Within the radiation treatment equipment, customized lead alloy blocks or a special Collimator device (a Multileaf Collimator) will shape the radiation beams to conform to the profile of the Head and Neck Cancer patient's Tumor, and will protect the healthy tissue that does not need to be treated. This sparing feature minimizes any potential damage to the healthy body tissue in the area of the Tumor.

- ## Additional Radiation Therapy Preparations

Concurrent with the development of the Radiation Therapy Plan, there are some further steps that will possibly need to be taken prior to the course of Radiation Therapy beginning. These activities will depend upon the patient's form of Head and Neck Cancer, and, its location in the head or neck. Such preparations may include:

- ### Inking of Tattoo Marks on the Patient's Skin

During a Head and Neck Cancer patient's planning phase in advance of their Radiation Therapy sessions, the Radiation Therapist will "ink" the patient with the equivalent of a *GPS coordinate.* That is, small, tattoo *dots* will be "inked" onto the patient's skin, usually on the chest area, which is where mine are situated. The purpose of these indelible dots is to provide the Radiation Therapy staff with a visible reference point that they can utilize each session to properly align the big Radiation Therapy machine. This, they do by centering a beam of light directly over the tattoo to ensure that the patient is in the exact same position on the table prior to each treatment session.

This tattoo process eliminates all guesswork with the process and makes sure that the strong beam of radiation is aimed precisely at the patient's Tumor each and every time, just as calculated by the Radiation Oncologist and the Radiation Physicist. The tattoos are about the size of a freckle and will remain on the patient's skin for the rest of their life. It's been almost nine years since I first received my Radiation Therapy tattoos and I can still see them in the mirror if I look extremely close. If "tattoos" make one "cool" as some people believe, then, these little *tat-dots* probably must make me *cool-ish.*

- ### Creation of a Head and Neck Mask

If the patient will be receiving radiation to the head, and/or, neck, there is a high likelihood that they will need to have a *"mask"* made. The mask is manufactured of *Aquaplast*, a mesh-like material that typically has a hole made for the patient’s mouth, and is formed with extra material that clamps to the table on which the patient will lay to receive their treatment. The mask is developed by placing the warm, soft, Aquaplast over the patient’s face, neck, and chest while they are lying perfectly immobile on the Radiotherapy table. While soft, the mesh is molded by Radiation Therapy staff to conform with the specific contours of the patient’s head, neck, and shoulders. An opening is made just outside the mouth, which will allow the patient to speak, and to suck on a tasteless, plastic “sucker” that is designed to stimulate saliva production. This helps to avoid mouth dryness.

After a few minutes, the mesh material will cool and harden into a mask that closely resembles the look of the sinister, protective headgear adorned by some Hockey Goalies. The mesh mask, when clamped to the table, helps hold down the patient’s head in the exact same location for each treatment. This consistent head placement is necessary, because it maximizes the effectiveness of the treatments, and helps to minimize any likely risk to the patient’s safety. When I originally started using the mask during my treatment sessions, to be perfectly honest, it did freak me out. There’s something really scary about having your entire head being immobilized and clamped down to *anything*, much less beneath a huge piece of revolving machinery. Nonetheless, I got used to it and found it to be slightly comfortable, even if those un-scratchable nose itches drove me crazy at times!

- ### Frequency of Radiation Therapy Administration

Typically, following completion of preparations for the Head and Neck Cancer patient’s Radiation Therapy Plan, the treatment sessions will start one to two days after. Usually, Radiation Therapy treatments are delivered once or twice a day, five days a week (i.e., business days – not weekends or observed national holidays) for five to seven weeks. The frequency, duration, and dosage of each of the treatment sessions will all be dependent upon the schedule and plan developed by the Radiation Oncologist. Generally speaking, for the first two to three days of Radiation Therapy treatment, the patient’s visits may take an hour or two to complete. This is simply because the patient may need some additional time to become familiar with the “daily drill” as the Radiation Therapy team explains the process and answers any questions the patient may have. Additionally, extra time may be needed by the staff to ensure that the radiation machine, the mask, and everything are working as designed, and as intended.

After the initial two to three sessions, each treatment should take 30 minutes or so, and the Head and Neck Cancer patient should be in and out of their session within 45 to 60 minutes, assuming that there are no holdups. Patients will then return daily, on-schedule, to complete the course of therapy. Patients will not feel or see anything bad during Radiation Therapy, and the ***treatment, itself, is painless.*** Any Side Effects resulting from the therapy usually take two to three weeks to become apparent. During the radiation course, patients are monitored by the Radiation Oncologist and Radiation Staff, and any adjustments are made as necessary. Patients should get plenty of rest and eat a well-balanced diet during the course of Radiation Therapy. Following the final treatment, the Radiation Oncologist will review any important instructions with the patient, and they will be given a follow-up appointment to check on the patient's status. Prior to the follow up visit, the Head and Neck Cancer patient might be asked to obtain a CT scan or MRI, so that the final results can be discussed.

- ### **National Cancer Institute Radiotherapy Book**

More information about Radiation Therapy is available in the NCI booklet ***Radiation Therapy and You: A Guide to Self-Help During Treatment.*** National Cancer Institute (www.cancer.gov) publications and materials can be obtained by phoning the Cancer Information Service (CIS) at 1-800-4-CANCER (1-800-422-6237), or through the NCI Publications Locator at www.cancer.gov/publications.

A Final, Brief Word About Radiation Therapy for Head and Neck Cancer Patients

If, as part of their treatment plan, the Head and Neck Cancer patient will be receiving Radiation Therapy near the Salivary glands, they may want to ask their Oncologist about the possibility of them utilizing the medication, Amifostine®. This drug, which is injected sub-cutaneously before Radiation Therapy sessions, has been proven to help protect the Glands from X-ray damage. I requested that I be approved for its use, which I was, and, thankfully, it worked great!

"When a person hears their doctor utter the words, 'I'm sorry but you have Cancer,' there will be an immediate mishmash of shock, fear, and disbelief coursing throughout the patient's mind, to which will also be added, uncertainty, resentment, and the warranted, unanswerable questions, 'How?,' 'Why me?,' and, 'Will I die?' These feelings and uncertainties are normal and inevitable, but, over time, they should disappear – hopefully, not unlike the patient's Cancer."

- Butch Sickler

Chapter Thirteen

Head and Neck Cancers – *The Treatment-Related Side Effects*

"While you're climbing out of the hole that was caused by your Cancer, be wary of those being dug by Doubt and Despair."

- Butch Sickler

As any reasonable person could sensibly assume, whenever one medically messes with the mouth, nose, tongue, esophagus, lips, throat, nasal cavities, or, any of the tissues in and around these very sensitive and fragile areas of the human body—and especially in the throes of Cancer Treatments—there will, in all probability, be some repercussions, and, most likely, they will not be good – at least for a certain period of time. So...*Drum Roll please*...welcome to the wild and less-than-wonderful world of *Head and Neck Cancer Treatment Side Effects*. This is the part where the patient *pays their dues.*

The Head and Neck: Full of Nooks & Crannies

Due to the elaborate nature of the anatomy in a person's head and neck areas, coupled with the forms of Cancer that can crop up in the numerous "nooks and crannies" in those respective locations, the challenges in successfully treating Head and Neck Cancers are very apparent, and the potentially *unconstructive* Side Effects from those treatments are an incessant reality. But, rest-assured, these Head and Neck Cancers, especially if detected and diagnosed early-on in their progression, are very treatable, and, many of the accompanying Side Effects can be minimized to the extent possible, if not eliminated.

It stands to reason that each form of Head and Neck Cancer is unique—as is the person that it "chooses" to serve as its host—so each manner of treating a patient's Head and Neck Cancer will also vary to some degree, depending on the patient's age and health state, their form of Cancer, its Stage and location(s) in the head and neck areas, and additional factors that physicians on the patient's Medical Team might consider. Then, after all of the evaluating, planning, and discussions are completed and the form(s) of Cancer treatment have been decided upon, the treatments will commence…and, yes, I hate to say it, but, most likely, so too will the accompanying Side Effects.

What are the Head and Neck Cancer Treatment-Related Side Effects?

The Side Effects that stem from the Cancer treatment(s) will, as anticipated, differ from one Head and Neck Cancer patient to the next, depending upon the mode of treatment(s) used, (i.e., common, conventional Radiation Therapy, Chemotherapy, and/or, Surgery), as well as on the durations, doses, and frequencies of the Radiation Therapy, and/or, Chemotherapy. All of this will feed into the extent and degree of severity of Side Effects realized by each patient. But, because all Head and Neck Cancer patients are different from each other, so too will their respective outcomes to the treatments differ, as will their body's responses to any treatment-related Side Effects. Additionally, there will be clear contrasts between each individual's responses to any efforts by the Medical Team and patient to mitigate their Side Effects. In other words, what affects one patient—either in a good or a bad way—may not affect another patient in the exact same manner. I guess that's why we're all called *individuals.*

The realistic bottom line is that there is no *"One size fits all"* treatment approach for all Head and Neck Cancer patients. Nor is there a "blanket" or a typical response on the part of Head and Neck Cancer patients to either the treatments performed, or, to the actions taken to help relieve or remove any resulting Side Effects. With this said, however, *it is safe to say* that the needs of each patient are very personalized, and that the patient's Medical Team will take all facts of the situation into account when working with the patient and their loved one, family or Caregiver, to develop the safest and most viable strategy for properly addressing each patient's Side Effects.

Cancer Treatment Side Effects – "The Price is Right"

In the interest of full disclosure, it must be stated that while the Medical Team will center its efforts on reducing or eliminating any negative treatment-related Side Effects realized by the Head and Neck Cancer patient, most treatments will result in some version of adverse physical, mental, or emotional impacts on the patient. These Side Effects might be minimal or severe, and they may be temporary or last forever, but, they all are part-and-parcel of the larger Cancer therapy attempt that's aimed at saving the patient's life. Essentially, they are what they are, and despite how much some Head and Neck Cancer treatment Side Effects could cause the patient some level of distress, inconvenience, hurt, or uneasiness, they are, in my personal opinion, at least a million times better than the alternative! This is one very good example of where ***strife can benefit one's life.***

Head and Neck Cancer Treatment Possible Side Effects – One-by-One

In most cases of Head and Neck Cancer, the most common, conventional treatments used to safely remove Cancers will include Surgery, Radiation Therapy, Chemotherapy, or two or more of these forms employed simultaneously, or sequentially, one after the other. As such, the realization of nasty Side Effects from one or all of these treatment modalities is a very real possibility, and one for which the patient, and loved one, family, and Caregiver should be prepared.

Unfortunately, it's true: Cancer Surgery, Radiation Therapy, and Chemotherapy can all induce much more than their fair share of uncomfortable and distressing problems. Honestly, the Side Effects that can be caused by each individual type of Head and Neck Cancer treatment are awful enough when experienced *alone.* But, combine two or three of the therapies at the same time, or, one after the other, and, it only stands to reason that any associated Side Effects will be compounded and intensified. As I've said before in this Book, *"No good deed goes unpunished,"* and so it goes with Cancer therapy.

☛ ***Authors Note:*** General and more detailed information about potential Side Effects that might be associated with the conventional five Cancer treatments—including for Head and Neck Cancers—is found in Chapter 7 of this Book, *The Cancer Treatment Side Effects,* under the heading, *Step 9 of the Cancer Journey,* and also in Chapter 11. And, as expected, a plethora of information regarding potential Side Effects of all conventional and alternative Cancer treatments is available in a multitude of resources regarding Cancer, including the National Cancer Institute online at www.cancer.gov, and, in hand-out materials provided to the patient by applicable members of their Medical Team. Following one's receipt of a Head and Neck Cancer diagnosis, it might be very beneficial for the patient, and their family or Caregiver, to research treatment selections for their form of Head and Neck Cancer, and to learn what they can about the treatments' success rates, possible Side Effects, and other pertinent information.

In all Cancer cases, however, the patient, and their family or Caregiver, will consult with applicable Medical Team members to determine—based on the patient's form of Head and Neck Cancer, its Stage and location, and the patient's general state of health—the most appropriate treatment(s) to be utilized to safely and (hopefully) completely eliminate the patient's Cancer. These individuals should discuss each type of treatment, the risks, benefits, and potential Side Effects, and how each form of Cancer therapy might temporarily or permanently alter the way the patient looks, talks, eats, or breathes.

During the actual Treatment Phase, and while the Head and Neck Cancer patient is recovering from their treatment(s), the patient, their loved one, family members, Caregiver, or Guardian, must inform members of the Medical Team when any distressing, painful, or uncomfortable Side Effects occur. This is so that the patient's health and comfort can be safely treated and monitored.

Adapted from the U.S. National Cancer Institute online resources at www.cancer.gov, my journaling notes, and materials provided to me by my Medical Team, following are descriptions of the prospective Side Effects that may come to pass either during, or after, the patient receives one or more of the three most widespread and conventional modalities for the treatment of Head and Neck Cancers:

- ## Surgery Side Effects - Head and Neck Cancer

Surgeries to remove Head and Neck Cancers will often cause Side Effects that impact the patient in a negative way. For example, contingent upon the patient's form of Cancer and its location and severity, and, depending on the invasiveness of the Cancer Surgery, the patient's ability to chew, swallow, speak, breathe, and perform other normal, *everyday* bodily functions may be slightly or severely affected. This can be true immediately during and after treatments, or, this may be the situation throughout the patient's life, long after their treatment(s) have concluded. Additionally, as with surgeries to any aspect of the body, surgeries to remove Cancers of the Head and Neck always run the risk of infection. However, much due diligence is performed by the Surgical Team to prevent this from occurring.

  - ### Pain, Swelling, and Discoloration at Surgical Site

For reasonable reasons, the larger the Primary Tumor and the greater is the area of marginal tissue (the potentially cancerous areas surrounding the Tumor) that has to be surgically removed, the more damage that could be done to the healthy, adjacent tissue. The same holds true for any surgeries to the head and neck area that are overly invasive. As an outcome of Head and Neck Cancer surgeries that are extreme in breadth and depth, the patient may appear different after surgery. Specifically, their face and neck may be swollen, painful to the touch, and colored pink to purple-ish, which is a typical reaction when there is trauma to, or laceration of, a specific area of the body.

Think about the last time you cut yourself with a knife, got a bad splinter, or maybe had a paper cut. It did not feel good after the act, and the impacted area of your body demonstrated its displeasure by hurting, swelling up, and turning any one of several shades, from *hot pink* to *aubergine.* Thankfully, in most cases, the discoloration, hurting, and swelling normally receded within a few days or weeks - again, depending upon how negatively the tissue was disrupted. The success of this healing process, however, assumes that the Head and Neck Cancer patient's Immune System is functioning properly and is able to battle off any potential infections. This also presumes that no other issues or complications come into play while the patient is recovering after the conclusion of their surgical procedure(s).

o Alterations in External Appearance

Early-Staged, localized Head and Neck Cancers can often be removed with less invasive surgical procedures. In these situations, the patient may be administered Local or General Anesthesia or they may be treated with Laser Surgery. In such cases, there, most likely, will be no need for an overnight hospital stay. However, in extreme instances of Head and Neck Cancer (that is, Cancers that are found in precarious locations, or, Cancers that are more deeply entrenched in the patient's head or neck areas), the Cancer Surgeon may have to perform what is referred to as a *Radical Dissection* to take away the Cancer and a considerable section of jaw tissue, and/or, neck muscle tissue with it, just to be certain that *all* potentially cancerous tissue is excised. This, certainly, is not preferred, but it may be necessary.

In more extreme cases of Head and Neck Cancer, the patient may stand a very realistic possibility of having the outward physical appearance of a part of their head or their neck altered for the rest of their lives. However, as I stated beforehand in this Chapter, Cancer Surgeons, in arrangements with other health care professionals, will do everything possible (within specified limitations) to diminish any drastic modifications to one's external appearance. And, in atypical and invasive surgical cases, Cancer Surgeons, or others, may be able to perform *Reconstructive Surgery* on the patient, and, as necessary, will design, develop, and fit Prosthesis to the patient in an effort to help them look as "normal" as possible following their Surgery.

During my Cancer pre-treatment preparations, my Surgeon told me that he would like to initially perform the Radical Dissection procedure on me to extract all cancerous tissue. But, thankfully (in retrospect), at that time, my Oncologist discussed this with my ENT Surgeon and convinced him to reverse his position on this approach. When my own Head and Neck Cancer treatment plan was ultimately developed and carried out, it called for *Neoadjuvant* Chemotherapy (delivered prior to Surgery), and Radiation Therapy, both of *which being followed by Surgery* to *clean up* any remaining cancerous cells from my Primary Tumor on the Base of my Tongue, as well as any potentially cancerous marginal tissue close to the Tumor. With that being said, the numerous Surgeries that I underwent (Biopsy tissue samples, Surgery to have Lymph Nodes removed, and Cancer tumor excision) all left me with temporary Side Effects, both inside and out. But, I've had no enduring negative affects to my head and neck functions and no permanent alterations to my outward appearance.

o Neck Lymph Node Removal – Possible Issues

In some instances, such as was the case during my own Head and Neck Cancer ordeal, if Biopsy tissue sample tests indicate that the Cancer has metastasized in Lymph Nodes in the patient's neck, Surgery will be utilized to remove the affected cancerous Nodes and any potentially cancerous marginal tissue in that vicinity. However, when this occurs, Lymphatic Fluid (also referred to as Serous Fluid) may accumulate in the tissues in the area after the Surgery, and may induce swelling and pain that could last for a considerable length of time. This, unfortunately, did happen to me, but, in retrospect, it did not have to be. Doctors, including Cancer Surgeons, do mess up.

When my Cancer Surgeon cut out the two cancerous Lymph Nodes and marginal tissues from my neck, he did not think to put a drain tube in the area. Such a device would have allowed the Serous Fluid to flow away from the surgical site, thus preventing any fluid build-up under the skin. But, because the physician failed to do that, I was forced to contend with a huge, ***very painful***, goiter-like growth on my upper neck for several days. *That was sure super attractive!*

The physician ultimately realized and mentioned his obvious oversight (*screw up?*) when I attended the subsequent appointment with him to have him take out the sutures from the surgical area. By then, though, it was much too late. My upper neck was already very swollen, shiny, tight, and had turned crimson red. And, believe me, it looked just as painful as it, in reality, was. If Lymph Nodes in the neck are taken out, hopefully the Surgeon will have the forethought to install a system of "wicking" fluid to prevent its painful collection under the skin. If he or she does not offer to place such a device, the Head and Neck Cancer patient should ask them to and insist upon it.

In any event, following the surgical removal of any Lymph Nodes, the shoulder and neck areas may become swollen, weak, and stiff, but these Surgery Side Effects should vanish over time, as did mine.

- ## Chemotherapy Side Effects – Head and Neck Cancer

Chemotherapy, as I've stated previously, is the use of potent, specially designed and administered medications to demolish Cancer cells within the patient's body. In general, anti-cancer Chemo drugs affect quickly growing cells, including the abnormal cancerous cells (which is good), and also normal cells (which isn't very good) of the Digestive Tract, Hair Follicles, Mouth, and Bone Marrow (which makes Red and White Blood Cells that help to fight infections). The Side Effects of Chemotherapy can depend upon the particular drugs that are given, as well as on their dosages and on their frequencies.

Generally speaking, Head and Neck Cancer patients who are receiving Chemotherapy could have Side Effects which will include: lower resistance to infection; painful sores in the mouth; Mucositis – inflammation of the membranes of the mouth and tongue; emotional distress; nausea; vomiting; loss of appetite; hair loss; pain; diarrhea; Anemia (a condition in which there aren't satisfactory healthy Red Blood Cells to carry sufficient oxygen to body tissues); and, changes in taste and hearing. Additionally, Chemotherapy may cause Cancer patients to feel abnormally fatigued, and, they might experience skin rash and itching, joint pain, loss of balance, and leg or foot swelling.

As has been mentioned before, Chemo Side Effects might be more extreme when the Chemotherapy is combined with Radiation Therapy, as was the case with my concurrent treatments. The good news—aside from the Chemo, hopefully, killing all of the Cancer in the patient's body—is that most Side Effects of Chemotherapy will, typically, be temporary in nature. As such, many of the Side Effects will eventually disappear after the treatments have concluded. Some Chemotherapy Side Effects, however, can manifest themselves for longer periods of time, and a few, I'm sorry to say, may continue for the rest of a survivor's life. My unhappy eyebrows sacrificed many hairs to the cause and have never regrown, but, that's how it goes.

Listed below are the potential Side Effects of Chemotherapy which Head and Neck Cancer patients might experience during and after their Chemotherapy. The following descriptions of Side Effects are from the National Cancer Institute (www.cancer.gov) resources, my journaling notes, and in materials given to me by my Medical Team.

- ## Neutropenia – Low White Blood Count (Reduced Resistance to Infection)

During the process of destroying quickly-multiplying Cancer cells, Chemotherapy can also reduce the quantity of rapidly-dividing *White Blood Cells.* White Blood Cells, which are produced in an individual's Bone Marrow, are critical to a person's health and well-being, as they help to recognize and fight-off infections. If a Cancer patient's number of White Blood Cells becomes too low due to their Chemo treatments, they have reduced resistance to infection, which is known as *Neutropenia.* Typically, this phenomenon begins about seven-ish days after each Chemotherapy treatment, and the patient's resistance to infection is usually at its lowest about 10 - 14 days after each Chemo session. Ideally, the number of White Blood Cells will increase steadily after that two-week period and will typically return to normal before the next cycle of Chemotherapy is due to begin.

Sometimes, however, due to Chemo-prompted Neutropenia, the White Blood Cell count *does not return to normal levels.* Should this occur, the Neutropenia can lead to possible health-related issues, and can cause Cancer treatment-related problems. Obviously, if the patient's White Blood Cell count drops to a perilously low level, the patient, the Caregiver, and the Medical Team will be very concerned about the susceptibility of the patient to any form of infection, which could put the patient's health at risk. Secondarily, low White Blood Cell counts might place continuation of the patient's Chemotherapy treatments in jeopardy, if only temporarily. In other words, there is a possibility that the patient's treating Oncologist would halt Chemo treatments until the White Blood Cell count returns to an acceptable level. This closely-monitored process could take some time.

To make sure that any potential infections are looked into as quickly as possible, and, to preclude the discontinuation of the Head and Neck Cancer patient's all-important Chemotherapy treatments, the patient should *speak to their treating Oncologist immediately if their body temperature exceeds 38°C (100.4°F), or, if they suddenly feel unwell, even if they have a normal temperature.* Head and Neck Cancer patients receiving Chemotherapy will commonly submit to a blood test before each successive Chemotherapy session in an effort to corroborate whether or not the patient's White Blood Cell count is above the required threshold. If the blood count meets or surpasses the tolerable and safe cut-off, the Oncologist will usually permit the Chemotherapy to continue. However, should the Cancer patient's White Blood Cell count fall below the prescribed level, the patient's Oncologist may postpone the patient's scheduled course of Chemo treatments until the established threshold is restored.

Thankfully, as one might come to imagine, medications exist for the purpose of stimulating the patient's Bone Marrow to produce additional White Blood Cells. Such medications can be prescribed by a physician if the patient's natural regeneration of blood cells is progressing slowly, and/or, if this obstacle is preventing the patient's regular Chemo regimen from moving forward on-schedule. During the administration of my own, quite intense Chemotherapy sessions, my White Blood Cell count did, occasionally, drop below acceptable and safe levels. When this occurred, my Oncologist would prescribe a drug to help my body "grow" more White Blood Cells. I was then provided with the medication, syringes, and other materials, and was instructed by the Oncology Nurses on the proper protocols for self-injecting the medication into my body. Subsequently, as applicable, each Monday and Tuesday before my Chemotherapy treatments—which typically were on Fridays, every week throughout my course of Chemo—I would inject the prescribed dosage of the medication into myself. Gratefully, the medication worked perfectly at restoring my White Blood Cell count, which enabled me to continue with my critical Chemotherapy treatments without interruption.

- ### Low Platelet Count – Lowered Ability of Blood to Clot (Increased Bleeding and Bruising)

Just as Chemotherapy can diminish the normal production of White Blood Cells in the Head and Neck Cancer patient, so, too, can

Chemo wreak havoc on the making of *Platelets*, which are the blood cells that help the blood to clot. Without the ability of the blood to clot, one can only imagine the risks involved with the Cancer patient who accidentally cuts themselves or sustains some type of laceration to their skin. It, therefore, is crucial that the Head and Neck Cancer patient inform their Oncologist or Oncology Nurses if they have any unexplained bruising or bleeding, such as from nosebleeds, bleeding gums, blood spots or rashes on the skin. The treating physician can order a blood test to determine if the patient's Platelet count is under tolerable levels. If a low Platelet level is confirmed, the Oncologist may order a Platelet Transfusion to help bring the important Platelet count back to a safe, normal level so that treatments can continue.

- **Anemia – Low Red Blood Cell Count (Reduced Energy and Increased Breathlessness)**

Okay, you knew that this one had to be next. Chemotherapy, being the *equal opportunity destroyer* that it is, wouldn't even think of screwing with the Head and Neck Cancer patient's *White Blood Cells and Platelets* without also messing with their *Red Blood Cells.* It is the Red Blood Cells that transmit that life-sustaining essential—Oxygen—throughout the body via the Circulatory System. Just like the other types of blood cells, Chemotherapy can drastically reduce the quantity of Red Blood Cells in the Cancer patient's blood. When this condition—known as *Anemia*—occurs, the patient may be tired and feel breathless. In such cases, the patient or Caregiver must tell their Oncologist or Oncology Nurses about their symptoms, so that a blood test can be given to evaluate the blood count levels. If the Red Blood Cell count is below the acceptable threshold, the doctor could order the patient to have a blood transfusion to bring their blood cell count—and, thus their body functions—back up to a normal level.

- **Nausea, Vomiting, and Diarrhea**

Man-oh-man, can I speak to this one! During the process of eradicating rapidly-dividing cancerous cells with Chemotherapy, the fast-dividing normal cells lining the patient's digestive tract will also be caught in the cross-fire and will be detrimentally affected by the potent drugs. Irritation to the sensitive cellular lining of the digestive tract will manifest itself in the form of persistent nausea, which may bring along with it some serious and insistent bouts of vomiting and diarrhea. A Head and Neck Cancer patient who is undergoing these symptoms during their course of Chemotherapy must bring them to the attention of the Oncologist and Oncology Nurses. The physician can prescribe anti-sickness *(Anti-emetic)* drugs to hopefully prevent, or greatly reduce, nausea or vomiting. If the sickness isn't controlled or continues, the doctor must be informed so that they can prescribe other anti-sickness drugs that may be more effective.

Throughout my entire life, B.C. (before Cancer), I had never experienced Nausea, and I had only vomited once, as an 8- or 9-year old, after eating some apparently nasty Chinese food *(yes, I do keep track of such things).* And, as long as we're being graphic, I will say that from a diarrhea standpoint, even though it happens to run in my family *(sorry, that's a joke)*, I don't remember ever being affected by it in a huge way prior to my Cancer experience. With that being said, I wouldn't go so far as to claim that I had a "cast-iron" stomach or digestive system. But, because my eating choices during my adult life have consisted of healthy, bland-ish, non-spicy, non-greasy and non-irritating foods, I have never consumed anything that has *pissed off* my internal gastrointestinal quietude. And, that also goes for any beverages, in that I don't savor the taste of alcoholic drinks (with the exception of some wines sipped in small amounts about once a year, if that), and thus, have never gotten drunk, nor had to suffer through the possible pain, misery, and vomiting associated with hangovers.

That all changed, however, when my Chemotherapy sessions kicked off in July of 2004. My Caregiver was driving me home from one of my medical appointments when I had to ask that she speedily pull off the road. For the first time in over 40 years I had to vomit, and I cannot begin to explain how painful that was to my throat that was already so raw and inflamed. Unfortunately, however, that was just the first of many such episodes in following weeks that I would be left with no choice but to bear. And, it was not only the irritation of my digestive system that would cause the queasiness and initiate the gag reflex responsible for vomiting. No, there was also the smell and taste of some foods and drinks; the salty taste that permeated the flavor of anything that I put into my mouth; and, the sickening taste of the thickened phlegm and saliva that formed naturally as one part of the healing process in my throat and on my tongue (exacerbated by the Radiation Therapy that I received concurrently with Chemo). As for diarrhea, I also suffered with periodic bouts of that, which, of course, helped to undermine all of my attempts to gain and maintain my crucial bodyweight. Physicians on my Medical Team prescribed medications to help reduce the Side Effects of nausea, vomiting, and diarrhea that I was experiencing, but, honestly, none of them worked well for me. That's not to say that they would not make a difference for others. My nausea issues finally went away after several weeks.

- **Loss of Hair**

Just as Chemotherapy pisses off the healthy, rapidly-dividing cells of the Head and Neck Cancer Patient's digestive system, some Chemo drugs will also attack the brisk-dividing cells of the patient's hair follicles. This sudden loss of head hair on a person is, perhaps, one of the most well-known, visible indications that the individual is most-likely a Cancer patient, and, if this is correct, that the person is being given Chemotherapy. Such is not always the case, of course, because there are other health conditions that can incite loss of head hair. And, nowadays, there are men—including countless that have a *full* head of hair—who shave their tresses to the skull for whatever reason. In any event, not all Chemotherapy medications prompt hair loss, but, most of the potent Chemo drugs will cause either total loss, or thinning of the hair on men and women, either temporarily (hair grows back after 3 to 6 months), or, for an indefinite period of time.

Head and Neck Cancer patients who will be participating in a course of Chemo should ask their Oncologist if the drugs they will be receiving are prone to cause loss of hair in patients. Once again, while each Cancer patient will vary with respect to their own body's response to Chemotherapy, the physician may be able to provide the patient with a "best guess," which is based on other patient histories. If the patient is concerned about their appearance in the event that they do forego hair during their Chemotherapy, the patient, and their loved one, family, or Caregiver can pursue the possibility of wearing a wig, hat, bandana, or scarf. The Oncologist and Oncology Nurses can steer the patient in the right direction to obtain these cover-ups. During my Chemo, my Oncology Nurses told me that my medicines would *definitely* cause me to lose my hair. *Surprise! They didn't!*

○ **Painful Mouth, Mouth Ulcers, and Throat**

While the Side Effects of Nausea can *really* suck for a Head and Neck Cancer patient who is receiving Chemotherapy, something that can hurt even worse (if that's possible), is the unbelievable pain that can be felt on the tongue, and in the mouth and throat. Each of these extremely sensitive tissues is susceptible—as are the patient's digestive system and hair follicles—to the Chemotherapy medicines. That is because these locations are lined with very similar, quickly-dividing normal cells that, regrettably, are targeted by the Chemo as if they were dastardly Cancer cells. And, at least for a period of time during and after the Chemo sessions, the damage sustained by all of the impacted healthy cells can negatively, and uncomfortably, affect the Head and Neck Cancer patient in terms of the uneasiness caused. To make matters even worse (yes, it is possible), if the patient is also being administered a course of Radiation Therapy (especially in the mouth, tongue or throat areas), concurrently with the Chemotherapy, the combined affect of both on the patient can be quite devastating.

I certainly do not mention any of this to frighten or stress the Reader, but, as I've pointed out many times elsewhere in this Book, when Chemo and Radiation Therapy are used simultaneously, they not only provide a much-improved and scientifically proven Cancer-killing capability as an advantage, but, risk-wise, they can also cause amplified levels of related Side Effects. These include: Mouth Sores and Mouth Ulcers (known as *Mucositis*) on the gums, tongue, cheek linings, and lips, dryness of mouth tissues, inflammation of mucous membranes, and, of course, any pain and discomfort in the patient's mouth and throat that are associated with the Chemo- and Radiation Therapy-induced Side Effects. The *"itis"* on the end of *"Muco"* in *Mucositis* refers to "inflammation," which is exactly what the raised, red, and painful mouth sores and ulcers are. Remember the last time that you bit your tongue or the inside of your cheek? That probably stung a lot. Okay, now envision you having several of those types of 3-dimentional and super-sore "blisters" going on at one time in your mouth. Got it? Okay, now imagine trying to eat and drink with that.

Thankfully, all is not lost to Chemo and Radiation Therapy, as there are many products and medicines that the Head and Neck Cancer patient's Medical Team will prescribe, administer, and train the patient to use at home, all in an attempt to minimize or eliminate, completely, as many of these discomforting Side Effects as possible. Many of these medications come in the form of gels, creams, pastes, mouthwash-type products and soft toothbrushes that the patient and Caregiver can try as one means of combating the treatment effects in the mouth and on the tongue. Typically, these products are specially made for Cancer patients suffering from Mucositis and other similar issues, and they can be helpful in many situations, depending on just how severe the Side Effects are. However, in more extreme cases of pain, the patient's Medical Team doctors may determine that one or more powerful painkillers are required, and will prescribe the drugs accordingly. Sometimes, but not always, the "big guns" will help.

The bottom line in addressing pain in the mouth and throat that's related to Chemo and Radiation Therapy treatments is that the Head and Neck Cancer patient must be *palliated* to feel as relaxed as possible. Whether this is achieved thru the use of over-the-counter oral-care products or the prescription of powerful Opioid painkillers, or both, it honestly doesn't matter. What does matter, though, is that the patient has the ability to eat and drink the necessary quantities of nutritious foods and beverages to help keep their body (and mind) as strong, energetic, and as healthy as possible. This is significant both during and after treatment, as the patient must ensure that they have the capability to complete their treatments, as scheduled. And, after their treatments have concluded, they must have the "right stuff" in their bodies to be able to recover as fully and suitably as possible.

If consuming nutrition is a problem for the Head and Neck Cancer patient because of mouth/throat pain or other circumstances, it is the responsibility of the Registered Dietician on the patient's Medical Team to modify the patient's eating plan to "work around" any debilitating Side Effects. This might include the intake of soups, pureed food, protein shakes, water and other *comforting, non-acidic, non-spicy, non-allergenic, non-irritating, non-hot* nutrients, that the patient can tolerate, swallow, ingest, eliminate, and enjoy (as much as possible considering the situation). The patient, their loved one, family members, or Caregiver must inform the Medical Team if the patient is experiencing mouth, tongue, or throat pain that is affecting the patient's ability to eat or drink. *Additional information regarding nutrition and Cancer can be found in Chapter 5 of this Book.*

I have mentioned numerous times within this Book how the Chemotherapy and Radiation Therapy treatments that I received for my Cancer wreaked havoc with my Digestive System (Nausea), and on my mouth and throat (Mucocitis). What's interesting is that I did not feel any negative Side Effects after my first few sessions of both treatments. I then became so daring as to ask my Oncologist and my Radiation Oncologist if I could have "extra" amounts of each just to make sure that we "got it all." They, of course, knew better and that I would eventually come to know the wrath of both therapies. *And, that, I did!* The combination of both forms of treatments kicked my ass, both in the *Nausea* and the *Pain* Departments, and, even though I had done all of my pre-Treatment homework and preparations for my mouth, the Side Effects eventually did hit me with both barrels.

Not only did I find it almost impossible to consume any food because my mouth and throat constantly felt like they were on-fire, but the nutrients that I *was* able to force down usually came back out the front door or went out the backdoor no sooner than they went in. I used a compendium of over-the-counter oral care products that my nurses had recommended, and *I also was taking as many as* ***five*** *very powerful prescribed Opioid painkillers at any particular time.* My nutritional plan consisted of high-calorie shakes, pureed food, soups, and water, and, as difficult as it was, I forced down a certain number of calories each day so that I could maintain my strength to continue with my critical therapies. I ultimately dropped just about 50 lbs. of hard-earned weight during the entire Treatment/Side Effect process. But since my Oncologist would not permit me to utilize the Stomach Tube (PEG, Gastrostomy Tube) for nutrient consumption, because of possible infection issues at the incision site, I had no choice but to live through the hell. Please note the operative word here is, *"live."*

- **Fatigue**

No matter how energetic and *go-go-go* of a person the Head and Neck Cancer patient may have been prior to their Chemotherapy treatment, the powerful Chemotherapy medications will potentially take their toll on the individual. Feeling tired is a typical Side Effect of Chemotherapy, probably because of the impacts that it has on the production of all the blood cells. But, fatigue might also be due to a combination of factors, not the least of which are a seemingly non-stop schedule, difficulty sleeping (for many reasons), painkiller pills which the patient may be prescribed, and the body's use of all spare energy reserves to help fuel the healing process. In between Chemo and Radiation Therapy sessions (as is applicable), the patient's body will expend thousands of calories attempting to do what it does best: *mend itself.* This process takes place most frequently at night for all people—including Cancer patients—but, the Cancer patient's body will try its utmost to shift its recuperative powers into hyper-drive at every chance it gets. As all Cancer patients will know based on any past injuries or surgeries they've had, healing is a natural occurrence that will happen, but, like most good things in life, it will take time.

Quite often, the most pronounced feelings of fatigue will be noticed by Head and Neck Cancer Chemotherapy patients especially towards the end of treatment and for some weeks after it's finished. If patients are feeling unusually tired, it's important that they pace themselves during the day, and that they attempt to get as much rest as they need. If the Head and Neck Cancer patient is still working or going to school while attending their Chemo (or Radiation Therapy) appointments, it is crucial that they attempt to balance their activities with gentle exercise, such as a short jog, walk, swim, yoga, or a bike ride, if physically able to do so, and, if their physician will allow.

If the Head and Neck Cancer patient feels sleepy during the day, it goes without saying that they should not drive or operate any machinery, thus placing themselves and others in harm's way. Some people aren't fatigued by Chemotherapy and are able to lead a semi-"normal" life during their treatments. Other patients realize that they become extremely tired and that they may have to take things a little more slowly. I've mentioned several times within this Book that all Cancer patients are different from one another, and so, too, are their responses to any of the Side Effects that may evolve. As such, all Head and Neck Cancer patients must do what functions best for their distinctive circumstances, and *do what their doctors recommend.*

During my own Cancer experience, I did start getting quite exhausted when I was about half-way along with my Chemotherapy and Radiation Therapy sessions. My Caregiver did accompany me to all of my initial Chemo and Radiation appointments, and to all of my early tests and meetings with my Medical Team physicians. But, after a while, I started going to these by myself, as she had her work and other obligations that she had to tend to. That all had to change, though, because, as I started the second half of my therapy regimen, I began getting so fatigued during the day—probably because of the Chemo and Radiation Therapy and the strong Opiate pain meds that I was on—that, for safety sake, we had no choice but for her to drive me to and fro again. Gratefully, she was able to get away from work to help me; otherwise, it would have been difficult for me to proceed with my vital Cancer-killing treatments, including daily Radiation.

- ## Numbness or Tingling in Hands or Feet

If the Head and Neck Cancer patient is being administered certain Chemotherapy drugs, they may become aware of changes in sensations in their hands and feet. This is due to the Side Effects that specific Chemo medications can have on the nerves and is known as *Peripheral Neuropathy*. The sensations may include numbness, and a tingling feeling, which could cause the patient to have problems in performing simple tasks that require nimbleness and dexterity of the fingers, such as buttoning and zipping garments, typing and writing, sewing, or, accomplishing similar fiddly jobs. Not all Chemotherapy medications will cause these “challenges,” so patients or Caregivers must notify the treating Oncologist or Oncology Nurse if the patient is experiencing these sorts of Side Effects. If the problem becomes overly troublesome, the physician may choose to lessen the dosages of the Chemo drugs in an effort to minimize the negative effects. As one might expect, changes in sensation can continue to get worse for 2-3 months after the patient’s course of Chemotherapy has finished, before slowly improving. Please be advised that it can take up to two years for symptoms to start improving, and that, sometimes, changes in sensations can be permanent. The *“Chemo Cocktail”* that I was administered was comprised of two medications—Carboplatin®, and Paclitaxel®—which were very effective in treating my Cancer. I did not feel any numbness or tingling sensations while using this combo.

- ## Changes in Hearing and Taste

Similar to the Numbness or Tingling Side Effects that can be originated by some Chemotherapy drugs, the Head and Neck Cancer patient may also become aware of alterations in their senses of Taste and Hearing – again, depending upon which Chemo medications are used. Ringing in the ears, known as *Tinnitus*, might cause the patient to lose their ability to hear some high-pitched sounds. Hearing losses may become more severe in instances where the patient is receiving higher doses and longer courses of Chemo treatment. Occasionally, because a person's ears and their sense of balance are so intertwined, the patient's ability to balance may become affected as well. Just as with most Chemotherapy Side Effects, any Tinnitus will tend to go away after the treatment stops. But, also like some Cancer treatment Side Effects, the Tinnitus may become permanent. During my entire Chemo treatment regimen, I did not have any ringing in my ears. If a Head and Neck Cancer patient begins to notice ringing in their ears, they should notify their Oncologist or Oncology Nurse immediately.

Not to be outdone, the Taste Buds on the tongue also have to get in on the Chemotherapy Side Effect activity. They deserve their *15 minutes of fame*, too! Like many of the Chemo Side Effects that are prompted by the specific Chemotherapy medicines that are used to treat the patient, many drugs can radically affect the sensation of *Taste.* I can definitely speak to this one, because the Chemo-induced tastes that I experienced *SUCKED!* Did I say they sucked? First of all, the most atrocious taste of all was the ubiquitous *salty flavor* of everything that I was able to swallow thru my excruciating, inflamed throat, including any saliva that I managed to conjure up. Seriously, no matter what I was able to put away—pureed foods, water, high-calorie protein shakes—all of them, no matter their intended flavors, tasted like eating or drinking 100% pure salt (and I know how that tastes, having swum in the ocean and inadvertently swallowed more than my share of saltwater). In any event, suffice it to say that salty taste made me sick, made me nauseous, and made me vomit. While the salty taste was horrific, there was also a very *metallic taste* that I noticed as my Chemo and Radiation Therapy continued. If one has ever tasted a penny (who hasn't?), they will have a good idea of this yucky Chemo-evoked flavor, which also made me feel very sick.

- **"Chemo Brain"** ***("Honey, I don't recall you asking me to…")***

Believe it or not, but the Side Effect, *"Chemo Brain,"* does exist, and, as far as I can remember, I did experience it and may still have it. Many patients who have accomplished their entire course of Chemotherapy do observe some temporary changes in their memory or thinking processes. Specifically, they find that it might be harder to do two things simultaneously; that they can't recall where they've placed things (what's new?); and, that they may have a difficult time holding things in their memories that they've recently heard or read. This concept of Chemo Brain is complicated to study and difficult to determine—compared to one losing their hair or having lower Blood Counts due to Chemotherapy—so, as I write this, the scientific and medical communities aren't sure how long the effect lasts, and what can be done to minimize its occurrence. Personally, I *will* attest to the fact that Chemo Brain is a real thing. I just can't recall why. ☺

Seriously speaking, Studies have noted that Cancer treatment as well as the Cancer, itself, can contribute to many of the symptoms that are described as "Chemo Brain." For example, Anemia (low Red Blood Cell count), sleep deprivation, depression, tiredness, and anxiety over a Diagnosis of Cancer can all affect the Head and Neck Cancer patient's concentration, and their ability to remember things. But, Medical Studies have found that Chemotherapy may also play a specific role in causing these symptoms. Neuropsychological testing has indicated that physiological changes in the brain do occur during a course of Chemotherapy. "Chemo Brain" is a relatively new term that refers to the cognitive changes that can take place in the Cancer patient as a Side Effect of receiving Chemotherapy treatments.

- ## Radiation Therapy Side Effects – Head and Neck Cancer

The prime objective of Radiation Therapy is to target Cancer cells in the Head and Neck Cancer patient by way of the delivery of calculated, powerful, and precisely directed X-ray beams, which are intended to eradicate the cancerous cells, while minimizing exposure to healthy cells. However, in addition to its desired effect on Cancer cells, Radiation Therapy will perhaps result in unwanted and painful consequences. These problems, known as Side Effects, will usually impact the patient's normal, healthy cells that are situated directly in the field of radiation, or, could encompass that healthy tissue that is located in close proximity (i.e., *"Margins")* to the malignant Tumor being targeted. The progress and the overall success of the Radiation Therapy Plan can be limited, based on the ability of the patient, and the patient's Medical Team, to minimize or get rid of these negative Side Effects to the extent possible. In other words, the complications of Radiation Therapy—especially if administered concurrently with Chemotherapy—can interfere with, and delay treatments, if they are not addressed quickly and completely by the physicians and patient.

The harshness of Radiation Therapy Side Effects to the Head and Neck Cancer patient is influenced by the variety of the patient's Cancer, and its Stage and location; the dosage and method by which the Radiation Therapy is given; and, the patient's general health and personal habits (i.e., is the patient continuing to smoke, and/or, drink alcohol?). Additionally, as stated multiple times within this Book, if the Radiation Therapy is administered concurrently with Chemo, the negative affects of the Side Effects could be magnified, compared to their relative severity were the treatments not given simultaneously. Further, a dose of radiation that might cause some discomfort in one patient, may elicit no Side Effects in another patient. With this being said, if Side Effects do evolve, the Head and Neck Cancer patient, or their loved one, family, or Caregiver, should report to the Radiation Oncologist or the Radiation Technologists or nurses, so that actions can be taken by the Medical Team and patient to reduce or remove these uncomfortable and stressful issues as quickly as possible.

From a general perspective, Head and Neck Cancer Patients who receive Radiation Therapy to the head and neck may experience *Mucositis* (inflammation of the mucous membranes of the mouth or throat, including redness, irritation, and sensitive sores in the mouth and on the tongue); *Xerostomia* (a dry mouth or thickened saliva); difficulty with swallowing; damage to the Salivary Glands; pain and discomfort; alterations in taste or loss of taste, which could decrease the patient's appetite, reduce their nutrient consumption, and lead to weight loss, nausea, and vomiting; *Dermatitis* (skin inflammation); fatigue and changes in sleep or rest patterns; earaches; diminution in White Blood Cell and Platelet counts; and, swelling or drooping of the skin under the chin, and alterations in the texture of the skin (the jaw may feel stiff and patients may not be able to open their mouths as wide as they could before treatment). To some extent, these Side Effects occur in most patients, and generally dissipate over time.

Another one of the frequently encountered complications of Radiation Therapy for Head and Neck Cancer is abnormally lower levels of Thyroid Hormone, which is referred to as Hypothyroidism. Signs and symptoms of Hypothyroidism may include unexplained or prolonged weight gain, fatigue, depression, constipation, pale skin color, and brittle nails. These symptoms are subtle and may happen later on in life. Therefore, it is important for Head and Neck Cancer patients who have received Radiation Therapy ask their physician to test them for low levels of Thyroid Hormone on a regular basis.

Finally, as much as I hate to say this (because I'm also in this same boat) a potential ***MAJOR*** Side Effect of Radiation Therapy is the development of a Second (new) Primary Cancer at some point in the patient's life. You would think that there would be some sort of *Double Jeopardy* law against things like that! Really, is one Cancer not enough for one person? Forming a Second Cancer is somewhat akin to being thrown in jail for killing the burglar in your own home. It just isn't right. But, in any event, treatment to the Head and Neck with Radiation Therapy can damage healthy tissues to such a degree that a new Second Cancer—completely unrelated to the Cancer that is being treated—may evolve in the patient's body. Second Cancers often take years to develop, which is precisely why Aftercare testing and monitoring are such critical components of the survivor's post-treatment follow-up care. The risks and benefits that are associated with Radiation Therapy should be carefully weighed. Patients, and their loved ones, family members, or Caregiver should discuss these issues with the Medical Team physicians when planning treatments.

Listed below are the possible Side Effects of Radiation Therapy that Head and Neck Cancer patients could experience during and after their Radiation Therapy. The following descriptions of Side Effects are from the National Cancer Institute (www.cancer.gov) sources, my journaling notes, and in materials given to me by my Medical Team. ***Note:*** Many are Side Effects also experienced with Chemotherapy.

- **Fatigue**

Head and Neck Cancer patients who are receiving Radiation Therapy experience some levels of fatigue during treatment. In fact, fatigue, which is a general feeling of being extremely tired, is one of the most common Side Effects of Radiation Therapy. Cumulative fatigue can be caused by Radiation Therapy, meaning that the level of tiredness increases over time, which is certainly what happened in my situation. Additional factors that contribute to fatigue onset are Anemia (Low Red Blood Cell count); prescribed Opiate painkillers and other medications; Hypothyroidism; the healing process; stress; depression; lack of sufficient good-quality sleep (Insomnia) and rest; a non-stop schedule; and, reduced food and liquid intake.

Fatigue usually lasts from three to four weeks after treatment stops, but may continue for more than two to three months following treatment(s). Because of safety issues with being fatigued, and, since recovery and energy conservation are crucial throughout the curative process both through and after treatment, it is particularly important that Head and Neck Cancer patients receiving Radiation Therapy try to rest as much as possible. This is the point when the patient should call for their Caregiver and their support network to assist them with chores, running errands, chauffeuring the patient to and from their medical appointments, and performing in any other roles, as needed. Taking short naps during the day, and getting uninterrupted sleep at night, can make a notable difference in the patient's energy levels.

☛***Authors Note:*** For further information pertaining to the Side Effect of *Fatigue* and its impacts to Head and Neck Cancer patients, please see the prior Section: *Chemotherapy Side Effects – Fatigue.*

- ## Skin Irritation and Redness – At Treatment Site

During the administration of Radiation Therapy to the Head and Neck Cancer patient, the potent X-ray beams will cause exposed skin (skin that is positioned in the field(s) of radiation) to appear red, sunburned, or irritated. While delivery, per se, of Radiation Therapy to the patient is not painful, the Side Effects of the radiation can lead to hurting of the skin that is covering the area of the targeted Cancer Tumor. And, unfortunately, but not unexpectedly, if the Head and Neck Cancer patient is also receiving concomitant Chemo with their Radiation Therapy, the skin reaction could be further aggravated. As such, the patient's skin will become sensitive, and the "sunburn-ish" look and feeling will typically reach its maximum during the closing week of Radiation Therapy treatment, and will continue into the first week, post-treatment. After that, it usually subsides fairly rapidly.

Because the patient's impacted skin can become sensitive to the touch as an effect of Radiation Therapy, it is vital that the patient and their loved one, family member, or Caregiver take precautionary steps to protect, and not worsen, the negative effects of the radiation. The Head and Neck Cancer patient can request special creams and gels from Radiation Oncologist or Oncology Nurse that are specially formulated to protect and relieve skin that is *in the line of fire* during their Radiation Therapy procedures. Patients on the receiving end of Radiation Therapy should also do their utmost to avoid scented body lotions, perfumes, tight-fitting clothing, and exposing the area to sun and wind (throughout treatment and for one year after – *best of luck with that!*). Additionally, it is advisable for radiation-treated patients to avoid touching chemical irritants, and use in the radiation field of lotion or ointments prior to Radiation Therapy that might change the depths of radiation penetration. During my Radiation Therapy and concomitant Chemo, I did realize the Side Effect of Skin Reactions in the area of my neck, but, it was manageable and not too severe.

- ## Nausea, Vomiting, and Diarrhea

Is there anything more debilitating, more miserable and more wretched than being nauseous, and, then, vomiting as a result of that nausea? Well, when speaking of Cancer Side Effects, the answer is probably *"yes,"* but, these two nasty Radiation Therapy Side Effects have got to be at the top of that list. For patients receiving Radiation Therapy to their head or neck areas, the severity of any nausea and vomiting Side Effects will depend upon many factors, including the patient's form of Cancer and its Stage (invasiveness in the body) and location, the patient's general health state, and the form of Radiation Therapy received and its dosages. And, as usual, the seriousness of these Side Effects will likely depend upon whether or not the patient is also receiving simultaneous Chemotherapy. If the Head and Neck Cancer patient is getting the *double whammy* of Radiation Therapy and Chemo, chances are pretty good that he or she is going to realize the wicked wrath of nausea. And, just as cookies and ice cream both go together, my apologies please, but so do nausea and vomiting.

By and large, radiation to the head and neck areas should not normally cause nausea, but some Head and Neck Cancer patients do experience nausea during Radiation Therapy treatment (especially in combination with Chemo). As I've stated multiple times within this Book, all Cancer patients are distinctive, as are the specifics of their Cancer situations, so what affects one person may not affect another. With that said, those patients who do experience nausea will usually notice it from two to six hours after their Radiation Therapy session, and they can expect it to last for about two hours. Again, if Chemo is involved, the feeling of nausea may be unrelenting, and it may or may not be accompanied by vomiting. *What an atrocious tag-team!*

As anybody knows who has ever had to *up-chuck*, *throw-up*, *toss cookies, vomit,* or, however one wants to exemplify it, persistent vomiting can result in the body's loss of excessive amounts of water and nutrients. If vomiting continues for more than three times a day, and, if one does not drink enough fluids, it could lead to dehydration and malnutrition, which could be devastating for any Head and Neck Cancer patient. The "other end" of this possible dehydration issue—both figuratively and literally—is that, generally, the Side Effects of nausea and vomiting could be joined by the third notorious member of this nasty gang: Diarrhea. When the Cancer patient is losing vital liquids and nutrients because of any of these Side Effects, the health complications could be very serious if left untreated. They, likewise, could reduce the effectiveness of anti-Cancer medications, as well as those drugs prescribed for pain or to counter any Side Effects.

If the Side Effects of nausea, vomiting, or diarrhea continue unaddressed, Radiation Therapy treatments (and, Chemotherapy, as applicable) may have to be discontinued temporarily by the treating Oncologists. Obviously, this is something that neither the Head and Neck Cancer patient nor their Medical Team want to occur. Patients and Caregivers must inform their Oncologists or Oncology Nurses if any of these Side Effects evolve. The Medical Team physicians can administer fluids and medications intravenously to the patient to aid the body in regaining critical nutrients and electrolytes. Medications can also be prescribed that could help to mitigate any nausea issues. During the last half of my Radiation Therapy and Chemo treatments and afterward, I realized sickening bouts of nausea, vomiting, and diarrhea. Regrettably, our efforts to tame them did not work well.

☛ ***Authors Note:*** For supplemental information pertaining to the Side Effects of *Nausea, Vomiting,* and *Diarrhea,* for Head and Neck Cancer patients, please see the previous Section: *Chemotherapy Side Effects – Nausea, Vomiting, and Diarrhea.*

o Mucositis (Inflammation of Mucous Membranes)

I've commented numerous times within this Book about the double-edged sword of concomitant Radiation Therapy and Chemo when the pair are used to treat Cancer patients. Well, for Head and Neck Cancer patients, the same *double-whammy* applies. On the one hand, the powerful combination of Radiation and Chemotherapy is very effective in exterminating numerous forms of Cancer. But, (and with Cancer, there is always a *"but"*), on the other hand, if there are any Side Effects that develop from the mixture, they could be pretty severe. And, when the regions being treated with Radiation Therapy are the patient's head and neck, that complicates things even further. This is because the Radiation Therapy (with or without Chemo) will cause damage to the Oropharyngeal mucosa, or, the sensitive linings of the mouth, tongue, lips, and upper throat. This painful and very disturbing inflammatory condition is referred to as *Mucositis.*

With Radiation Therapy, Mucositis will, on average, develop gradually over a period of 2-3 weeks after commencing the radiation treatments. The Mucositis Side Effects will typically show up in the form of blister-like, red, and painful mouth ulcers on the Head and Neck Cancer patient's inner cheeks and lips, and small *"white-ish"* and red bumps on the tongue. To make matters even worse (that ***is*** possible), secondary Bacterial Infections, Viral Infections *(Herpes),* and Fungal Infections *(Thrush)* are all probable too. The occurrence and harshness of these Side Effects will, in general, depend upon the field(s) of radiation, the region(s) of the head, and/or, neck that were targeted, and, the cumulative dosage and duration of the treatments. Because most Head and Neck Cancer patients will receive delivery of radiation to the location of their Primary Tumor on a daily basis (except weekends) through the complete course of their therapy, any healthy tissue exposed to the X-ray beams will have extremely little time to recuperate before being *zapped* yet again. And, wouldn't you know it, we just happen to need our mouths to eat and drink. *Darn!*

Mucositis can be enormously painful for the Head and Neck Cancer patient, and can hinder food and fluid intake, which can then lead to nutritional deficiency and potential weight loss. But, before any Readers start thinking that this is the solution to meet their New Year's Resolution weight-loss goals, think again. Believe me, this is ***not*** how you want to go about it. Nutritional food and fluid intake is one of the most vital considerations for ***all*** Cancer patients, but, for the Head and Neck Cancer patient, it is even more critical. This is because the region(s) of the head and neck being treated and harmed by Side Effects are the very areas utilized by the patient to consume essential food, water, calories, other nutrients, and medicine. Unlike a Prostate Cancer patient or a Breast Cancer patient, whose mouths and eating abilities may be influenced minimally or not at all during their respective Cancer therapies, the Head and Neck Cancer patient, regrettably, *gets nailed right where it counts – in the ole' smacker.*

As is the case with all detrimental Side Effects, if the patient is experiencing significant weight loss or dehydration, they, or their loved one, family members, or Caregiver must alert their Oncologist or their Oncology Nurses or Registered Dietician. In extreme cases of malnutrition and weight loss, the physician may order a surgically placed Enteral Feeding Tube (Gastrostomy Tube) to deliver the food and water (typically temporarily) directly into the patient's stomach by by-passing the sensitive and throbbing mouth. The Medical Team may also recommend prescription pain medications (including very strong Opiate- or narcotic-based drugs) to help minimize discomfort. Additionally, the doctor, nurse, or Registered Dietician may propose specific over-the-counter products that may help to mitigate some of the Side Effects of Mucositis. They also may provide the patient and their Caregiver with instructions on how to maintain meticulous oral hygiene, and to modify the patient's nutritional plan to ensure that spicy, acidic, sharp, and hot foods and alcohol are removed from the patient's diet. During my Cancer ordeal, I did have major Mucositis as a result of my Chemo and Radiation Therapy, but, we did our best to manage the pain. My Mucositis Side Effects did disappear after my treatments ended, which usually happens with most patients.

☛***Authors Note:*** For supplemental information pertaining to the Side Effects of *Mucositis* for Head and Neck Cancer patients, please see the prior Section: *Chemotherapy Side Effects – Painful Mouth, Mouth Ulcers, and Throat*. For additional material regarding Enteral (Non-mouth) Gastrostomy Tube Feeding, please see Chapter 5, *The Cancer Patient's Nutritional Plan.*

o Xerostomia (Dry Mouth – Lack of Saliva Due to Possible Salivary Gland Damage)

So, you assumed after reading about the cruel Mucositis Side Effects, that things would lighten up – right? Well, sorry to break it to you, but right along with Mucositis (inflammation of the mucous membranes in the mouth and upper throat), Radiation Therapy could also screw up the Head and Neck Cancer patient's mouth by literally reducing the patient's abilities to produce saliva, either partially, or totally. In medical terminology, the condition of dry mouth / loss of saliva is known as *Xerostomia*, and believe me, it's properly labeled. If one has ever worked outside, or participated in a tiresome sporting or recreational event where no water or fluids were available to "*wet their whistle,*" they will have a good idea of how the Cancer patient will feel after receiving Radiation Therapy to their head and neck. The dissimilarity being, that with the Head and Neck Cancer patient, this lack of saliva production to moisten the mouth may, perhaps, be permanent, whereas, the worker, athlete, or hiker will, hopefully, be able to soon relieve their dry mouth with water and other fluids, and thus return their mouth and saliva levels to their normal condition.

The saliva production scarcity for the Head and Neck Cancer patient will normally start becoming apparent to the patient after the first two to three weeks of Radiation Therapy. But, worse yet, what saliva the patient is able to conjure up may be very thick (mucous or phlegm) and can become extremely sickening if swallowed and not expelled. The loss of saliva production is directly related to the form of Radiation Therapy used, the whereabouts of the patient's Primary Tumor, the irradiation dose and duration, and, most importantly, the amount of salivary tissue (Salivary Glands), that were exposed to the extremely powerful X-ray beams. While state-of-the-art technology, and accurate, well-calculated Radiation Therapy treatment plans are designed and used by the Radiation Oncologist, Radiation Physicist, and Radiation Technologists to carefully, safely, and effectively aim the radiation beams directly at the targeted Primary Tumor, there is a lot of other healthy tissue, including the Salivary Glands, that can find themselves directly *in the line of fire.* It is this incidental harm to normal, non-cancerous tissue that can result in nasty Side Effects.

When considering Salivary Glands while treating the Head and Neck Cancer patient with Radiation Therapy, the regions of the head and neck are *virtual minefields of Salivary Gland activity.* For example, there are three pairs of primary Salivary Glands found on both sides of the head in three different regions: The ***Parotid Glands*** are the largest Salivary Glands, and are underneath, and in front of, each ear; the ***Sublingual Salivary Glands*** are found just beneath the tongue in the mouth; and, the ***Submandibular Glands*** are positioned just underneath the lower Jawbone (Mandible). But, that's not all: In addition to the three pairs of superior (Major) Salivary Glands, there are also hundreds of smaller (Minor) Salivary Glands that line many parts of the mouth, nose, and the Larynx (Voice Box). These small, minor Glands can only be seen under a microscope. As can be easily gathered from this information, it would be nearly impossible for an external beam of radiation (no matter how precisely directed) to *not* impact one or more of the Salivary Glands to some extent.

In a situation whereby the Head and Neck Cancer patient has *Bilateral Radiation Therapy* (radiation administered to *both sides* of the patient's head, and/or, neck), the threat of *totally* losing Salivary Gland production of saliva is much greater than if the irradiation is given to the patient unilaterally (from only one direction). When the radiation is directed to the patient's tumor from one aspect only, it is very likely that only those Salivary Glands directly in the path of the radiation may sustain harm, whereas the Salivary Glands on the non-irradiated or opposite side of the head will suffer little or no damage. But, no matter how or where the Radiation Therapy is directed to the Head and Neck Cancer patient's Primary Tumor, it is critical that as much salivary tissue be spared as possible. Whether individuals give it any thought or not, saliva is essential for good dental health, and is vital to assist in the breakdown of foods for better digestion. Since saliva is the first line of defense against cavities, the drier the mouth, the greater the risk for cavities, tooth decay, and other issues. Head and Neck Cancer patients who are experiencing the Side Effects of Xerostomia must inform their Oncologist as quickly as possible.

☛***Authors Note:*** Because of the gravity of Xerostomia resulting from Radiation Therapy, ***prior to*** a Head and Neck Cancer patient beginning their Treatment Phase – as was explained in Chapter 4 of this Book, *Preparing for Cancer Treatment, Step 6 on the Journey* – it is very significant that the patient obtain a pre-Radiation Therapy dental consultation and treatment (as necessary) with a dental expert familiar with Radiation Therapy issues. Problematic teeth within the radiation treatment region may need restoration or, if not restorable, may need to be extracted ***prior to*** commencing Radiation Therapy to moderate later risk for jaw problems. One of the most grievous Side Effects that can develop is Osteoradionecrosis of the Jaw (Literally, *"Death of the Jawbone caused by Radiation").* This nasty condition is discussed in greater detail in a following Section in this Chapter.

At a bare minimum, all Head and Neck Cancer patients and survivors could need daily life-long fluoride treatments, along with a supervised rigorous dental hygiene regimen, in an effort to minimize any degradation of their oral health over time. Artificial saliva and constant wetting of the mouth with water and other liquids may also be helpful in generating *"spit."* Although Xerostomia Side Effects may improve in many Head and Neck Cancer patients and survivors with time, in other survivors, they can be *for life.* But, that does not have to be: I "discovered" a medication—Amifostine®—during my pre-treatment research, that gratefully salvaged 100% of my salivary function on both sides of my head, despite being bilaterally radiated.

- **My Use of Amifostine® to Salvage my Salivary Gland Functions During Radiation Therapy**

Talk about serendipity! Following my Cancer diagnosis, but before my initial meetings with the physicians on my Medical Team, I and my Caregiver thoroughly researched all elements of Head and Neck Cancers, including all of the latest and greatest scientific and medical tools that could potentially be used to eradicate the disease. Then, after I received a 2nd Opinion from an Ear, Nose and Throat doctor and Cancer specialist who was the first to expose my Primary Tumor on the Base of my Tongue, I was able to narrow the focus of my research to that specific form of Cancer. And, that's when it all came together. Not only did I identify two Chemotherapy drugs that had the most successful "kill rate" for my form of Cancer (which my Oncologist ended up utilizing), but I also found out that the Intensity Modulated Radiation Therapy (IMRT) machine was, at the time, the most precise and successful means of accurately delivering radiation to kill Base of Tongue Cancers. (Which, thankfully, it was for me).

Another one of my more key research "finds," however, was information regarding the drug, Amifostine, which, according to the documents I read, could help to reduce most Salivary Gland damage caused by Radiation Therapy to the head and neck areas. In most of my research on the use of Radiation Therapy to treat Head and Neck Cancer patients, I learned that the powerful radiation can really do a number on the Salivary Glands located in the field of radiation, and that the nasty Side Effects of Dry Mouth (Xerostomia) could result, as well as other unfavorable late effects. Further, I learned that the Salivary Glands exposed to Radiation Therapy could lose the ability to produce saliva for the rest of the Cancer survivor's life. I had read numerous accounts about Cancer survivors whose saliva-producing functions had been damaged forever by Radiation Therapy. And, I also listened to the stories told by survivors during some of the Head and Neck Cancer Support Group meetings that I attended when they related how difficult it was to not be able to generate "spit" because of radiation harm to their unprotected Salivary Glands. All of these survivors always had a bottle of water handy to moisten their mouth and to help them swallow. There was no way that I was going to let that happen to me if there was any way that I could possibly avoid it.

I learned during my research that Amifostine is a medication that was originally developed for use as a Radioprotective agent in a classified project to protect soldiers against chemical warfare during WWII (*Both Chemotherapy and Amifostine got their unlikely starts due to the use of chemical warfare by the Germans in the Great War – who would have thunk it?).* In any event, after declassification of the secret project, Amifostine was evaluated for use within the U.S. as a protective agent against the toxic Chemotherapy drug, Cisplatin, which can cause damage to the Kidneys in patients being treated for Ovarian Cancer. Amifostine was further analyzed for its abilities to protect Salivary Glands of Head and Neck Cancer patients receiving Radiation Therapy. In 1995, the FDA approved Amifostine for use as a *Cytoprotectant* during the treatment of some forms of Cancer.

Amifostine comes as a powder to be mixed with liquid that is injected intravenously (into a vein), or subcutaneously (just beneath the skin into the abdomen), by a physician or a nurse (or under their guidance) in a medical facility. When Amifostine is used to preserve the Kidneys against the damaging effects of Cisplatin, it is normally given over a duration of 15 minutes, starting 30 minutes prior to the start of Chemotherapy sessions. When Amifostine is utilized to save Salivary Gland function from possible Radiation Therapy damage, it is typically administered for a period of three minutes, generally 15 to 30 minutes before the start of the Radiation Therapy treatment.

Amifostine is a prescription medication that must be utilized only under the supervision of a physician. In terms of negative Side Effects of Amifostine, it could cause dizziness or drowsiness, which could be exaggerated with certain other medications, so care must be applied for the patient to not drive or operate any machinery if these symptoms evolve. Amifostine can also cause low blood pressure and shortness of breath, so these concerns must be directly monitored in Head and Neck Cancer patients using the drug. Further, Amifostine can prompt nausea and vomiting immediately after injection, so, the Head and Neck Cancer patient must be aware of this possibility.

After I "found" this *wonder-drug* while conducting my pre-treatment research, I contacted the ENT physician whom I saw for a Second Opinion about my diagnosis (and who located the site of my Tumor) to ask him if he thought that the use of Amifostine might be advantageous in my circumstances. The doctor expressed his dismay that I actually came across such information, and told me that I was doing the prudent thing by looking at all possible solutions. He then shared his professional opinion that he would recommend use of the medication to help spare my Salivary Gland functions if my Medical Team concurred. Having this endorsement in-hand, I contacted my interim Oncologist and my treating Radiation Oncologist to get their opinions. Both of the doctors were somewhat hesitant to give me the go-ahead, which, honestly, surprised me. My Radiation Oncologist told me that she ***would not disallow its use***, but, she added that she had not seen any definitive Studies that found that Amifostine would be beneficial in preventing radiation-induced damage to the Salivary Glands. My initial Oncologist (not my ultimate treating Oncologist), however, had a different rationale for his reluctance: He told me that it would be really expensive to use the drug and, that he didn't think that my insurance would cover the cost. *Oh yeah? Wanna bet?*

When my original Oncologist told me that Amifostine would be, *"Very expensive and might not be approved."* I could not believe my ears. As soon as this physician told me that, I immediately asked him, *"If Amifostine could help save my Salivary Glands, what better time to approve it and use it, no matter how much it costs?"* With my first Radiation Therapy appointment just days away, I asked him to at least endeavor to get the medication approved by the HMO for my use. It took about two long weeks, but around 10:00 one evening while I was sleeping, the Oncologist called me at home to inform me that the Amifostine had been authorized. *Thank the Good Lord!!* On July 14, 2004, I had my very first Radiation Therapy session, but, I wasn't informed by my Oncologist of the Amifostine approval until July 21, after I had already had six Radiation Therapy treatments.

Upon receiving notice of the drug's approval, my Radiation Oncologist immediately put a plan in motion, whereby she acquired the Amifostine for me. She then held a training session in her clinic for all of the other physicians, the nurses, and me, on the proper and safe method for me to inject myself subcutaneously with Amifostine in the clinic prior to delivery of my Radiation Therapy. Along with this was the need for the nurses to scrutinize my blood pressure very closely after each injection, and to cope with any nausea issues that may arise. Since I was the first Cancer patient to receive Amifostine for Cancer treatment at this large Northern Virginia hospital, none of the staff were familiar with the protocol. But, beginning on July 26, 2004, we all came together for my initial injection. Following that first day, all went well with ensuing injections, with the exception of nausea that I experienced on occasion. The bottom line and the most significant outcome of all of this is that I, *"stuck to my guns,"* and I succeeded: I now have complete Salivary Gland function, *and spit!*

o Mouth and Throat Pain – Inadequate Nutrition

Welcome to the epicenter of Radiation Therapy Side Effects. *Pain in the Mouth and Throat,* figuratively speaking, are the *Mother and Father* of all Radiation Therapy Side Effects. Yes, regrettably, Nausea, Vomiting, Diarrhea, Mucositis and Xerostomia can all seem malevolent enough because of the pain and emotional suffering that they can incite, *individually,* with the Head and Neck Cancer patient. But, *collectively,* each of these Radiation Therapy Side Effects, and others, can create an unspeakable tenderness and burning sting to the patient's mouth and throat that can be just about unbearable. I know, because I lived with that agonizing feeling for quite some time, even though my physicians did their very best to limit my pain with a host of prescription Opioid (narcotic) pain killers. My mouth and throat discomfort truthfully felt as though someone had poured lighter fluid into both of those areas, and then followed that up with a lit match.

Generally speaking, mouth pain and throat tenderness caused by Radiation Therapy are the primary Side Effects that give this type of Cancer treatment such a negative rap – at least for Head and Neck Cancer patients. Yes, regrettably, mouth discomfort, to some extent, is extremely universal in patients with Head and Neck Cancers that are treated with radiation. In fact, more than 80% of Head and Neck Cancer patients experience mouth and throat pain *during* treatment, and 30% of Head and Neck Cancer patients continue to undergo the same Side Effects of mouth and throat pain for six months *after* their treatment has ended. Concurrent Chemo contributes to these stats.

The most excessive Side Effect of Head and Neck Radiation Therapy for most patients is soreness inside the area of the mouth or throat in the place where it is being treated, combined with increased production of phlegm, and/or, thick mucous. As a person might have experienced during a bad Chest Cold or the Flu, the viscous phlegm and mucous are formed as part of the body's natural healing process. But, these two gooey body secretions can cause their own nasty Side Effects such as incessant coughing (to clear them from the mouth or throat), which could exacerbate the pain in the throat; nausea (due to their *"gross"* consistencies, especially if they are swallowed), which may lead to vomiting, which can, likewise, aggravate the sting in the throat; and, difficulty breathing, especially when the patient is lying down, because the discharges will collect and "pool" in the throat.

The mouth and throat pain problems usually begin about two to three weeks after first receiving Radiation Therapy treatment, and will normally increase in intensity throughout the treatment duration and after the therapy has stopped. This excruciating pain will usually dissipate in some Head and Neck Cancer patients over a period of 4 to 8 weeks following the completion of Radiation Therapy. But, the Side Effects can persist for many more months in other patients. As with other Cancer Treatment-related Side Effects, there is no way to predict how each Head and Neck Cancer patient will respond to the treatment or its effects. But, one thing for certain is that all Head and Neck Cancer patients realizing radiation-induced pain in the mouth and throat will be observed very closely by members of the Medical Team, who will take all necessary actions to resolve any pain issues to the extent possible, as quickly and as safely as possible.

As deemed necessary by the Medical Team Oncologists, the patient's doctors will, as a rule, prescribe powerful narcotic (Opiate) painkillers to help alleviate any discomfort. These medications will, in all probability, be of the fast-acting and long-acting types, but, all of them will likely cause the patient to get ***Major Constipation.*** As such, it will be essential that the patient also be administered a Stool Softener of some variety to help alleviate that painful and dangerous predicament. During the worst of my Cancer therapy Side Effects—when I found it almost impossible to swallow any food or fluids due to the intense pain in my mouth and throat—I was on as many as 4 or 5 of the Opioid painkillers at any one time. Despite the two Stool Softeners that I was consuming, I realized—for the first time in my life—the most agonizing and humiliating constipation ever. Without going into graphic detail, let's just say that I had to get quite creative with my hands to *work things out.* It was immediately following that awful experience that I contacted my physicians and asked them to prescribe a better Stool Softener that would thwart such a thing from happening again. My Oncologist prescribed a sugar-based laxative, which, thankfully, worked perfectly from that point on. Up until my experience with constipation, I'd never had to *give birth* before. But, after that, I acquired a newfound respect for the Moms of the world!

Because of the sickening tastes, the dry mouth and the sting of the inner membranes of the mouth and throat that will accompany Head and Neck Cancer Radiation Therapy, many patients may lose a good deal of bodyweight, both during and after treatment. This may happen because they find the food or liquids to not be palatable (i.e., they could taste salty, bland, or be of a sickening consistency), or, it could be because the distress of physically chewing and swallowing the food or fluids may be too hard to bear. This can cause the patient to either not consume nutrients at all, or, to eat and drink very small quantities each day. In either instance, of course, both scenarios are a recipe for disaster in that inadequate and irregular intake of proper nutrients, fluids, and calories may be harmful to the patient's health, as well as their capability to proceed safely with their Treatment and Recovery phases. The patient's physicians and staffs and others on the Medical Team will work with the patient, their loved one, family members, or Caregiver, to try to minimize any malnourishment and dehydration Side Effects caused by Radiation Therapy – especially if the radiation is delivered concurrently with Chemotherapy.

In cases of severe mouth and throat pain, the patient's health care professionals will provide the Head and Neck Cancer patient with dietary advice as well as symptomatic medical management. A Registered Dietician will be involved in the patient's care during the course of Radiation Therapy to help them maintain satisfactory daily intake of calories, water, and other fluids. If the patient is unable to consume enough food and fluids *by mouth* to maintain their strength and bodyweight, or to prevent dehydration, the patient's physicians may have to order the patient to receive food thru alternative means. In such cases, a Surgeon may insert an Enteral feeding tube into the patient's stomach through an incision in the patient's abdomen. This typically, temporary tube (known as a Gastrostomy tube or a PEG), will allow liquefied foods to be physically pumped into the patient's stomach, which will facilitate proper nutrition without causing more pain to the patient's sensitive, and inflamed mouth and throat. *It is important, though, for patients to continue swallowing, even with a Gastrostomy tube in-place*. Otherwise, the swallowing muscles may atrophy (swallowing is not an automatic process), which could cause permanent swallowing problems and make it difficult for the Head and Neck Cancer patient to wean themselves off of the Gastrostomy tube, even after the course of Radiation Therapy has concluded.

When the radiation-induced Side Effects of mouth and throat pain occur, it may be tempting for the Head and Neck Cancer patient to want to take a break from treatments. This is not a good idea. The normal, "collaterally damaged" tissues—i.e., the skin and the linings of the mouth, tongue, and throat—that are responsible for most Side Effects during Radiation Therapy, tend to respond to radiation as do the cancerous cells. So, logically speaking, if the Radiation Therapy (and Chemo) treatments were so comfortable to the patient that they did not produce acute Side Effects to healthy, normal cells, it stands to reason that the treatment(s) would not be effective against Cancer. Therefore, the treatment of most Head and Neck Cancers represents the classic *"no pain, no gain"* situation that I have alluded to several times within this Book. Any cessation of the therapy to decrease the Side Effects will afford the Cancer an opportunity to proliferate and spread in the body, and will radically reduce the likelihood of a cure.

During my own Cancer experience, as I've mentioned many times in these pages, the Side Effects of mouth and throat pain were probably some of the most torturous aspects of my journey. My pain issues made it just about impossible for me to eat or drink anything, and, as a result, I lost roughly 50 lbs of bodyweight both during and after my courses of Chemo and Radiation Therapy. I wanted to try to use the Gastrostomy Feeding Tube to give my mouth and throat a break, but my Oncologist did not approve it due to the potential for infection and swallowing problems during and after its use. She did, however, require me to consume a minimum of 3,000 calories every day, using both liquefied foods and high-calorie protein shakes. She told me that I must force down that many calories to make sure that I would be able to maintain the strength and endurance to continue with my treatments, and to facilitate a successful recovery. So, I did what I had to do, and, according to my journal, gutted down 2,750 to 3,000 calories each day. As for the Feeding Tube, in retrospect, I am very happy that I did not use it. A friend and fellow Head and Neck Cancer patient with my same form of Cancer ***did*** use the PEG Tube, but, he could not re-train himself to swallow again. Regrettably, he had to continue to use the Feeding Tube to eat for the rest of his life.

☛ ***Authors Note:*** For supplemental information pertaining to the Side Effects of *Mouth and Throat Pain* for Head and Neck Cancer patients, please refer to the prior Section: *Chemotherapy Side Effects – Painful Mouth, Mouth Ulcers, and Throat*. For additional guidance regarding Enteral (Non-mouth) Gastrostomy Tube Feeding, please see Chapter 5, *The Cancer Patient's Nutritional Plan.*

o Alterations in Taste

If Salivary Gland tissue is impacted by the Radiation beams, the Head and Neck Cancer patient will normally realize a dry mouth and altered taste. These Head and Neck Cancer Side Effects usually appear within two to three weeks after beginning Radiation Therapy. The patient's capability to taste will typically return gradually over a period of several months during their recovery, after completion of the Radiation Therapy. Radiation can induce changes in taste as well as tongue pain. Such Side Effects can further decrease food intake, which could detrimentally reduce the patient's bodyweight, and their ability to continue with their treatments. Although in most Head and Neck Cancer patients the altered taste will gradually dissipate six or so months after therapy, in some patients, regaining taste may never normalize. Yes, several individuals realize a permanent alteration in their abilities to taste, which can definitely cause issues if the patient happens to be a food or drink connoisseur, or a lover of chocolate or other delicacies. Personally, the only modifications to my taste that I noticed both during and after my simultaneous Chemotherapy and Radiation Therapy, was that all the food and drink tasted sickeningly salty, and that some had a peculiar, metallic taste, almost as though I was sucking on nails or coins. Thankfully, a few weeks after ending both courses of therapy, the crazy taste issues slowly went away.

☛***Authors Note:*** For supplemental information pertaining to the Side Effects of *Alterations in Taste,* and how they impact Head and Neck Cancer patients, see the previous Section: *Chemotherapy Side Effects – Changes in Hearing and Taste.*

o Loss of Appetite – Loss of Bodyweight

Not unlike some other Side Effects resulting from Radiation Therapy, the loss of appetite in a Head and Neck Cancer patient may lead to fatigue and nutritional deficiencies. Whether caused by pain, nausea, terrible palatability, or strange tastes, the lack of appetite can lead to some serious problems for the Cancer patient. It is important for the patient to take care of their strength, energy, bodyweight, and physical and emotional endurance during their entire Cancer journey because, the patient's life, literally, might be hanging in the balance.

Consuming sufficient healthy food, fluids, and calories are vital, and health care specialists on the patient's Medical Team, along with a Registered Dietician, will work with the patient and their loved one, family members, or Caregiver, to develop a personal nutritional plan for the patient. The plan will feature healthy foods and fluids, while at the same time, be designed to get around any Side Effects caused by Radiation Therapy (and Chemotherapy). Eating more little meals throughout the day, instead of three square meals, may help, and the patient will want to shun spicy, salty, hot, crunchy, and acidic foods, while consuming foods and liquids that are rich in nutrients, such as veggies and fruits. In general, appetite will increase when treatment ends and the mouth and throat pain wounds have had an opportunity to heal, and, after the taste buds return to normal. It took me quite a few months to get my full appetite back when my therapies stopped, and it took a little over a year to reclaim the almost 50 lbs. I had lost.

- ### Hair Loss – At Treatment Site

Not like Chemotherapy, which can cause the Head and Neck Cancer patient to lose hair on their head (and, perhaps, other areas of their body), hair loss caused by Radiation Therapy occurs *only at the site of the Primary Tumor that is being treated.* In other words, if the patient's treatment plan calls for radiation to their pelvic region, they would not the lose hair on their head (unless the loss is prompted by concomitant Chemo). If the patient is to be administered Radiation Therapy treatment for a Head and Neck Cancer, however, there is a good chance that they will experience hair loss on the face, scalp, or neck – *wherever the X-ray beam is directed.* The good news is that in *most* cases, one's hair will grow back after treatment is complete. But, there are some instances, such as my own, in which the affected hair does not grow back – *ever.* As an example, the whiskers on my neck, cheeks, and jaw line that were directly in the *line of fire* of the radiation targeting the Tumor on my tongue have never come back. It's actually a mixed blessing, though: On the one hand, if I wanted to grow a beard, it would look shabbier than Abe Lincoln's. But, on the bright side, at least I don't have to shave as much, or as often.

☛ ***Authors Note:*** For supplemental information pertaining to the Side Effect of *Hair Loss,* for Head and Neck Cancer patients, please be directed to the previous Section in this Book: *Chemotherapy Side Effects – Loss of Hair*.

o **Late Effects (Delayed Side Effects)**

According to the National Cancer Institute (www.cancer.gov), the number of Head and Neck Cancer patients who win their battles against Cancer and live for numerous years after Radiation Therapy treatments have ended, has increased. That’s a wonderful thing. But, regrettably, as I’ve stated many times in this Book, those *“numerous years”* may have a “price tag” attached, and that outlay will come in the form of not-so-good Side Effects. Thankfully, most Side Effects will come and go when the Radiation Therapy has ended. In some patients, however, Side Effects will not dissipate after treatment, but will continue from one day to the next, or they will initially manifest themselves in the survivor, many months, or maybe, years, down the road after the final Radiation Therapy session. Delayed Side Effects that materialize at least 6 months after Radiation Therapy has ended are referred to as *Late Effects*. Yes, in some Head and Neck Cancer survivors, their past Radiation Therapy will bequest to them the *non-gift that keeps on giving.* In many Head and Neck Cancer patients, Late Effects will be minimal in nature, but, per the National Cancer Institute, www.cancer.gov, more than 5% of patients will experience Late Effects that could be classified as, *“severe,”* or *“life-altering.”*

Radiation typically affects only the area(s) of the body being targeted, so any immediate or delayed Side Effects will generally be limited to those regions of the Head and Neck Cancer patient’s body that were exposed to the radiation during their treatments. Normally, whether or not a patient will realize Radiation Therapy-related Late Effects will be dependent upon:

- The specific area of their body that was irradiated
- The dose and duration of their course of Radiation Therapy
- If the patient received Chemotherapy before, during, or after their Radiation Therapy

Late Effects from Radiation Therapy are atypical in Head and Neck Cancer survivors, but, they *do* rear their ugly heads on occasion, and when they do, they are usually permanent. As I've mentioned many times in this Book, the Aftercare monitoring of Cancer survivors is vital to their sustained health and survivorship, and, this is especially true for Head and Neck Cancer survivors who did receive Radiation Therapy. Preceding, during, or after the patient's Radiation Therapy treatments, the treating Radiation Oncologist or Nurse will talk with the patient, their loved one, family, or Caregiver about the likelihood of Late Effects in the patient's case, and will chat about ways to help prevent them, symptoms to be watchful for, and how to treat them if they occur later in life. Survivors should not fear Late Effects, but, should accept them as an adverse part of the Cancer-killing process.

Following are Late Effects that could be realized by Head and Neck Cancer patients and survivors who've received a course of Radiation Therapy as one part of their Cancer treatment plan. The information below has been adapted from my journal notes, materials from my Medical Team, and the National Cancer Institute (www.cancer.gov):

- **Fibrosis**

High doses of radiation for a prolonged period of time, such as during an entire course of Radiation Therapy to the head and neck areas, can result in the condition, *Fibrosis*. Fibrosis is the formation of a large amount of fibrous tissue (scarring) in organs or other parts of the body as the result of inflammation, irritation, or the process of healing. The Side Effect of Fibrosis might become aggravated in a Head and Neck Cancer survivor who received Cancer Surgery in the head and neck areas. In such cases, the neck may develop a "woody" texture, become "stiff," and have restricted movement. Late onset of Fibrosis may also happen in the survivor's Pharynx and Esophagus, leading to stricture (closing off, or constriction) of those organs that are essential to the consumption of foods and liquids, and, of course, necessary for the breathing process. As is usually the case, Fibrosis, Edema (tissue swelling), exasperating discomfort, and Lymphedema (swelling of the Lymph Nodes) are possible in many Head and Neck Cancer survivors who received Radiation Therapy to the neck area.

If the Head and Neck Cancer survivor or their Medical Team believes that the person may possibly be at risk for the Late Effect of

Fibrosis due to Radiation Therapy, there are several actions that the patient / survivor can take in an effort to help prevent, or reduce, the lack of movement and any discomfort created by the condition. As one example, exercising the muscles of the neck can help to reduce neck tightness and will also help to facilitate an increase in the range of motion of the neck and head. The individual will need to perform these exercises for the remainder of their life to maintain ample neck mobility. Additionally, receiving treatment by Physical Therapists who have a proficiency in addressing Cancer-related Side Effects in patients and survivors can help to "break down" the stubborn tissues affected by the Fibrosis, and, thereby, potentially relieve associated discomfort and stiffness. These exercises should also help augment the strength and ranges of motion of the impacted neck muscles.

As is generally the case, the earlier the intervention, the more successful the result will be for the patient. A newer modality using an external laser is also available to help reduce swelling, and, there are also medical means of dilating or enlarging any constrictions in the Esophagus or Pharynx. Swallowing dysfunction due to Fibrosis will often require a change in the patient's/survivor's eating plan, as well as Pharyngeal Strengthening Therapy, or Swallowing Therapy. This is especially true for those Head and Neck Cancer patients who have had Surgery, and/or, Chemotherapy. Swallowing exercises are increasingly utilized as a preventive measure, because, unbeknownst to many people, if a person does not continue to swallow, the body will forget how. Swallowing is a learned behavior – not automatic.

As for my own *Fibrosis* situation, I'm on the fence right now as to whether or not I'm affected by this particular Late Effect. I say this, because, roughly two years ago, in 2011—about 7 years after I completed my Radiation Therapy—I started experiencing a tingling and numbing sensation in the area of my left shoulder and neck. The left side of my neck and throat, of course, is where I had the Surgery to eradicate my cancerous Lymph Nodes and Primary Tumor, and is precisely where the Radiation Therapy was focused to eradicate the tumor and any suspect, surrounding tissues. The strange feeling that I continue to experience in my left shoulder and the left area of my neck is actually pretty creepy. First of all, as I said, the area is numb to the touch, in that I can pinch it as strongly as I possibly can, even with just my fingernails, and I feel absolutely no twinge at all. To be honest, I think I could slice myself with a knife there or poke myself with a fork, and I wouldn't feel a thing. It's almost like rubber, but, the reason I don't know if this is a symptom due to Fibrosis or not is because my neck, shoulder, and chest muscles are as strong, mobile, and robust as always. The doctors I've asked also don't have a clue.

▪ Osteoradionecrosis of the Jaw (Death of the Jawbone Caused by Radiation)

For most Head and Neck Cancer patients who realize nasty Side Effects from Radiation Therapy, the Side Effects are short-term and will usually appear within six months of their final exposure to radiation. Contingent upon the form of the patient's Cancer, as well as its location and Stage, and, depending on the patient's sensitivity to Radiation Therapy, including the type of treatment and its dosage and duration, patients may experience Side Effects of the short-term variety. But, also probable, is that the Head and Neck Cancer patient receiving Radiation Therapy may realize longer-term or Late Effects which includes scarring and narrowing of the blood vessels *(Intimal Proliferation in the Arterioles)* within the treatment area(s). This can lead to inadequate blood supply, and can result in chronic, long-term Side Effects, to include damage or death to the soft tissues or bones. Scientifically speaking, these occurrences are referred to as Necrosis ("death"), Osteoradionecrosis *("death of bone due to radiation"),* or Radionecrosis *("death due to radiation").* Lack of satisfactory blood flow to tissues can also contribute to inferior healing of wounds, and related problems such as life-threatening infections (no White Blood Cells circulating at the affected body location to fight off invaders).

As many as 10 to 15% of Head and Neck Cancer patients or survivors who received higher dosages of Radiation Therapy as one vital element of their treatment plan, will experience the potentially deadly Late Effects of Radiation Therapy that impact the survivor's Circulatory and Skeletal Systems. The risk of Osteoradionecrosis is directly related to radiation dosages and durations, and the degree of tissue getting radiation. Usually "in the line of fire" during Radiation Therapy to the neck or lower head are the jaw bones – in particular, the Lower Jawbone *(Mandible),* and the Upper Jawbone *(Maxilla).* The greatest peril of post-Radiation Therapy Osteoradionecrosis lies with the Mandible, because each plane of the jaw receives ***one-sided*** or independent vascular circulation. The Maxilla, however, receives collateral blood supply that circulates between ***both sides*** of the jaw.

Osteoradionecrosis of the Jaw is usually characterized by the following symptoms or physical conditions in the treatment area(s):

- Systemic infection
- Difficulties with tasting, eating, drinking, and speaking
- Pain and ultra-sensitivity to hot and cold foods and drinks
- Fistula formation (a passage caused by disease, or injury)
- Diminished or complete loss of nerve sensation
- Deterioration of gums to expose Teeth Roots and Jawbone
- "Death" and loss of bone in the Mandible in extreme cases

Ideally, as I've mentioned previously in this Book, steps will have been taken by the Head and Neck Cancer patient ***prior to their Radiation Therapy treatments*** to prepare their mouth and teeth for the onslaught of Side Effects that can accompany such treatment. It is of utmost importance that the patient obtains comprehensive oral and dental care ***before Radiation Therapy begins*** in an effort to help prevent, or at least to minimize, problems popping up after treatment is underway. In so doing, the teeth and linings of the mouth, tongue, and inner cheeks should be thoroughly examined to identify any oral disease, which could lead to serious infections that could necessitate post-radiation surgical therapy. All oral disease should be eliminated pretreatment, and any teeth that will be within the fields of radiation and are too decayed to preserve via fillings or Root Canal, ***should be extracted before*** the commencement of Radiation Therapy. Tooth extraction and dental disease in irradiated areas are major features in the development of Osteoradionecrosis of the Jaw. This is because an unhealthy tooth can serve as a source of infection to the Jawbone, which can be particularly difficult to treat after radiation. Ideally, at least 7 to 14 days should be allowed for healing after any significant dental work is done before the initiation of Radiation Therapy.

As for the treatment of Head and Neck Cancer patients and survivors who have developed the Late Effect of Osteoradionecrosis of the Jaw, doctors can address the problems with topical antibiotics, antiseptics, and pain medications. Treating physicians will probably also take steps to eliminate any trauma to the affected area(s) of the Jawbone, and will recommend that the patient avoids all removable dentures if the denture-bearing area is within the Osteonecrotic field. Additionally, the health care professional will possibly take steps to ensure that the patient is receiving sufficient nutritional intake, and, if the patient is a user of tobacco or alcohol, that they put an end to these behaviors as promptly as possible, as they will only make the condition worse. In extremely severe cases of Osteoradionecrosis of the Jaw, surgical intervention and reconstruction of the lower jaw, or Mandible, may be necessary for aesthetic and functionality reasons. In such situations, a multidisciplinary Cancer Team could be formed that will address the patient's issues. This team might be comprised of Oncologists, Maxillofacial Prosthodontists, Dentists, Hygienists, Surgeons, Nurses, Physical Therapists, and others, as necessary.

Finally, as both a proactive and a reactive measure to counter the Late Effect of Osteoradionecrosis, treating physicians may order the Head and Neck Cancer patient/survivor who received Radiation Therapy to submit for a course of *Hyperbaric Oxygen Therapy*, also known as, *HBOT*. Over the last few years, HBOT has proven to be an effective treatment for some Head and Neck Cancer patients who previously had few chances of recovering from the Late Side Effects of Radiation Therapy. HBOT increases the amount of oxygen in the blood by exposing patients to pure oxygen within a sealed chamber set at pressures greater than the ambient atmosphere. Experts believe that HBOT helps patients heal by stimulating growth of new blood vessels in the treatment area following radiation-induced damage.

- **Hyperbaric Oxygen Therapy – Major Defense Against Osteoradionecrosis of the Jaw**

More than 14 million individuals alive in the U.S. today have been treated for some form of Cancer, and about half of these have received Radiation Therapy in an effort to help abolish their disease. While improved Radiation Therapy equipment and techniques have increased treatment precision and reduced disparaging Side Effects caused by the Head and Neck Cancer patient's exposure to radiation, the high doses of radiation used to destroy cancerous cells might still cause long-term or delayed damage to adjacent healthy cells in some patients. Hyperbaric Oxygen Therapy (HBOT) has proven effective to help decrease the Late Effects of Osteoradionecrosis (*death of the Jawbone caused by radiation)*, by helping the blood to carry more of the healing oxygen to the affected areas in the patient's head.

Hyperbaric Oxygen Therapy sessions, which require a Head and Neck Cancer patient to lie in a see-thru, particularly sturdy and sealed oxygen chamber (that is similar to those utilized by Deep Sea Divers to preclude them from realizing *"the Bends"* when surfacing after an incredibly deep dive), are recommended for management of Osteoradionecrosis of the Jawbone. According to Scientific Studies, Hyperbaric Oxygen Therapy has been found to increase the oxygen saturation of irradiated tissue, promote the formation of new blood vessels and capillaries in the treatment area(s), and, also, to augment the repopulation of *Fibroblasts* (cells in the body which manufacture connective tissue) in the treatment area, and *Osteoblasts,* which are cells that create bone (that have actually evolved from Fibroblasts). All of this contributes to the body's ability to strengthen and heal.

Prior to any Dental Surgery being accomplished, HBOT is typically prescribed for those Head and Neck Cancer patients whose Jawbone has been irradiated. The HBOT consists of 20 to 30 *dives (you've gotta love that terminology!)* of 100 minutes each, at 100% oxygen, from 2 to 2.5 Atmospheres of pressure. If Dental Surgery is then needed, ten dives of ***post-surgical*** HBOT are recommended. As for the Side Effects of HBOT, patients may experience ear-popping (think of the last time you traveled by plane or drove your vehicle at lower/higher elevations), mild sinus discomfort, claustrophobia (the oxygen chamber is relatively small and enclosed, but, thankfully, is transparent), and temporary (or, so they say) short-sightedness when completing more than 20 HBOT sessions. Most patients do not have any symptoms after HBOT and can return to work the same day.

During my own Cancer experience, I found out, while at my pre-treatment Dental visit, that one of my teeth needed a Root Canal. I worked with my Medical Team to have that done. Then, following my Cancer-killing treatments—including Radiation Therapy—I was going to have that tooth pulled. I had not been advised about HBOT by my Medical Team during my Cancer treatment, so, thankfully, I wrote on my Health History Form that I had had Radiation Therapy, and the Oral Surgeon caught it. He asked if I had had HBOT, which I had not, so I submitted to a total 40 *dives* from April-July of 2005, with 30 sessions before I had my tooth pulled, and 10 after. Luckily, my tooth extraction went perfectly, and while the Oral Surgeon was standing above me and heaving on my tooth with all his strength, he yelled, *"I see blood!"* It was almost as though we had struck oil. I had no issues with the HBOT treatments, with the exception of my eyesight. While any vision changes caused by the extreme pressure are supposed to be "temporary," mine have lasted until now. Prior to my HBOT, I could view distances perfectly, but had to wear reading glasses for any close-up viewing. Now, I have the exact opposite of that problem, in that I can read even the smallest type with no help at all, but, I've had to get glasses to clearly see long distances. The moral of this story, I guess, is that you can't believe all your doctors tell you. But, do believe this: ***Get HBOT PRIOR to Dental Surgery!***

- **Secondary Cancers**

I will end this Chapter on Head and Neck Cancer treatment-related Side Effects on a somewhat somber note, but, only because I must point out the insidious reality that Radiation Therapy has been known to lead to the Late Effect of developing a Secondary Cancer. A Secondary Cancer is another form of Cancer that can occur that is unrelated to the patient's first, Primary Cancer, and, that can develop many years after the original Primary Cancer was treated and killed. The National Cancer Institute (www.cancer.gov) found that *Cancer Survivors* have a ***14% higher risk*** of developing a *new Cancer* than people who have never been diagnosed with an initial Cancer. That possibility increases with Cancer survivors who received Radiation Therapy for their first Cancer, and, for those survivors who received Radiation Therapy as children. All the more importance, as specified numerous times within this Book, that *all* Cancer survivors actively participate in post-treatment monitoring and Aftercare. Thankfully, Secondary Cancers are rare, but they do occur. Should the Head and Neck Cancer patient experience a Secondary Cancer diagnosis, as one can anticipate, they will be just as well-supported as they were during their initial Cancer battle by their Medical Team, loved ones, family, and Caregiver. It is important for the patient to consult with their doctor about the potential risks, and to weigh them against the benefits to be derived from Radiation Therapy as a treatment option.

"Cancer patients are never alone on their brave journeys. Not only will they have their loved ones, families, Medical Teams, and friends to help them along the way, but, they are walking a path well-worn with the courage of millions who have successfully traveled this way before. One's Cancer journey may be long or short, tough or easy, or a little bit of both, but in every case, the Cancer patient, with their support network, will do all they can to beat their own Cancer, and, in the process, will inspire others to conquer theirs."

-- Butch Sickler

Chapter Fourteen

The 5-Month Saga to Find my Neck Issues – *A Medical Mess!*

"All patients—but especially Cancer patients—must "own" their medical care. Doctors are invaluable, but not infallible. It is up to us small fish in a very big sea to float any mistakes to the top."

- Butch Sickler

When I received my Cancer Diagnosis on June 7, 2004, I, quite honestly, was fortunate that I received a diagnosis of Cancer at all. I know, that sounds like a peculiar thing to say, so let me phrase it another way: The only reason I found out that I had Cancer doing its contemptible deed within me was because I had to assert myself and stand my ground with a few doctors who either didn't care that my throat and neck were hurting continually for a long time, or, who overestimated their own capacities to provide high-quality customer service and health care for their patients. Thankfully, I was alert and took my health into my own hands, because, God knows what would have happened had I not done so, and simply gone with the doctors' incorrect opinions. That may have led to no diagnosis, no treatment, and possibly, no life. However, before I get down to the nitty-gritty of what went wrong thru the 5-month-long search for the root of my neck tribulations, I'll furnish a little background about my past, and explain what caused me to seek medical attention in the first place.

My Lifelong Quest for Health and Fitness

During my entire teen and adult life, I have taken exceptional care of my body by doing, or not doing, most of the numerous things that medical, scientific, and nutritional "experts" recommend, in an effort to stay healthy, and, to help prevent the invasion of infections, viruses, and diseases—including Cancer—within my body. This, I have done (and continue to do), by not smoking or drinking alcohol; by only consuming healthful foods and drinks; by exercising almost daily; and, by ingesting vitamins, minerals, anti-oxidants, herbs, and nutritional supplements that have been found, via scientific research, to help keep a body healthful and fit. But, as with so many things in life, the only guarantee is that there are no guarantees. I guarantee it.

While the delivery of my Cancer Diagnosis by my physician did mark the beginning of my protracted and, ultimately, rewarding, Cancer journey, my story actually starts much further back, when I was a young teenager. It was when I was roughly 14 years old that I made a conscious decision to live as healthy of a life as I could from that point forward. As I think about it now, there were influences in my life at that time which encouraged me to make such an ironclad commitment to myself at that very young age – my Dad's smoking, drinking, and obesity being three of them. I wanted none of that.

Choosing the Healthy "Road Less Traveled"

When I around 14, ironically, I sold high-calorie donuts each day before school in an effort to earn enough money to buy my first barbell set. It was in my initial year of Junior High School that I first realized how naturally physically strong I was, especially because I was a pretty skinny teenager. My coaches and classmates were also amazed at how much weight I could lift, which, in many cases, was greater than many "jocks" who weighed much more than I did. As time progressed, during the 1960s, I started reading the only muscle-building "literature" that was available at the time: Cultish, ad-filled, *"Muscle Mags."* These former versions of the more polished fitness magazines of today, featured articles on weightlifting and nutrition, as well as being chocked full of pictures of enormous Bodybuilders, invariably posed on a California beach and surrounded by throngs of bikini-clad beauties. The colorful periodicals were created to inspire skinny young guys like me to lift weights, and to become bigger and stronger so that that mean bully wouldn't kick sand in *my* face as he did the scrawny dude in the old Charles Atlas ads. It worked for me, and ignited a fire within my being that has burned until present day.

Reading and re-reading these magazines, I developed a plan for my weightlifting workouts, and, also, did my best to stick to the nutritional suggestions featured in the dog-eared *mags,* which, for a teenaged boy, is asking quite a lot. My progress was slow—genetics always has a habit of dictating things contrary to our best-laid plans and wishes—but, after several months, bulk started to manifest, and, eventually, I began putting some meat on my bones. I continued my strict workout and eating regimen throughout my high school years, and, as time went on during my 4-year enlistment in the Navy and at the university after that, I continually stepped-up my weight training by using heavier weights, different exercises, and an array of fitness equipment. Also, as time progressed, more and improved nutritional supplements started to appear as more companies joined the fitness craze that hit America in the 1970s and 80s, along with Arnold-you-know-who, and a host of other male and female fitness experts. I, for one, was certainly hooked on the training, the food, the friends, and, most of all, the health benefits that I derived from the entire process.

Taking My Love of Fitness to Another Level

As I steadfastly refined my fitness regimen for health's sake, I also, coincidentally, started taking the "fruits of my labors" into the competitive arena and began participating in a host of weightlifting activities and events. Commencing in the mid- to late-1970s while at New Mexico State University, I started competing in Bodybuilding, Olympic Lifting, and Power Lifting Contests, which I continued to do well into the 1980s. I also performed "Strongman"-type feats of strength which included: Bending 3/8" steel reinforcement bar ("re-bar") while clamping it in my padded teeth and pulling down on the ends with my hands; lifting cars off of the ground by their bumpers; pushing two coupled, empty Railroad Box Cars over 50 feet on level tracks from a dead stop; and, heaving very heavy semi-truck tires to a rack over 10' off of the ground. The guys at the lumber yard where I worked part-time during college called me, *"The Human Forklift."* Essentially, from the time I was 14 years old, when I bought my first barbell set, until today, when I work out with my own home gym, I have been involved in one way or another with the "Iron Game."

In addition to involving myself in the "physical" elements of physical fitness via my own training and participation in competitive events, I have, over the years, also delved deeper into the managerial and educational facets of the "fitness business." This, I did in 1978-1979 by instructing "Weight Training and Fitness" classes at New Mexico State University for two semesters as a paid Undergraduate Instructor. While a Naval Officer stationed in Alaska, from 1981 to 1982, I taught a "Weightlifting for Women" Continuing Education class on-base, and, I also designed, built, and outfitted a state-of-the-art weightlifting and aerobics gym on-base for use by all personnel. Throughout the years, I have also been a Certified Personal Fitness Trainer; a designer and Manager of many Health Clubs; a Strength Event Judge at various contests; and, while working with the Federal Government in Washington, DC, the National Fitness and Wellness Coordinator for the entire U.S. Customs Service. I also earned a BS degree in Biology and a Minor in Physical Education to top it all off.

During the approximate 45-year span that I have been lucky enough to have been involved in the health and fitness world, I have also been extremely fortunate to have met some of the kindest, and most down-to-earth, humble, and authentic men and women that I have ever known. Also, at times during these numerous years, I have had the wonderful opportunity to help countless individuals improve their health, strength, and fitness levels. I have also helped them lose weight and change their appearance for the better; assisted them in boosting their confidence and self-esteem; and, have, likewise, aided them in retaining their statuses in the military or in "salvaging" their marriages. In the 4+ decades that I have been involved in health and fitness in one form or another, I have seen and heard it all. But, at the very hub of what these individuals have desired, and what I have endeavored to give to them, has been the motivation, the inspiration, and the enlightenment to help them enhance, extend, and enjoy their lives. What better gift is there to give, *and* to receive?

Good Health + Good Fitness = Bad Cancer So Much for Doing all the "Right" Things!

As you may have gathered while reading this Book, and, as I have addressed in the preceding Section, as a teenager and an adult, I have taken excellent care of my body from a physical standpoint in the interest of keeping it healthy, fit, and strong. In staying fit, the muscular might that I have developed within my body has translated into a heightened state of mental strength and higher self-confidence as well. *"Strong body, strong mind,"* was, and is, my credo, and I have endeavored to live my life by those words for the last 45 years. Because of the many precautions I have taken with my body and my health during that time, I, admittedly, had developed sort of a sense of invincibility about my being. In other words, I felt strongly—but not in a pompous, arrogant way—that my body was protected from, and impervious to, almost any inward or outward health threat to its well-being. With the veracity of my Cancer diagnosis, however, that delusion would come crashing down. Yes, much to my surprise, my "suit of armor" allowed the Cancer to penetrate and hit its mark.

Me coming face-to-face with a Cancer diagnosis was quite a leap for me, considering my major run-ins with hospitals through the years had consisted of a Tonsillectomy when I was seven years old; some stitches in my rear-end when I was about 14 after my brother, Buz, pushed me off the couch back and through a glass end-table top while we played "King of the Mountain;" a broken shoulder blade, ribs, and toes as a result of a Rodeo accident when I was in college; the reattachment of my right Triceps muscle ripped from the elbow while lifting heavy weights, as an adult; and, some plastic surgery of my face to erase some of the disfigurement caused by some awfully nasty acne that I experienced as a young adult. So, how does one go from all of this to a Diagnosis of Cancer? A good question, and the very same one that is probably asked by many Cancer victims.

Any individual who has never experienced a showdown with Cancer—either personally, or through a loved one, family member, or a friend—might, initially, have no idea how, when, why, or where Cancer "decides" one day, out of the clear blue, to begin mutating, growing, multiplying, and spreading within one's body. I was one of those people who was actually pretty "clueless" about Cancer, even though I had had a limited involvement in dealing with my Mom's, Grandmothers', Aunt's, and several of my friends' personal Cancer occurrences. But, unfortunately, I *was way too familiar* with the not-so-good outcomes of a bunch of those Cancer experiences. With the advent of *my own* Cancer diagnosis, however, I would immediately immerse myself in books, materials from my Medical Team doctors, and online resources, in an effort to learn what I could about Cancer in preparation for what would ultimately become a very demanding, protracted, and, fulfilling Cancer journey. My learning about Cancer began the instant I received my diagnosis, and, it has not stopped.

How it All Began: Throat Pain & Neck Swelling

In January of 2004, I had come down with a real bad case of something, which would just not go away. I treated the symptoms—which included a bad fever, stuffiness, headache, coughing, difficult and painful swallowing, and a bad sore throat ***only on the left side***—with the typical over-the-counter medicines. With no relief in-sight, however, in late January of 2004, I scheduled an appointment to see a doctor on February 26, 2004, to determine if they could figure out what was ailing me. For almost four weeks, between the time I made the appointment, and when I actually saw the doctor on February 26, I did everything I could to treat my sore throat, from gargling with salt-water, taking sore throat lozenges, and spraying my throat with the typical numbing Lydocaine sprays, to ingesting over-the-counter aspirin and painkillers, and other anti-inflammatory medications.

Unfortunately, all of my attempts to get rid of the sore throat symptoms were in vain. The common lozenges, sprays, and "magic elixirs" on the drug store shelves—which typically helped to relieve "ordinary" throat pain—did absolutely nothing to help eliminate the discomfort that I was realizing with my throat. Additionally, during this interlude of waiting for my doctor's appointment, my girlfriend told me that she noticed some unusual swelling on the left region of my neck, just below my ear and jaw line. She was correct. My neck on the left side *was* pink and swollen. Both of these symptoms were not typical for me as I rarely got the Flu or Colds, much less a non-stop sore throat. But, the left-side throat pain and swelling were very real and had to be checked by a doctor – the sooner, the better.

Doctor No. 1 - Incorrect Medical Opinion No. 1 – Not a Good Start

My doctor's appointment on February 26, 2004 finally rolled around, and none too soon. By the time of my doctor's visit, the pain in my throat and the swelling in my neck were very pronounced. As

I described my situation to the physician, she attempted to assess my condition, and soon thereafter came to a conclusion. After her quick evaluation, she told me that she was sure that I had Bronchitis, and she prescribed a "Z-Pack" (a 5-day course of a common antibiotic) to see if it may help to reduce the fever, pain, and inflammation. She further suggested that I follow-up with my Primary Care Physician in two-to-three days if I noted no improvement. Well, Z-Pack or no Z-Pack, things only got worse with my bad throat pain, so I took the doctor up on her proposition that I go to my Primary Care physician. I scheduled an appointment to see him on March 2, 2004.

Doctor No. 2 - Incorrect Medical Opinion No. 2

In retrospect, the appointment on March 2 with my physician turned out to be another *"Red Herring"*-type of opinion / diagnosis. A *"Red Herring,"* or "false indicator" type of diagnosis, means that my doctors initially thought that my ongoing, severe throat pain was being caused by a condition other than Cancer. In fact, my Primary Care doctor also pinned the "Bronchitis" label on my symptoms, but he additionally added "Sinusitis" to the post-visit notes. He thought that my cough and sinuses were causing my aching throat pain, but I told him that no matter what I tried, the pain would not go away. As for the neck swelling, he attributed that to a reaction by my Lymph Nodes as a result of the inflammation within my throat (*you think?*). He prescribed a codeine-based cough syrup and sent me on my way.

Obtaining absolutely no relief from the narcotic cough syrup that my Primary Care Physician prescribed, and, with my throat pain and neck swelling becoming ridiculous (not in a funny way), I called his office again, and I insisted that I be seen by the doctor as quickly as possible. For obvious reasons, I was extremely concerned about my non-stop signs as I had not experienced anything like this in my life. I knew my body *very well,* and certainly well enough to know when something extremely wrong is going on with it. Unfortunately, the office couldn't schedule me in for two weeks, but, on March 16, 2004, I finally did get in to see my Primary Care physician – again.

This time around, my doctor knew by my voice and the look on my face that I meant business and that I was not going to agree to any slapdash, come-what-may opinions from him. I told him right-off-the-bat that ***I DID NOT have any Bronchitis or Sinusitis,*** and, I reiterated to him for the third or fourth time that my sore throat pain was ***located only on the left side,*** and, that no matter what I used to relieve the pain, nothing worked. I told him that his and the previous physician's opinions were simply that – *opinions* – and I steadfastly insisted that he order a CT Scan, an MRI, or any other scan or image that could help to identify what might be causing my throat and neck problem. I also told him that I wanted a referral to an Ear, Nose, and Throat (ENT) doctor who would know more about throat and neck problems. He did as I requested, I thanked him, and I left his office.

ENT No. 1 – Incorrect Medical Opinion No. 3 – A Shameful, Unprofessional Medical Debacle

I managed to get an appointment to see an ENT physician on March 24, 2004, which was almost 2 months after I first sought help from doctors for my one-sided sore throat aches and swelling on the left area of my neck. When I saw—who I will call *"ENT No. 1,"—I* had been scheduled for the CT ordered by my Primary Care doctor, but, I had not yet obtained the Scan. Upon meeting ENT No. 1 in the hospital on the morning of March 24, suffice it to say that I was not impressed. To be honest, I was very insulted. For starters, this doctor didn't look at me when he entered the room, but, looked down at the folder he held in his hands. Equally, he never introduced himself, or offered his hand to shake mine, which is typically normal procedure. I found that to be extremely strange. Even more offensive is that the only time he looked in my direction was when I pointed to the left side of my throat and neck when I showed him where my pain and swelling were. Other than that, he did not once look me in the eyes.

Secondly, ENT No. 1 was either very scatter-brained or had Attention Deficit Disorder because he didn't listen to anything I was repeatedly telling him during our discussion. For example, he asked me three times, *"Do you smoke?"* or, *"Are you a smoker?"* when I had already responded to him, *"No I don't."* and, "*No, I'm not.*" two previous times during the same conversation. And, finally, ENT No. 1 did not have one clue when I asked him what could be causing the hurtful throat pain ***on only one side of my throat,*** and why my upper neck was so swollen on the same side. In fact, as outright insane as this sounds, this ENT doctor—who's treated several Head and Neck Cancer patients as a part of his practice, and whose job it is to know Cancer-related symptoms and to recognize the disease—shamefully went with my prior two physicians' notes, and attributed my swollen neck and one-sided sore throat to *Bronchitis* – not something serious like *Cancer. Looking back at this, you have GOT to be kidding me!*

This pitiful, snobbish excuse of a doctor told me that he was certain of his opinion and that he was dead-set on not pursuing it any further. That made me feel ***very*** uncomfortable, so I told him that I did not agree with his opinion because I knew my body, and I knew that this had to be something else. Just as I expected from his body language and demeanor, he gave me that "holier than thou" look and questioned how I, a patient, could question him, a doctor. Needless to say, when this fiasco ended, I marched straight up to the Medical Director's office and reported his disgraceful behavior, told her that I wanted him removed from my case, and I insisted that I see the Head of the Ear, Nose, and Throat (Otolaryngology) Department.

ENT No. 2 Introduction and My CT Scan Results

On March 29, 2004, I finally received the CT Scan that my Primary Care doctor had ordered two weeks earlier. Also around the end of March, the Hospital Medical Director contacted me to tell me that, per my request, she had reassigned my case to the Head of the Otolaryngology Department, a doctor whom I shall refer to here as ENT No. 2. Soon after, on April 9, 2004, I attended my appointment with ENT No. 2. In contrast to ENT No. 1, ENT No. 2 was a very personable, congenial, and respectful professional, and, he was sure to introduce himself, shake my hand, and give me his total attention while we spoke. He told me that he was aware of my bad experience with the prior ENT doctor, and he offered his apologies on behalf of the Department for the other doctor's behavior. Following that, ENT No. 2 said to me, *"You look like you're in great shape at 52 years of age."* He then asked what I do to take care of myself, after which I told him that I lift weights each day, eat only healthy foods, and that I don't smoke or drink alcohol. He then told me, *"Good for you, it shows."* I thanked him for both his apology and the kind words.

Subsequent to our introductory conversation, ENT No. 2 and I got down to discussing my medical issues, during which I told him about the symptoms of my ***left-sided sore throat*** and neck swelling that I had endured since January, three months previous. I then told him that I was very frustrated because the physicians I had seen kept trying to pin my condition on either Bronchitis or Sinusitis, when I knew that it had to be something else. After listening to me, he said that he understood my concerns and told me that we would try to get to the bottom of it. ENT No. 2 then mentioned that he had received the results of my CT Scan, and he explained that among other items, the report indicated, *"Necrotic Lymphadenopathy in the left Anterior Cervical Triangle with two enlarged necrotic Lymph Nodes between 12mm and 2cm in size."* (Translation: Necrotic Lymphadenopathy is a term meaning "disease of the Lymph Nodes," and is typically used with swollen or enlarged Lymph Nodes. The causes could be due to infection, auto-immune disease, or Cancer malignancy). ***Ding, Ding, Ding, did you catch that? – "Cancer malignancy."***

Two enlarged Lymph Nodes on my neck was not surprising, as I knew that they had been causing my neck to swell up. But, the *real* question was, what was causing my Lymph Nodes to increase? When I asked this question of ENT No. 2, he could not give me an answer. However, he did tell me that he wanted to schedule me for a Laryngoscopy (a diagnostic procedure to view my Larynx (Voice Box) with a lighted scope). He stated that he also wanted to perform Biopsy Surgery on me, as he wanted to obtain some tissue samples of my neck areas in an effort to verify what may be causing my one-sided, persistent sore throat. Before I departed his office, ENT No. 2 wrote me prescriptions for an antibiotic and a painkiller in the hopes that they would help bring me some relief. After my office visit with ENT No. 2, it took awhile for the hospital to fit me in to their packed Surgery docket. Finally, on April 23, 2004, under the knife I went.

My First Biopsy Surgery with ENT No. 2

When I had Biopsy Surgery on April 23, 2004, it had been three months since I first sought medical attention, and two months since I saw my initial doctor. Yet, I still had no medical explanation, nor a diagnosis as to what might be responsible for my throat pain or the reason for my enlarged Lymph Nodes. My Caregiver drove me to the hospital that morning, as frustrated as me, that with all of the skilled physicians, advanced medical techniques, and state-of-the-art equipment at their disposal, after three long months of searching for the "smoking gun," we were no nearer than we were on day-one. We hoped that the tissue samples that ENT No. 2 was going to take from my neck ***(from my throat and Lymph Nodes on the left side, I had presumed)*** that morning would help point us in the right direction.

The Biopsy Surgery that I had on April 23 would be the first of numerous such surgeries that I would have throughout my Cancer journey. When the patient is already suffering from immense throat pain, the last thing they need is some sort of invasive trauma to that area. But, thankfully, the tissue removal is performed under General Anesthesia, and the sampling *must* be accomplished to verify either the presence or absence of many diseases within the body, including Cancers. A doctor's opinion can be suitable for identifying *possible* medical conditions, based on physical exams, blood tests, images, and other diagnostic tools. But, *proof-positive diagnoses can only be obtained thru microscopic laboratory examination of actual tissue samples* removed from suspect areas within the patient's body.

Thankfully, my initial Biopsy Surgery went well and without complications. The next step would be for me to wait for the Biopsy results, which I gradually learned would be one of the most difficult, worrying, and frustrating elements of my entire Cancer journey. It's actually very similar to the, *"She loves me, she loves me not"* games we played as kids with the petals of a flower. However, the, *"I have Cancer, I don't have Cancer"* feelings I experienced while awaiting the results of each of my Biopsy Surgeries were much more difficult because there was just so much at-stake. In any event, following my initial Surgery, ENT No. 2 scheduled me for a post-Surgery visit in his office for May 6. It was during this consultation that he would be sharing with me the results (dated April 26) of my Biopsy exam.

My Biopsy Results – ENT No. 2's Big Mistakes!

On the morning of May 6, 2004 when ENT No. 2 entered the examination room where I had been waiting, we both exchanged our pleasantries, and then, with a big smile, he said, *"I've got good news for you Butch! The Laryngoscopy results were clear and the Biopsy Pathology came back Benign." "'Benign,' as in not Cancerous?"* I asked him. *"Yes,"* he said, *"there was no Cancer." "What a relief,"* I responded, *"because my family has a history of Cancer and this is such a strange set of symptoms that I was actually starting to worry that I might have something serious like that." "You have nothing to worry about, Butch,"* he reassured me, *"you're as healthy as can be."* I thanked him for his optimism and told him that that news was good to hear. But, I then asked him how he took the Biopsy samples from my swollen Lymph Nodes, because I told him that I didn't see any external indications of surgical incisions, nor, did I feel any new tenderness or pain on the inside of my throat. Then, I inquired—as I had asked all of the doctors whom I had seen for these issues—*what the heck was causing the throat pain on my left side, and why were my Lymph Nodes swollen?* At this juncture, ENT No. 2 sat down in a chair, thought a moment, and responded to each of my questions.

ENT No. 2 began, *"The reason that you don't have any signs of surgery near your swollen Lymph Nodes or on the inside of your throat on the left side, is because I only took tissue samples from the right side of your throat."* I listened very attentively so that I didn't miss or misunderstand anything he said. He then said, *"The CT Scan you took on March 29th indicated that you had an uncharacteristic Right Vallecula, so I took tissue samples from that area in an effort to determine what may be the cause."* (Translation: A Vallecula is a depression just behind the root of the tongue that's between the folds in the throat. These depressions serve as "spit traps," where saliva is temporarily held to prevent initiation of the swallowing reflex). He followed that up with, *"I didn't take any tissue samples from the left side of your throat as nothing abnormal was indicated on the CT."*

"As for what might be causing the pain on the left region of your throat and what is responsible for your swollen Lymph Nodes," the doctor added, *"we're not sure."* Talk about a swift kick in the balls! How I wished that my Caregiver were with me at that time to listen to all of that with me, and to corroborate that this was actually taking place. I honestly felt as though I were in a parallel universe, a bad nightmare, or, down an *Alice in Wonderland* rabbit hole, but, I was definitely listening to these incomprehensible words coming out

of the doctor's mouth. When ENT No. 2 finished speaking, my jaw dropped. I was in complete skepticism of what I was hearing, and I, without a doubt, could not make a bit of sense of what he was telling me. *"Doctor,"* I told him very emphatically, *"if you are only going by what the CT Scan results said, remember that they also indicated that I have two* ***very enlarged Lymph Nodes*** *on the left region of my neck, which are also very visible, as you can see."* with me pointing to them. *"Not only that,"* I said, *"but* ***all*** *of my throat pain—as I've told you and all of the other doctors all along—is only on my* ***LEFT*** *side,* ***NOT*** *the right. Knowing this, why in the world would you* ***only*** *sample the* ***right side*** *of my throat while you had me in the operating room, when I've been telling you clearly that my* ***left side*** *has been in pain and swollen these last four months?"* ENT No. 2 could tell that I was pissed off, and rightfully so. There was no excuse for this.

You could hear a pin drop, the exam room was so quiet. The doctor, with his head drooped within his hands, stared at the floor as I waited for his response to my intense—but justified—questioning. I am no doctor, but, doctor or not, I have the common sense to know that if the left side of a person's throat or neck is hurting for four or so months, that, most likely, something not-too-good on the left side is causing it. I know about "referred pain," but, I knew for a fact that nothing on my *right side* was creating soreness and swelling on my *left.* Unquestionably, the source of my intense pain had to be located on the left side of my neck, but, somehow, ENT No. 2 missed it.

Just how bad ENT No. 2 blew it during my Biopsy Surgery and Laryngoscopy on April 23, 2004, was further evidenced by the notes that the physician entered into my medical record on April 27. By his own account, ENT No. 2 wrote, "*A complete Laryngoscopy was performed examining the patient's oral cavity, Glottic Regions, Oropharynx, Hypopharynx, Supraglottic Regions, Vallecula, and Periform Sinuses. The patient had some inflamed looking tissue in the right Vallecula that corresponded to an abnormality on his neck CT scan. This was biopsied and sent to pathology. The remainder of the tissue was normal in appearance. A bimanual palpation was performed and his Nasopharynx and* ***<u>his base of tongue were clear.</u>*** *The CT scan also showed* ***<u>evidence of a cystic mass in patient's left cervical region</u>.*** *This was palpable with intraoral bimanual exam."* (The highlights of the text in these last three lines are mine).

ENT No. 2, in his post-procedural notes, states erroneously that, ***"his base of tongue was clear,"*** when it was not. The Base of my Tongue was, ultimately, where my cancerous Tumor was located when a doctor that I saw for a Second Opinion discovered it a short while later. Secondly, while ENT No. 2, did correctly note that I had a, ***"cystic mass in patient's left cervical region,"*** he failed to act on that fact in the operating room by not taking any Biopsy samples of tissues from the mass. That "mass," by the way, just so-happened to be my Lymph Nodes that had been distended for about four months. For obvious reasons, these two grave oversights by ENT No. 2 could have cost me my life. They didn't, only because I took him to task.

ENT No. 2's Admission of Mistakes and Apology

"I'm sorry, Butch," ENT No. 2 spoke, as he raised his head from his hands, *"you are correct. I should have biopsied the Lymph Nodes on the left side of your neck. I took samples based on the CT scan of the questionable areas on the right side of your throat, but, I also should have taken tissue samples from the left side. Again, I am very sorry and I can completely understand why you are upset."* I could see the sadness in ENT No. 2's face as he apologized, but, the fact of the situation is that he *F'd up* big time. A person can be given a lousy haircut by their stylist, or, maybe, served a hamburger with onions after they ask that they *"hold the O,"* but, those mistakes can be righted and are not life-threatening. Physicians, however, must be held to a much higher standard because, quite frankly, they can hold a person's life in *their* hands. One screw-up with them, and it could be "lights out." And, unfortunately, that occurs much too often, even in this country. *"Doctor, I appreciate your apologies,"* I responded, *"and I'm glad you realize why I am frustrated and upset. I have had these problems for four months now, and you're the fourth doctor I have seen, but, none of you can figure out what's going on with me. What I want to know is when are we going to test the left side of my neck or throat, because it* ***really*** *hurts and nothing is helping?"*

Before I gave ENT No. 2 a chance to answer my question, I told him, *"Unfortunately now doctor, I don't know if I have faith in you. I mean, I requested that my case be assigned to you because, as you know, I had no confidence in ENT No. 1 due to his dishonorable behavior. And, now, here I am with you, the Chairman of the ENT Department, and you do this. Now I don't know what to think." "I can completely understand why you would feel this way, Butch,"* the doctor said to me, *"but, I promise you that if you continue with me, I won't let you down again. We will locate what is causing your pain and swelling, and, once we do, we will do what we can to fix it."* At that moment, I was a complete mess, and my mind was plagued with disbelief, coupled with confusion as to what I should do next. First of all, I was a *healthy* guy, which made the relentlessness of the pain and the swelling of my neck, all the more abnormal and significant. Secondly, I was facing a cumbersome, impersonal *medical machine* and a doctor who is the Head of the Department in whom I have lost all confidence. *"I appreciate your commitment to find whatever it is that is causing my problems, but, before we do anything else on this, I would like to speak once again with the Medical Director." "Of course,"* ENT No. 2 said, *"I completely understand how you feel."*

My Second Meeting with the Medical Director, and Proceeding with ENT No. 2 &Biopsy No. 2

Subsequent to my disappointing discussion with ENT No. 2 on May 6, I saw the Medical Director of the hospital facility where I had seen both ENT doctors. ENT No. 2 had already approached her to tell her what had occurred following his and my visit, and she was kind enough to provide her apologies on behalf of the hospital. I told her that I had reservations about continuing with ENT No. 2 on my case because of what had taken place, and I said that the only way I would stay with him is if the HMO and ENT No. 2 commit to do the best job possible to determine what was causing my pain and to help me get over it. The Medical Director told me that she understood my apprehensions, but, assured me that ENT No. 2 and all hospital staff would do their utmost to get to the bottom of my medical condition, and to treat it accordingly once it was discovered. I thanked her for the commitment, and told her that I would continue with ENT No. 2. She said she would have ENT No. 2 contact me to schedule my pre-op visit for my second Biopsy Surgery procedure, which he did. My pre-op was on May 28, and I had my Surgery on June 1, 2004.

Little did I know how that day was soon to change my life…forever.

Fighting Words

By Butch Sickler ©
June 2004

Looking beyond my eyes
as if to summon my Soul
my Doctor speaks softly
harboring the accumulated pain
of many to whom he has
given this news

The cold dark-alley ambush
of the messenger's words

shock
frighten
anger

and well-intentioned consolation
falls deaf upon a mind clouded
by the unanswerable questions

when?
why?
how?

But there is no time for that now
We have Cancer to kill

My fearful but confident Soul responds –
What do we do and when do we start?

Chapter Fifteen

"D-Day" – My Cancer Diagnosis – *Day-1 of My 3+-Year Cancer Journey*

"Think of a Cancer Diagnosis, not as a Sentence to die, but, as an opportunity to live, once again."

- Butch Sickler

A Cancer Survivor, unless they were a very young child or quite elderly when their Cancer was first diagnosed and disclosed to them, will forever remember the date and location that they received their threatening news. Some of these individuals might accidentally overlook some birthdays, the occasional Wedding Anniversary (God forbid!), or, maybe, even their son's or daughter's recitals or soccer games. But, I assure you, they will *always* be able to recall the day that the extremely heavy weight dropped out of the sky, and, without warning, landed abruptly on their head. From the very moment that the health care professional delivered the news of malignant Cancer to the man, woman, teenager, or child, their world—and that of their loved one, family, and friends—was turned upside down, and would remain forever changed. But…not always changed for the worst.

My "D-Day"

In U.S. history, *"D-Day"* was June 6, 1944. That is the well-known day when Allied forces launched the Invasion of Normandy, which eventually contributed to the overthrow of Nazi Germany and the beginning of the end of World War II. ***My*** *"D-day"*—the date of my Cancer Diagnosis—was just over sixty years later to the day, on

June 7, 2004, and ***my*** *Omaha Beach* was a medical clinic located in Northern Virginia. Even as I write this in 2013—almost nine years later—it's almost like yesterday that I listened to my Ear, Nose, and Throat (ENT) physician utter those fateful words to me: *"I'm sorry, Butch, but you have Cancer."* With those seven troublesome words began a seemingly non-stop journey for over three lengthy years that was, without question, the most challenging, the most agonizing, the most emotionally distressing, and, in the end, the most humbling and rewarding undertaking that I've ever experienced in my life. And, not unlike those victorious American heroes who stormed the deadly beaches at *Colleville-sur-Mer* in France on that unforgettable day in '44 and survived *their* war, I, also, am very grateful to God that I am alive, and that I am able to talk about *my* personal war with Cancer – a conflict in which I eventually became triumphant.

This, then, is the account of how my roughly 3+-year Cancer journey "officially" began after a protracted and frustrating 5-month personal and medical search for the source of my throat pain and my neck swelling. Following a few incorrect opinions and diagnoses on the part of doctors, finally, on June 1, 2004, I went in for my second Biopsy Surgery. It was the outcomes from this Surgery that I hoped would once-and-for-all be able to tell us what had been eliciting the extreme sore throat and Lymph Node swelling on the left side of my neck for over five months. And, sure enough, Life was all too eager to deliver. As it turns out, Life had a very big surprise waiting up its sleeve, and my physician had to be the one to pull it out and discuss it with me. While his responsibility was not too easy to be sure, I'm guessing that my role was just a little bit harder to play. Here is how it all unfolded when I showed up at his office on June 7, 2004, to get the results of my June 1 Surgery, and, to have additional work done.

Biopsy No. 2 Follow-Up Exam with ENT No. 2

My "D Day" actually began as just another ordinary day for me, aside from the excruciating tenderness I was experiencing at the location of my Biopsy Surgeries on my upper left neck area, and, the persistent throat pain on the same side that had been disturbing me for over five months. I attended this appointment with ENT No. 2 for the purpose of him providing me with the outcome of my Biopsy

Surgery that he had performed on June 1, just a few days prior. He also would be taking out the sutures and relieving the swelling that had developed in the Lymph Node region of my neck, just below the jaw line. During the June 1 Biopsy Surgery, ENT No. 2 had cut out some tissue samples and two Lymph Nodes from the left side of my neck in an effort to determine what might be responsible for the sore throat pain that had distressed me for several months. It was my due-diligence and insistence that ENT No. 2 Biopsy my swollen Lymph Nodes that resulted in me having this second Surgery to begin with. He had blown the original Biopsy Surgery on April 23 by not testing the Nodes on the left side of my neck, and, as a result, I had to have a second Surgery on June 1, over one month later. That was a lot of vital time wasted because of ENT No. 2's error in judgment, and, it allowed my Cancer to progress undetected for five additional weeks.

When ENT No. 2 performed this Biopsy Surgery, he did not insert a drain tube as he should have to permit the Lymphatic Serous Fluid to draw off. As a result, the surgical area became unbelievably distended due to the collection of the fluid, and equally as agonizing. Doctors are only human, right, but, common sense (there is that term again) would dictate that if you close off something that you know is going to fill with fluid, more than likely it will swell and grow. And, once it does, it will either explode, or, in the case of people, will hurt like hell until it's relieved. I would be in that latter group. But, even though my horribly swollen and painful neck definitely needed some fast attention by the doctor, it was the Biopsy results that captivated *my* interests. To be frank, I was anticipating that the physician would give me what I fully expected to be the *favorable* outcomes from the tissue Biopsies that he had performed, as well as some insight as to what may be causing my throat pain and my Lymph Nodes to swell.

After ENT No. 2 entered my exam room on the morning of June 7, I observed that he was unusually reserved and appeared to be deep in thought. *"Possibly, he has something heavy weighing on his mind."* I reflected to myself. *"Whatever it is, something isn't right. He's not his usual smiling, talkative self."* I secretly wondered if he still might be feeling considerably ashamed about his oversights that occurred with the initial Biopsy Surgery. After we greeted one other when he first came into the exam room, his eyes and facial reactions revealed how astonished he was to see such a massive protuberance bulging from my neck. And, he appeared to be equally as perceptive when he observed the discomfort that I was realizing because of the violent swelling. The doctor continued to remain extremely quiet as he carefully evaluated and palpated my neck bulge, but, I broke the silence by asking him how he was going to relieve the swelling and pain. He told me that he would first take out the stitches, and then he would aspirate the fluid, which he would do by first preparing the site antiseptically, and deadening the area with local anesthetic.

Following standard out-patient surgical procedures, ENT No. 2 methodically removed the sutures from the laceration, and he then proceeded to empty the big, hurting bulge with a *super large syringe with an extremely large needle.* Quite honestly, I was amazed at the extraordinarily large quantity of Lymphatic Fluid that he sucked out of me with that "mother of all syringes." Finally, with that avoidable procedure having been accomplished, the swollen area continued to remain extremely tender and painful. But, at least, thank God, I felt confident that my neck was not going to *detonate.* However, I was still quite concerned that the doctor had not yet given me my Biopsy results; nor, had he attempted to explain the source of my sore throat or the cause of the swollen Lymph Nodes that he had biopsied.

Dropping the "C Bomb" on Me

After the doctor had drained the fluid from my smarting neck growth and covered the region with some sterile gauze dressings, he continued to be surprisingly withholding of information. That is, he spoke very little unless I asked him specific questions about what he had just done with my swollen neck. I still had not asked him about the outcome of my Surgical Biopsies, as I figured that he would tell me in due time – that was, after all, the reason for the appointment that morning. However, I would quickly find out the rationale for his restrained demeanor. He would be informing me of the not-so-good results of my Neck Lymph Node Biopsies from the piece of paper—which I soon found out was a Laboratory Pathology Report—that he was holding in his hands. A paper that would soon change my life.

When that moment-of-truth finally arrived, ENT No. 2 sat down in front of me, glanced up from the report he was holding, and looked me squarely in the eyes. With no further adieu, he eventually mustered up the personal compassion and the professional sense-of-duty to deliver the message that he had certainly been dreading since first receiving the Pathology Report, himself. With the soft but firm voice of someone who has said these words to no-telling-how-many-patients, ENT No. 2 uttered them to me: ***"I'm sorry Butch, but you have Cancer."*** His matter-of-fact, but concerned, words kept ringing in my ears. Then, recounting directly from the Pathology Report, he further elaborated on the Biopsy Surgery findings to tell me that my Cancer had been categorized as a, ***"Metastatic Poorly Differentiated Squamous Cell Carcinoma with Unknown Primary Site."***

While delivering those words, the doctor seemed to look past my eyes, as if trying to peer deeply into my soul. He knew too well, based on my excellent health history, that my insides were churning by what he had told me and he did his best, with his earnest focus on my reaction to the news, to summon any sort of resolve that I could muster. *"Based on what we know right now, Butch, you have what is considered to be a Head and Neck Cancer, and it appears to be advanced."* ENT No. 2 continued, as he seriously overestimated my ability to make any sense of, much less to comprehend, what he was telling me. This was information that I could have lived my full life without, and, this stark disclosure was even more troublesome when I thought of the discussion ENT No. 2 and I had on April 6 after my first Biopsy Surgery when I expressed my uneasiness about Cancer. During that conversation, ENT No. 2 clearly told me, concerning my potentiality for Cancer, *"You have nothing to worry about, Butch, you're as healthy as can be."* Obviously those former words of his were not backed up, completely erroneous, and would come back to haunt him with the revelation of my Cancer diagnosis. *"This is why he was so quiet when he first came in the room."* I soon realized.

Shock, Questions, and Fear, but No Logical Explanation for My Cancer

"Head and Neck Cancer?" I loudly questioned ENT No. 2 as I conjured up scenarios in my mind of what exactly was meant by that term. I had never heard of that type of Cancer before, and, quite truthfully, just the sound of it scared me half to death. Let's see, the

neck envelops the throat, tongue, esophagus, wind pipe, spinal cord, vocal cords, nerves, major arteries, and a bunch of other goodies that are necessary to help us breathe, eat, drink, taste, talk, swallow, and, well…live, in general. And the ***head***? Well, that's also pretty darned essential because it happens to enclose the brain, eyes, mouth, nose, glands, ears, a few marbles in my case, and, all the *wiring* for God-knows-what-else is pretty compulsory for living a normal life. Now, low-and-behold, I find out that I have Cancer somewhere within that miraculous mixture of critical body parts. *"What a great reward I've received for my years of eating healthy, working out daily, not using tobacco or drinking alcohol, and not taking baths downstream from the discharge of a radioactive chemical plant."* I thought to myself.

To say that I was blind-sided by my Cancer diagnosis would be the definitive understatement! Never in my wildest dreams did I ever expect those words to come out of my physician's mouth *to me, about me.* I would have understood just about anything else but that. But, he did say I had Cancer, and I was left to sit there and process thoughts so unbelievable that they were instantly incomprehensible to my logical mind. These were the same "2+2 = 5" type of thoughts that one may have when something completely illogical takes place, such as a pig dropping from the sky, or a politician actually keeping his campaign promises. This was ludicrous and would have been my worst nightmare had I actually been sleeping. But, I was very wide awake, and ENT No. 2, having duly informed me of my fate, did what he could to console me. My brain and my heart, however, were racing a million miles an hour, hearing, but not listening.

I was thoroughly bewildered on one hand, frightened on the other, and I even felt very angry – angry at not only the Cancer for violating my body—as would be expected—but also terribly upset at my body for allowing the Cancer to occur. How a person who takes fantastic care of their body for most of their life like me gets Cancer, was unfathomable to me. As much as I attempted to pay attention to ENT No. 2 as he tried to reassure me with his words, my mind was much too active processing the information and attempting to make sense of something that, truthfully, defied practical explanation. The questions, *"Why?" "What?" "How?"* and *"When?"* all came very quickly to my mind, but, of course, there were no answers to be had. Even though I had many questions that I wanted to ask him, I was so busy thinking of possible causes and my unknown fate that I found it hard to speak. It's like winning the Lottery, but just the opposite.

A Family History of Cancer, but It Didn't Directly Cause Mine

Having been entirely shocked by ENT No. 2 with the mind-boggling news of my Cancer diagnosis that morning, my mind spun in all different directions trying to sort out what might have caused it in the first place, especially considering my allegiance to health and fitness. Drawing blanks, and thinking of no reasonable place, thing, or occurrence that may have led to my Cancer, I did eventually think back to some members of my extended family—both Grandmothers, my Aunt, and my Mom—all of whom came down with varied forms of Cancer. Each of these brave women gave their Cancers the fights of their lives. Unfortunately, for our Grandmothers and for my Aunt, their brave efforts weren't quite enough to ultimately win their wars. It was extremely devastating to lose our Nana and Momo, and Aunt Connie, but, we were truly blessed that our Mom, Betty, thankfully, survived her Cancer for over 38 long, but content and hopeful years. When Mom passed on April 13, 2012, it was not due to Cancer, but, was caused by some other natural body processes that just gave out.

Nana, our Grandmother on our Mother's side of the family, unfortunately perished from Pancreatic Cancer, while Catherine and Connie, my Grandmother and Aunt on my Dad's side, did ultimately give way to their Lung and Breast Cancers, respectively. Regardless of this apparent family history of Cancer, however, and, despite the fact that I did not know much about heredity and Cancer when ENT No. 2 gave me the bad news on June 7, 2004, I do know now that I did not come into my Head and Neck Cancer from my ancestors – I, in reality, did that all on my own. However, that is not to say that the influence of my relatives' Cancer incidences may not have played a role in the development of my disease. While there was assuredly no direct link between my relatives' Cancers and my own, perhaps, any cancerous genes passed down thru my family have placed me (and, possibly, my Brothers and Sister, for that matter) at a greater risk to contract *any form* of Cancer, assuming that additional Risk Factors may have come into play. To be honest, however, there is no way of knowing either way, so, I have resigned myself to the belief that my Cancer was caused, not by my heredity, but by something—or some things—that occurred in my own past, and, even, Random Chance.

Quiet Time to Think

Realizing that I might require some time alone following our brief discussion after the diagnosis, ENT No. 2 left me by myself in the exam room for quite awhile to reflect upon the words that he had just delivered. Prior to leaving the exam room, the doctor patted me on the shoulder and told me that, *“Everything is going to be okay.” “Easy for him to say.”* I recall thinking, as I continued to sit in utter amazement and stare aimlessly at the cream-colored walls and pink cabinets that had surely borne witness to this grim situation so many times before. On his way out of the room, the doctor handed me my Pathology Report, which, in vivid black and white, and, as casually as if it were a flier advertising cookies and brownies at a Bake Sale, told me that patient, *Ronald C. Sickler,* was found, thru biopsy tissue sampling of the Neck Lymph Node area, to have been diagnosed via Pathology, with a ***“Metastatic Poorly Differentiated Squamous Cell Carcinoma with Unknown Primary Site.”*** In retrospect, I was very grateful that ENT No. 2 had permitted me those few minutes in the room alone after he informed me of my diagnosis. That brief respite of “alone time” gave me a very important opportunity to think things through, to get over and past my initial emotional responses, and to pull myself together, both physically and mentally.

While the description of my Cancer on the Pathology Report sounded very frightening at face value, I did entirely comprehend—reluctantly—the part about me having malignant Cancer somewhere in my body. But, what *really* horrified the heck out of me were the words on the report, ***“Unknown Primary Site,”*** and the physician’s judgment regarding my Cancer most likely being a ***“Head and Neck Cancer.”*** *“What if the Cancer started in my Brain, or my Lungs, or my Pancreas?”* I dreadfully pondered in my mind, as I, expectedly, thought the worst of my predicament. I had so many questions and so few answers – at least right then. A person usually doesn’t give these sorts of things much thought until it is *their* turn in the Cancer hopper. I was both disorientated and frightened for a significant time after ENT No. 2 delivered the revelation to me. To the physician's credit, though, before he departed the exam room minutes earlier, he did aim his best to tell me what he could, to answer my questions as best he could, and to console me to the best of his ability. However, without the doctor around, the brief recess that he permitted me was just what I needed to reassess the situation, and to think more clearly about the questions I wanted to ask and the attitude I needed to have.

Transformation from 'Victim' to 'Victor' Mindset

When ENT No. 2 reentered the exam room to look in on me following my personal, introspective moments, he found me to be a completely different person than the one he had left just a short time before. I then felt confident and in-control, and I knew that I could tackle this Cancer challenge just as I did so many other things in life – I considered it simply as another "project" that I would undertake, systematically and consistently, until I could bring it to its successful conclusion. In the case of my Cancer, of course, this meant that the "project" would not be "completed" until my Cancer was thoroughly destroyed and eliminated from my body. In other words, not unlike my Mom, who was a 32-year Breast Cancer survivor at the time of my diagnosis, I, too, could only see myself as a survivor when this was all said and done. When the doctor left the exam room earlier, I was confused, worried, and, pretty much a sobbing basket-case, not really knowing which way to turn. Then, within the period of just a few minutes, he saw a person who had transformed into an unafraid, more self-assured individual, who was prepared to do whatever was necessary to meet this Cancer thing head-on. Still sitting on the chair when ENT No. 2 reentered the room, I got up, stood in front of him, and looked him squarely in the eyes. Without any hesitation, I then stated to him, very matter-of-factly and to his surprise, *"This Cancer picked the wrong person to fuck with. I'm going to kick its ass!"*

No-doubt astonished by my sudden sense of bravado and my obvious change in demeanor, a small smirk came across the doctor's face. He nodded his agreement with my bold prophecy, and uttered softly, *"It is good to be strong and optimistic. That's half the battle won right there."* While I still had the doctor's undivided attention in the exam room, and, despite my new-found self-confidence, I told him that I had read the Pathology Report, and that I still had a few additional questions I needed to ask him. ENT No. 2 welcomed my inquiries. First, I told him that I was still very concerned about the words, ***"Unknown Primary Site"*** that stood out in large, bold letters on that life-altering piece of paper. I asked him what, precisely, was meant by those three words, even though I had a pretty good idea of what he was going to tell me. And, secondly, I asked him to clarify what, ***"Advanced"*** meant, relative to my own Cancer diagnosis.

Don't Know Where the Primary Tumor is, But Do Know That It's Advanced

Concerning my question about that terminology, ***"Unknown Primary Site"*** on my Pathology Report, ENT No. 2 explained that while malignant Cancer was identified in the Biopsy samples that he had taken and submitted for examination from the Lymph Node area of my neck following the June 1 Surgery, the results did not indicate conclusively where within my body the Cancer had originated. The doctor suggested that the Cancer had probably spread to my Lymph Nodes from another location in my body—and most likely from the area of my head or neck—but with only Biopsy tissue sample results solely from my Lymph Nodes to use for confirmation, he concluded, *"There is no way of identifying the specific location of the Primary Tumor in your body without additional testing and examination."*

I grabbed onto the words, *"Primary Tumor"* while he spoke, as that was the first time that ENT No. 2 had uttered that term during our discussions. Just hearing the mention of that word, *tumor,* raised my "fear factor" a few more degrees. Of course I had heard the word *"tumor"* spoken in conjunction with Cancer before, but that's when the realization actually hit home for ***me***: *"I have a tumor just like all those other people with Cancer. My God, I have a Cancer Tumor!"* I reflected to myself. In relation to my question about his statement that my Cancer is, ***"Advanced,"*** ENT No. 2 told me that Cancers are Staged, Graded, or Classified by medical scientists and physicians, based on their level of progression and spread within the body. He stated that the Staging system being used typically classifies Cancers from Level 0 to Level 4, with Level 0 referring to those pre-Cancers that could become cancerous if left ignored. Level 1, he said, is the least invasive and localized (hasn't spread to other parts of the body) and, that Level 4 Cancers are the most intense and, usually, the most difficult to treat. Level 2 is less severe than Level 3, and so on. He said that physicians and scientists utilize the Stage of the Cancer, in addition to other diagnostic information, to determine the most ideal methods for treating each individual's particular form of Cancer. In the instance of Head and Neck Cancers like mine, the doctor told me that if the Cancer spreads to the Lymph Nodes, it typically is graded as a Stage 3 or 4, and is classified as an, *"Advanced Stage Cancer."*

"Just great," I thought to myself, *"not only did I get Cancer from out of nowhere, but **MY** Cancer just has to be on the scary end of the grading scale." "Stage 4 Head and Neck Cancers,"* ENT No. 2 added, "*are generally those Cancers that initiate somewhere in the mouth, nasal area, or throat, and can spread through the Lymphatic or Circulatory system and metastasize in the Lungs. Brain Cancers are not considered as Head and Neck Cancers,"* he stated, *"as those Cancers have their own classification."* When ENT No. 2 told me about Stage 4 Head and Neck Cancer progressing to the Lungs, I did feel an ironic, but nevertheless, authentic, sense of relief, because it meant that my *advanced* Cancer had apparently not made it that far. Had the Cancer manifested itself in one or in both of my Lungs, I'm sure that one of the various diagnostic scans or exams to which I had submitted over the last many months would have indicated any such activity, and, that it would have been "discovered" by some medical professional at some juncture (one can only hope!) and I would have been notified. Thankfully, that was one phone call I *did not* receive.

The Tumor's Not in the Lungs, and Probably Not in the Brain – So, Where Is It?

From what I knew and had heard about Lung Cancer, it was typically one seriously tough cookie to crumble. My specific Cancer was apparently the equivalent of me being shot with a bullet that just missed my vital organ (my Lungs), with me surviving the potentially fatal wound. Close, but, thankfully, not close enough. I was further privately relieved by the words of ENT No. 2 that Brain Cancers are not included within the "Head and Neck Cancer" family. That news seemed to me like yet another bullet dodged. These two providential revelations made me realize, right then and there, that I will need to start counting my blessings when and where I can get them. *"As bad as things may seem with Cancer,"* I reasoned, *"they can always be much worse."* My questions having been answered, I knew that my situation was just as I had surmised: The physicians had no definite idea where my Cancer initiated, but, they did know that it was in an "advanced" phase, rather than, *"fresh out of the box,"* and, that there was a pretty good likelihood that its originating location might be in my mouth, nasal area, or throat, vs. in other areas of my body.

Going out on a limb, and, as expected, thinking the worst, as people are often prone to do when dealing with "unknowns," I asked ENT No. 2 if it were possible that the Cancer could be elsewhere, in another critical organ within my body. Being the tactful diplomat he was, who had, most likely, been down this very road with numerous previous Cancer patients, he opted not to speculate in answering my question. He also probably recalled the grave disservice he did to me when he incorrectly stated during my prior post-Biopsy consultation that *I was much too healthy to get Cancer.* However, ENT No. 2 did reassure me, that, most likely—and considering the symptoms in my throat and neck—my disease did originate in that location. ENT No. 2, aware of the concerns in my voice and questioning, tried to assure me, *"Your Primary Tumor will definitely be located through further examination and testing, and once it is identified, it will be treated aggressively." "Okay doctor,"* I said, *"I'll trust you on this one."*

ENT No. 2 Exam of My Throat Comes up Empty

Thinking logically (which is one of my biggest faults), I then asked ENT No. 2 if it was possible that the tumor could be what has been causing the pain on the left side of my throat for several weeks. He said, *"That scenario is a definite possibility, but, I will first have to perform a physical examination in the office to help determine if that might be the situation."* ENT No. 2 did follow-through with a physical exam of my throat by using a tongue depressor and a mini-flashlight that morning, and he did palpate the rear end of my tongue as far as he could with gloved fingers (which, of course, stimulated my gag reflex). He then told me that he did not see or feel anything irregular. And, because he viewed or felt nothing out of the ordinary during this basic, physical diagnostic exam, ENT No. 2 all but ruled out the likelihood of my Cancer being the culprit responsible for my sore throat. Which begged the question, *"If you feel or see nothing wrong down there, what **IS** the cause of my constant sore throat?"*

Still Throat Pain and Swelling – Still No Answers

When I asked ENT No. 2 what could be responsible for the persistent sore throat pain that I had suffered on ***only*** the left side of my throat for the former five months, he honestly could not come up with a reasonable or meaningful explanation. I remember thinking to myself, *"This is not just an ordinary MD. This is an Ear, Nose, and Throat Specialist who certainly deals with these signs and symptoms as part of his regular daily practice, and yet, he cannot explain why I have had unrelenting pain on the left side of my throat, or, why my Lymph Nodes had been so swollen."* I was literally dumbfounded by this realization. At first, I had to convince a doctor back in March of 2004 to order a scan of my neck, and then, there I was that June with the ***Head*** of the ENT Department—after I had had to suffer with one slip-up after another—and he hadn't noticed anything new about my throat pain since my first appointment with him in April. I've heard that Medicine is not an exact science, and this made me a believer.

As exasperating and unbelievable as this crazy scenario was beginning to become, I truly felt in my heart-of-hearts that my throat pain and my Cancer were somehow connected. I mean, it only made sense, for what other explanation could there be? *"If I can see it so clearly,"* I asked myself, *"why in the hell can't these doctors, whose job it is to notice such things?"* My logical line of thinking was that if 2 + 2 = 4, then, Cancer + tumor = left side throat pain. But, despite my mounting exasperations, I was left with no choice but to defer to the physician's knowledge and expertise before drawing any of my own conclusions. So, I took ENT No. 2 at his word that my Primary Tumor would be located and treated, and I told myself I would hope for the best. Following this personal commitment, I then asked the doctor, *"What do we do now, and how soon can we start?"* I didn't realize it at the time, but it was at that very moment that the planning process for my Cancer treatment got underway. It also was when I reaffirmed my personal commitment to *kick my Cancer's ass.*

Important Next Steps – First, Find My Tumor

In response to my questions about our next steps and when we could get started taking those steps, ENT No. 2 told me that his initial recommendation would be that I submit to further testing and examination in an effort to locate the Primary Tumor, which, in his professional judgment, was situated somewhere within my Head and Neck regions. *"Nothing can happen to properly address the Cancer until we can determine where it formed to begin with. We must first identify the Primary Tumor so that we will know where to direct our attention."* said the doctor. For once, something sounded sensible to me, which prompted this reflection, *"Just like any other problem in life, you must first determine the source before you can take steps to fix it. What pertains to a toilet leak apparently also holds true for Cancer."* I sadly lamented to myself. *"Once the tumor is located,"* ENT No. 2 continued, *"I may have to first perform a Radical Neck-Dissection Surgery as a precaution to remove any cancerous tissue remaining in the Lymph Node area on your neck just below the jaw line, where I had taken the biopsy samples." "OK – makes sense."*

Continuing with his extemporaneous explanation of potential treatments to get rid of my Cancer, ENT No. 2 told me, *"Following your Surgery, I will recommend that you receive Chemotherapy and Radiation Therapy, either in combination with one another, or, only Radiation alone, to help eliminate the Cancer."* The Chemotherapy, he mentioned, would be administered intravenously, and should kill any cancerous cells that the Surgery didn't remove, as well as any stray Cancer cells elsewhere in my body. Before I could receive any treatments, however, he stated again that the Primary Tumor would first have to be found, as the Surgery and radiation would have to be directed at that specific site to destroy the cancerous cells, and to be of any benefit. ENT No. 2 then told me that our next step would be to begin scheduling more diagnostic tests to try to locate the tumor, and, consultations with an Oncologist and a Radiation Oncologist.

My Turn in the Cancer Hopper

I acknowledged what ENT No. 2 told me, and, actually, was somewhat familiar with the three treatment modalities he mentioned, because I clearly remembered my Mom having to submit to Surgery for her two Breast Cancer Mastectomies during the 1970s, and, to a course of Radiation Therapy for the subsequent treatment of Cancer metastases in bones in her back and her ribs in later years. I also had friends whose family members, including young children, had to run a very similar treatment gauntlet during their own conflicts with the disease. During those experiences, I had been out on the "sidelines" looking in, observing and helping those courageous individuals with their Cancer experiences as best I could during their times of need.

In previous instances when I have been involved with others affected by Cancer, I remembered feeling in my heart and mind, not only the sadness and anxiety that came along with a revelation of the disease—especially when it affected family members and friends—but also the strong hope of a potential victory and the possibility of a full life after. But now, with *my own* Cancer occurrence, it was *my* turn to play in the game. This time around, I would be on the *inside looking out*, and my new perspective, while certainly very scary and unnerving, did, ultimately, give me a good vantage point from which to view the entire "playing field" for my upcoming battles. It would be within this stadium that I, and my support team, would ultimately prepare and carry out my plan to beat and survive my Cancer.

Positive Words and Follow-on Appointments

Before I left the exam room on June 7, 2004, ENT No. 2 told me that his staff would be in touch with me regarding my upcoming consultation appointments that they were going to make for me with an Oncologist and a Radiation Oncologist. Both of those physicians, along with ENT No. 2, would become the "Charter Members" of my Cancer Treatment Medical Team. *"During the interim,"* ENT No. 2 urged me, *"try to think positive and don't be too tough on yourself. That strong body that you've taken such good care of over the years is what's going to help you get through this. Your body will pay you back. You just wait and see."* Finally, the doctor advised me, *"You will have a large team taking care of you every step of the way, but you will also need either a family member or a friend to assist you. There will come a time when you will need their help, so you might want to start thinking of someone who can provide that for you. The role of a Cancer Caregiver isn’t easy,”* he insisted, *“and it takes up lots of time on their part. But, in the end, their assistance will prove invaluable to you.” “I understand completely.”* I told the doctor.

After I sat listening to, and processing in my mind, the vital wisdom and the suggestions that ENT No. 2 had presented to me, I thanked him for his reassuring words and advice. I confessed to the doctor that it would take some time, but, that I was sure that I would eventually get past my feelings of disloyalty and distrust about my body that were bewildering me at that time. I felt that my body had betrayed me after I had taken such good care of it for over 40 years, and, honestly, that hurt. But, I knew that for me and my body to be able to prevail against my Cancer, I would have to rely on both my strong body and my mind to get me through it. *“Knowing myself as I do,”* I told ENT No. 2, *“I will study and consider all the facts-at-hand, and I will do everything that I can to try to turn this negative situation into something positive and favorable. I’ve done it all my life with other things, so I don’t see why I can’t do it with my Cancer as well.”* ENT No. 2 acknowledged my positive words, and voiced his concurrence with my optimistic affirmation. I also mentioned to ENT No. 2, in response to his advice about me getting a Caregiver, that I had a girlfriend who may want to be my Caregiver to help and provide me with support during my Cancer predicament. “*Good, you will need that.”* he said, *“She will become a very important lifeline for you as time goes on. At some point you will need some help.”*

“Sounds good, but, how about the additional diagnostic tests to try and find my Primary Tumor, doctor? When will we do that?” I asked, making sure that we did not forget that important step. *“We can do two things.”* ENT No. 2 presented, and then, continued, *“We can schedule you for some additional exploratory exams and testing within the HMO, and, you also have the option of seeing physicians outside the HMO for a second, third, or fourth opinion about your diagnosis.” “Okay doctor,”* I responded, *“I definitely want to have additional testing, and, probably, the sooner the better.”* I asserted. *“But, I also like the idea of getting additional doctor opinions. How does that work?” “For outside opinions,”* ENT No. 2 answered, *“I must first have them all approved so that your health insurance will cover them for specific physicians, and, then, it will be up to you to schedule them.” “But, how will the doctors know what I’m coming*

in for, and how do they let you know what they find?" I asked him, being the clear Cancer virgin that I was. *"Good questions, Butch." "Actually, because I will be the Lead Physician on your case, I will provide your medical information to the doctors you select, and they will correspond back to me with each of their findings. It's standard practice and it works very well."* ENT No. 2 concluded. *"All right, thanks, doctor,"* I replied, *"I'll take you up on both of those offers."*

After this exchange with ENT No. 2, it suddenly dawned on me that the gears were already turning, and that things were speedily taking shape in an effort to track down my Cancer so that we could get down to the business of eradicating it from my body. In the brief amount of time that the physician and I had shared with one another on that morning of June 7, we had accomplished quite a lot. But, I was still as extremely puzzled as ever that I had developed Cancer to begin with, and, that the location of my Cancer Tumor—and, in my opinion, the source of my sore throat—still had yet to be discovered. As I was leaving ENT No. 2's office, I shook his hand and told him, *"I will do anything that needs to be done, and as often as necessary, if it will help me get rid of my Cancer." "That's good,"* he said, "*as there will be a bunch to do to prepare for treatments when the time comes. But, we will take care of everything one piece at a time."* I acknowledged his words, and I told him that I would be waiting for his calls regarding my next round of diagnostic tests and my follow-up appointments with the members of my Medical Team. I also told him that I would research the "Second Opinion" possibility with an outside doctor, and would let him know what I was going to do.

Our Mom's Inspiration – My Beacon of Hope

When I exited ENT No. 2's office on the morning of June 7 with proof-positive medical authentication of my Cancer diagnosis in-hand, I departed with a relatively optimistic, but, nonetheless, still disorientated and troublesome state-of-mind. Other than being told that I had Cancer, not much else of what had happened in the exam room that morning made a lot of sense to me. But, after I got over my initial doubts and the surprise of the "ambush," and, when I was afforded some personal time by the doctor to come to grips with the news, I told myself that I would no longer ask why and how this had happened to me. That nature of thinking, I realized, would get me nowhere, because, truthfully, there were zero answers to be had – at least not then. Instead, I convinced myself that I would focus all of my efforts on getting through this, no matter what it would take. I had an understanding that it would be rough-going, based on what I knew about Cancer, but, I also knew myself and that I don't back down to most things without first giving them an honest fight.

We all know the adrenaline rush we get when we undertake or do something we haven't done for quite some time, or at all, such as shoveling the winter's first heavy snow, exercising our bodies for the first time in a long awhile, doing back-breaking, blister-forming yard work, or, going dancing all night in a classy new pair of stiletto high heels (sorry, but I can't personally attest to *this* one!). A person undertaking these activities and others may not perceive the ensuing aches and pains when they are in the center of them. Our minds and bodies get so preoccupied with the fun or the labors at-hand that we often may ignore or disregard any associated discomfort. When we wake up and get out of bed the next day, however, it's a *completely* different story: Without fail, good ole' Mr. Pain comes a-knockin', and sometimes, *very* loud! I believe that this same sort of suffering certainly applies to a Cancer patient upon receipt of their unwanted diagnosis. The way that I can best describe how my body and mind reacted to the unpredicted, back-handed slap of my Cancer diagnosis on the morning of June 7, is to say that I immediately felt physically violated, emotionally devastated, and unbelievably confounded. This stark revelation sent both my mind and body reeling, and without a question, these feelings came with their own respective versions of anguish and pain. And along with that, came a huge load of fear.

Yes, the feelings of confidence I felt after the visit with ENT No. 2 didn't cover the fact that I was very frightened, and rightfully so—bearing in mind that nasty Cancers had been responsible for the much-too-early demise of quite a few of my earlier family members and friends—but, I also clung tightly to the hope that everything was going to be okay, just as ENT No. 2 had told me it would be. And, I needed to search only as far as my Mom, Betty, for that bright ray of hope. In 2004, the year of my diagnosis, my Mom had already been a 32-year Survivor of Breast Cancer, and, thankfully, had lived thru two Mastectomies and three other Cancer metastases in her bones –

all of which she was able to defeat. So, with our Mom, and the quiet courage that she had exposed throughout the many years of battling Cancer and its after effects, also came the inspiration that I knew I would need to, hopefully, conquer my Cancer as well. *"If Mom can do this,"* I advised myself, *"so can I."* This encouraging reflection would be the beacon to which I would steer, and the lifeline which I would hold, as I navigated the treacherous waters ahead.

Trying to Make Sense of a Dark Alley Ambush

As I continued to walk away from ENT No. 2's area through the hospital halls, I could not help but reflect back upon the outcome of my meeting. I recalled that immediately after the doctor gave me the results of my diagnosis, my mind was racing a million miles an hour, as was my heart. The hurricane of questions, explanations, and frightful thoughts became one constant, energizing blur. Even after I had some time to myself to think about what had happened and to finally pull myself together after receiving the unfavorable news, my focus was aimed so intently at the physician and everything he was telling me, that I had no means of doing or thinking of anything else. I was, for quite some time after delivery of the cancerous revelation, that proverbial "deer caught in the headlights." The predicament was actually quite intense, as things can often be when one is shockingly attacked or blind-sided by something that is potentially destructive. An unanticipated diagnosis of Cancer—the medical equivalent of an ambush in a dark alley—is definitely no exception. But, after things settled down in the exam room, and, when I later exited the doctor's office, the adrenaline rush that had consumed me earlier and that had helped me cover-up much of the anxiety and fear I felt when I first received the diagnosis, was no longer there to help protect me from the truth. Then, it was just my body, my heart, and my mind: Raw, exposed, unfettered emotions, coupled with dread and confusion.

That day, June 7, 2004, was a day that I was certain I would always remember, and one that certainly opened my eyes to some of the sad realities of life, and, that lent credence to that age-old adage, *"Shit happens."* The more that I attempted to make sense of it all, the more frustrating it became. Being an individual who has always attempted to err on the side of caution, rather than undergo a *laissez-*

faire, "come-what-may" approach to live my life, I was thoroughly confounded by what had just happened to me. *"Darned if you do; darned if you don't."* I recollect thinking to myself as I continued to slowly wander through the immense building and towards my car in the parking structure. Entering the elevator, I wondered what I had done, or not done, in my life, to "induce" my Cancer. It also dawned on me that I was due back at my job in the U.S. Government for the rest of the day, and, I knew that my girlfriend would certainly want to hear what she, no-doubt, was thinking would be the *"good"* news about my Biopsy outcome. I considered calling my girlfriend on my cell phone to break the report to her, but, then, told myself that this sort of blockbuster news must be delivered in person, as crazy as it is. *"All of that would take place in due time."* I reasoned, but, first, I knew that my mind had to try to digest the aftermath of the "freight train" that had just hit me head-on. Having in-hand, the convincing, verified proof of the Cancer diagnosis that I had received not more than an hour ago, I felt compelled to take a little time to sit and think about what had just occurred, and, to ponder what may lie ahead.

Taking Time to Sit, to Think, and to Wonder

When I finally made it to the lower level of the hospital after I left ENT No. 2's office that morning, I slowly wandered past the large waiting lobby adjacent to the pharmacy and I rounded a corner into a hallway that led to the garage. Just as I did so, I came across a very delightful and bucolic appearing, "indoor-outdoor" spot that the hospital had provided for all patients and their families. While I had attended prior doctors' appointments at this same facility, I normally scurried right past this area and had never taken the time to explore it and enjoy it for what it was. This was a place in which folks could sit and read, meditate, and talk in peace-and-quiet, removed from the hustle-and-bustle of the hospital's inner sanctum with the television racket and repetitious and annoying P.A. announcements. The area was a pretty large, square atrium that was surrounded by brick walls on two sides, and by two ground-to-ceiling walls of windows on the others. The designers of this unique, peaceful space had also situated four strategically-placed stone-like benches among and below some very beautiful, but geographically-challenged, "jungle"-type plants. It wasn't Hawai'i, but a pretty nice substitute for the time-being.

The enclosed area was additionally capped with a very large, semi-transparent roof, which resembled a solid skylight that allowed the filtered sun to bathe both people and plants alike, while keeping out the Spring and Summer rains and Winter snows. One certainly would not expect to see a semblance of the Rain Forest in Northern Virginia, but this area was a very nice touch, and was just the space that I needed to reflect and attempt to make sense of my new Cancer situation. Slowly surveying the Zen-like surroundings, I walked the circular gravel path and selected a bench near the brick walls on the farthest side from the entrance. I hoped that I would have a bit more privacy there, away from any potential "gawkers" and distractions in the crowded waiting room just beyond the glass partitions.

When I sat down on the warm bench in this lovely, tranquil oasis, it didn't take long for it to slam me again: *"I have Cancer!"* I reminded myself, as I began sobbing quietly, my head cupped in my hands. *"Of all people, **ME**!"* I mused, as if I were trying to extract some sort of sense out of the nonsensical situation. ***ME:*** *Mr. Fitness, Mr. Healthy-Eater, Mr. Vitamin- and Anti-Oxidant-Taker, Mr. Non-Smoker, and Mr. Non-Drinker.* I thought about all of the things that I had done (and not done) for most of my life so that I wouldn't get Cancer or any other destructive diseases. But there I sat, *Mr. Cancer Victim,* Pathology Report in-hand, that, for all intents and purposes, blew all of that "good," healthful, well-intentioned stuff right out of the water. *"Cancer Prevention,"* I recognized right then and there, *"was not quite all that it was cracked up to be, at least in my case."*

The reality of the situation—as unreal as it was—came as an extremely harsh blow, not only to my super-fit body, but also to my typically resilient mind. For the very first time in my life, I began to question and doubt the same body that I had worked so diligently to strengthen and protect. *"If I have done all the 'right' things with my body and life and I **still** got Cancer,"* I attempted to reason, *"how do I keep it from coming back if I am able to overcome it?"* Being the analytical person I am, I tried to take this scientific revelation apart, piece-by-piece, in an effort to come up with coherent answers, or, at least a sensible explanation for it all. But, as I would soon come to realize, there are no logical answers, because, this nasty disease, by its very nature, is not rational or reasonable. It is extremely efficient, and it is very persistent, but, it doesn't make the least bit of sense.

Getting It Together – Thinking Like a Survivor

Still camped beneath the large-leafed umbrella of a splendid palm tree that briefly evoked fond memories of the several beautiful beaches I had visited during my life, my thoughts soon drifted back to the exam room and what had happened just minutes before. In my mind, I began reliving the moments, scene-by-scene, almost as if I were being forced to sit through the twinges caused by a low-budget horror flick. *"How do you prepare for such news?"* I asked myself, as I sat frustrated in the stillness of the peaceful space and attempted to derive some sort of response. *"You don't."* I realized. *"Life serves us surprises like this, and worse, all the time,"* I thought, *"but then it leaves you hanging to fend for yourself." "Do or die," "Life or death,"* I lamented, *"why do so many things have to be so black and white?"* There is no getting Cancer halfway. It's all or nothing.

My thoughts again turned to my courageous Cancer warrior, Mom. I had attempted to be beside my Mom as best I could—even via long distance—during her, then, 32-year battle with the disease, and I recalled how devastating and unforgiving Cancer can be. But, the moment that ENT No. 2 gave me ***my*** shocking news about ***my*** Cancer, much of the knowledge and the experience that I had gained from my Mom's Cancer ordeals, all but evaporated in my mind with ***mine.*** This was ***me*** to whom the doctor delivered the report. Now, it was ***my*** life or death we were talking about. I had taken the news of my diagnosis personally and very hard at the onset. However, I did recollect that after ENT No. 2 had delivered his message to me, and when he had afforded me quiet time to try to comprehend the reality of what had just happened, I stopped asking myself and the doctor, the *"How?"* and *"Why?"* questions. At that juncture, earlier in the exam room, I had managed to muster up the nerve that soldiers often use to disguise their own worries prior to going into battle. Instead, I asked my doctor, *"What do we do, and when can we start?"*

I continued to hang around within the serene confines of the Japanese-style garden without interruption for several introspective minutes. I again started thinking about what may have happened to prompt my Cancer. I also began to speculate on what the future may hold – for me, for my body, and for my life. But, after replaying the proceedings of my appointment in my mind, time and time again, I repetitively came right back to the very same conclusions: *"It didn't matter how, when, or why I got Cancer,"* I reassured myself, *"if the Pathology Report is correct, which I'm sure it is, I **have** Cancer, and there is nothing I can do to change that fact, other than to rid it from my body."* I told myself right then and there that I was not going to dwell on the past or censure myself or my body. *"It is what it is,"* I reasoned, *"and the most important thing that I can do right now,"* I convinced myself, *"is to focus on the future, and to think only about how I'm going to beat this Cancer and become a survivor." "I am a Cancer survivor."* I kept saying to myself, as my mind attempted to wrap itself around this new—and at least for me–unfamiliar concept. With that solemn commitment "carved in stone" in my mind and my Pathology Report clutched firmly in my hand, I raised my chin, left the tranquility of the garden, and exited the hospital to the mixed-up world outside. My next stop would be my place of work to inform my girlfriend and my co-workers of my unbelievable fate.

Life is Simply Not Fair (Alert the Media!)

When I left the hospital on the morning of June 7 after what had seemed to be an eternity, I had about an hour's drive back to my place of work, and to my girlfriend's office just down the street from mine. And, like it or not, that commute gave me another 60 minutes or so to ponder over what had transpired earlier that morning, and to wonder what the next few months might have in store for me. *"One thing for sure,"* I told myself, *"my life is absolutely going to change very quickly."* If the preliminary couple of hours since receiving my diagnosis were as tumultuous as they had been, I could only imagine the roller-coaster ride that was still to materialize. I also realized, as I drove south on the Interstate, how very little I knew about Cancer, even though I had been somewhat involved with my Mom's Cancer experiences, and those of my friends', through the years. Of those occurrences, however, all of which were several years ago, I thought optimistically to myself that, *"The therapies, medicines, techniques, and equipment employed in 2004 have got to be much different, and much more advanced and safer, than those used many years ago."* I remembered back to our Mom's first of two Mastectomies she had in the early 1970s for her Breast Cancers. At that time, Surgery (that is, the complete *amputation* of the breast to eradicate the Cancerous tumors) was just about the only alternative available, as Chemo and Radiation Therapy commenced being commonly used to treat Breast Cancers a few years later. Things *had* changed, and for the better.

Granting the matter of Cancer some additional contemplation as I navigated the Virginia highways, I continued thinking that I did lack knowledge of what Cancer was (other than knowing the harm it can create), where it comes from, how it occurs, how the treatments work, or, how and why the disease occurs in some people and not in others. What I *was* aware of, however, and, *"What really sucks,"* I thought to myself as I started getting closer to my place of business, *"is that people like me who have made an attempt to do the 'correct' things, health-wise, and who are in otherwise terrific shape, end up getting Cancer, while several people who are morbidly obese, smoke two packs of cigarettes a day for their entire adult life, or, who drink beer and other alcoholic beverages day and night, never come down with the disease."* I certainly was not drawing this comparison in my brain to *desire Cancer* upon any smokers, alcohol drinkers, or obese, unfit people, as I would never think such a thing. But, to be honest, the obvious inequality did piss me off, and it proved to me, yet, once again, that life is just not fair. Life, for all intents and purposes, is simply a matter of every individual doing what they believe is most appropriate for them, taking their chances, hoping for the best, and living with the consequences of their decisions and actions, be they good or bad. In other words, no matter what you do, the possibility of getting screwed in life is pretty damn good. *Que sera, que sera.*

Sharing the News of My Diagnosis

Just about an hour after I departed the hospital, where I had received the surprise of my life earlier that morning, I finally arrived at the multi-building U.S. Government office complex where I and my girlfriend worked. Passing my office facility on the left, I drove directly to the building in which her workstation was positioned. She knew how much I've cared for my body and how fit I have been all my life, so, I anticipated that she would probably be expecting me to *phone her* or *email her* with my Biopsy findings when I got back to my office, rather than me delivering the outcomes to her in-person. I presumed, of course, that she would be presupposing that all would be fine and dandy with my lab results, exactly as I had miscalculated earlier in the day when I thought that the doctor would be providing me with nothing but rave reviews. *This news,* however, I knew was going to shock the heck out of her, just as it did me when ENT No. 2 stunned me that morning with my out-of-the-blue diagnosis.

Informing My Girlfriend (And Soon-to-be Caregiver)

When I parked my car and sauntered into the building where my girlfriend worked and up the stairs to her workspace, the reality and seriousness of the moment suddenly nailed me like another 2x4 across the head. I knew that she would, most likely, be just as dazed, and just as skeptical, as I had been upon first learning of my destiny. But, she was also a strong, optimistic, and level-headed woman who had been thru some similar medical adversities with her father in the previous year. Her father had regrettably, and unexpectedly, passed away because of a Heart Attack in his wife's and his home, and, my girlfriend, being the oldest sibling in her family, became the rock to which her other family members looked for strength and consoling. Because of this, I hoped that after this initial surprise I was about to deliver to her, she would be able to bounce back after processing the information, and, that she would in some way, be able to make some sort of sense of the illogicality of the situation – something that I, up until then, had still not been able to do. *"And better yet,"* I carefully hoped, when I approached the landing at the top of the stairwell not too far from her desk, *"possibly, she will want to be my Caregiver,"* just as ENT No. 2 had suggested, *"to help me thru my Cancer when the going gets tough."* I was soon to learn of her responses.

Exiting the stairwell, I entered the hallway and walked a few more feet before turning left into the spacious office space where my girlfriend's cubicle was located. *"Here goes nothing."* I commented to myself as I circled back behind the walls of her cubicle. She was there, working diligently at her computer with her back towards me and the opening of her workspace. She had affixed a small convex "rear view" mirror on her PC monitor so that she could see who may be approaching her from the back, and, it seemed to do its job well that morning. No sooner did she see my small reflection in her little "fish eye," than she spun around in her chair and jumped up to greet me. From the looks on her face, she was both happy and surprised to see me standing there, but she knew me well, and could read me like a book. It didn't take but a couple of seconds for her to notice that I was not my usual cheery and goofy self. She knew by my demeanor that something was definitely not right – and she was right.

We approached one another and gave each other a hug and a kiss, as boyfriends and girlfriends might, including in the office. She held both of my shoulders and then took a couple of steps rearward as if to assess the damage. *"Oh my God, Butch, your neck still looks so painful. It's still so red and swollen. Did the doctor drain it and take out the stitches? Is that's what's causing you to look so sad?"* she asked. She could gather, even underneath the cumbersome gauze dressings applied by my ENT, that the huge, distended growth up on my neck was still causing me excruciating pain. My girlfriend had been with me every step of the way since we first observed the sore throat pain and neck swelling in January of that year. And, she had shared with me for five months after, the absolute frustrations of an exceedingly clumsy, bogged-down HMO medical system, and a few seemingly incompetent or indifferent physicians who didn't appear to have any clues as to what might be causing either problem.

After she asked her questions about my neck tenderness and my appointment that morning, I held back my tears about the truth and told her, *"Yes, the neck swelling is part of the reason that I am feeling bad, because it does still hurt like hell."* I then followed that declaration up by telling her further, *"But, there actually is another reason that I'm not being my 'happy-go-lucky self' right now. If you don't mind, I'd rather discuss it with you in private than out here in your cubicle."* That's all that it took – when I mentioned the word, "private," she knew that something extremely untoward was going on. She also started to look very worried and frightened as she tried her best to understand and interpret my face and my emotions.

My girlfriend's boss had a large office just around the corner from her work cubicle, so she suggested that we could use his space for privacy, as he was out of the office for the day. Holding hands, we silently walked side-by-side to his office, and, upon entering, we gradually closed the door behind us. With just the two of us standing there in that large space, dark except for the few rays of sunlight that slivered thru the blinds, the silence shortly became overwhelming. I realized then that there would be no easy means to tell her about my Cancer diagnosis. Rather than get into a lengthy explanation of what had transpired that morning with ENT No. 2, I thought that it might be best to tell her the news directly, exactly as the doctor had earlier done with me. Facing one another, eyeball-to-eyeball, with our arms outstretched and our fingers entwined, I attempted to speak, but my words froze in-place and were soon overcome by my emotions.

Despite my most heartfelt efforts to put on a strong front for my girlfriend's sake, I soon began to cry. Observing my agony, she pulled me closer to her, and held and comforted me, as she, herself, began to well-up with tears. Still not knowing what was causing my suffering, she looked me in the eyes and gathered the strength to tell me, *"Whatever this is, Butch, you are going to be okay. We won't let anything happen to you, and we both will take care of whatever it is that's causing you this pain."* Upon hearing her reassuring words, I nodded my concurrence in the affirmative, and told her how much I appreciated her positive outlook and support. At this point, knowing that my girlfriend would help me get through this ordeal, my resolve strengthened, and I once again felt self-assured and in-control of the dire situation. Then, with me looking into my girlfriend's, and soon-to-be Caregiver's, eyes, I managed to muster up the will to give her the news. *"As hard as it is to believe,"* I told her, *"I have Cancer."*

Completely surprised to hear that "C" word come out of my mouth, the stunned expression on my girlfriend's face was probably identical to the look of disbelief that I had on my own face when the doctor had delivered the diagnosis to me earlier in the morning. *"My Biopsy results showed Cancer in my Lymph Nodes where the doctor performed this surgery,"* as I delicately patted on the gauze dressing and then dropped another bombshell on her, *"but, the physician said that they don't know where the Primary Tumor is."* My girlfriend continued to look totally perplexed by the shocking news, but stood silently as she allowed me to continue speaking. *"I asked the doctor if he thinks all of this is responsible for my sore throat pain, and he doesn't know that either."* *"But, what does this mean – what do we do now?"* my girlfriend asked, obviously just as confused as I was after ENT No. 2 had blown me away with this identical, unfamiliar information. *"The doctor told me that I will have to get more tests to determine where the Cancer started,"* I told her, *"and to see if it's what's responsible for causing my non-stop sore throat."*

My girlfriend's and my tears had mostly dried by then, and she continued focusing very carefully on all of my words as I spoke, realizing that her own life was getting ready to change quite quickly, as would mine. *"My ENT doctor did not know for sure, but he told me that I will most likely have to have Surgery, Radiation Therapy, and Chemotherapy to treat my Cancer. His office is going to begin scheduling consultations with both an Oncologist and a Radiation Oncologist so that they can determine what I will need. They will be giving me a call soon to let me know what will be next."* With that, my girlfriend hugged me once again and told me that we would get through this. I told her that I had already made up my mind, earlier that morning, that I would definitely be a survivor, and I told her the same thing that I had exclaimed to the doctor a few minutes after he had given me the bad news: That *"My Cancer had picked the wrong person to fuck with,"* and that, *"I'm going to kick the Cancer's ass!"* With these thoughts, and with her knowledge that I mean what I say, we both smiled, and walked out of the room with the realization that we both would have our work cut out for us. Unbeknownst to us at that time, however, was what exactly that work was going to entail.

Having our wits about us following our brief discussion just moments before, my girlfriend walked me down the stairs and out of the building to my vehicle. It was a beaming, sunny day, with just a hint of the hot, humid, Northern Virginia summer-to-come, and, it definitely was in stark contrast to the "foggy, and somewhat freezing and tumultuous weather system" that I had brewing within my body. Like most hurricanes, I was hoping and praying that the one which unexpectedly blew into my life would continue to carry right on thru and fade away completely from the radar. I was no Meteorologist, but, I was giving the prospect of this "weather report" around a 99% probability. After getting to my car, my girlfriend and I hugged and shared our "good-byes," and I told her that I would be seeing her at home later on that evening. Just a few months before, she and I had moved into a brand-new home that we had custom-built on top of a hill, on a gorgeous 3-acre wooded property bordered on two sides by creeks. It was such a beautiful place both inside and out. But, a big batch of *home-baked Cancer diagnosis* was not the type of house-warming gift that either one of us had planned on receiving.

Sharing the News With My Boss

Waving "good-bye" to my girlfriend one final time, I drove out of the parking lot and down the street to deliver my next round of notifications – this time, to my boss and co-workers in my office building. On the occasion of my Cancer diagnosis, I was employed with a Federal Agency that was accountable for protecting the U.S. homeland (where I still work in 2013 in Albuquerque). In my job as a Team Leader for two divisions, I managed in the region of twenty government and contract employees who encompassed my groups. While all of us were predominantly professional in our dealings in the workplace, we also were awfully close with one another; much like a bunch of family members, as some well-formed teams can be. At that same time, I was also the Chairperson of a sizeable Working Group that was formed at the direction of the Commissioner of our Agency. That group was made up of roughly twenty-five individuals from multiple organizations within the Agency, and, at the point of my Cancer diagnosis, we had already been meeting on our project for numerous months. Just like all the members of my regular teams, several of us on the Working Group had also professionally bonded with one another during the course of our official undertakings.

All of the people with whom I worked were well aware of the goiter-like growth beneath my jaw-line on the left region of my neck that had been painfully building in size over the previous two weeks. Out of respect for my privacy, however, no one asked what had caused the distension, but, a few did inquire if I was okay, or if I was experiencing any pain. I had been telling them the information as I knew it at the time insofar as the inflammation and bulge being the result of the Biopsy Surgery I had had a few days prior. And, I did answer their questions about pain by reassuring them that the large protuberance was awfully sensitive to the touch, and, that it did *"Hurt like hell!"* On this day, the day of my diagnosis, however, I would be giving much more detailed news to my boss, those on my team, some Working Group members, and other co-workers within the building. I was well aware that word of my diagnosis would no-doubt circulate throughout the building, and, with all of my friends knowing what a "health nut" I am, would come as a huge shock to each of them. I also knew that in the aftermath of my Cancer, some changes would have to be made within the groups that I was leading to accommodate my uninvited, new, number-one priority.

My office was positioned such that it faced the parking lot to the West, and was directly around the corner on the right-hand side from the entry doors and the hallway in the front of the building. As such, when I entered the facility, I greeted the Security Guard at the front desk with a, "Hi," but then quickly entered my office without seeing anyone else. I was thankful for that, because I knew that I would not be able to cover my visible anguish from those who knew me well. My plan was to settle in my office, door closed, for a few minutes to once again "decompress" in the peace and quiet. The last thing I felt like doing at that juncture was facing a lot of people—especially the close associates that each of them had become—but, I did know that I'd have to *"let the cat out of the bag"* at some point. There was no way that I would *not* tell these individuals about my Cancer, but, I chose to first gather my thoughts, and to contemplate what I was going to tell them, and how I was going to say it.

I did ruminate in my office for a few quiet moments prior to me calling my boss to ask if she was in her office and could meet up with me. She would be the original co-worker with whom I would share the news. After discussing everything with her, I would then call my team together for an impromptu meeting so that I could tell everybody at once. As for me updating the Working Group members and the executive managers to whom I reported for that endeavor, I would do that before the next meeting, which was scheduled a few days out. I determined that there was no other way to inform my co-workers of my diagnosis than to, essentially, be straightforward with them about the medical findings, and to advise them of what may be coming down the line. Nothing extreme would need to be done at that point-in-time, work-wise, because, on day-one of my journey, I honestly did not know what would be required of me from a "time" standpoint. Nor, was I aware of how I would be feeling physically and emotionally once the "Cancer ball" started rolling, or what sort of shape I would be in to continue working in my position full-time. All of that information, I assumed, would be coming in due-time.

My boss was in her office and available to meet, so I told her that I would be down in a moment or two, as I had something that I needed to share with her. When I entered her office, she looked up at me and saw me amble in with the prominent, red "growth" in the area of my upper neck. The mega-sized "boil" had not deflated that much, even after the doctor had drained the fluid that morning, and the inflammation was still readily visible, despite the tape-and-gauze dressing applied by the doctor. I did notice my boss's eyes wincing as we greeted each other – her grimace, no doubt, in solidarity to the pain she presumed that I must be feeling thanks to the swelling. She knew that I had had neck Biopsy surgery a couple weeks earlier, and she was also aware that I had a follow-up appointment that morning to have the stitches removed from the surgery site. What she did not know, though, as I walked into her office and sat down on a chair in front of her desk, was that my day was turning out to be shockingly different than I ever could have imagined in my wildest dreams.

"You're not looking too good there, Butch." my boss quickly conjured up after I took a seat in front of her. *"Nothing like stating the obvious."* I thought to myself, and then I jokingly responded to her statement by firing back, "*Thanks for the vote of confidence. I appreciate it.*" Following that brief exchange, she and I talked for a couple of minutes about the freakish-looking and still ***very*** sensitive growth that dominated my upper neck. *"Well, the reason I wanted to speak with you,"* I mentioned to her, *"is because I've got some not-so-good news to share with you."* This really got her attention, as the expression on her face changed from one of inquiring interest, to the look of authentic concern. Not wanting to beat-around-the-bush, I continued, "*As hard as it is to believe, I just found out that I have Cancer.*" I somehow managed to relay to her just before my voice started to waver beneath the weight of saying that damned "C" word again. She didn't offer anything in reply, but just stared at me with eyes wide-open as if I had just told her that I had seen Elvis having breakfast with Jimmy Hoffa. *"These Lymph Nodes here in my neck tested positive for Cancer,"* I told her as I tenderly patted my gauze dressings, *"but, the bad part is, my physician told me that they don't know where the Cancer started within my body. He told me that the Cancer formed somewhere else, and then migrated to my Lymph Nodes. They'll have to do more exams and tests to find that out. He did say that he thinks it may have begun in my head or neck."*

My boss could tell by my words and the look on my face that I was in conspicuous anguish, both physically and emotionally, and although it was exceedingly difficult for her to process the shocking news—knowing how health-conscience I am—she did proffer some empathetic words, and, affirmed to me, *"If anyone can beat Cancer, Butch, you can."* My boss knew me too well, and was well aware of how I had, without fail, thrown my heart and soul into my work and everything that I did in my life. She knew, as I did, that I would be dedicating the same levels of passion, commitment, and energy into combating and overcoming my Cancer that I have done with all of my many work projects and other undertakings. *"I'm sure that you will have a demanding schedule ahead of you once things kick-off, so do what you need to do and don't worry about your work here."* she reassured me. *"You've got some good teams and they will cover for you. The most important thing now, Butch, is that you get well."*

"Thanks very much," I responded, *"but, I will try to work as long as I can until it becomes too difficult for me. I'm sure that the distractions and keeping busy will do me some good." "That would be fine,"* she said, *"but, make sure not to overdo it." "By the way,"* she asked, *"have you told anyone in the group yet?" "No, that's my next stop,"* I responded, *"but, I did want to share the news with you first." "I do appreciate your understanding and for supporting me throughout this,"* I added, *"because I don't know what to expect. I will beat it though,"* I confirmed, *"I do know that!"* With that, we both stood up and gave each other a professional "good bye" hug, at which instant she asserted that, *"Everything is going to be okay."* I thought to myself as I departed her office, *"She's the third person to tell me that today."* With that nature of positive energy surrounding me, there was no way that Cancer was going to get the best of me. It was then time to deliver the news to the folks on my teams.

Notifying My Co-Workers

After I finished meeting with my boss, I breathed a big sigh of relief as I returned to my office. It felt somewhat therapeutic to be able to unburden myself of the weight of my Cancer diagnosis by sharing the surprising news with my girlfriend and co-workers, other friends, and, when the time came, with my family. It is these people that would become the support network to whom I might have to look should things start getting tough for me. I sat in my office for a few moments once again to regroup, and to gather my wits about me before calling my many team members together for a group meeting. There were twenty people on both teams that I hoped would be there that day so that I could share the news with them in a single attempt. Once I felt prepared to face the gang, I called my assistant and asked her if she could have everyone on the teams meet me in one of the large conference rooms for an impromptu team meeting.

A few moments later, at the appointed time, I left my office and walked down the hallway to the meeting room. The members of my teams were used to having spur-of-the-moment meetings due to the nature of our work, but, as they would soon find out, this was not going to be just another ordinary meeting. I entered the room to find almost the inclusive bunch assembled around the table. Some of the team members weren't at work that day, so they would learn of my situation in due time. As I entered the room, I said "Hi" to everyone and I made some "small talk" and joked around with them for a few moments. Feeling nervous once again, I did this in an effort to help soften the blow of the shocking revelation I was about to announce. The tables in this conference room were positioned in the shape of a large square with an opening in the center, and every seat was filled, in addition to some people sitting around the periphery of the room. All awareness was on me to learn what "curve ball" the government had thrown at us this time. Curve ball – yes; government – no.

"You all are probably wondering why the sudden meeting." I said to them, looking around the room at each man and woman as they sat focused on my words, and, no doubt, on the large puffiness on my neck that was impossible to dodge, despite the gauze dressing masking its surface. *"As several of you know, I've had a sore throat for quite a few months,"* I continued, *"and, this swelling on my neck is the result of Biopsy Surgery that I had a few days ago. They took samples of tissue from there thinking that it may reveal the cause of my throat pain. Unfortunately, the doctor didn't place a tube in during the surgery to permit the fluid to drain, and what you see is the result of that."* I mentioned as I gently patted my fingers on the swelling on my neck. *"But, to be honest with you, right now, that's the least of my worries. Unfortunately, there's more to it than that."*

By this stage in my announcement, the folks had placed their pens down on their notepads, realizing that this was not going to be an ordinary business meeting and that there would be no noteworthy points to record. I began, "*Well, this morning at my surgery follow-up appointment,*" my voice becoming tentative as it had earlier with my girlfriend and my boss, *"I got hit with a wicked 'curve ball.' In fact, there was no way on earth I could have seen it coming."* My cryptic words, I knew, were raising their individual curiosities, but, as I sat there looking at these co-workers who had also become my good friends, I was finding it a little difficult, once again, to actually come out and say that iniquitous and cumbersome word, *"Cancer."*

Taking a deep breath to maintain my self-control, I looked at the three men and the three women seated directly across the square, donut-shaped tables from me, and I decided that I might just as well get directly to the point. So, that's what I did. *"Gang,"* I uttered, *"I found out just this morning that I have Cancer."* There, I said it – just like that, the cat was out of the bag. You could have heard a pin drop, and a few of the individuals' jaws actually *did* drop, as all of them looked at me in absolute disbelief of what I just said. I was a known practical joker and pulled off many a prank during our team meetings, but, they could surely tell by the inflection and sincerity of my voice that there would be no remote-controlled farts emanating from beneath the table on this day. Nope, this was no joke.

All of the people in the room knew how "picky" I was with my eating, and that I worked-out and took great care of my health and body every day. When they heard the word, *"Cancer"* come out of my mouth, it, naturally, caught them completely by surprise, and they did not know how to react. Basically, it was the same response that I had experienced personally that morning when the doctor told me, and the precise reaction displayed by my girlfriend and my boss when I shared it with them. I did notice that all those present looked at me with expressions of concern and empathy, and that two of the women in the room teared up. But, most of them shook their heads and looked at me, dumb-founded, as if simply to say, *"No way."*

My co-workers appeared to find it troubling to vocalize their feelings, because, understandably, it was a pretty awkward moment for them. I had experienced very similar types of sentiments in the past—as do most people—when bad news is shared about a loved one, family member or a friend, especially when the news concerns their health or their life. With a surprise of Cancer, it is exceedingly tough to communicate one's feelings, because one wants to express their sorrow to the victim or family without it sounding too negative. But, at the same time, they want to articulate their positive thoughts and prayers that things will turn out okay, all the while *not knowing what the future may hold for the person.* It is that wicked fear of the unknown that can paralyze and frighten the heck out of most people.

Unfortunately, almost every individual knows, or is related to someone who has had to suffer through Cancer, and, they are well aware of the challenges and potential outcomes with the disease. As such, they know that each Cancer victim is—for lack of a better way of saying it—"playing with a loaded gun," and they're not quite sure what to say or do about it. Of course, the patient's family members and close friends will classically step in and do and say those things that will be the most beneficial, the most encouraging, and the most supportive for their Cancer Warrior. Others, including those further removed from the patient, will also usually offer their positive words and acts to the person, but will, hopefully, steer clear of conveying any defeatist or "doomsday"-types of thoughts. That's not good.

In the conference room, after I disclosed the revelation of my Cancer diagnosis to my co-workers, I broke the silence by telling the group, *"According to the physician, my Cancer is pretty advanced. This, they determined from the results of the Biopsy Surgeries in my Lymph Nodes. The bad part is,"* I added, *"they're not sure exactly where my Cancer started in my body."* Going into a tad more detail, I told them, *"My Pathology Report said that the Primary Tumor site is unknown, so additional testing will need to be done to determine that."* I concluded the brief meeting by telling the group that I had already spoken to our boss about my circumstances, and that we had agreed that I would continue to work while I was still capable for an undetermined length of time. I told the men and women that I would doubtless have a busy schedule attending medical appointments and Cancer treatments, and that at some point, I would probably have to stop working to center all of my energies on beating my Cancer. To this, they all nodded, and assured me that they would all continue to make me proud, and that they would hold down the fort for me.

Telling My Mom and My Sister – My Concerns

When I got home on the night of June 7, 2004, my girlfriend-turned-Caregiver and I had a bunch to talk and think about. She was already home when I arrived, and, after a huge hug of a greeting, she told me that she had informed all of her family members and friends of my Cancer diagnosis, which, she mentioned, thoroughly shocked all of them. She also relayed from them, their thoughts, prayers, and encouraging words, as well as their offers to assist us with anything we might require. I was unbelievably moved by everyone's kindness and selflessness. The immediate and heartfelt outpouring of love and support that I had received from everyone on *just the first day* of my Cancer journey told me that my Cancer *would not stand a chance!*

At this juncture, most of those close to me were aware of my Cancer news, with the exception of the people who were the closest to me of all – my own family. I knew that I would have to tell them, but, I also was aware that the process of doing so would be "dicey," especially with my Mom and my Sister, Vikki. As for Vikki, I was very concerned that letting her know about my Cancer may possibly throw her into a deeper depressive state than she was in much of the time. Vikki, bless her loving heart and kind soul, had fallen prey to the ravaging scourges of alcohol, cigarettes, (and most likely drugs), and, as a result, our typically beautiful, fun-loving, outgoing, happy, and loving daughter, sister, and mother, had depreciated—physically and emotionally—into a frightened, cloistered, and very unhealthful version of her former self. Our Mom, Buz, Rich, and I had all done our best to help her rid herself of these demons, but, in the end, it all came down to Vik doing it for herself. Sadly, she was never able to do so. For these reasons, I chose not to tell her the news right then.

I knew that I would have to inform Mom of my Cancer, but, the more that I thought about it, the more apprehensive I got about letting her know. This was because Mom was a "worrier" by nature, and she was always very concerned about her kids and our health. I knew if I told her about my diagnosis, that she would take the news very hard, and, worse, that she would unquestionably blame herself for "passing" her Cancer on to me. I figured that that possibility was probably not true, but, I also knew my Mom very well and how she thought. I was certain that my brothers, Buz and Rich, would be able to process and understand the revelation of my diagnosis, albeit with sorrow and concern. With our Mom, however, I knew that I would have to address my Cancer with her very delicately, as the last thing I wanted to do was to cause her stress that could affect *her* health.

My Tumor is Located and I Inform My Family

I began my Cancer journal on June 7, 2004—day-one of my Cancer journey—and, on June 8, I wrote, *"I will tell Buz and Rich when I know more."* My new Caregiver and I hit the ground running on June 8 to start the scheduling of meetings and other appointments with physicians and clinics for consultations and tests. One of these appointments was with another ENT physician (who I will refer to as "ENT No. 3") outside of my health plan, who I arranged, through my HMO, to see for a Second Opinion. This outside opinion, which took place on June 10, proved to be a very necessary next step. This is because, during a regular, 30-minute outpatient Endoscopy Exam of my throat and neck, *ENT No. 3 found the Primary Tumor* further down on the Base of my Tongue. *Finally, after* ***five long months****, we I.D.'d the damned culprit responsible for my non-stop sore throat!*

Initially, ENT No. 3 graded my Cancer as a Stage III, but he reassessed it as a Stage IV. When ENT No. 3 told me that, I recalled what ENT No. 2 had told me about Stage IV Cancers. While this did scare the hell out of me, at least we knew where the Cancer was and what form we were dealing with. That meant that my Caregiver and I could begin our research, and work with the Medical Team on my Cancer-killing treatment agenda. Per my journal, on June 17, I knew enough about my Cancer to tell Buz and Rich, which I did. They felt very concerned about me, but they both gave me the same brotherly encouragement that we always shared in difficult times. I eventually did inform my Mom and Vikki of my Cancer in January 2005, when I flew back to New Mexico. I wanted to tell them in-person after all of my treatments had ended so that they could see that I was healthy. When I walked into Mom's Nursing Home room, though, she knew immediately by my weight-loss that something was not correct, and she was fretful. When she asked me why I had not told her earlier, I lovingly responded, *"Mom, I'd much rather have you mad at me for five minutes, than worried about me for several months."* To that, she gave me the *"Mom"* look, and was just thankful that I was alive.

Cheating Death

By Butch Sickler ©
November 2006

The dark voice beckoned
like a cold harsh wind
it pierced my chest
razor-sharp talons
pulled at my beating heart
but I did not go
it wasn't time . . . and yet it called

I looked its way
but for a moment
it knew I would
and so it pleaded
again for me to come
but I did not go
it wasn't time . . . and yet it called

My tear-filled eyes
turned away
looking to my soul
for strength
but my ears did not listen
except to my beating heart
and I refused to go

it wasn't time . . . and it stopped calling

Chapter Sixteen

My 3+-Year Cancer Journey From Diagnosis to "Cancer-Free" Survivor – *My Journal Month-by-Month Summary*

"Everything in life has a weakness. Where you locate its weakness, you will find your strength."

- Butch Sickler

*Say there Pardner...*have you heard the one about the guy who was fit as a fiddle, strong as an ox, happy as a lark, healthy as a racehorse, and tougher than nails, and then, one day out of the clear blue, he was advised by his physician that he has Cancer? Well, that certainly is an extremely terrible joke, and, unfortunately, the punch line doesn't get much better: Yes, over 1.7 million men, women, and children in the U.S. fall prey to the ubiquitous and horrendous health threat—Cancer—each year, as do over 6 million people, worldwide. And, the real irony here, is that all too often, many individuals who have taken extensive precautionary measures to help prevent, or, at least minimize, their risk of developing Cancer by living a healthful, stress-free, and fitness-oriented lifestyle, end up becoming hapless victims of the parasitic, and sometimes deadly, disease, nonetheless.

Darned if You Do – Darned if You Don't

Much to my surprise, and to the astonishment all those who know me, I am one of those people who has done all of the "correct" things for most of my life to remain healthy and fit—physically and mentally—yet I suffered the cancerous onslaught nevertheless. *And to think that during that time, according to what I was reading and hearing from all the so-called "experts" on the subject, I was doing all the right things that made me practically invincible – a veritable Superman® of sorts. Well, that was until Kryptonite came along!*

All joking aside, despite my 40+ years of continuous weight-training and cardiovascular exercise routines, my incessant healthful nutritional regimen (including consuming only healthful foods and beverages, ingesting every Vitamin and "Free-Radical-killing" Anti-Oxidant supplement known to humanity), and my life-long aversion to tobacco and alcohol, in June of 2004, I received the shock of my life: I received a diagnosis of Stage IV Head and Neck Cancer. That certainly wasn't my Plan A, and it darn sure was not in my Plan B. I mean, seriously – who in the world would even think for one second that a diagnosis of Cancer is in the cards for them, especially if they have taken great care of their body throughout their lives? Definitely not me. But, apparently, that's where Plan "C"—as in "Cancer"—comes in. I've said it before in this Book, and I'll say it again: *With Cancer, you're damned if you do, and damned if you don't.*

My fate, though, not to be taken lightly, reminds me of some humorous words spoken by Mark Twain in which he advocated, *"Be careful about reading health books – you might die of a misprint."* As I write this in 2013, I am, thankfully, very much alive following my unexpected encounter with Cancer. But, Mark Twain's prophetic advice, when translated figuratively, can't help but place a sobering spin on the reality that poor health, or, God forbid, even death, may be as close as an unpredicted "misprint" away. I had been extremely conscientious and responsible in my "reading" all of my life, but life decided to throw me a misprint in the form of Cancer, nonetheless.

When I first received my Cancer diagnosis on June 7, 2004, I joined a very select group of approximately 1.37 million Americans at that time who were afflicted annually with this redoubtable threat to human life. Both back in 2004, and today in 2013, chances are almost 100% that you, or someone you know—be they a loved one, a family member, relative, friend, co-worker, or an acquaintance—either has Cancer now, is a survivor of Cancer, or, will contract the disease at some point during their lifetime. It is not my intention to frighten or alarm you with my candor, but the eye-opening statistics do speak for themselves. After I was smacked squarely between the eyes on the unfortunate day of my Cancer diagnosis with the crystal-clear reminder that, *"Shit happens,"* I remember thinking to myself, ***"If this can happen to me, as healthy as I am, it could happen to anyone."*** And, yes, sadly it does—every day—thousands of times a day, to men, women, and children, all around the globe. In the U.S., alone, just four Cancers—Breast, Lung, Colorectal, and Prostate—account for over *750,000 new diagnoses each year.* Add to that the diagnoses from the other 200+ forms of Cancer, and, the number of Americans affected each year adds up to about 1.7 million. *Yikes!*

Let My Cancer-Killing Begin – My New World

After receiving my fateful Cancer diagnosis on June 7, 2004, I started my original Radiation Therapy sessions and Chemotherapy treatments a little over a month later – on July 14, and July 15, 2004, respectively. In between the acknowledgment of my diagnosis and the commencement of my treatments, I and my Caregiver did all we could to prepare me for the known inevitabilities and the prospective unknowns that were associated with the forms of Cancer treatment I was due to receive. When all was said and done, treatment-wise, I finally watched as the last drop of powerful Chemotherapy medicine slowly entered my body on August 27, 2004. I had my final Cancer-killing Radiation Therapy session on September 2, 2004.

In the period of just a little over three months, I transitioned from being an individual with an unalleviated sore throat which was *caused by my Cancer*, to becoming a confident Cancer survivor with an extraordinarily painful mouth and throat that were *caused by the therapies used to eradicate my Cancer.* It was the horrible ache that evolved from the combined treatments of both Chemo and Radiation that "fried" my incredibly sensitive and stinging tongue, mouth, and throat tissues. And, it was the accompanying nausea, thick mucous, constipation, diarrhea, and difficulty I had with eating, drinking, and sleeping, which materialized into the initial feelings of malaise and hopelessness that I experienced soon after my treatments had ended.

When I first started my Cancer treatments, I was continuing to work full-time at my job within the U.S. government, working out with weights every day, and, even shuttling myself to my treatment sessions and other medical appointments. I wasn't feeling too much soreness or any other Side Effects from the treatments, initially, so I continued with my customary, run-of-the-mill routine for some time. My Caregiver—my girlfriend, Joanne–had accompanied me to all of my pre-treatment appointments and to my first bunches of treatment sessions. But, with me feeling physically able, and, with her having to work, herself, she was not able to attend all of the weekly Chemo or daily Radiation Therapy appointments with me. As time wore on, however, and, as both the treatments and powerful pain medications started affecting my ability to safely transport myself all alone, my Caregiver had to step in to ferry me to my various meetings with my Medical Team members, and to my Chemo and Radiation sessions.

Eventually, when it became too much for me to handle *both* my Cancer program needs and my work responsibilities, and, after the treatment-related Side Effects and other issues started interfering with my standard routine, I had to cease doing some of the "normal" things. Most notably, I had to stop working at my job and I went on Sick Leave. Additionally, I had to restrict lifting weights every day. This, my doctors told me I needed to do, so that I could safeguard all of my calories and energy to remain internally strong, and to be able to heal from each of my Cancer-killing therapies. I certainly did not miss not going to work, but, having worked out almost every day of my adult life, it was difficult for me to give up that important part of my day, if only temporarily. I did feel confident, however, that if all went well with things—Cancer-wise—I would be resuming both my work, and my workouts, at some point in the not-too-distant future.

Like probably a bulk of Cancer patients who have stared the "evil monster" in the eye and battled it with every ounce of strength they could muster, when I completed my various Cancer-eradicating treatments, I felt a huge sense of both *relief*, and of *accomplishment*. I knew in my heart-of-hearts that I had done everything I could do in advance of the treatments to get ready for them, and, I was thankful that my body had reacted well to the Cancer-removal effects of the Surgeries, Chemotherapy, and Radiation Therapy – at least based on what my doctors had told me. Additionally, I felt rather empowered by the fact that I had successfully—although painfully—stood up to the many uncomfortable Side Effects that had evolved as a result of those treatments. Or, so I erroneously thought – as it turns out...

Bye-Bye Cancer Treatments – Hello Side Effects

Some time after my Cancer therapies had ended, I remember thinking to myself, in retrospect, *"The Side Effects have been bad—REAL bad—but despite the intense pain in my mouth and throat, the immeasurable sickening nausea and mucous, the lack of sleep, and the surprising amount of weight and strength I have lost the last few months, I am still alive, and all the pain and suffering will soon be behind me. We have destroyed my Cancer . . . now it's time to get better and get on with my life."* Not so fast Cowboy... As I would swiftly learn, both to my dismay and my further discomfort, that line of thinking was not only extremely naïve, but, it was also incredibly premature. As it eventually came to pass, unbeknownst to me at the time, I actually had a sizeable quantity of unfinished Cancer-related business with which I still had to contend over the next few months.

After the conclusions of my Cancer treatments, the follow-on symptoms of the Side Effects were definitely testing my will from a physical standpoint, but, they soon started to wear very thin on my classically optimistic emotional state as well. For over three lengthy years subsequent to my Cancer Diagnosis, I wrote in a daily journal, in which I recorded anything and everything of importance that had to do with my Treatments, my Side Effects, and, my Recovery and Aftercare. Among many other entries in my journals, I kept track of the intensity of physical pain that I felt I was experiencing on a daily basis. This I did by assigning a subjective number using the typical Pain Scale of 1 to 10, with "1" representing the least discomfort, and "10" being the most extreme. As it turns out, 10 was ***way*** too low.

According to my daily Cancer journaling, when I first started my Chemotherapy and Radiation treatments, and mid-way through, I was experiencing pain levels from one end of the scale (1.5), to the other (10++), depending upon a variety of factors on any given day. In an effort to help relieve the pain, physicians on my Medical Team had me on at least five high-powered Opiate pain killers at any one time, including the Fentanyl ® Patch, which is 80 times stronger than

Morphine, and which delivers medication through the patient's skin. However, despite the very potent pain and anti-nausea medications I was taking, and, in spite of the nutritional plan I was on, which was custom-formulated to minimize my eating and drinking difficulties, my *physical* problems gradually began to develop into *mental* ones.

Stated pervasively throughout my journal entries for the next few months after finishing my Cancer treatments are my ubiquitous mentions of the following nonstop problems that I was experiencing frequently at that time: Me, having chilling, horrible dreams at night about drowning and not being able to breathe, being in car accidents, and people trying to kill me; me, soaking the bed sheets and pillows completely with sweat every night; me, not being able to sleep very much because of the extremely insufferable coughing induced by the constant flow of healing mucous that formed in my mouth and throat day and night; and me, getting sick and vomiting repeatedly because of the incessant nausea caused by the Chemotherapy, as well as the sickening salty and metallic taste of most foods and beverages.

I also found myself starting to become particularly miserable because I could not work-out, and, due to pain, I could not consume satisfactory quantities of calories each day, thus prompting my body, which I had worked so many years to build and protect, to become a slim, frail, shadow of its former self. Further, for all of my merciless mouth and throat pain, I was employing so many prescribed narcotic pain medications that they were creating painful constipation issues, and, they caused my brain to "space out," mentally and emotionally, including during my dreams each night. And again, throughout most of this same occasion in time, the physical pain level measurements that I noted in my journal were "10+++++" – *on a scale of 1 to 10!*

Coping with the Nasty Pain and Depression

When the bottom fell out of my world, emotionally, after I'd concluded my Cancer treatments, it was not something that abruptly altered my life one day as had my Cancer diagnosis. In other words, I didn't wake up one morning and then utter to myself, *"I really feel mentally like shit today. These must be the emotional problems that all of those people in the Support Group were talking about."* It was nothing close to that. My post-Cancer treatment emotional issues, as honestly surprised as I was to fall victim to them as had many other patients/survivors, came upon me very steadily over time. And, they were persistent. Once my mental demons started to rear their wicked heads, they slowly, but surely, kept rearing, and rearing, and rearing. And, while I was well aware that the *possibility* of me experiencing some form of mental and emotional problems was very real after my Cancer treatments—based on what I had read and heard from those who had "been there"—I was completely not ready for the excessive depths to which my own mental feelings would eventually plummet.

My first mention of having post-Cancer treatment emotional complexities in my daily journal happened on September 18, 2004, a bit over two weeks after my ultimate Radiation Therapy session, and just three weeks following my finishing Chemotherapy drip. On that particular day, I wrote, *"I am very depressed today because of pain and inability to swallow and eat. I'm trying to think positive, but it is difficult when I watch my body withering away, and the pain not getting any better. Pain level is '10++.'"* This pain level, and these sentiments, pretty much summed up my world for several months – again, with some days and nights being better or worse than others. Things did get worse when I entered myself into Drug Detox to get over my dependence on prescription painkillers in February of 2005. As time went on, I also started rating my anxiety levels from 1 to 10.

As the weeks progressed following completion of my Cancer therapies, I continued to have the same daily and nightly issues with eating and sleeping difficulties, terrifying dreams, weight loss, throat and mouth pain, nausea, and the deepening, seemingly never-ending anxiety. Gratefully, all of my Medical Team members, as well as my Caregiver, were assisting me in dealing with these Side Effect issues in every possible way as they evolved. My physicians addressed my physical and emotional problems through the prescription and use of different—and greater dosages of—medications for treating nausea, mouth, tongue, and throat soreness, sleeping disorders, constipation, anxiety, and other upsetting symptoms. Additionally, my Registered Dietician modified my Nutritional Plan to eliminate all whole foods that I found too agonizing to eat, and recommended the ingestion of only healthy, liquefied foods, warm water, and high-calorie protein-rich shakes. Essentially, I was a skinny, hurting, pill-popping mess.

Staying the Course to Beat My Cancer – A Month -by-Month Summary of my 3+-Year Journey

During my three+-year Cancer ordeal, my Caregiver ensured that I took my medications on-time every day and night, and she did her very best to prepare liquefied meals for me that were appetizing, non-irritating, nutritious, and, as easy to consume as my enormously sensitive mouth, throat, and tongue tissues would stand for. And, of course, she continually encouraged me and provided to me the moral support that I needed through it all. I attempted to do *my* part to cope with the physical discomfort and mental anguish I was experiencing by attempting to be as physically and mentally strong as possible; by consuming as much water, liquid food, and calories as possible each day; by taking each of my medications on schedule; by attempting to get as much rest as sufficient, both day and night; and, by trusting in my faith and hope, and in my strong commitment to apply the power of *"Mind over matter"* to get past my Cancer-related obstacles.

My support team and I tried to manage the various persistent Cancer treatment-related Side Effects immediately after my therapy, but, in months following, I would be blindsided by additional health issues—such as *Pneumonia* and *Prostatitis*—that added more fuel to the fire. All of these would end up challenging my mettle, but, as my Dad once told me, *"Anything is possible, but you must make it so."* So, that's just what I did. Eventually, throughout weeks of enduring excruciating physical pain by way of utilizing powerful medications and my own God-given strength; dealing with, roughly, two years of overcoming extreme anxiety and depression thru Psychotherapy and my own fortitude; and, bolstered by the unending love, support, and encouragement from my loved ones, family, Caregiver, and friends, and the help of my doctors, nurses, and other professionals, finally, at the end of over three long years, I came out of it all, ***Cancer-Free.***

Following, in this Chapter, is the story of what I did after my Cancer Diagnosis, and what I, my Caregiver, and my Medical Team did for the next three+ years to help me overcome my disease and to become a Cancer-Free survivor. Included within the Sections of this Chapter are ***several highlights and lowlights from each month*** that I logged in my Cancer Journal for three+ years after my Diagnosis.

☛***Authors Note:*** In the following Sections of this Chapter, I've briefly summarized the essence of many of the entries in my Cancer Journal between June 8, 2004, and December 2007, when my doctor had declared me to be "Cancer Free." Because the following journal notes are regarding ***my own*** personal Cancer diagnosis, preparations, treatments, Side Effects, pain levels, medicines, recovery, aftercare, diet, survival, and other facets of my program, the Reader should be mindful that such references pertain to ***my*** Cancer journey, and may, or may not, apply to other Cancer patients and survivors. I provide this ***"window to my world"*** for informational purposes only, so that it may assist others impacted by Cancer—including Head and Neck Cancers—in comparing their own journeys. In all instances, Cancer patients and their loved ones, family, and Caregivers, should always defer to the professionals on their Medical Team for assistance.

June 2004
The Month of My Diagnosis

*On June 8, I rated my throat and tongue pain as a "7," and, on June 30, it was a "9." With my physician's approval, I continued taking my usual vitamins, minerals, and anti-oxidants, and, I added others to help boost my Immune System. On June 10, I and my Caregiver saw ENT No. 3 for a Second Opinion. During an Endoscopy exam, he located the Tumor at the Base of my Tongue and graded it as a **Stage 3**. ENT No. 3 recommended a combination of Chemo/Radiation with Surgery as necessary. The next day, ENT No. 3 called to tell me that he reassessed my Cancer as **Stage 4.** My Caregiver and I began researching Cancer, Head and Neck Cancers, and Base of Tongue Cancers, to learn about them, what it takes to kill them, and any other beneficial information. On June 14, my bodyweight was **177.5,** and, on my doctor's orders, I started a weight-gain diet with high-calories and double portions. I got unbelievably sick after wolfing down two hamburgers and a milkshake. By June 20, I weighed **185.5**. During the month, my Caregiver and I met with three Oncologists and my Radiation Oncologist for consultations and planning. All of them recommended the Radiation/Chemo combination with Surgery only as necessary. They each also warned of the significant Side Effects of Chemotherapy and Radiation Therapy. My Radiation Oncologist explained the process and said she will use the very precise IMRT machine. I had a CT Scan of my chest, which, thankfully, indicated no Cancer presence in my lungs. On June 18, I had Biopsy Surgery of my throat and tongue. Results found Cancer only on the left side of my tongue where my tumor was located. I had a pre-Radiation Therapy dental exam and fluoride treatment on June 24. On June 25, I had* *a PET Scan, which found no Cancer in my body except on the Base of my Tongue. We scheduled my Chemo and Radiation Therapy starting dates in July. I was still consuming normal food and drink, and I was still working out. The pain in my throat and on my tongue was getting much worse. I was prescribed Percocet® and Vioxx® for pain, and Valium® for sleep.*

July 2004

Month 1 of Treatments – Month 1 since Diagnosis

*On July 1, my throat and tongue pain was a 9.5, and on July 31, was a 7.5. My research on pubmed.com indicated the most effective Chemo drugs for Base of Tongue Cancer were Carboplatin® and Paclitaxel®. On July 2, I contacted ENT No. 3, the 2nd Opinion doctor who found my tumor, to ask him if he would agree to the drugs I found for treating my form of Cancer. He told me that he concurred with me on the medications, when used in combination with Radiation Therapy. On that same day, I contacted my treating Oncologist and told him I wanted to use these Chemo drugs – he agreed and planned my Chemotherapy accordingly. I also told my treating Oncologist that I wanted to take Amifostine®—which I had located during my research—to salvage my Salivary Glands during Radiation Therapy. On July 22, the doctor called me at home to tell me the Amifostine® had been approved, and I first injected it into myself with doctor supervision on July 26. My Caregiver and I went on a pre-Cancer Treatment vacation for 4th of July, but it was cut short due to a tooth issue. I had a Root Canal on July 6, and got a Radiation Therapy Tattoo and had my Mask made on July 8. On July 9, I had a Surgery to implant my Chemo Mediport in my chest. My Radiation Therapy Simulation was on July 12, and Radiation Testing and a CT Scan on July 13. My daily Radiation Therapy began on July 14, and my weekly Chemotherapy started July 15. My first Chemo dose was three-week's worth. As I watched the first drop of Chemo enter my body, I said, "Fuck you Cancer! You are dead!" On July 19, I met with my Registered Dietician to design my eating plan. On July 25, foods began tasting weird and salty. I was still eating whole foods and taking vitamins /minerals. The following were prescribed for nausea: Anzemet®, Ativan®, Zofran®, and Phenergan®. I was still working at my job and working out. On July 23, my bodyweight was **198**, but eating whole foods was starting to hurt. On July 25, it was difficult to swallow due to throat pain. I started self-injecting Neupogen® on July 26 to improve White Blood Cell counts.*

August 2004

Month 2 of Treatments – Month 2 since Diagnosis

My pain level on August 1 was 8, and on August 31 was 10++ -- basically, off the chart. My daily Radiation Therapy, and my weekly Chemo sessions *continued on-time, as did my Amifostine® and Neupogen® (as necessary) self-injections. August is when many of my radiation- and Chemo-related Side Effects started kicking-in in a big way. I became nauseous after each Amifostine® injection, so I had to be treated with nausea medications each day. My energy levels began dropping and I became very tired every day, for which I needed to take naps. My sleep at night was very difficult as I coughed incessantly due to formation of thick, salty-tasting mucous in my throat. I continued to eat softer, healthy, whole foods, but, was a very slow process each meal, and it was almost unbearable to swallow due to throat and tongue pain. I continued taking vitamins/minerals and working out, but, my workouts had become very slow due to lower energy. On August 2, I was prescribed liquid Percocet® (Roxycet®), which helped reduce some pain. On August 6, I saw my Oncologist to ask if I could have the feeding tube. She abstained, stating that there could be infection and swallowing issues. Throughout the month, I continued to work some days, but had to take off others due to tiredness. My Caregiver had to take me to treatments on those days. On August 11, I attended my first Head and Neck Cancer Support Group – I found it very discouraging to hear some of the patients' Side Effect stories. On August 13, my weight was **184**. I had to start using Magic Mouthwash® and Gelclair® products to help decrease excruciating mouth and tongue pain, and, I used Fluoride Paste in tooth trays two times a day. On July 17, my doctors prescribed MS-Contin® and the Fentanyl® duralgesic patch for throat pain. Fentanyl® is 80 times more powerful than Morphine. At this point, I was on 4 prescription drugs for pain, three of them narcotics. On August 26, my Radiation Oncologist called me, "The Poster Boy for Radiation Oncology," because she told me how well I was handling all of my treatments and Amifostine® self-injections. On August 27, I had my last Chemotherapy – **Yea!** – I took flowers for the nurses. It became hard to swallow my pain pills and food. My thick, salty, sickening mucous began to make me nauseous day and night. Outpourings of love, prayers, and support from friends and family continued to come in daily. On August 30, I had to stop working due to pain, nausea, and fatigue.*

September 2004

Month 1 of Recovery/Aftercare – Month 3 since Diagnosis

My throat and my tongue pain continued to get worse. On September 1, I rated it a 10++, mid-month, a 10+++++, and, then, on September 30, a 10+++++. I had my final Radiation Therapy session on September 2 – ***Yea again!*** *During the entire month, I was nauseous and queasy, due to Chemo and radiation, and sickening, thick phlegm. Prior to my Cancer, I had only vomited once in my life; in September, I vomited a total of nine times, which made the pain in my already raw throat incredibly worse. My physicians prescribed another pain pill, Dilaudid®, which brought the* *total of pain medications I was on to five. My physicians continued to increase the strength of my Fentanyl® patch to help me manage my non-stop pain. September 4 was my most painful day yet. I was miserable as I found it nearly impossible to swallow any food, drink, or pills. My tongue started developing white lesions and fungal Thrush due to Mucositis, which added even more pain. I could not sleep at night as I had to get up every five minutes to get rid of large amounts of thick mucous. I continued to eat very soft, pureed foods per my Registered Dietician, but it took me <u>two hours to get down one meal</u>. My Caregiver was unbelievably helpful trying to prepare food I could eat and trying to make me as comfortable as possible. On September 10, I could only eat 1,000 calories per day, and by September 16, I only weighed **157 lbs**., down almost 30 lbs. from one month ago. Per my Oncologist, I had to increase my daily caloric intake to 3,000 calories (with the help of Boost® shakes), which I did on September 15, but, it took MAJOR willpower for me to force it down. All of the food and drinks tasted sickeningly salty and metallic. By September 17, I had not had a BM for six days, due to the five prescription narcotic painkillers I was on. That day was "my most miserable day thus far." I was incredibly depressed as my constipation was excruciatingly painful. Because my stool softeners weren't working, I asked my doctor to prescribe something else. She put me on Lactulose®, which worked very well. I had not been out of the house for over two weeks, so was very depressed. I felt well enough on September 19 for my Caregiver to take me out for a wonderful drive in the country on a sunny day – thank God! My doctors put me on prescription Diflucan® for Thrush (a Mouth Fungus similar to Mucocitis), Vicodin® for pain, and Amoxycillin®, an antibiotic to minimize infections.* ***<u>My total of painkillers was then six, and my total number of prescription drugs was 16.</u>*** *From September 11 through the end of the month, I did not workout, as my doctors told me that I must conserve my energy to assist the healing process. My doctors also asked me to stop taking nutritional supplements.*

October 2004

Month 2 of Recovery/Aftercare – Month 4 since Diagnosis

My pain level was 10+++++ on October 1, and the same on October 31. Throughout the entire month, the Side Effects of pain, nausea, fatigue, Thrush, Mucositis, salty and metallic tasting food and drink, anxiety, lots of thick, sickening phlegm, vomiting, and others, continued day and night. I got some temporary relief with my painkillers and my personal diet plan, but, I was very miserable most of the time. On October 3, I started noticing pain when I urinated, and on October 4, I woke up in bed soaked in sweat. On October 4, I had a CT Scan of my neck. On October 6, I threw up due to nausea, and, for several days I ran a slight fever and continued to sweat abundantly at night. With my doctors' approval, I again started taking my vitamins, minerals, and anti-oxidants on October 9, but I still was not able to workout. My urinating pain continued through October 10, so I visited my Primary Care doctor on October 11. He diagnosed me with Prostatitis, and prescribed Cipro®, an antibiotic. On October 13, I vomited because of nausea on my way to CT Scan follow-up appointment with ENT No. 2. He had no CT Scan results, but, did a physical exam of my tongue that found a very agonizing, red, swollen region on the left base of my tongue. I asked him to arrange for me to go see an outside ENT for a second opinion at another hospital, which he did for me – for November 2. On October 14, I vomited again due to nausea and salty tastes. On October 15, my pain was unbearable when urinating, so my Caregiver rushed me to a clinic for an evaluation. My temperature was 102 degrees, so an ambulance took me to the hospital for in-patient monitoring and care. My Oncologist was then notified and she asked the hospital to hold me due to my low resistance to infection. The hospital hydrated me and pumped me full of antioxidants and released me on October 18. My weight on October 18 was ***153 lbs.*** *I continued antioxidant Zosyn® via IV at home for Prostatitis. Finally, my urination pain went away. From October 20 to 23, I continued to sweat and cough profusely at night, and my tongue and throat continued to hurt incredibly. For the first time, on October 23, I had a very horrible dream at night that I was suffocating. On October 24, I had a very difficult time breathing. My Caregiver rushed me to the hospital, where I was diagnosed with Pneumonia and given an IV drip of Levequin® antibiotic. October 25 was "My worst day yet," as I still could not breathe and was cold. I had a very scary dream on October 25 that I was drowning. My Caregiver took me to the Oncology Clinic, where I was put in a bed and hydrated for over 4 hours. The physician put me on Diflucan® again for Thrush and oral Levequin® for Pneumonia. The remainder of October didn't get any better. My sleep was interrupted each night with coughing thick mucous from my throat and lungs. My throat continued to burn uncontrollably and I kept getting very nauseous, for which I took Phenergan® semi-successfully. My nutritional plan still consisted of high caloric, but healthy, pureed foods. I was still not working. On Halloween, October 31, the weather was nice, so I and my Caregiver and the pups took a walk in the woods near our home.*

November 2004

Month 3 of Recovery/Aftercare – Month 5 since Diagnosis

I was so glad to see the end of October as it was a most miserable month from start to finish, but, November would be almost as unbearable. I was still taking the same, numerous prescription painkillers, but, my physicians had to keep upping the dosages to reduce the continuous pain in my throat and mouth. My pain levels on November 1 and 30 were again 10+++++. I was also still on Diflucan® for Thrush, Levequin® for Pneumonia, and all of the same anti-nausea meds. I still found it almost impossible to swallow food, drink, medicine – anything! On November 2, I had my appointment with an ENT at an outside hospital that ENT No. 2 had scheduled for me on October 13. This physician performed a Laryngoscopy (flexible tube with a light and camera directed down my nose and throat) and a physical exam, both of which found no evidence of residual tumor on the base of my tongue. He said I did not need biopsy surgery. Thank God – another bullet dodged. My sleeping at night was horrible, with thick mucous, dry throat, Thrush, and horrible dreams. I had to get up several times a night to spit, drink water, and pee. I was taking Mycelex® lozenges and Diflucan® for Thrush, but didn't help much. I was still taking vitamins and minerals, and drinking pureed, healthy food and drink, but it took two hours per meal for me to consume 3,000 or more calories. On November 14, I weighed ***151****. I was uplifted by the overwhelming kindness, encouragement, support, and prayers pouring in from my Caregiver, family, friends, and co-workers. As the physicians kept raising my painkiller dosages, I became more lethargic and nauseous if I didn't take my meds precisely on time – I think my body was becoming dependent on the Opiates and reacted very harshly when I did not "feed my need" regularly. I believed the high amounts of narcotics I was taking, along with my difficulty breathing at night, were responsible for my unbelievably bloodcurdling dreams while sleeping. My doctors prescribed Ambien® to help me sleep, but, it didn't work. On November 15, I had a good day physically, mentally and emotionally for the first time in a very long while. My nausea continued to cause stomach aches almost every day, and I was so fatigued from not being able to sleep at night, that I took naps whenever I could during the day. November 19, my Birthday, ended up being nice as my Caregiver decorated the home, got me presents, and took me to a restaurant for REAL food for the first time in months. It took me forever to eat, and I looked and felt horrible, but the day and night were special, and I was very grateful. I continued to attend all of my many follow-up appointments with my Oncologist, ENT No. 2, Mediport flushes, and other exams and tests. My food continued to taste salty and metallic. I saw my Oncologist on November 23 and asked if she would order a PET Scan for me, which she did. On November 25, Thanksgiving, I gave thanks that I was alive, but, felt horrible and celebrated it in bed. On November 26, my Caregiver took me to the hospital because my throat hurt so much and my neck swelled up on both sides. The doctor treated me for Thrush, which was still kicking my ass. I had a very scary dream on November 27 in which I was hurt real bad in a car accident. What the hell is up with the horrible dreams?! On November 29, when I was driving home from one of my medical appointments with my Caregiver, we were in a car accident (just as I had dreamed two nights before), but, thankfully, we weren't hurt. On November 30, we picked up a rental car to drive in the meantime.*

December 2004

Month 4 of Recovery/Aftercare – Month 6 since Diagnosis

I continued to replace my Fentanyl® patch every two to three days during the month so that I would stay ahead of the pain curve and not experience the dreadful feelings of withdrawal if I replaced it too late. But, despite the regular and higher dosing, my throat and tongue burned all day and night. My pain levels had not changed and were still 10+++++ throughout the month. On December 1, I was driving to an appointment with ENT No. 2 when a huge tree blew down across the road and landed right on the hood and engine of the rental car I was driving. One second faster and it would have come through the windshield and possibly killed me. Okay God, what have I ever done to you or anyone to deserve all of this? Good grief! How about spreading this shit around a little?! Enough is enough! To make matters worse, I didn't buy the rental car insurance (who does?), and it ended up costing me. I got another rental car and bought the insurance, but, just my luck, nothing hit me after that. On December 2, I was a mental and physical mess, so took lots of Valium® to "Wipe my head clean of all that was happening to me." I had my rescheduled visit with ENT No. 2 on December 3, during which his physical exam found my throat very red and swollen, which I fully expected. I asked the doctor if he would prescribe Trazodone® for me to help stop the terrible dreams I was having, which he did. Trazodone® is an antidepressant used to treat depression and anxiety disorders, and used off-label for insomnia. On December 4, after taking Trazodone®, I had the best night's sleep in weeks, with no bad dreams! I continued to experience awful Thrush for which I took the same meds with no noticeable results. I was still consuming pureed foods and drinks, but very slowly, due to intense throat and tongue pain. I also continued to take vitamin/mineral supplements. On December 9, I got a very painful Cold Sore in my mouth (Why not? I've had every other issue in my mouth, so why not add another problem to the mix?) My Caregiver took me to the doctor to get a prescription for Acyclovir® to treat the sore. At this point, I was taking so many different medications, I was happy that my Caregiver was keeping track of them all. I started back to work on December 15, in afternoons only, for the first time since my treatments. It felt weird to be working again, but all of my co-workers were glad to see that I had pulled through. I thanked all of them for their kindness and support. The second half of December, I was feeling very abysmal, mentally, emotionally, and physically, including having scary dreams again, so I took a multitude of meds to deal with each of those Side Effects. I continued to have very bad nausea, as well as headaches so I was taking three different medications to get to sleep. December 20 was a big day for me as I started working out again for the initial time since September. I had missed my workouts very much. On December 22, I had my first post-Cancer treatment PET Scan that, on November 23, I had asked my Oncologist to schedule. I took lots of meds and tried to get some good sleep in preparation for our Christmas party at our home with my Caregiver's family and our friends. It was a lot of excitement and was very tiring, but this was the first time in months that I was able to see family and friends and for them to see me. The gathering helped to encourage me and give me hope that there would be more to life after I got past my Cancer situation. On December 27, 28, and 29, I had three good days in a row, where my ability to eat and drink had improved, as had my nausea, but, it was probably due to me replacing my Fentanyl® patch every day instead of every three days. I continued using Diflucan® and Magic Mouthwash® to deal with the endless Thrush. On December 30, my Oncologist called me late at night about my PET Scan results. She told me that the scans revealed, "An increase in Glucose uptake by my cells in my throat which may indicate Cancerous activity, but that only a Biopsy Surgery would be able to tell us for sure." She also said that the indication could be "healing healthy tissue" instead. OH CRAP!! Just when I thought that things couldn't get any worse, I had to worry about the possibility of still having Cancer until I could have Biopsy Surgery. Good bye, 2004!!

January 2005

Month 5 of Recovery/Aftercare – Month 7 since Diagnosis

January 1 – Happy New Year or something like that. It was last January that I first noticed my sore throat and neck swelling. This January 1, I felt very fatigued and nauseous, and my throat hurt and was very dry, and my voice was raspy – the price that I had to pay for enjoying a few better days previously, God forbid. On January 2, I saw ENT No. 2 for a check- up, and we discussed my PET Scan results. I told him how worried I was after my Oncologist had given me the news, and he said he understood. He told me that he would schedule me for Biopsy Surgery on January 14 so that we could see what was causing the PET scans to "light up." I continued working afternoons at my job when my medical schedule and physical and mental states permitted. Because my throat and mouth soreness was slowly diminishing, I finally was able to start eating soft foods again (instead of pureed), such as soups, oatmeal, poached eggs, mashed potatoes, rice, and ground turkey, etc. On January 7, on my way to the office, I got so tired that I pulled off to the side of the road to sleep for awhile. On January 8, I flew to Albuquerque, New Mexico so that I could visit with my Mom, my Sister, Vikki, and my Brother, Buz, and to break the news to my Mom and Sister. I had hidden from them that I had Cancer, as I did not want their health to falter due to their worries about me. I met Buz for breakfast at IHOP® on January 9, and we went to Mom's Nursing Home to see her. As I expected, Mom was devastated by seeing my weight loss and hearing my voice, and she became upset that I had not told her about my Cancer. I told Mom that I'd rather have her mad at me for five minutes than worried about me for several months. She understood and told me that she was so happy that I was alive and that she would be there for me. I was so blessed that Mom took it so well and that she did not hold herself responsible for "giving" me her Cancer. On January 10, I broke the news of my Cancer to my Sister, Vikki, who came to Mom's Nursing Home. Vik, who had her own emotional and physical health problems, was upset deeply when I told her about my Cancer. I told Vikki that some good should come out of my experience by her going to the doctor and attending Alcohol Detox. She scheduled an appointment for January 13. I had a very wonderful time in Albuquerque with Mom, Buz, and Vik, and I was so happy I made the trip. It was very hard to say good-bye to everyone on January 11 for my trip back to Virginia on January 12, but we all got through it. Little did I know it at the time, but when I gave Vikki a "good-bye" hug in the parking lot of Mom's Nursing Home and pleaded with her to help herself, that it would be the last time I would see my Sister alive (Our Dear Vikki passed away on June 3, 2005). By January 13, I had tried to wean myself off of as many of the narcotics painkillers as possible, because my throat and mouth pain was starting to subside. I was having difficulty with the Fentanyl® patch, so I asked my Oncologist if she could help me taper off of the patch. She told me that I could, "Bridge it with Ativan®," but, that didn't help me one bit. On January 14, my Caregiver taxied me to my long-awaited, post-Pet Scan Biopsy Surgery. ENT No. 2 took 6 tissue samples from my throat and tongue and sent them to Pathology for evaluation. That's when the REAL worrying began. On January 15, my Caregiver left on a one-week vacation with her girlfriend. I was sad to see her go, but very happy for her, as she needed a fun break in the worst way. The last 12 months had been just as harrowing for her as they had been for me. By January 19, I was taking many Percocets® for the pain resulting from my surgery. On January 20, I was very depressed worrying about my biopsy results, and on January 21, I had my post-surgery visit with ENT No. 2, during which he delivered the results. During my appointment, ENT No. 2 told me that the results of my PET Scan were negative, and that the "lit up" areas on the scans were all "false positives." I was so relieved, and wrote, "Thank God, this is one of the best days of my life." I called everyone I knew, including my Caregiver on vacation, and told them the great news. They were all so excited for me. On January 23, I was getting VERY stressed at work because of a change in our group and some weird personalities, so I started looking for another job in our parent organization. On January 24, my Caregiver, thankfully, returned. That same day, I got another job working for one of the nicest women I had known in my Government career. What a huge relief, which helped to reduce my stress a lot. On January 26, I called my HMO to see if someone could help me get off of the narcotic painkillers. They scheduled me to see a Psychiatrist on February 1. I stopped taking Percocet® for my post-surgery pain on January 27, and started on Extra-strength Tylenol® and Motrin® for pain. Whenever I would not replace the super-powerful Fentanyl® patch or try to reduce the dosage, I would go into a really dark place, which I attributed to withdrawal symptoms. As usual, my tiredness, bad dreams, and nausea persisted. My workouts, though, were going well.

February 2005

Month 6 of Recovery/Aftercare – Month 8 since Diagnosis

*If I thought my Cancer journey to this point had been crazy and difficult, I was soon to add to that mess in a very big way. On February 1, I saw the Psychiatrist to talk about my narcotic painkiller dependency that my other doctors could not help me overcome. He was a highly esteemed and a very compassionate man and told me, "Physicians try to help but hand out pain pills like candy, and they teach patients how to fly, but not how to land." I asked if he could help me, and he told me he would enter me into a Detox Clinic at a hospital the following day. I told my new boss that I would not be in the office for some time, and, on February 2, my Caregiver drove me to the Detox Clinic at a northern Virginia hospital. They peeled off my last Fentanyl® patch and began weaning me off Opiates with decreasing doses of Methadone®. I had no idea what to expect, but on the first day I went to many lectures and I found myself among many street cocaine and heroine users and alcoholics, all in for help to get over their addictions. I wrote on February 3, "I am nauseous and anxious most of the day, but am receiving Methadone® many times a day, so my withdrawal symptoms have not been as intense. I am finding the discussions, classes, and meetings beneficial, but it is the interactions with the other group members that I find the most helpful, heartwarming, and eye-opening. I am thankful for them and the entire staff. Most of the participants have lost their jobs, families, money, and other things because of their addictions, but, they are asking for help. God bless them all!" During my 9-day stay at Detox, I received the same meds for sleep and nausea and ate soft, whole foods. By February 8, I was down to just one Methadone® a day and felt very horrible physically and emotionally, with very bad anxiety, a headache, feeling cold and achy, and debilitating nausea. I was discharged from Detox in the late afternoon of February 9 because insurance would only pay for nine days of Detox care. I was so glad to see my Caregiver when she picked me up, and so happy to return home. Upon discharge from Detox, I weighed **164 lbs**. When we got home, however, a new set of problems began. On February 10, I wrote, "I had the worst night ever, with sweating, nausea, anxiety and a horrifying dream that a guy was trying to kill me." I spent the entire day in bed after, feeling miserable. On February 11, 12, and 13, I also stayed in bed all day* *because I was anxious, tired, nauseous, and had bad headaches, and body aches – withdrawal symptoms, still, without a doubt. I was taking several prescribed sleep, anti-nausea, anti-anxiety, and pain medicines including Ambien®, Trazadone®, Serex®, Motrin® Compazine®, Valium®, Ativan®, Phenergan®, and Catapres®, which I continued throughout the month. I had to force myself to eat any food as it made me sick to my stomach, and I started losing bodyweight again. On February 16, I called the department where I received Radiation Therapy and suggested to them that they speak with patients about the possibility of narcotic painkiller dependency, and that they assist their patients in addressing such issues. During my check-up with my Oncologist on February 17, I also recommended to her that the Oncology program include patient education regarding Opiate painkiller addiction and dependency, and how to get help if needed. She told me that that was a great idea and said that they would consider that for the future. I told my Oncologist about my horrible anxiety and nausea and asked if she could suggest something for them, as I was still going thru withdrawal. She recommended Acupuncture, and set an appointment on February 23. On February 19, I restarted my workouts and slept with a heating pad on my stomach to help with nausea. On February 20, I began writing a book of my poetry to help keep my "mind over matter," and to distract me from my severe anxiety and nausea. After my beginning Acupuncture session on February 23, I seemed to notice anxiety and nausea relief, though, the next night I got absolutely no sleep, and my Acupuncture on February 24 didn't seem to help. On the same day, I had a check-up with ENT No. 2, who did an Endoscopy and physical exam of my throat and tongue. He told me that all looked and felt well – finally, some good news. He also referred me to get a blood test for my Thyroid. On February 25, I saw a Psychotherapist associated with the Oncology Clinic. I explained my intense anxiety issues to him. He told me, "Cancer, like a snake molting its skin, made you very vulnerable. That vulnerability scares you, as you are now afraid of what is around the corner, when you used not to be." He added that that image of myself can be changed, but that it could take significant time. My weight dropped to* ***158****, and my anxious worries continued thru February 26 when I wrote, "Now that I've gotten through my treatments, recovery, and detox, I think all the activities of the last year are finally hitting me. I must think about NOW and not worry." On February 27, I wrote, "I still have to deal with 3 things that I think are causing my anxiety: the fact that I spent years protecting myself and still got sick; my fear of protecting myself again and it not being good enough; and, that I need to 'remake' myself so that I will understand that I can't always control what happens with my health." On February 28, I listened to the self-help tapes my brother, Buz, gave me to help with my anxiety. My Caregiver also did what she could to comfort me. I finished February by writing, "I hate feeling like this. I want* <u>*me*</u> *back."*

March 2005

Month 7 of Recovery/Aftercare – Month 9 since Diagnosis

By March 1, my body told me that I had finally conquered my narcotics withdrawal. I started out March by returning to work again for half-days, but still with days and nights full of non-stop anxiety. Thankfully, though, my work-out strength was improving, and I was slowly gaining back my weight. On March 2, I saw a dentist about getting a permanent crown for the tooth in which I had received a Root Canal last July before my Cancer treatments started. The dentist told me that my tooth was cracked down to the root, so a crown would not work, and I would have to have the tooth pulled. I continued to take the same prescription sleep, anti-anxiety and anti-nausea medications and, with greatly reduced throat and tongue pain, was now eating a larger variety of healthful, whole foods, as well as still taking all of my vitamins, minerals, and workout supplements. On March 6, I wrote, "My anxiety is not as bad as yesterday, but still right around the corner, ready to strike. I kept busy writing, working out, and helping clean the house. Thank God that I am feeling better physically, and all of my workouts, my bodyweight and appetite are improving, but, mentally, it's going to take awhile. I want so much for the anxiety to go away soon so that I can enjoy life again." On March 9, I went back to the Head and Neck Cancer Support Group at the hospital for the first time since August, and I benefited from the experience by listening to others as they related their accounts, and, I also shared my stories for new patients and others still in recovery and aftercare like me. On March 10, I had my Mediport flushed – my bodyweight had increased to ***163 lbs****. I continued to work on my Poetry books before work and after I got home to try to keep my mind occupied, and to reduce my anxiety by thinking only positive thoughts. I tried not taking a Trazadone® or a Serax® on March 11to see if it affected my anxiety. My experiment backfired – my anxiety came back ten-fold, so I quickly took both medications, which helped a little bit. On March 12, my anxiety was extremely nasty and I wrote, "I worry about everyday things that never fazed me before, but, I'm mostly bothered about what happened to me and what I can do so that it doesn't take place again." My workouts continued getting stronger, thanks to me being able to swallow more whole foods again, take my protein and weight-gain supplements, and lift weights everyday. I started gaining back that hard-earned muscle that I had lost over the last few months. On March 14, I had a visit with the Psychiatrist that helped me get to Detox on February 1.We talked about my anxiety and that I blamed my body for letting me get Cancer after I had taken excellent care of it all my adult life. The doctor told me, "You need to continue to be you and not blame yourself for your Cancer, because no one knows what caused it." His words took a large load off my shoulders. My anxiety kept* *coming mid-month—sometimes worse than others and mostly in the AM—but, I was usually able to mitigate it with medications. I had another visit with the Oncology Psychotherapist on March 16, who told me, "We don't have control over much in our lives, including you getting Cancer, so, just let God control things, because He will anyway." His wisdom helped me very much. My throat continues to get a little dry while sleeping, so I drink water, suck on lozenges, and spray Salavert®, which helps keep it moist. I continued gaining bodyweight and on March 24, weighed in at* ***173.5 lbs***. *I had my monthly follow-up visit with ENT No. 2 on March 25, and, he told me that my prior blood test results came back perfect. The physical exam and Endoscopy of my throat, tongue, and neck Lymph Nodes also showed no issues, thankfully. He was very happy with my weight gain and overall look, and he told me, "Your tongue feels like a baby's butt. You're back!" I asked ENT No. 2 if I should return to work full-time, and he told me that I should continue with half-days for some time. I and my Caregiver had a wonderful Easter Dinner out on March 27, and I was so grateful that I was able to eat "real" food again. I also was happy that my Oncologist had decided for me not to get the Stomach Tube, as one of my friends with the same type of Cancer as me did get the tube, and he couldn't consume food without it – he couldn't teach himself how to swallow so he must always pump liquid food into his stomach through the tube "to eat." It is sad. My friends and people at work who I speak with are noticing my weight gains, and congratulating me on safely getting thru my treatments, trying to keep a positive state-of-mind, and trying to reclaim my life. I noticed on March 30 while brushing my teeth, that I cracked one piece of my tooth off and it was hanging by some gum tissue. I would have to see an Oral Surgeon.*

April 2005

Month 8 of Recovery/Aftercare – Month 10 since Diagnosis

April 1: April Fools' Day, my Mom's Birthday (God bless her), and a very busy day for me attempting to find an Oral Surgeon who would accept my insurance that could pull my bad tooth. I scheduled the appointment for April 4. My anxiety levels were already high enough, but increased when I knew I'd be getting my tooth pulled – an anxious moment no matter what. I and my Caregiver went for dinner on April 2 to the home of a friend who also had Base of Tongue Cancer. He was dependent on the Stomach Tube to eat, and was also addicted to Percocet® painkillers, but was not using them for pain. I suggested that he do all he can to wean off of both, or else his life would be miserable forever. He was seeing a Speech Pathologist to try to learn how to swallow again, but to no avail. I told him that I would do what I could to help him get off of the narcotic painkiller, which he told me he appreciated. On April 4, at the Oral Surgeon's office, I completed the health history paperwork and when I sat down in the surgery chair, the

Oral Surgeon, who was reading my health questionnaire, asked me if I had received Radiation Therapy to the jaw / neck area for treatment of my Cancer. I said I had, to which he said that we couldn't do anything to my tooth until I receive a full course of Hyperbaric Oxygen Therapy. When I asked him what that was, he explained that the radiation to the jaw bones will eliminate blood flow, and that Hyperbaric Oxygen Therapy will force oxygen into the body at high levels, which will help healing, and help form new capillaries in the jaw bones. Without the therapy, he told me I could suffer from Osteonecrosis of the Jaw, or "ONJ," ("death of the jawbone") when I get a tooth pulled, which would be disastrous. He told me that my Cancer physicians should have informed me about this condition and the precautions, but, I told him that I didn't remember them covering that, nor did I see anything about it in the research that I had conducted. He gave me the name and phone number of a Hyperbaric Oxygen Therapy Center in Northern Virginia. After my visit, I contacted my Radiation Oncologist on the phone and informed her about the oxygen treatments. She said she concurred with the decision. I next got ahold of ENT No. 2, to tell him of the development, and to ask if he could refer me to the Hyperbaric Oxygen Therapy Center for treatment. He did, and I was approved. My beginning "HBO" diagnosis session was scheduled for April 14. On April 11, I had my Mediport flush and met with the Oncology Psychotherapist to discuss my anxiety. He asked how I was coming and I told him that I was feeling better, as I was working very hard on focusing on positive, creative things, keeping my mind occupied, eating more food, having stronger workouts, regaining back my lost weight and muscle, going on day-trips with my Caregiver, and working part-time at my job. He told me that he was very impressed with my progress since our last meeting. Nevertheless, I still had intense anxiety every morning, which I treated daily with Ativan® and Trazadone® with some success. By April 12, I was drinking five protein shakes a day and eating three large meals a day. I had my HBO diagnosis consultation on April 14, and I was told by the doctor that I would receive thirty 2-hour sessions prior to having my tooth pulled, and then ten 2-hour sessions after. They introduced me to the imposing, clear, cylindrical tube in which I would be sealed each day to receive my treatments, and set up my first session for April 27. As if I were not anxious enough already, the thought of being cooped up in an enclosed chamber for two hours each day made my worries even worse. On April 15, I and my Caregiver left on a small three-day vacation to get us out of the house so that we could both decompress from the unbelievable, and at times, unbearable, last one-and-a-half years of non-stop medical commitments and one thing after another. At this point, my weight had increased to ***175 lbs.*** *– hallelujah! I was once again able to sleep all night without any bad dreams, sweating, coughing, mucous build-up, or other problems, which was a great reprieve. For some* *reason, on April 18, the day after returning from our vacation, the bottom fell out of my life, emotionally. On that day, I wrote, "I don't know why, but for some reason, I feel overwhelmed, I'm not speaking comfortably, and I don't feel happy. I feel negative and that something bad is going to happen, but I don't know what or when. I only pray that it's not true." The uneasy, self-doubt feelings persisted for the entire next week, with little or no relief. I tried to think positive and keep busy, but it didn't help much. I attended my first HBO Therapy session on April 27. It went well, as did the April 28 and 29 sessions, with no noticeable Side Effects other than being claustrophobic – two hours is a long time to be cooped up! I also had an upset stomach and anxiety, for which my doctor now prescribed Xanax®.*

May 2005

Month 9 of Recovery/Aftercare – Month 11 since Diagnosis

For once, a month started out uneventful, other than me experiencing the intense negative, anxious, and depressing feelings that had resurfaced two weeks prior. On May 2, I began week-two of my HBO Therapy, and still noted no Side Effects. My workouts were getting stronger and my appetite larger. On May 3, I started being very quiet and subdued due to anxiety. Thankfully, on May 4, I had something to cheer me up: My physical exam and Endoscopy with ENT No. 2 was favorable, as were the results of my latest CT Scan, which indicated no issues with my throat, tongue, or lungs. During that May 4 appointment, I told ENT No. 2 about the resurgence of my severe anxiety, and that I didn't know what was causing it. He told me, "It's not uncommon to have such feelings after what you've been through. Be prepared because they may continue for a very long time." On May 6, I wrote, "My anxiety or depression and feelings of uneasiness and sadness have lasted all day today. I have a horrible feeling in my stomach and I feel withdrawn, and I am not joking or talking with people like I normally do. I can't shake the anxiety, but I'm getting good at hiding it." I was still working on my Poetry Books, but, even that wasn't helping my depression or anxiety. On May 8, I wrote, "I have a very uneasy feeling in my entire body and head. I feel panicky and don't feel much self-confidence. I think I feel so uncertain about my future." On May 9, I got to play Caregiver as I drove my Caregiver to the hospital because she had been having pain in her stomach. Thankfully, it was a treatable ulcer, no-doubt exacerbated by all that she's been subjected to during my non-stop Cancer ordeal. My sleeping at night was okay, thanks to Ambien®, Trazadone®, Valium®, and Zanax®, and, my workouts and eating continued to improve. On May 13, I had my worst day of depression yet, and I was overwhelmed by things that I would not normally think twice about. Thinking positive and staying busy didn't help like they did previously. On May 15, my Caregiver and I had a talk about my depression, and I thanked her for her understanding, help, and patience, and I told her that if she ever needed to talk with me about it to let me know, because I knew how much my feelings and status affected her. That day, I wrote, "We also talked about the potential causes of my depression including my surprise diagnosis with excellent health, my fear of the unknown in the future, the restrictive oxygen treatments, and, if I'll be able to do anything to prevent a Cancer relapse. Any or all of those could be responsible for my depressive state." It made me feel bad that I could not be happier for my Caregiver, because I knew that my feelings brought her down. On May 16, I started week 4 of my HBO, and, for the first time, I started noticing a Side Effect of the therapy: My long distance vision started getting blurry. I was told that that might happen, but, I was assured by the physician that changes in eyesight are "only temporary." Thank God that I was still only working half-days at the office, because there was no possible way I could have handled the high-pressure stress of full-time work in my mental state. I had a follow-up appointment on May 17 with the Psychiatrist who'd entered me into Detox four months prior. I told him about my depression and that I thought I was holding myself, and my body, responsible for my Cancer. He told me, "You had your legs cut out from under you. You used to think, because you took care of yourself, that you were in a different category than everyone else, but, your Cancer made you realize that you're the same as obese people who smoke." The doctor also said to me, "You can't put a timeframe or deadline on getting over the problem. It will take some time. But, just as you've attained your fitness goals, so, too, will you reach your mental ones." He further offered, "When you're used to winning all of the time or being in better physical shape than a majority of people, especially your age, it was a tremendous blow to your ego and your self-image when the Cancer attacked you, of all people, especially with so many out there that have much higher risks than you." This very wise, experienced Psychiatrist hit the nail on the head. My problem was, how and when I would come to grips with the many truths he presented? My sleep continued to be okay, but my anxiety worsened over the next few days, for which I continued to take Trazadone® three times a day. On May 21, my close-up vision, which used to be very bad, was now much better and clearer – a Side Effect of the HBO. On May 22 and 23, my Caregiver and I took a mini-vacation to "get away from it all." The "distractions" during the trip helped, but, after getting home, on May 24, I wrote, "I have HORRIBLE anxiety, so bad that it turns my stomach, my heart races, my breathing is deeper, and it lasts all day, despite taking 3 Trazadone®." Also on May 24, I started week-5 of HBO Therapy. My Caregiver, always looking to help me in any way possible, bought me two books on Depression and Anxiety, which I started reading. Being worried about my Caregiver, on May 30, I wrote, "My Caregiver and I have been having lots of talks about my depression, anxiety, and my panic attacks, as

I am just as concerned about how this affects her as it does me. I know that this is very tough on her, and I don't take it for granted. She's very strong and holding up, thankfully." Finally, the month of May concluded on a very bad note: In my journal, I wrote, "MY ANXIETY/DEPRESSION TODAY WAS THE WORST YET! I started week 6 of HBO Therapy, but, it was a horrible session. I had a panic attack in the O2 chamber and started crying for no apparent reason. I also got very sweaty and my heart raced out of control. It is one of the worst and most helpless feelings ever." My Caregiver and I discussed this and determined that I must see a therapist more often. Thank God my workouts and appetite were still getting better.

June 2005

Month 10 of Recovery/Aftercare – 1 Year since Diagnosis

My 1-year anniversary of my Cancer diagnosis, and what a long, horrible, but, grateful, year it has been. On June 1, I contacted ENT No. 2 to get an appointment to talk with him about my depression and anxiety, which we scheduled for June 7. He called in a prescription for Klonopin® for me to help treat my anxiety, which I started taking. I had my Mediport flush on June 2, and discussed my depression with my Oncologist. As if things were not bad and stressful enough, on June 3, I wrote in my journal that it was "...the most horrible day of my life, because Buz just called to tell me that our wonderful, caring, compassionate and kind Vikki, passed from this life to the next. My problems are nothing compared to that. God bless her and Mom. We love and will miss her so much." I later learned that Vik passed away while visiting Mom in the Nursing Home, and that nurses and EMTs came to her side immediately. If God wanted Vik's life to be spared, that was the perfect time and place to save it – but He wanted her with Him, as she had experienced far too much pain here on earth. She is at peace, and that is what's most important. Her passing, though, did cause my anxiety to go from bad to worse. Thankfully, my brother, Buz, stayed with Mom to help comfort the loss of her only daughter. On June 5, Mom and Buz took care of Vik's cremation arrangements, and I wrote and sent Vik's obituary to them for publication in the Albuquerque paper on June 6. I started my sixth week of HBO Therapy on June 6, and was still experiencing the Side Effects of horrible distance vision, but perfect close-up vision, the opposite of what I used to have. The doctor told me that these symptoms would go away, but, I doubted it. I visited ENT No. 2 on June 7 to have my monthly Cancer check-up, and to talk about my depression. Thankfully, my throat, tongue, and neck exam results were favorable. Because the Klonopin® was making me sleepy during the day, he prescribed Zoloft® for me to treat my anxiety. I flew to Albuquerque on June 10 and was so happy to see Mom, and brothers, Buz and Rich, who had been going through Vik's personal effects prior to my arrival. Our Dear Vikki's service was on June 11, and *was attended by 50+ people in Mom's Nursing Home. It was beautiful and family and friends had so many wonderful things to say about her and her life. I stayed to comfort Mom and to help clean out more of Vik's things on June 12, but had to return to Virginia on June 13. The Klonopin® seemed to help me sleep better around mid-month, but it was too early to know if the Zoloft® was going to work I had my final "pre-tooth extraction" HBO Therapy session on June 16, and on June 17, I contacted the Oral Surgeon to make an appointment to have my tooth pulled; however, he told me that he had not received a letter from the HBO doctor stating that my thirty sessions had been completed. On June 18, I noted that for the first time, my upper and lower gums were very tender, and my lower right jawbone was hurting for some reason. My gum and jawbone pain hurt for several days, so I made an appointment to see the HBO Therapy doctor to see if he knew why this was happening. On June 22, I saw the physician and he told me that my X-rays were fine, and that he didn't know what was causing the pain. He did provide me a prescription for the antibiotic, Clindamyacin®, which I started utilizing, along with the mouth rinse, Chlorohexadine®. I stopped taking Zoloft® because it seemed to be making my face and body "puffy." I was still working at my job part-time, and my co-workers were so thoughtful to me, and they provided flowers for Vik's service, for which I was very thankful. On June 25, I had "<u>very bad panic attacks</u>," but my gums and my jawbone were feeling much better. I resumed taking Zoloft® to see if it would help my anxiety. The Oral Surgeon scheduled me for my tooth extraction on June 28, as he had received word that I completed my thirty HBO sessions. Thankfully, the tooth extraction went well, and the Surgeon, while pulling my tooth with all his might, yelled, "I see blood!" meaning that the HBO Therapy had done its job. I was thankful for that very important blessing. The Surgeon gave me a prescription for Vicodin® for pain, and the anti-biotic, Amoxycillin®, to help stave off infection. My sleeping was starting to become difficult toward the end of the month, even though I was taking multiple sleep-inducing meds. On June 29, I started my ten post-tooth-extraction HBO Therapy sessions. Anxiety was having its way with me, and on June 30 I wrote, "The Zoloft® doesn't seem to be reducing my anxiety or depression. I can't be happy or playful, as usual."*

July 2005
Month 11 of Recovery/Aftercare
1 Year/1 Month since Diagnosis

I continued with my HBO Therapy on July 1, and continued reading Self-help books, listening to the tapes Buz had loaned to me, and started doing relaxation and visualization techniques I had been given, but, none of them seemed to help me diminish or eliminate my depression, anxiety, and panic attacks. On July 2, I started getting very bad diarrhea, possibly because of my upset stomach and anxiety, or, due to the huge volume of various drugs I was using, or both. I stopped taking Valium® for sleep on July 4, and was still not realizing any relief from Zoloft® for anxiety. The Zoloft® product literature said it may take up to six weeks to start working…WTF? I had a follow-up appointment with my friend, the very helpful and knowledgeable Psychiatrist, on July 5. We discussed my depression and anxiety and we talked about my anti-anxiety meds. He told me that the dosage of Zoloft® I was on was too low, so he discontinued that and prescribed a higher dose of Prozac®. He also prescribed Compazine® for nausea. Finally, he told me that I should obtain regular and frequent Psychotherapy to help me get over and past my mental issues. He gave me names of Psychotherapists who have worked with Cancer survivors and who are aware of emotional issues that Cancer patients and survivors face. I called a therapist on the list, and scheduled my first Psychotherapist appointment for July 25. The next day, July 6, I had the customary diarrhea, upset stomach, and nausea in the morning, but, thankfully, the Prozac® and the Compazine® seemed to help me later in the afternoon and evening. This pattern continued until July 11, and, then, on July 12, I wrote, "Thank God, I did not wake up with nausea or diarrhea for the first time in ages" On July 13, I had my tenth and final HBO post-tooth-extraction therapy session, and was happy to put all of that behind me. Things seemed to improve a little on July 17, when I entered in my journal: "Prozac® does seem to help make me feel more like my old self once again – happier, playful, more positive, energetic, and optimistic. It feels nice." My workouts, my appetite, and outdoor physical activities, such as my ability to work in the yard, all continued to improve and recapture some normalcy back into my life. My Caregiver and I also started doing more things out of the house, such as going to restaurants, the movies, and visiting friends and family, which helped us take our minds off of my anxiety and negative stuff and keep them on positive, optimistic things. On July 20, I accompanied my friend and Base of Tongue Cancer patient (who was addicted to Percocet® and the Stomach Tube, and who I promised to help him come off of the drug) to a meeting with a drug detox doctor. All went well with the consultation, and, thankfully, over time, he managed to come completely off of the medication and his life improved tremendously. He told me that he very much appreciated my help and my inspiration, because I had successfully beaten my painkiller dependency. My bodyweight on July 21 was ***183.5,*** *an increase of 7 lbs. since April 15. Not very much, but every hard-earned pound counts. On July 22, I wrote, "Today, my anxiety and diarrhea are worse than normal and the Prozac® didn't seem to help much. I felt pretty bad most of the day and didn't even have a good workout." Things continued the same for the next few days from a physical and a mental standpoint, including my messed-up eyesight,* *the diarrhea, anxiety, nausea, and queasiness. On July 25, I had my first appointment with the Psychotherapist, and I really liked him and felt very comfortable with him from the start. I prayed that he would be able to help me break the deadlock that I had been realizing for months with my nasty anxiety and depression. My therapy sessions were to be weekly. The more I used Prozac®, it seemed like the weaker I was in my workouts, and I also seemed to be losing muscle size. But, I had no choice but to continue using it to battle my anxiety. My Caregiver and I finished out July with a mini-vacation out of town, again, designed to help us give our minds a break. I continued keeping my mind busy writing the two volumes of my poetry.*

August 2005
Month 12 of Recovery/Aftercare
1 Year/2 Months since Diagnosis

August 1 was a very busy day for me: I started working 7-hour days vs. 5-hour days. Plus, I had appointments with both my helpful Psychiatrist, as well as ENT No. 2, for my monthly Cancer check-up .Gratefully, my check-up went perfectly, and I asked ENT No. 2 if he could order a chest X-ray in addition to my regular PET Scan of my throat and neck. He said he would. During my visit with the Psychiatrist, I told him that I had done research on Prozac®, and I had found that it has several negative Side Effects, and, that a person can experience withdrawal when coming off the drug. I told him that I would like to stop using it and asked him if I could use natural St. John's Wort, instead, to better my mood. He told me, "Because of your lifestyle and your natural approach to wellness, you should probably not take Prozac® anymore." He said that he did not see any problems with me using alternative medicine, and provided me with tapering-off instructions. He also told me to wait for two weeks after quitting Prozac® before I start the St. John's Wort. August 2 and 3 were pretty good days with no nausea, diarrhea, or anxiety, but, on August 4, it was a different story, as I had all of the above – again. Also on August 4, I had my monthly Mediport flush, blood test, and Thyroid test. My bodyweight that day was ***185,*** *barely up since July. I had my second Psychotherapy appointment on August 5 with the man whom I entrusted implicitly my mental state. Essentially, I turned my heart and mind over to him so that he could help me mould both back into pre-Cancer shape. During my appointment, he told me, "You've dealt with the panic of death – now you need to deal with the panic of life. That will take some time, especially considering the ways you have reevaluated and reprioritized many of the things in your life." That one made me think. By August 6, I was off of Prozac® and Zoloft® totally as I did not want to become dependent on them and have to go through withdrawal – again. I still was having the "big-three" every morning: nausea, anxiety, and good* *old-fashioned diarrhea. By August 7, I was only using ONE prescription medication—Ambien® for sleep—as I had successfully gotten myself off of all other drugs. My eyesight also continued to be messed up as I thought it would be, despite the HBO doctor's claims to the contrary. On August 8, I started taking St. John's Wort, a natural herb used for treating anxiety and improving one's mood. On August 10, I was feeling less apprehensive and anxious, and on August 11, I went to see my Primary Care doctor about my persistent diarrhea. He attributed it to Irritable Bowel Syndrome (IBS) based on what I had been going through. My Caregiver and I attended a birthday party on August 13, and afterward, I wrote, "I was surprised with how positive, talkative, and happy I was." On a roll, I wrote in my journal on August 14, "I am starting to feel much better, physically, mentally, and emotionally, Thank God! I pray it continues." For the first time in a long time, on August 15, I woke up with a horrible dream and couldn't get back to sleep. For the remainder of August, I slept well with Ambien®, but did continue to wake up each and every day with the horrendous diarrhea and anxiety. I had Psychotherapy sessions on both August 15 and 19, and also had a PET Scan of my throat and neck on August 19. My appetite and food intake was excellent during the month, as were my workouts. My weight on August 23 was* ***188.5*** *– slowly but surely creeping up. Finally, after a year, I started working full 9-hour days at my government job again. That felt a little strange, but, since I had been working part-time for so long, it wasn't too bad. I had Therapy again on August 26, after an entire day of nausea and horrible anxiety. During therapy, we talked about guarding my heart from pain and trying not to internalize all of the hurt that I was feeling. I summed up my situation on August 27, when I wrote, "I woke up with huge anxiety and diarrhea, and I was not happy all day or night, and my workouts aren't too good either. Basically, I'm a big mess, but, thankfully, I'm now Cancer-free and healthy, thank God." I took my Caregiver on August 29 to her Endoscopy procedure for her ulcer. Thankfully, all looked well and her results were favorable. August would end like many other months with non-stop anxiety and never-ending diarrhea. My depression took a new turn on August 30, when I wrote, "For some reason, I am viewing the world, politicians, and many people with a very skeptical eye, and I allow myself to get very upset and frustrated with what I see. I have to not allow myself to get all worked up by all the things that are beyond my control."*

September 2005
1 Year/1 Month of Recovery/Aftercare
1 Year/3 Months since Diagnosis

The month of September began with my eyesight still being messed up from the HBO Therapy, and me hoping that it would some day return to my pre-

*Cancer and pre-HBO levels. September 1 started with a semi-full schedule as I had a Mediport flush and my monthly Cancer check-up with ENT No. 2. Thankfully, the flush went well, but my follow-up appointment with ENT No. 2 – not so much. The doctor gave me the frightening results of the PET Scan I had gotten on August 19. He told me that an area on the back, left side of my tongue, where my Primary Tumor was located, "lit up" on the scan, meaning that it found activity (possibly Cancer) due to the uptake of Radioactive Glucose by cells in that area. I asked the doctor if it was my Cancer coming back, and he told me that he could not answer that without a Biopsy of the tissue in that area. I told ENT No. 2, that I definitely would agree to another Biopsy Surgery and asked him how quickly we could get it done. He told me he would schedule within the next two weeks, which he did. On that day, I wrote, "I feel optimistic and positive about the outcome of my biopsies, but, I am guarded because of the possibility that it may be Cancer." I told ENT No. 2 that I was having real bad dreams again, so he prescribed Trazadone® for me again. My Oncologist was also informed of the scan results and my upcoming Biopsy Surgery. September 2, I wrote, "<u>I feel very depressed</u>." and on September 3, I continued to have non-stop anxiety and diarrhea. My bodyweight on that day had increased to **191.5,** and two days later was **193.** My body was soaking up long-lost weight like a sponge, despite my incessant "runs." My sleeping at night was difficult, despite taking Ambien® and Trazadone®, because of my overworked mind thinking all the time, and because of my dry throat, for which I sucked on Salavert® lozenges. I continued to attend my weekly Psychotherapy, but, I did not have any breakthroughs, as my high anxiety levels persisted. My scary dreams did, thankfully, diminish with the Trazadone®. On September 13, I wrote in my journal, "I am <u>very nervous</u> about the upcoming Biopsy Surgery, although I am thinking and acting positive. I pray to God that all is well." Very early in the morning, on September 14, my Caregiver and I arrived for the Biopsy Surgery. Thankfully, the surgeries went well and the doctor told me that the PET Scan "hit" may have been due to healing scar tissue. He told me that he would contact me immediately when he had my results. ENT No. 2 prescribed Vicodin® painkiller for the intense pain in my throat and tongue caused by the multiple biopsies. He also prescribed the antibiotic Amoxycillin® to help prevent infection. On September 16, I stayed home from work because my throat and tongue hurt so much. I also had to eat soft foods again and could not workout. I received great news in the evening when ENT No. 2 called to tell me that all of my Biopsy results came back favorable – there was no recurrent or new Cancer, thank God! "False Positives" again. That was the second time that my PET Scan had scared me to death by indicating that I possibly had Cancer. That sucks! On September 17, 18, and 19, I started tapering myself off of the narcotic drug, Vicodin®, because I was very fearful of painkiller dependency. I did* *start having nauseating and painful withdrawal symptoms which dredged up my past, horrible experiences. On September 18, I wrote, "When I woke up today, I felt horrible due to my withdrawal from Vicodin. My stomach is upset; I have a headache and diarrhea. I feel foggy, and feel like I have the flu. My whole body aches. I feel overwhelmed and just want to sleep. There is nothing that I can do but tough it out. My body is now ultra-sensitive to Opiates." I had my Biopsy Surgery follow-up appointment with ENT No. 2 on September 21. I told him I was still feeling very depressed, anxious, and nauseous. Trazadone® was making my mouth and throat very dry. By September 27, my mental state continued to deteriorate with no relief in sight. On that day, I entered in my journal, "My worst day in a long time, I felt so depressed and worthless and my scalp is breaking out with bumps." My vision issues due to the HBO persisted and weren't getting any better as the doctors told me they would – surprise, surprise. In my final therapy session of the month, my Psychotherapist told me he thought I was doing well, considering the surgery and narcotic withdrawal I had been through. Amid all of my problems, I could not believe the consistent outpouring of support that I continued to get from friends and family, even this far out from my diagnosis. And, of course, I knew that I would never be able to repay my Caregiver for all that she had done and sacrificed over the last one-and-one-half years to encourage, comfort, support, and care for me.*

October 2005

1 Year/2 Months of Recovery/Aftercare
1 Year/4 Months since Diagnosis

Thankfully, October began uneventfully, but, with the ordinary anxiety and nausea. My anxiety was becoming so persistent and very depressing, so I started to rate it on October 3, on a scale from "1" to "10,"with 10 being the best, and 1, the worst. I had my monthly Mediport flush on October 3, as well as my check-up with my Oncologist. All went well with those, and I rated my anxiety a "5" on that day. On October 4, I felt overwhelmed and frightened, but, on October 6, I wrote, "I didn't feel good, psychologically, but my Caregiver and I had a long talk last night with her trying to help me see that everything is going to be okay, which I know in my heart it is." On that day, I gave my anxiety level a 3, for "very poor." I was continuing to work, full-time at my job, and was also working out and back to eating my normal three large meals a day, along with lots of healthy snacks, and protein shakes, vitamins, and minerals. It was all paying off, as my weight had jumped to ***197 lbs****. by October 6. At least the physical part of me was starting to feel "like me" again, even if my mind was not. I continued to take Trazadone® and Ambien® to help me sleep, and Salavert® lozenges to moisten my dry mouth and throat caused by the Trazadone®. I attended my* *weekly Psychotherapy sessions, and benefitted by sharing my life story and my feelings of being betrayed by my body that I had taken such good care of through the years. He was an extremely attentive listener, and was very familiar with the problems faced by Cancer patients and survivors, and he offered heartfelt ideas and suggestions to me for overcoming my fears. On October 7, 8, and 9, I rated my anxiety much better with a 7 and an 8. On October 9, my bodyweight had jumped to* ***198 lbs****., just shy of the weight I was before Cancer pulled the rug out from under me over a year before. I wrote on October 11, "Today was a* <u>*very bad*</u> *day. I felt overwhelmed and depressed most of the day," and on October 12, "I had another bad day. I have a lack of self-confidence and I'm thinking negative thoughts about my past Cancer problem, and am worried about it repeating in the future." I continued with my "future fears" for several days, and prayed that I could have more faith in God and myself that everything would work out okay. I and my Caregiver continued to keep busy doing outdoor projects in hopes that my anxious mind would get a break while doing physical things. This strategy seemed to work well, as I rated my anxiety with an 8 on weekends, and, typically, a 5 or 6 during the week when working or staying inside the house. I had a very good day on Sunday, October 16, when I wrote in my journal, "I had little, if any, anxiety or feelings of lack of self-worth. I felt pretty positive and self-confident today, thankfully. We worked outside all day, which wiped me out physically, but, I felt good otherwise." I felt not too bad, mentally, on October 18, when I wrote, "I had a good day with no real anxiety or negative feelings. I'm doing everything I can to try not to dwell on future challenges, fears, and unknowns. I must be happy for now and today." These were some of the self-help lessons that my therapist had given me in our last session. October 19 was a banner day, weight-wise, as I finally broke the 200 lb. barrier at* ***200.5 lbs****! It took me well over one year of working out hard and eating lots of nutritious food to finally get it all back. Most people try to lose weight – I have to fight to keep it on. On October 20 and 21, I noted that I began to really feel the stress of full-time work, as the projects I was working on were very high-level and important, and, as a result, extremely overwhelming for me. My anxiety levels were very high, and at my therapy appointment on October 21, my therapist told me that I will have to learn how to say "no," so that I don't take on more than I can handle. My therapist also suggested that I begin writing all of my worries, concerns, fears, and thoughts down on paper so that it would make it easier to get them off my chest and to confront them, one-by-one. His suggestion led to me writing so many thoughts, that I decided to put them all in a book, which I ultimately did and had published, along with my two poetry books. On October 22, my Caregiver left for her annual trip to visit her girlfriend, which left me alone and caused me to be even more anxious. But, she did need to get away from it all for a little bit to recharge* *her batteries, and I was so happy she did. I rated my anxiety a 5 that day. On October 26, I had a very bad day at work. I didn't want to talk with anyone, so closed my office door, and stayed to myself. Later, I wrote, "I tried to adjust my attitude and kept telling myself that this is all BS and to try not to take it all too personally or seriously." I regrouped the next day, and on October 27, in my journal, I noted, "Today was much better than yesterday, thank God, because I forced myself to not let the job frustrate me. It is definitely not worth it. I want to stay healthy." On October 29, my Caregiver returned to Virginia, which helped to decrease my anxieties. I ended October on a positive note (and an anxiety rating of 9), for which I wrote on October 31, "Actually, had a very good day, mentally speaking, and felt comfortable having fun and telling jokes. Unfortunately, both have been rarities lately." My workouts were great, but my eyes still had issues.*

November 2005

1 Year/3 Months of Recovery/Aftercare
1 Year/5 Months since Diagnosis

My anxieties and depression were getting very old, as I started yet another month with more of the same. On November 1, I woke up with anxiety, but it lessened during the day, as it did on most days, especially if I kept myself busy. Work continued to depress me, but, I appreciated my job and I gave it my best despite my emotional problems. My Mediport flush on November 1 went well. As for my job, on November 2, I wrote, "I think that being at work is depressing me more than anything." My anxiety on November 3 was a 6, and I wrote, "Today was okay, but I still have periods during the day when I have panic attacks and I start breathing heavily and feeling overwhelmed. Generally, I will relax and close my eyes, and these feelings sometimes go away." My sleeping was getting better on most nights as I was on Ambien® and Trazadone® at this point, but, daily, the anxiety was there to greet me when I woke up each morning. I wrote on November 4, "I started off the day at my work with anxiety and feeling gloomy, but, I relaxed my mind for a period and slowed down my breathing, which did help. I do seem to have a real problem being happy, whatever that is." My Caregiver and I continued to take day trips to get out of the house that, as beautiful, bright, and spacious as it was, seemed at times like a dungeon with walls that kept closing in, the longer we stayed inside. After almost 2 years of dealing with my throat, Cancer, and depression issues, everything connected with these problems unfortunately became guilty by association. And, unfortunately, that included our beautiful home on 3 wooded acres that was bordered on two sides by lovely creeks. What a shame. During the next few days, from November 5th thru the 10th, my anxiety levels were somewhat stable as I rated them as a 6. I did my best to try to get securely *through each day at work without panicking or feeling too overwhelmed. My weekly Psychotherapy sessions continued to be very eye-opening and helpful. My therapist's primary objective was to try to ease me back into Life, and to equip me with the proper tools and defense mechanisms that would better facilitate my abilities to withstand and safely cope with Life's occasionally cruel realities. In so doing, his main intention was to prepare me psychologically for any unforeseen challenges that might be lurking around the various corners—figuratively speaking—that I may possibly be encountering during what I hoped would develop into a very lengthy and successful life. Throughout my Counseling sessions, my therapist typically would give me a few "homework" lessons, which he recommended that I accomplish in between our weekly appointments. Some of his assignments encouraged me to concentrate on the "here and now," and to minimize my "anticipatory" thought patterns and needless worrying. Other coursework encouraged me to trade in all of my negative "what if" thinking for that of a more optimistic, constructive kind. My therapist also recommended, and we discussed at great length during some of my sessions, that I actively practice "Self-Help" behaviors to assist me in eliminating, or, at the very least, minimizing, the intense anxiety and significant depression that I had experiencing for the last several months. I was well aware that any form of distress plays havoc with one's Immune System, and that a weakened and compromised Immune System is Cancer's best friend. Having recovered completely from my nasty Cancer from a physical standpoint, my primary objective at this time was to maximize my mental well-being. This meant that I would have to do everything within my power to diminish stresses in my life, and, consequently, to facilitate my emotional stability. First and foremost on my list of things to do was to stop watching the News on TV, listening to it on the radio, and reading it in newspapers or magazines. I found the News to be invariably bad, and overwhelmingly frustrating and anxiety-inducing. My second ambitious objective in attempting to remove unnecessary tension from my life was, contrary to all of my past practices and experiences, to try not take my job in the government too seriously or too personally. Both the news and my job added fuel to my depression fire. I began my news moratorium after my Psychotherapy visit on November 11, and I had already begun working on relaxing my mind at my job the first week of November. I was bound-and-determined to defeat my anxiety, just as I had beaten my Cancer and my dependency on the prescription narcotic painkillers. I also continued to work on my poetry and "self-help" books at home, which kept my mind occupied in a positive way. I sent my poetry books in for final publication on November 17. November 18 wasn't a good day, emotionally, but, November 19, my Birthday, was much better, because my Caregiver and I enjoyed a night out for dinner, and she got me very thoughtful gifts. I got another gift on November 21, during my check-*

up with ENT No. 2. Following my physical exam and Endoscopy, he told me that my throat and tongue looked perfect. Thank God! On November 23, I flew out to Albuquerque to celebrate Thanksgiving with my Mom and my brother, Buz. I stayed in Albuquerque until November 29, and I was so thankful I made the trip so that Mom could see my physical improvements, and, so that I could spend some important quality time with her and Buz. The only bad part of the trip was that I was eaten by Bed Bugs in the hotel. I hated to leave, but, I was happy to get back home and to my Caregiver. My eyesight didn't return to pre-O2 levels. The changes were permanent.

December 2005

1 Year/4 Months of Recovery/Aftercare
1 Year/6 Months since Diagnosis

My newfound physical problem, which helped take my attention off of my usual anxiety, were the Bed Bug bites with which I had to contend, that I had gotten in Albuquerque. I took Benadryl® for the unbelievable itching that persisted until December 13. On December 3, my Caregiver and I worked on the yard, again, to do anything that got us out of the house and kept my mind constructively occupied. I had a great day, emotionally, on December 6, when I rated my anxiety a high 9 and wrote, "I felt very good today for some reason," almost as though it was such an anomaly to have a favorable day (which it was) that I had to rationalize it somehow. I again addressed this conundrum on December 8, when I wrote in my journal, "Today was another good day, physically, emotionally, and mentally, for which I am very grateful. It is a strange feeling to feel good, and to not feel bad about feeling good." I had my weekly Psychotherapy appointment on December 9, during which I gladly told my therapist the progress that I had made by using his suggestions and advice. I told him that I could trust my body and mind again, and that I had gotten past blaming my body for my Cancer. I mentioned to him that I felt much stronger, both physically and mentally. He was very pleased with my transformation, which he had been aiming towards, and observing, over the last several months. I boldly told the therapist, "I'M BACK!" I continued to have good days, mentally, from December 10 to the 14, but went a little off-track on December 15. I wrote that day, "I woke up feeling very strange for some reason, and felt strange all day but never knew exactly why. I could not get back on-track all day. Had some anxiety and diarrhea, for the first time in a long while." I started gradually tapering off of Trazadone® on December 16, as I didn't think I needed it to ward off bad dreams or the monsters under my bed at night anymore. Further confirming the "new me," I noted in my journal on December 17, "I felt pretty good today overall. Thank God I have my life back, physically, mentally, and emotionally. It is so nice to be happy again and to not be expecting or anticipating something bad to happen. I'm not feeling overconfident – just comfortable one day at a time." On the 18th and 19th of December, I felt so-so, mentally, for no-telling what reasons. I did feel better on December 20 and 21, and rated my anxiety with excellent 9 and 9+ ratings, respectively. I continued to feel great, and to count my blessings. It was both a sad and a happy day on December 23, because I had my final Psychotherapy session with my therapist. I hated to tell him "good-bye" because he had helped me so much. He wished me well and told me that should I have any emotional relapses (which he said can be normal with Cancer patients and survivors), I should come see him again. My workouts, eating, and all other basic life necessities were going well, and, I truly felt like my pre-Cancer self once again, inside and out. I had received my published books about poetry from the publisher just in time to send my books out to family and friends as Christmas gifts. That was such a wonderful feeling, and the writing of the two books helped me thru some really tough times during the preceding months. My Caregiver and I shared a low-key, but very festive and nice Christmas in our home, which we had decorated to the hilt for the holidays. I had a very heartwarming call with my Mom, who was experiencing her first Christmas without Vikki by her side. She was so sad, but I was proud of how strong and content she was on the phone, considering. Of course, we all missed our dear Vikki. I had good days after Christmas, which continued throughout the rest of the year. I summed it all up on December 29, when I wrote in my journal, "I woke up feeling good and it continued all day, physically, emotionally, and mentally. I pray that it all continues. It would be so wonderful to end 2005 and begin 2006 on a very positive note, and I pray that that happens. We have all been very blessed, and I thank God for it." And, finally, on New Year's Eve, I wrote, "Thank you God for 2005 ending positively, with all of us being healthy." Good night, Tiny Tim, and to all of us, a good night.

January 2006
1 Year/5 Months of Recovery/Aftercare
1 Year/7 Months since Diagnosis

This was, indeed, a Happy New Year, which I celebrated with my January 1 entry in my journal, "Thank God we concluded 2005 with all of us being healthy, and that we are starting 2006 the same way. I pray that all things good continue." I did, however, still, have some lingering emotional issues that did impact me for several days following. I wrote on January 3, "For some reason, I did feel a little "off" all day, and not very fun or talkative. I don't know why." On January 4, I followed with, "Today, I woke feeling really bad and off-balance inside for some reason, just like yesterday. I'm not sure why, but I am not happy emotionally. It may just be my 'time of the month.'" By this juncture, I had not totally stopped taking Trazadone®, which I began tapering off of on December 16, so, I thought that the lower dose may be contributing to my anxiety. I decided to up it to a full dose to see if that could be contributing to my bad anxiety ratings of 4, and 5 that I gave myself from January 4th through the 15th. I wrote on January 6 in my journal, "I feel like crap emotionally and mentally. I feel okay, physically, but for some reason, I'm losing size and bodyweight, and my strength is less than normal. Oh well, at least I'm healthy, so I shouldn't complain." January 8 and 9, which I gave sad anxiety ratings of 3 and 4, respectively, were, likewise, just as devastating on me emotionally. January 8: "I woke up feeling totally horrible – the worst I've felt in weeks for some reason. I don't know for sure what's going on with me, but, I feel down emotionally and mentally. Nothing I would do or think about would bring me out of my funk. Time will tell what it is." January 9: "I am back to taking a full dose of Trazadone® to see if that helps. I just can't shake whatever it is. I felt especially fragile today and started crying when I thought about Vikki. I didn't get any better during the day or evening. I'm just not able to have fun or be happy." I thought that if I went to the Head and Neck Cancer Support Group that it might help my mental state, so, on January 11, I did. At the end of the evening, the only way it helped me, as sad as it sounds, is that I listened to other patients and survivors who told stories of their own experiences and problems that were so much worse than mine. Everything in life, I guess, is relative. Another good thing that came out of the evening was that I got to see my Radiation Oncologist, who told me that she could not believe how good I looked. I needed that. On January 13, I noted that my distance vision was continuing to get worse, while my up-close vision was improving – the polar opposite of my pre-Cancer/pre-HBO vision. Oh well, it is what it is. It became just another aspect of my "New Normal" way of life. My Caregiver's birthday was on January 16, so we celebrated that with dinner and gifts, which was nice. By January 18, my emotional state began improving, when I wrote, "I worked on my Cancer book most of the day. I felt good in all ways, thankfully, and am much happier and enjoying life more. I don't know why I felt so down last week, but, it's great to be back. I'm grateful that my life has taken a more "normal" and even-keeled turn, and I pray that it continues." There is a possibility that the full dose of Trazadone® was responsible for my mental turn-around, but, whatever it was, I needed it in a bad way. I had another mood-lifter on January 18 during my check-up appointment with ENT No. 2. After a physical exam and Endoscopy of my throat and tongue, he told me that everything looks excellent, and, that my tongue "Is as smooth as a baby's butt." ENT No. 2 also scheduled me for a PET Scan on January 20. I did have the PET Scan on January 20, which went well. The hard part, for me, once again, was the fear of the unknown while waiting for the results. January 21st thru the 26th were, thankfully, above average days, physically, mentally, and emotionally, with no major issues. I rated my anxiety levels at 6 and 7 during those days. On January 27, I had my monthly Mediport flush, which went well, and I also had my follow-up appointment with my Oncologist that went exceedingly well. She told me that my PET Scan results came back favorably. Thank God, no "false-positives" again like the prior two PET Scans, which meant no follow-up Biopsy Surgery. It also meant that I was one step closer to being Cancer-free. Talk about an anxiety killer! The stronger I got, mentally, during the month, the easier it was for me to stomach work and the news. I controlled my work – not the other way around, and, I kept up with the current news to the degree that it didn't depress me. January 2006 was the Second Anniversary of me first experiencing throat and tongue pain, which led to the detection, diagnosis, and eradication of my Cancer. It had been one hell of a ride to get there!

February 2006
1 Year/6 Months of Recovery/Aftercare
1 Year/8 Months since Diagnosis

My "New Normal" way of life, it seemed by February 2006, was to expect that each day, it would be a crapshoot as to how I would feel emotionally. Physically, I was holding my own each day, because of my healthy eating and strong daily workouts, but, emotionally, I seemed to be far from out of the woods. On February 4, I rated my anxiety a so-so 5, and I wrote in my journal, "Today, I feel pretty good physically, but, mentally, I'm not too happy or positive. I'm feeling out-of-sorts for some reason. Didn't get any better in the evening." My sleep continued to go well as the Trazadone® seemed to be doing its job, but I needed a kick-start every morning to pull ahead of my residual anxiety before it could slow me down. On February 7, I had an eye exam appointment with a doctor, who I asked to check my eyes. I told him about the HBO Therapy, and how the vision changes that I experienced were supposed to be only "temporary," per the doctors, did, in fact, turn out to be permanent. He said that I did not have Glaucoma or any other eye problems, but, that the HBO Therapy did change the shape of my lenses and corneas in both eyes. He measured my right eye at 20/60 and my left eye at 20/40, far from where they were before my Cancer. He told me that I would need to get glasses for my distance vision, which I did for the first time in my life. On February 8, I went to the monthly Head and Neck Cancer Support Group at the hospital where I received my Radiation Therapy 1 ½ years prior. The group helped me a lot with their accounts of problems and victories during their own Cancer journeys, and I relayed to them the physical and emotional lowlights and highlights that I had known up until that time. It was an extremely productive and wonderful meeting of numerous patients, survivors, and their loved ones and family members, *who, like me, were fighting with everything they had to reclaim their pre-Cancer lives, or, as much of those lives as they could. On February 10, I noted that I had a good day at work as I was very busy, and on February 11, I awoke feeling pretty good and had a nice day, physically, with a very strong workout, and, emotionally, with no anxious or negative thoughts. I continued to work on my "self-help" book containing my thoughts, quotes, and opinions, almost daily after work and on weekends, to keep my mind occupied. Simultaneously, I worked on my first iteration of the book on my Cancer story, the beginnings of what became this book. On February 15, I had a very good day, mixed with concerns about my vision, when I wrote, "I woke up feeling good in all respects, gratefully, but, my vision continues to be a problem. I can read the smallest print with no glasses, but, I can't read anything past 3 to 4 feet as it's blurry." I never had that issue prior to my HBO Therapy, as my distance vision was always 20/20. February 17 was another nice day. I wrote in my journal, "Today was a good day in all respects and I was relaxed at work, thankfully. I feel pretty good physically and mentally, and am grateful that all continues to go well." On February 19, I, once again, began to taper off of Trazadone®, which I was taking to help me sleep and to decrease my anxiety. I hoped that doing so would not mess up my sleeping or emotional state. From the 22nd to the 24th, I started having small withdrawal symptoms from coming off the Trazadone®. On the 22nd I entered, "I am noticing some small withdrawal Side Effects from tapering off of the Trazadone®. I feel less happy, more under the weather, and I'm timid." On the 24th I noted, "<u>I feel like crap</u> today emotionally and mentally. Not very happy or excited and feeling very timid with complete lack of self-esteem." Thankfully, I ended the last few days of February with no noticeable signs of withdrawal. I went from a full dose of Trazadone®, to ¾ of a dose, but still had 75% to go. I had to take it very slowly. Other than that, my work, workouts, eating, and I and my Caregiver, were well.*

March 2006

1 Year/7 Months of Recovery/Aftercare
1 Year/9 Months since Diagnosis

March 1 got off to a good start in all respects, which I noted in my journal as follows, "No noticeable Side Effects due to tapering off of Trazadone®. In fact, I'm having a good day, Thank God, mentally and emotionally. I'm also doing good physically, and my workouts are excellent and strong." I was still on a ¾ dose of Trazadone®. My good sleep, reduced anxiety, and good appetite and workouts continued for the first few days of March, but, I did have a bad day at work on March 2 due to my anxiety. On March 3, I was much stronger emotionally, and I wrote, "I had a good day today, and much better than yesterday. I was able to shake off all the crap at work yesterday and turn my attitude around." Things continued to go good for me, when I wrote on March 7, "No withdrawal from Trazadone® tapering, so I may be ready to drop down to half a dose in a couple of days. Work is bearable and thankfully going well. I'm so fortunate to have the job, the boss, and the office I do." Because my Trazadone® tapering had gone so well for three weeks on a ¾ dose, I decided on March 11 to lessen the dose to one-half, once again, hoping that it would not have any negative affects. As of March 14, things were going well with the tapering, as I wrote, "No noticeable Side Effects from tapering down to a ½ dose on Trazadone®. I really have been feeling much better physically, mentally, and emotionally than I have in a long while. Plus, my body, skin, and hair are feeling and looking better than they have been." My Caregiver and I continued to give our minds a break by keeping busy working in the yard on weekends, and going out to eat, run errands, going to movies, visiting friends, and other distractions. These sorts of things were very important in helping both of us inject some normalcy back into our lives – the pre-Cancer lives that we both had to put on-hold almost two long years ago. By March 2006, I was seeing ENT No. 2 every two months for my follow-up examinations instead of once a month. I had my 2-month check-up on March 20, and, gratefully, my Endoscopy and physical exam went very well. "ENT No. 2 told me, "It looks like nothing ever happened to your throat and tongue." but, boy, did it! The half-dose of Trazadone® seemed to be working okay, but, on March 21, I was having emotional issues when I wrote, "Today, I didn't feel too confident or positive about things, and, actually, was pretty tentative and quiet. I don't know why." My gloomy mental state continued on March 22, when I entered, "I felt even worse today, emotionally and mentally, than I did yesterday. I am very thankful to be happy and healthy, which I am most of the time, but, I'm having a pretty bad couple of days for some reason." I had my monthly Mediport flush on March 24, which went well, and, all of my days from March 25th to the 29th were pretty even-keel. But, on March 30th, I had a very bad day. I wrote in my journal, "I had a very lousy and short night's sleep. The day continued to be horrible, and was one of the worst in a long time due to stupid shit and idiotic people at work." I rated my anxiety as a very, very poor 3 on that day – the lowest in several weeks. Thankfully, I ended the month uneventfully, and had a better day at work.

April 2006

1 Year/8 Months of Recovery/Aftercare
1 Year/10 Months since Diagnosis

On April 1, I wished Mom "Happy Birthday," but, for some reason, I was not happy. On that day I wrote, "I started worrying about stuff today, and I had real bad diarrhea. It's been months since I've felt like this, and I'm not sure what's causing it." My emotional problems persisted to April 3, when I wrote, "I took ½ Trazadone® and I feel mentally lousy again today with upset stomach and diarrhea. I just pray to God that everything turns out alright, in all respects. My body feels so yucky." And, the emotional downturn continued on April 5, which I rated an all-time low of 2 on the anxiety scale. That day, I wrote, "I had another horrible day emotionally. I felt like crap, and I am finding it very difficult to be happy and joyful. I am pretty much negative and pessimistic about things, and I hate that. It's not me!!" Things turned around slightly for me on April 7, when I wrote in my journal, "I had a better day today, emotionally. I don't know if it's that I'm worrying less or what, but I wasn't in the same dark shell that I've been in for the last two weeks. I hope I can start seeing better in distances, because that is affecting me physically, also." On April 8, as much as I did not want to, my doctor recommended that I raise my Trazadone® back to a full dose to help with my new anxiety issues. What a shame – I thought that I was successfully tapering off of the drug. I also switched from taking the St. John's Wort to improve my mood, to another natural mood-enhancing supplement, 5-HTP. On April 9, 10 and 11, my anxiety problems appeared to decrease, possibly due to the Trazadone®, the 5HTP, or both. On April 12, I volunteered to coordinate, facilitate, and host a fishing event for the very first time ever in Northern Virginia, during which local children with disabilities and their parents are paired up with bass boat fishermen for a day of fishing and fun. I wanted to give back for all of the wonderful help, kindness, love, and encouragement that people had given to me during my Cancer journey, so I got a hold of the Cast for Kids® organization, a non-profit in Washington State, to volunteer to organize and host the Virginia event. They had never had an event in Northern Virginia, so, they told me that they would love for me to do it. For the 2006 event, I personally lined up over 50 corporate and government sponsors, 150 volunteers, and over 30 bass boat fishermen from four bass fishing organizations, to provide a very special day of fishing and fun for over 30 disabled children and their parents at a lovely park on the Potomac River. (I also organized an even larger event in 2007, and, when I left Virginia to come to New Mexico in 2008, I turned over the annual Virginia Cast for Kids® event that I founded to the State Parks and Recreation Department, who has held it ever since). My Caregiver thought I had a few screws loose by taking on such a large responsibility, thinking that it would add to my already anxious mind. But, it turns out that it actually helped, because it kept me VERY busy for many months, and, my Caregiver even became one of the event volunteers. She had an incredible time, as did all of us, providing an exciting day for those very special kids and their families, both in September of 2006 and 2007. I noted on April 15 and 16, that for some reason, I was again losing weight even though I had been eating and working out the same as I had been. On April 17 and 18, I suffered another emotional downturn. On April 18th, I wrote, "I slept well, but, I'm still not feeling like myself emotionally. Work was okay, but, I wasn't able to be happy about things. I'm not sure what is causing my negative feelings, but they are definitely kicking my ass." April 19th, 20th, and 21st were some of the worst days I had had in a long while, and I rated my anxiety as a lousy 2 on those days. On the 20th, I entered, "I took a full Trazadone®, but, it was not good because I still feel like crap. I feel as though I have absolutely no self-confidence to do things, and I have no self-esteem. I feel very timid and when I'm at work, I just close the door and like being by myself. I'm nice to people, but I just don't feel like going out of my way to interact with them. I definitely feel like a shell of who I really am." My mental issues ran over into the 21st, when I wrote, "I woke up feeling pretty blah. Today at work was horrible and I got to feeling very down about myself and great decisions I've made in my past that had such horrible outcomes, such as me losing so much of my money and real estate in divorce. My Mediport flush didn't go very well either, as they weren't able to draw any blood. It was clogged and took the Oncology nurses over two hours to clear it with blood thinners." From April 22nd to the 24th, my days were still bad anxiety-wise, but, not as terrible as the 25th. I wrote on that day, "I woke up feeling bad today, and work was horrible and I got so stressed out! I had to work until 8:30 p.m. on a project." I rated that day an all-time low 1 on my anxiety scale – my worst anxiety in months. Things did turn around for me on April 28th, when I jotted, "I felt quite a bit better today, and, thankfully, had a very relaxing day at work to make up for the hellish days I had earlier. I feel a little better emotionally, and physically, too. I have to focus on definitely not being stressed, because my health is the most important thing of all." Thankfully, I concluded the roller-coaster month of April with a nice anxiety rating of 7, and a good day on April 30. I wrote, "Today was a good day for me. Thank God. I needed it badly."

May 2006

1 Year/9 Months of Recovery/Aftercare
1 Year/11 Months since Diagnosis

During May 2006, I continued with my ***daily*** *journaling only for the first week of the month. Then, for the rest of May and subsequent months, I just captured some of the more noteworthy things that occurred each month in my journal. This is because, as I neared the two-year anniversary of my Cancer diagnosis, things were beginning to quiet down a tad—medically speaking—and I actually had little to write about on most days. With that said, however, I did continue to track and rate my trusty, longtime friend, Anxiety, which I did through the month of August 2006. So, getting back to the first week of this month, I continued to take Trazadone® and Ambien® to help me sleep, and, it did help me. My anxiety levels on May 1st and 2nd were a 6 for both days, but, on May 3rd, it dipped to a very low 2. I wrote on that day, "Today was a very stressful day today, and I got overwhelmed* *by my thoughts and everything I have to do." Things improved for me on May 5th and 6th, when, I graded my anxiety levels a 7+, and captured in my journal on the 5th, "Today was a much better day with little stress, and not too much work." and on the 6th, "I had a good, strong workout, and a very successful morning. Thankfully, I continue to feel encouraged and positive about everything." During the week of May 8, my anxiety levels fluctuated from a 7 to a 2, and the week of May 15, my I rated my anxiety level at a horrible 1 to a better 6. Because of the see-saw, up-and-down emotional roller coaster I had been on the prior two weeks, I scheduled a follow-on session with my Psychotherapist, who I had not seen for about five months, since December 2005. For some reason, I could not, for the life of me, get past my depressive, anxious state, although, everyday, I did my best to put on a smile and give it my best shot. I attended my Psychotherapy session on May 22, and explained my continued emotional problems with which I was still challenged. He listened to my explanation and, as he had done in our prior sessions, suggested that I continue to focus on the here-and-now, not on what the future may or may not hold for me. Additionally, he tried to convince me to believe in my body and mind, and to not second-guess or blame either one of them for my Cancer. And finally, he told me, "You just wait and see – your strong body that you've worked for years to protect, is going to repay the favor." I left his office with renewed faith, but, knew I was not out of the woods just yet. The week of May 22, I rated my anxiety levels in the 5 and 6 range, but did get some very good news on May 25, when I had my monthly Cancer check-up with ENT No. 2. I wrote, "Thank God everything looks and feels good in my throat and on my tongue." The doctor scheduled me to get a regular, post-treatment CT Scan on July 14. I finished out the month of May with anxiety ratings from 2 to 5. Not good*

June 2006

1 Year/10 Months of Recovery/Aftercare
2 Years since Diagnosis

This is the ***Big Second Anniversary of My Cancer Diagnosis!!*** *Kind of a weird thing to celebrate, but, it's a million times better than* **not** *having a second anniversary of a Cancer occurrence to celebrate. On June 1, I had a follow-up visit with my Oncologist, who said she was pleased with my progress, but, I told her that while I felt terrific physically, and that I was able to eat, exercise, and do other things just fine, I was still having issues with anxiety and mild depression. She asked if I was seeing a therapist and was happy when I told her I had restarted my sessions. She told me that she would see me again in August after I had my July 14 CT Scan, and my CT follow-up exam with ENT No. 2. At that time, she said, she would make a decision about whether or not to have my Mediport surgically removed. On June 5, I attended my Psychotherapy appointment, but, I still suffered* *mild anxiety during the entire month of June, as hard as I tried to put all of my therapy tools to work. During June, my anxiety averaged from 5 to 7.*

July 2006

1 Year/11 Months of Recovery/Aftercare
2 Years/1 Month since Diagnosis

This was the two-year anniversary of the start of my Cancer treatments. I could not believe how fast, but slowly, the time had passed during the last 2 years. I started out July with a very high (and good) anxiety level of 8, which was a very welcome change from the last several weeks. On July 4th, I left on a cross-country trip to New Mexico to move my household goods to Albuquerque, where I would be moving in January 2008, to take care of my Mom in her Nursing Home. I pulled in with the moving truck on July 6, and my brother, Buz, and I, moved all of my stuff into a storage space. It was so fantastic to surprise my Mom with my visit and to see Buz. During the week of July 10, I rated my anxiety levels a very high and happy 9, and I returned to Virginia from NM on July 11. On July 14, I had the CT Scan that ENT No. 2 had scheduled in May as a normal procedure to verify that my neck and chest were clear of any unfavorable-looking tissues in those areas. I began attempting to taper off of Trazadone® for the third time on July 16, but noted in my journal on that day that my anxiety level had sunk to a very miserable rating level of 1 for some reason. That severe anxiety persisted the entire week of July 17 and into the week of July 24. On July 25, I stopped using Ambien® to help me get to sleep, but, I started using Melatonin, which put me to sleep, but came with a night-full of crazy (but not frightening) dreams. I had a successful Mediport flush on July 27, and on July 29, I stopped taking Trazadone® for the first time in almost two years. I ended the month of July with some wonderful news when ENT No. 2 called me on July 31. He told me that my head and chest CT Scan came back clear. Despite that favorable news, though, my anxiety rated a low 1. I continued to visit my therapist each week, but the turn-around was slow.

August 2006

2 Years of Recovery/Aftercare
2 Years/2 Months since Diagnosis

According to my journal, I started out the month of August on a high note, mentally-speaking, as I graded my anxiety the highest 10! This continued into the week of August 7. On August 8, I had my post-CT Scan follow-up appointment with ENT No. 2. He had already phoned me with the terrific news of my CT results in July, but during this appointment, he performed a physical exam of my throat, tongue, and neck Lymph Nodes, and this exam also was favorable. I continued having one successful test after another, so, slowly-but-surely, I began feeling more comfortable about my health at the time, and also about my prospects of having a future life. I had a very good feeling that that "great unknown," and not knowing what the future held for me, was probably what was responsible for most, if not all, of the anxiety and depression that I had been experiencing for the last two years. On August 11, my Oncologist contacted me to tell me that she had decided to have my Mediport removed. She told me that she had reviewed my very good July 14 CT Scan results, and that she felt that I would no longer have a need for the Mediport for Chemotherapy or blood drawing purposes. She told me that the Mediport removal surgery was scheduled for August 28, but that I would have to have a pre-surgery blood test on August 25. I continued to have very positive days during the weeks of August 14 and 21, and on August 25, right on-schedule, I attended my pre-surgery blood test. Prior to arriving at the hospital for my Mediport removal surgery, I wrote the word, ***"NO"*** *onto a large bandage and placed it over my right nipple. The Mediport was surgically implanted about 4-5 inches above the nipple, so I wanted to have some fun with the doctor and make sure that he didn't try to extricate the wrong "device" during the surgery (ala stories about doctors who have amputated or operated on the wrong appendage). After I arrived at the surgery clinic on August 28 and took off my shirt, both the surgeon and nurse caught sight of the "warning label," and, after staring at it for a few moments, cracked up, and could not stop laughing. Luckily, when the time for the scalpel came, they had regained their composure, and both my nipple retention, and the Mediport removal, went off without a hitch. I completed the month of August feeling much more self-confident, and much less anxious. I stopped seeing my therapist as I was feeling more optimistic about my future, my body, and my health, just as he had said.*

September 2006

2 Years/1 Month of Recovery/Aftercare
2 Years/3 Months since Diagnosis

This September was a good month for me as I had no major events with my health, my work, or my life. My Caregiver and I had finally settled into the "New Normal" way of our life, that, for all intents and purposes, was like our pre-Cancer life, except that I was "walking on egg shells" much of the time – at least for awhile. This is because I didn't know from day-to-day, whether I would feel confident or not, frightened or not, or happy or not. Over time, these questions, doubts, and apprehensions would give way to a more optimistic approach to my life and higher levels of self-esteem. This was a very welcome change and something that I had not known for over two long years. My Caregiver, and my family, friends, and co-workers let me know how great it was to "have me back." I could not agree with them more. The first and second weeks of September found me experiencing no anxiety of any significance, and my eating, working out, and work were all going very well. On September 7, I had my stitches removed from my chest Mediport removal site, and I still carry that scar like a badge of honor on my right Pec. The weeks of September 11th, 18th, and 25th, were all pretty uneventful with very little anxiety, which was precisely how I liked them.

October 2006

2 Years/2 Months of Recovery/Aftercare
2 Years/4 Months since Diagnosis

October turned out to be another "slow" and very run-of-the-mill month for me as far as my Cancer recovery was concerned. What a blessing that nothing unfavorable was happening with my body and my health, and that I was still successfully rebounding from an emotional standpoint from the horrible depression and anxiety that had plagued me for over two years. It was, indeed, a breath of fresh air, for both me and for my Caregiver. Bless her heart, she had endured the worst of times with me for what seemed like an eternity, and she did it with no complaints or apprehension whatsoever. For that, I will always be grateful to her. The weeks of October 2nd and 9th were good weeks for me and almost anxiety-free. On October 16, I saw my Oncologist for my monthly check-up. She, likewise, had noticed the lively spark in my step and the calm in my emotional state. I told her that therapy had made a huge difference in my life, and that I probably would not have crawled out of that never-ending depressive spiral without the professional help of my talented Psychotherapist. I mentioned to her that I was getting to a point where I trusted my body again, and that I was grateful that I was in such good physical shape before I got Cancer. I told her I knew it was one of the things that helped me to survive both the Cancer treatments and all of the horrible Side Effects. She agreed with me that my being healthy prior to my Cancer was very important to my treatment and recovery, and she told me that my body should continue to strengthen over time, which should help my overall outlook on my future to become more optimistic. I thanked her for all of her help and encouragement over the last two years. The weeks of October 23rd and 30th were, thankfully, uneventful for me.

November 2006

2 Years/3 Months of Recovery/Aftercare
2 Years/5 Months since Diagnosis

The first week of November was good in all respects with my life, and from a physical and an emotional standpoint. I was recapturing my confidence, regaining my bodyweight and my strength, and, reclaiming the life that my Caregiver and I had had to sacrifice for over two very long years. Things were once again, beginning to come together and make a little sense. With each successful follow-up medical exam under my belt, I actually began to convince myself that things might turn out okay, after all, in the end. I had never given up hope that I was going to survive my Cancer, but, its awfully nasty reputation of doing serious damage to people—or worse—does have a way of seriously screwing with a Cancer patient's or survivor's mind. Definitely, the very real possibility of Cancer-caused mortality was forever on my mind, and is surely what helped to cause the horrible, debilitating depths of depression and anxiety to which I had fallen for the two years following my treatments. The weeks of November 1st, 6th, and 13th, had no significant ups or downs that I had noted in my journal, but, I did have a wonderful time celebrating my Birthday on November 19th. On that day, I noted in my journal, "Today is my Birthday that I did not know that I was going to have, but, I am so grateful to God that, here I am, writing this as a Cancer Survivor. I realize that every one of my Birthdays—in fact, every Cancer Survivor's Birthdays—are one of the best, most meaningful gifts that I, or they, can possibly receive. No longer will I take for granted, or lament, the act of becoming one year older." On November 21, I had my bi-monthly follow-on Cancer screening visit with ENT No. 2. Thankfully, this physical exam of my neck, throat, and tongue went well, as the doctor noted no new activity, redness, or swelling. As the doctor had done the last few exams, during this one, he once again told me, "Your tongue is as soft and smooth as a baby's butt." That's what I needed to hear, and once again, helped my self-esteem. It was time for my next follow-up PET Scan, so he scheduled me for December 8. I ended November with a Physical Exam on November 28 with my Primary Care Physician, which went well.

December 2006

2 Years/4 Months of Recovery/Aftercare
2 Years/6 Months since Diagnosis

The end of another year, and a much better year than the previous two, for which I was very thankful. The month of December started out just as well as November had ended, and continued through the week of December 4. On December 8, I attended my fourth post-treatment PET Scan, which was a regular precaution to confirm that the "coast was clear" with my throat, tongue, neck, and upper body areas, including my Lungs and other organs. Because of Cancer's nasty habit of spreading to-and-fro within the body, I was very happy to submit to my bi-weekly physical exams with ENT No. 2, and my regular, but less-frequently scheduled, CT Scans and PET Scans. For obvious reasons, if cancerous cells from a recurrent tumor or a new Cancer were alive within my body, I would want to know about it as soon as possible, so that I and my doctors and Caregiver could begin taking fast actions to safely eliminate the disease. But, what I **did not** *like, however, was waiting, and waiting, and waiting for the damn results, which, in some cases, could take upwards of two weeks. This PET Scan went off without a hitch, but, it wasn't until December 18, ten days after the Scan, that I got a VERY scary telephone message from my Oncologist regarding the results of the Scan. In her message to me, she said, "...you have a technicality on your PET Scan results that I will need to speak with you about. Please call me back as soon as you can." Okay, now if that wouldn't scare the shit out of a Cancer survivor, I don't what would. Of course, as luck would have it, I got the message in the evening, after the Oncology Clinic had closed, so, I had to stew on that news the entire night. Both my Caregiver and I were frightened that the Scan revealed more "highlighted" tissue, which could mean that I might have some sort of Cancer presence. "Obviously if it was good news," I told my Caregiver, "she wouldn't have left such a message with a request for an urgent call-back." Nevertheless, I called the number to the Oncology Clinic that evening and left a message that I received her message, and I asked her to call me back the following day. On December 19, my Oncologist did call me back to give me the very frightening news. I wrote in my journal on that day, "I got a call from my Oncologist who told me that there is an area of activity on my Liver that appears different than it had on prior CT Scans. She said that the growth may not be consistent with my type of Cancer, but, that we will want to check it out thoroughly so that we will know for sure. She ordered a CT Scan of the Liver and asked me to schedule an appointment for the Scan, which I did." What definitely sucked, though, was that due to the Christmas and New Year holidays, the earliest I could schedule a CT Scan was January 8, 2007. It goes without saying that I had one hell of a miserable Christmas and New Year while I was waiting, worrying, and wondering what was going on with my Liver, one of the most vital organs in the body. Good-bye, self-confidence; hello, depression and anxiety, all over again. And, this is how I rang in 2007.*

January 2007

2 Years/5 Months of Recovery/Aftercare
2 Years/7 Months since Diagnosis

Of course, the first entire week of January was horrible from an emotional standpoint. I couldn't sleep, concentrate at work, or function as normally as I had been for the last few months. All of the adrenaline and self-esteem that I had accrued during the last several weeks with my favorable exams, and CT Scans, my weight gain and strong workouts, and my positive frame of mind and quasi-normal life with my Caregiver, was, in a matter of one Scan and one short phone call, all but wiped off the slate. Although I tried to think positively that everything was going to be all right, all of the scary memories of my first two years following my Cancer diagnosis continued to swarm, uncontrollably, in my mind. God, how I wanted to get past that PET Scan, and how I prayed that the results would, once again, be okay. I did submit to the follow-up CT Scan on January 8, as scheduled, and then, had to wait for almost another two weeks for the Radiology results to come back. I had heard other Cancer patients and survivors that I had met use the term, "Scanziety," to express the mental torment that they had to suffer while waiting for their test or exam results to return. Without question, I had also been overwhelmed with the same emotions after almost every test, but, especially after I had had so many PET Scans come back with "False Positives." I could only hope that ***this*** *PET Scan was not a "true positive." So, I waited for almost* <u>*eleven excruciating days*</u>*, until January 19, when, finally, ENT No. 2 called to give me the good news – yes, another "False Positive" of something that looked like Cancer, but, thank God, was not. I entered in my journal, "ENT No. 2 called to tell me the great news that the "highlight" on the PET Scan of my Liver was NOT Cancer. I am VERY relieved, but, I honestly don't know how many of these up-and-down roller coaster rides I can take with the False Positives. Out of 4 PET Scans, this was False Positive number 3. If Cancer doesn't get me, the False Positives will!!" After dodging yet another bullet on my long Cancer journey, I then came down with a super-nasty cough, headache, congestion, sore throat, and runny nose. As horrible as I felt, I was thankful that the condition was not related in any way to my Cancer. This was the* ***normal*** *Flu, which my Primary Care doctor treated with antibiotics and other drugs. What a way to end the 3- year anniversary of my suffering the cancerous sore throat!*

February 2007

2 Years/6 Months of Recovery/Aftercare
2 Years/8 Months since Diagnosis

I ended January with the horrific Flu, and it continued well into February. In fact, I kept having the unremitting and dreadful cough, runny nose, sore throat, congestion, and headaches, up to the 22nd of February, which was 5 weeks since it began, and, I still saw my Primary Care doctor for check-ups and medications. It had been almost 2 ½ years since I completed my Cancer treatments, so, I knew that this terrible bout of the Flu was not due to my lowered resistance caused by Chemotherapy. But, it was obvious to me that my Immune System had suffered some sort of major breach so that the Flu could invade my body and move in for such an extended length of time. On, February 6, when I was in the midst of my Flu, I got a call from my Oncologist, who provided me with an update on the follow-up CT Scan that I got after my most recent PET Scan scare. ENT No. 2 phoned me on January 19 to tell me my results were negative for Cancer (Yes!!), but that my Oncologist had more exact information. On February 6, I wrote in my Journal, "My Oncologist called regarding my follow-up CT Scan. She said that the "activity" and growth on my Liver was a 1cm Cyst that is nothing to worry about. Thanks God!!" I thanked my Oncologist for following up with me and told her, "It is better to be safe than sorry, and, I was grateful that it was nothing more serious." After finally getting over and past the Flu on February 22, I finished out February with no other major events.

March 2007

2 Years/7 Months of Recovery/Aftercare
2 Years/9 Months since Diagnosis

March began rather quietly from a physical and mental standpoint, and I got some very good news during my bi-monthly physical exam with ENT No. 2 on March 6. He once again told me, "Your tongue is as smooth and soft as a baby's butt." and the Endoscopy of my tongue and throat showed no new redness, or swelling. He told me that everything was healing well, considering all of the Radiation Therapy and surgeries that I had had over the course of my Cancer program. On March 6, my weight had dropped to ***188 lbs.,*** *as I had not been able to consume the quantities of calories and foods during my five weeks of Flu that I would normally have eaten. Also, I had to stop working out while I had the Flu, so that, likewise, contributed to my loss of weight. Finally, on March 7th, I was able to resume my work-outs, which I greatly needed. All continued to go well during the weeks of March 12th and 19th, but, on March 25th, unbelievably, I again came down with coughing, stuffiness, sneezing, congestion, and a horrible headache. On March 30, I once again saw my Primary Care doctor, who diagnosed me with Sinusitis and Bronchitis, and, once again, prescribed some heavy-duty antibiotics for me. It had been a month and a week since I had had my prior issues with these same symptoms, so, when this hit me again, my body was still in the process of recovering from the last round and was not fully healed. Thankfully, however, I was able to thwart this episode in one week, and I concluded the month of March feeling stronger and healthier.*

April 2007

2 Years/8 Months of Recovery/Aftercare
2 Years/10 Months since Diagnosis

Thankfully, the month of April went smoothly throughout. I started off by calling Mom on April 1to wish her "Happy Birthday." Thankfully, she was doing quite well and staying as healthy as possible, considering the many medical issues that she had going on at any given time. She was so strong and such a trouper no matter what, and always was more concerned about my health and my Brothers' health—as thoughtful as she was—than about her own problems. She was such an inspiration to all of us, and her love certainly helped me get through my own Cancer ordeal. The week of April 9th went very well, and on April 18th, I had my bi-monthly follow-up visit with my Oncologist. We talked about the PET Scan results and the cyst on my Liver, which she again told me will not present any health problems to me. We also discussed the nasty Bronchitis and Sinusitis and the Flu that I had had the last two months. She agreed with me that both incidences had come around on their own, as they would for any person, and that neither were the result of my anti-Cancer care. She commented that I looked very healthy and she asked how my Caregiver was doing, as she had met her many times prior to, during, and after my Cancer therapy. I told her that my Caregiver was doing well, and that both of us had gotten our lives back on-track in all respects. I added that she and I were both so grateful for the efforts of everyone in the Chemo and Radiation Oncology clinics, as well as my Cancer Surgeon, for helping me to get my life back. April ended up without any health issues, and with me finally feeling like myself again.

May 2007

2 Years/9 Months of Recovery/Aftercare
2 Years/11 Months since Diagnosis

Finally, a month without any emotional or physical health problems for a very welcome change. I, certainly, had earned a break, and my body and mind were responding happily to the unexpected "vacation" from physical challenges and mental stressors. My eating, workouts, and work continued to go well, as did the other things that I and my Caregiver did in our "New Normal" way of life. I had no medical tests or examinations during May, so, status quo with my health prevailed, and the month ended as smoothly as it had begun. I started telling myself at that point, that I would never, ever, take "nothingness" or "slow times" for granted again, as I had done in my pre-Cancer life. My Cancer experience taught me that "Stopping to smell the roses" is not just an overused saying – it is an absolute necessity.

June 2007

2 Years/10 Months of Recovery/Aftercare
3 Years since Diagnosis

3 YEARS DOWN, forever to go, I hoped!! As with the month of May, June was also pretty low-key in terms of medical situations with my body and mind. Physically and emotionally, I was doing very well, although, on the 3rd of June, I, of course, was extremely sad of the anniversary of my Sister, Vik's passing. I called Mom to talk with her so that both of us could offer our support to one another. Mom was still so saddened about the loss of her only daughter on this day two years ago, as were my brothers, Buz and Rich. The weeks of June 4th, 11th, and 18th, all went very well. On June 22,

I had my bi-monthly follow-up Cancer Screening Exam with ENT No. 2, who performed the usual Endoscopy of my throat and tongue, a physical exam of my tongue base and beneath my tongue, and, felt my Neck Lymph Nodes to check for any abnormalities. Thankfully, all went well with all tests, which helped, once again, to bolster my self-confidence. The month of June slipped unceremoniously by with, thankfully, no health problems.

July 2007

2 Years/11 Months of Recovery/Aftercare
3 Years/1 Month since Diagnosis

July made it three months in a row with me having what most people may consider a boring, uneventful life, and I loved it! Boring was good for me, because it meant that all of my "systems were go," and that I had no fires, figuratively speaking, that I had to put out. I was contacted by ENT No. 2 on July 3rd, who told me that he had scheduled me for another CT Scan on August 9. The CT Scans and PET Scans seemed to come around often, but, honestly, I loved going in for both because it meant that if there happened to be any nefarious, clandestine Cancer cells hanging around in my body, they would be immediately uncovered and dealt with appropriately. That is not to say that I wasn't still getting bad cases of "Scanziety" prior to the exam and while awaiting the results, but, with so many favorable outcomes (including negative "False Positives") it was getting easier to calm myself down both before and after. July rolled into August, very happily for me.

August 2007

3 Years of Recovery/Aftercare
3 Years/2 Months since Diagnosis

August 27, 2004 was when I had my ending Chemo session, and it seemed like SO long ago. So much had happened—both good and bad—since that time, that it was almost mind-bogging to think of what I had been through, all due to a cancerous lump on the lower reaches of my tongue. From that single Tumor and the incessant sore throat and swollen Lymph Nodes that ensued, after three prolonged years, here I was, healthy, strong, and happy once again. The first week of August went very well, as did the second. On August 9, one day before my Sister, Vikki's birthday, I submitted for my CT Scan. The Scan, itself, went well, but, as usual, I had to wait on, and worry about, the results. On August 15th, I had my follow-on, check-up visit with my Oncologist. It was too early for her to go over my CT Scan results with me, but, we did talk about general things regarding my physical status and my emotional situation. I told her that since the last time I had seen her in April of this year, that I had had three great months without any health or other problems. She was very happy to hear that and told me that she was so pleased with my progress and overall attitude. By the 27th of July, which *was 19 days after I had gotten my CT Scan, I still had not heard about my Scan results, so I called ENT No. 2 and left a message to ask him about it. I didn't hear back from ENT No. 2 on the 27th or the 28th, so I called back on the 29th to speak with him. His Medical Assistant told me that she had not gotten my message that I left on the 27th, which I didn't believe for one minute. I asked her to have him call me back because it was already three weeks, and I still had not yet received my CT Scan results and I was very concerned. I also called and left a message for my Oncologist on the 29th to ask her if she knew where the results may be. I received a call back from my Oncologist on July 30th, who left a message to tell me that she was not able to see my results in their system, and she recommended that I follow-up with ENT No. 2. Finally, on July 31, 5 days after my initial message to him, ENT No. 2 called me back. He told me that, even though he was the doctor who had ordered the CT Scan, he had not yet received my results. I reminded him that it had been 23 days since I had my Scan, and that I was going crazy waiting for the results. I told him this was unacceptable. He agreed and apologized, and told me that he would do his best to run down my results. The "fires" that I didn't have to put out in May, June, and July were burning very wildly and out of control in August, all compliments of my HMO, who could not locate my latest CT Scan results. Not a good way to end the month, because **I** was the one doing all the work to locate them.*

September 2007

3 Years/1 Month of Recovery/Aftercare
3 Years/3 Months since Diagnosis

Not surprisingly, the first week of September, no one from the HMO called me about my CT Scan results. I was hoping that ENT No. 2, would have let me know what was going on, but I didn't hear from him for six days, so I, once again, had to be the one to instigate contact. I was extremely upset and frustrated that no one seemed to care about a Cancer survivor having to wait for a month for their CT Scans results—which could be either bad or good—so, I contacted the Member Services Supervisor at the Corporate Office to express my complaints and dissatisfaction with what I was going through in attempting to locate my Cancer test results. The Supervisor told me that she would attempt to locate the problem. I told her that I wanted to write a letter to the CEO of the HMO to explain what had happened to me, to lodge a formal complaint with the HMO, and to ask for answers. The Supervisor gave me the name of the CEO, as well as her mailing address at the HMO Corporate Office for the East-Central Region, which included the Northern Virginia, Washington, DC area. After my phone call with the Supervisor, on September 6, she called me back later on in the day. In my journal on September 6, I wrote, "The Member Services Supervisor said she contacted the Ear, Nose, and Throat Department at ENT No. 2's office *to try to find about the results. She said she had been told that the Scan was preliminarily read on September 4th, and that ENT No. 2's Assistant said she would send a message to ENT No. 2 to call the Supervisor. ENT No. 2 called the Supervisor and told her that the preliminary results of the Scan were entered on September 4, but, that the final results were not yet in, and he will call her when they come in." What an F'ing 3-Ring Circus! How something like this could occur in this day of computers and modern medicine was beyond me, but I knew that I would make sure that the CEO was well aware of this major "F-up" by someone or some thing within her HMO organization. On September 6, I received another call from a person in the HMO Corporate Office regarding my Scan results. I wrote, "...from the corporate office called to tell me that she had spoken with the Imaging Center Radiology Tech, who told her that the Radiologist read the film, but that the final report will be read on Sep. 8. He said that he will request the film be sent directly to me. She also said that ENT No. 2 will give me a call when he gets the results." Three years of me receiving CT Scans and PET Scans without an issue (other than the three "False Positives"), and, then, out of nowhere, this absurd and uncalled-for circumstance. And, it was **me** who had to unnecessarily spend time doing the HMO's job for them trying to find my CT Scans. On September 7, I wrote and sent a 3-page letter to the CEO of the HMO in which I expressed how upset I was that I had to be the one to investigate my missing CT Scan results for several days, when that clearly should have been my doctors' or their staffs' responsibility. I also stressed that as a Cancer survivor, not only is it a very difficult thing to have to wait for scan results to begin with—because of the associated worries that Cancer might be found—but for the results to be "lost" for an entire month is totally unacceptable and in excusable. Further, in the letter I specified four things that I demanded from the HMO, and, I also offered a recommendation in the letter in the interest of preventing something like this from happening in the future to other Cancer patients and survivors. I told the CEO of the HMO that I insisted on receiving the following: **1)** My CT Scan results; **2)** An apology written on HMO letterhead and signed by the CEO for the stress and suffering that I had experienced during the last month waiting for my Scan results, and for the time, effort, and frustration that I had to experience to insist that HMO personnel locate my results; **3)** An "unvarnished explanation with no cover ups so typical in the Medical industry" of what happened to prevent me from receiving my results for an entire month; and, **4)** What lessons had the HMO learned, and what action would the HMO take, as a result of this issue, to prevent such a thing from happening in the future to other patients and Cancer survivors? Finally, in the letter to the HMO CEO, I also offered a suggestion that might help fix the problem of test results becoming lost or ridiculously delayed after they are ordered by a doctor. I recommended in my letter that the HMO use an* *automatic, "red flag"-type of notification that the system would send to the doctor who ordered a test, or scan, if the results were not delivered to his or her computer dashboard or email within a specified time frame, such as a week or the standard ten days. With this automatic alert, the physician would be reminded that the test results they ordered had not been received and that **they, not the patient**, would then have to request their status, and attempt to locate their whereabouts. That reminder would also, hopefully, cause the doctor to update the patient in a timely manner of the situation. Having mailed my letter to the HMO CEO on September 7, on September 10—exactly one month after my CT Scan—I received calls from both ENT No. 2 and my Oncologist. Both of them gave me the FANTASTIC news that my Scan results were favorable. While the news was indeed great and very welcome, it was also somewhat anti-climatic after what I had been through to get my results. Nevertheless, while I did get my CT Scan results, as I'd demanded from the HMO CEO, she still owed me three other things, which would manifest themselves in October. But, as for September 2007, I put that month behind me with, thankfully, no additional "fires" to stomp out.*

October 2007
3 Years/2 Months of Recovery/Aftercare
3 Years/4 Months since Diagnosis

*I began October with an optimistic perspective, because I was feeling good from both a physical and an emotional standpoint. The debacle that I had experienced in August and September with my CT Scan results had really taken its toll on me then, but, by the first week of October, I had to let that go, and was simply focusing on enjoying the gift of life that I had received following my Cancer treatments and recovery. My positive outlook became even brighter, when on October 5, I received a very astonishing phone call at my work office. When I answered the phone, the caller identified herself as the CEO of the HMO, and she was actually **crying** while she spoke with me. She told me that she was reading my letter that I had sent, and that she could not find the words to apologize to me for what had happened to me, especially as a Cancer survivor, with my Scan results becoming lost, and, with me being the one that had to do all the work to locate them. She told me that while she did want to apologize to me in-person on the phone, that she would also be sending me a formal written apology as I had requested. The CEO, who was incredibly nice, professional, compassionate, and very humble, told me that she would have one of her Vice Presidents call me in the near future to provide me with an honest explanation of what happened with my Scan results, and why it took four weeks for me to receive them. And, finally, the CEO thanked me profusely for sending her the suggestion on how to fix the problem. She told me that when she received my letter, she immediately called together her Medical Director and her Director of*

Information Technology (IT), and she told them that she wanted them to design, develop and implement the automated "red flag" alert process that notifies physicians who order tests when the results of those tests are not delivered in a pre-determined time period. The CEO told me that she thought that was a great idea, and again expressed her gratitude for me suggesting it in the interest of helping patients down the line. The CEO and I ended our conversation with her giving me the phone number to her direct line, and, once again, her heartfelt apologies. One week later, as the CEO had promised, I received the official written apology from her. Three weeks after that, on October 26, I got a call in my office from the HMO Vice President of Clinical Operations. In my journal on that day, I wrote, "...the Vice President of Clinical Operations called and apologized for my experience, and told me that my delayed CT Scan results were the result of both human and systematic errors." She stated, very candidly, that HMO personnel, including my ordering physician and his staff, did not do their job in researching or locating the missing results, or, in keeping me aware of status. She also pointed out that the Imaging Center did not do the job they should have done in hurriedly reading and entering the Scan results into the system. I also entered into my journal that the Vice President had stated, "Mr. Sickler, because of your letter and recommendation, the HMO has enacted procedural reporting changes, including the automatic system notification that you suggested, that will preclude this type of thing from ever happening again. Again, we thank you for your advice." And, finally, the VP of Clinical Operations for the HMO hit me with information that I definitely did not expect. She told me, "This is such a strange coincidence, because my husband, who is in his early 50's, was recently diagnosed with the exact same type of Cancer you had – Cancer at the Base of the Tongue. Hopefully, because of lessons we've learned about your recent experience and the actions we've taken as a result to fix the problems, my husband, as well as other patients and Cancer survivors, will never have to go through the bad experience that you did." I responded by thanking her for sharing that personal information with me, and for her kind words. I also wished her husband and her well with his Cancer, and I told her that I simply did what I thought was right for everyone involved, and that I did hope that my experience would help others. I was so pleased that this process had come full-circle, and that the month of October ended on such a positive note.

November 2007

3 Years/3 Months of Recovery/Aftercare
3 Years/5 Months since Diagnosis

After the craziness that was August, September, and October insofar as my "CT Scangate" was concerned, the month of November was a nice change and a welcome opportunity to lay low and look forward to what I hoped would be a very relaxing, fun, and festive holiday season. The first week of November, as well as the weeks of November 5, 12, 19, and 26, were just as I liked them – nothing stressful or overwhelming at work or in my life. I was back to living as normal of a life as possible after surviving Cancer, in that I was able to do all of the things that I did in my pre-Cancer life. But, my "New Normal" life came with "fine print" that clearly stated, "Don't ever take your life, your health, your family, and your friends for granted, and, don't ever be too proud or sure of yourself, because you know that it can be taken away from you in an instant." I celebrated my nice Birthday on November 19 with my Caregiver and her family, and we also had a fun Thanksgiving. I ended November on a very positive note with yet another favorable physical exam with ENT No. 2 on November 30. The doctor also scheduled me for another Cancer screening PET Scan, on December 11.

December 2007

3 Years/4 Months of Recovery/Aftercare
3 Years/6 Months since Diagnosis

December 2007 was my last month in Northern Virginia, as I transferred in January 2008 with my government job to my hometown of Albuquerque, NM, so that I could take care of my Mom in her Nursing Home. Needless to say, December was a very busy month because of all of the preparations for my move, and saying good-bye to all of my friends and co-workers. I believe the most difficult thing of all was to say good-bye to my Caregiver and her family, all of whom had taken such unbelievable care of me during the almost four years of my Cancer journey. My Caregiver gave so much of herself to help me get through some incredibly rough times, and for all that she so selflessly did, I will always be exceedingly grateful. I also made the rounds to each of my Cancer doctors during the month to say my good-byes to them, to thank them for all they did to help save my life, and to get copies of each of my medical records, so that I would have a complete set for the physicians in Albuquerque. I also attended my fifth and final post-Cancer treatment PET Scan on December 11th. I felt very confident that I would get my results on-time, and that they would be favorable, not "False Positives" again. About two weeks following, I went to see my Oncologist for my final visit, and ENT No. 2 for my final physical exam with him. She gave me the great news about my PET Scans, but it did bring tears to my eyes to say my "Good-byes" to my Oncologist, and to all of the Oncology Nurses. I also had a hard time saying good-bye to ENT No. 2, as we had both been through so much together during the last 3 ½ years. This was a ***<u>VERY TERRIFIC</u>*** *appointment, because, not only was my Physical Exam favorable, but ENT No. 2 told me,* ***"Congratulations Butch, you are now 'Cancer-free!'" Thank you God!*** *I had been waiting for 3½ years to hear those words. What a wonderful way to begin the next Chapter of my life!*

One Way

By Butch Sickler ©
October 2011

It is a long road to be sure
but it is not a pathway to nowhere

This route has many known obstacles
with rises and dips and hairpin turns
scattered about its demanding length
and peppered with perilous drop-offs
that await the unaware on either side
or any who might lose sight of their reachable goal

As you travel on your critical journey
go slowly and stay close to the center
keep your eyes open but don't look down
glance rearward only to see how far you've come
but then promptly look ahead again
to focus carefully on your attainable destination

Millions have safely gone this way before you
and millions more will follow after
but it is up to you and those around you
to cautiously navigate the hazards
and to celebrate the achievements
as you steer courageously to that well-earned place

Cancer survival

It is a long road to be sure
but it just happens to be going your way

Chapter Seventeen

Fast Forward...to 2013 – *I'm Still Striving, Thriving, & Surviving!*

"The most important day of my life was when my doctor told me that I was 'Cancer-free.' The next most significant day has been all of those since."

- Butch Sickler

As I write this in 2013, a lot of water has passed under the bridge since Cancer first called my number over 9 years ago. Within this book—among various other things—I have attempted to capture my Cancer-related experiences that transpired during the first three+ years of those nine, beginning with my freaky Diagnosis, proceeding through Treatments, and finishing with my Recovery and Aftercare. But, the truth of the matter is, Aftercare for me, and for every other Cancer survivor, never really concludes – that is, unless the survivor opts for whatever reason(s) not to participate in the follow-up health monitoring process. But, for those Cancer survivors who *do* wish to have a say in their health and in their future, as I've alluded to many times within these pages, they will be watched more closely than a field mouse at a Barn Owl Convention. And, that's for life.

New Cancer Happens – As if One is Not Enough!

A Cancer survivor doing their due diligence during Aftercare is highly recommended, of course, because some Cancers are prone to recur a second or a third time, and, occasionally, completely new Cancers have been notorious for ambushing some who have already survived one or more prior rounds with this despicable disease. It's been said that lightning doesn't strike twice in the same place, but, I know a few Cancer survivors who may beg to differ with that view. Aftercare follow-up exams are prescribed to confirm the continuous absence of one's Cancer in a best-case scenario, or, to determine the presence of recurrent or a new Cancer, in a worst-case. During each instance, however, whether one's Cancer is a first Primary, a second Primary, or the recurrence of an initial Cancer, earlier detection, safe and appropriate treatment, and regular post-treatment monitoring are fundamental in beating the odds for continued survivorship.

Doing MY Post-Treatment Due Diligence

It is for the scary facts that recurrent and new Cancers evolve (and because I love my Life so darn much) that I diligently attended all of my regular Monthly, Bi-Monthly, Quarterly, and Semi-Annual Check-ups throughout the first eight-or-so years of my survivorship. Now that I have, thankfully, transitioned into my ninth year of being Cancer-free, my Ear, Nose, and Throat (ENT) doctor has me seeing him once a year for my follow-up exams. His line of thinking is that while I may not be completely "out of the woods" with my *Cancer-free* condition (no Cancer survivor actually *ever* is), I am far enough beyond the most vulnerable years (the first five), that he believes the threat of recurrence has diminished to a level whereby more frequent medical scrutiny is unnecessary. I'm comfortable with that opinion.

Every year currently, right around the anniversary date of my Cancer Diagnosis each June, I submit to my twelve-month follow-up exam. The annual check-ups that I presently receive consist of a physical exam, which includes an Endoscopy (a lighted camera tube that is guided by the ENT doctor thru my nostril and down my throat for a good look at the Base of my Tongue); the physician's palpation of my Neck Lymph Nodes and beneath my tongue with his fingers; and, best of all, the doctor "walking" his heavenly-tasting *(gag me!),* vinyl-gloved fingers way down my throat for a few moments to feel the Base of my Tongue for any possible new tumor activity.

Additionally, on a yearly basis and usually at my request, the ENT physician will order some X-rays of my Lungs. This is because the Lungs, strangely enough, are one of the body locations—besides the Neck Lymph Nodes—where my form of Head and Neck Cancer has been known to metastasize in later Stages. One can never be too cautious about keeping tabs on the locations where these types of Cancers prefer to hang out. Thankfully, though, over these last nine+ years, my due diligence has paid off in the form of favorable follow-up physical exams and clear Lung X-rays. And, gratefully, both of these conclusions have contributed to a heightened state of my well-being – both physically and mentally. Just knowing every day that I am remaining Cancer-free takes a big load off of both my body and my mind, as one can imagine. In other words, I realize that I have been blessed, because I know that my body is healthy, and I am very well aware of just how fortunate I am, considering the alternative.

Living with Treatment Side Effects and a Possible Late Effect – Nine Years Later

Thankfully, each of my post-Cancer monitoring exams have gone well, but, I must confess that I am still living with a few of the Side Effects from my Cancer Treatments that have persisted during the last nine years. Additionally, I very well may have a Late Effect that evolved around three years ago with which I must now contend, but, the "jury is still out" on that one because no one knows for sure. As for my persisting Side Effects, one that resulted from Chemo did affect my eyebrows, which still have not grown back in to their pre-Cancer volume. My head hair and eyelashes are as thick as before, but, my eyebrows are lacking. No big deal, though, because I'm not planning to do any Calvin Klein® photo shoots anytime soon.

Speaking of Chemotherapy Side Effects, I would like to be able to invoke the *"Chemo Brain"* defense for every instance when I don't recall something important. In the interest of being forthright, though, I'll blame my lapses in memory on plain ole' forgetfulness. But seriously, from a Radiation Therapy Side Effect standpoint, I'm still "paying" for that treatment in a quite a few ways. For one thing, I'm still not able to grow many whiskers in the areas on the left and right sides of my cheeks and neck that were exposed to the field of radiation. Those hair follicles apparently got fried, right along with the Cancer Tumor on my tongue. But neither has come back, so I'm definitely not complaining in either case. Besides, I'm not a beard-type guy, and I'm perfectly happy with my little Soul Patch.

As a result of radiation exposure to my jaw bones during my Cancer-killing therapy, I had to receive Hyperbaric Oxygen Therapy (HBOT) to help prevent the prospect of getting Osteoradionecrosis, or *"death of the jaw bone due to radiation."* But, because the HBOT *force-fed* me with pure oxygen in a sealed chamber at awfully higher pressures for many weeks, it, somehow, reshaped my eye lenses and caused my eyesight to change from being far-sighted (I used to need glasses for *all* reading) to being short-sighted (I can now clearly read the smallest type *without* glasses). All of my physicians told me that this vision changes would be "temporary," but, obviously, they were wrong and are here to stay. I've learned to live with my new vision, and now have glasses for seeing distances. Honestly, it is what it is, and I'm happy that I no longer need glasses to read the small stuff.

As for the potential Late Effect (a Side Effect that manifests itself many years after treatment) that I've mentioned prior, from out of nowhere in 2010, I started feeling a constant numbness of the skin and a prickly, nagging pain on the left region of my neck. This area just happens to be "Ground Zero" for the Radiation Therapy which I received in 2004. The numbing and pain also impacts my chest and shoulder area on the left side, but, mercifully, this condition does not impact the function of my shoulder, chest, or neck muscles, as they are as strong and as functional as ever. However, the numbed skin in those locations feels weirdly *rubber-like,* and the underlying prickly pain is persistently troubling. I don't have any clue what this is, and neither do my doctors, but, I think that it may be Fibrosis, which is a Late Effect associated with prior Radiation Therapy. Time will tell, I guess, whether it is something dangerously bad, or just something uncomfortable that I'll have to continue to live with and endure.

Finally, to conclude this Section about my continuing Cancer Side Effects on a positive note, because I took earlier steps to protect my Salivary Glands from radiation beam exposure during my course of Radiation Therapy, luckily, my Glands are still totally functional, and my saliva production is just as terrific as my pre-Cancer levels. I'm thankful for that, and it goes to show you – people should never take anything about their bodies for granted, including their *spit!*

Living My "New Normal" Life – Better to be Safe than Sorry

I've made mention in former Chapters of this Book about the frightening Laboratory reports I received following three of my five post-treatment PET (Positron Emission Tomography) scans in which the images "lit up," and indicated that I still *might* have cancerous activity taking place within my body. Thankfully, those PET results were ultimately determined to be *"false positives,"* due, possibly, to my healthy tissue healing at the site. But, as one might imagine, just the *thought* of me having an additional Cancer freaked me out, much less having to struggle through additional treatments to kill the beast a second time. Now, about 7 to 8 years since those scary scans (and, in-part, because of them), I am living a *"New Normal"* way of life.

I obviously can't speak for every Cancer survivor alive (13.7 million in the U.S. alone!), but, I *can* vouch for myself when I state that I do still periodically *look over my shoulder* for that most evil of medical menaces – our Cancerous Archenemy. Not all the time, of course, but whenever something in my body just doesn't feel right, and, especially if it hangs on for more than a few days. In my pre-Cancer life, I would certainly take serious notice of any questionable symptoms or conditions in my body that came out of nowhere. And, not like several men (or so I've heard), I would eventually have the signs checked out by a doctor if they didn't go away on their own. In 2004, I made such a judgment to obtain medical intervention for my unrelenting sore throat symptoms, which, thankfully, is what led to us finding, treating, and successfully eradicating my Cancer.

In my pre-C days, though, if I was having some sort of issue with my body and my health, I would never automatically think to myself, *"Uh oh, this quirky thing I'm feeling could be really serious and might be something that could snuff my life."* In fact, when I received my Cancer diagnosis in 2004, honestly, this vicious disease was the *furthest thing* from my mind. *But, Surprise, Surprise, look what life had cooked up for me!* Nowadays, however, with my post-Cancer *New Normal* way of looking at, and living, my life, while I definitely don't think "the sky is falling" every time that something seems askew with my body, I certainly don't disregard the feelings.

Actually, to the contrary, I give any peculiar symptoms very serious attention – almost as though my life depends upon it – which it *does.*

Nowadays, if I notice that any out-of-the-ordinary symptoms are continuing for very long, I don't waste any time getting down to business: Depending upon the degree of pain or perceived urgency, I will schedule an appointment and go to see a physician as quickly as possible. Or, I will first conduct research on the internet, including use of the *Symptom Checker* features of various medical websites, to try to pinpoint the culprit(s) that may be causing the problem. Then, depending on what my research turns up, and, as appropriate, I will schedule an appointment to visit my Primary Care physician or my ENT doctor, or, I will go to the Emergency Room (ER) so that I can have things checked out in person. And, of course, I will also rely on my God-given intuition and my lifelong familiarity with my body to perform my own self-assessments when trying to determine how possibly serious, urgent, and harmful the condition(s) may be.

When Status-Quo is a Good Thing

As I have mentioned multiple times within this Book, I took excellent care of my *pre-Cancer* body during my teen and adult life thru my exercise workouts and healthful eating habits, and, by not smoking or drinking any alcohol (with the exception of a sip of wine maybe once or twice a year – *whoopee!).* In any case, at 62 years of age as I write this, my lifestyle has stayed unchanged to this day. For example, my low-fat, low-sugar, low-salt *post-Cancer* nutrition plan continues to be terrific (thanks to my disciplined eating regimen and Jayni's wholesome and scrumptious cooking!); my weightlifting and cardiovascular workouts are as powerful and as productive as ever; I continue to consume the full variety of vitamins, minerals and some herbs, as well as all of my protein-packed, muscle-building workout supplements; and, to the extent possible, I attempt to keep my stress levels as low as I can (which, admittedly, is *NOT* an easy thing to do when working with the Government…but, I digress). I also continue to take exceptional care of my oral health and teeth with twice daily brushing, flossing, and fluoride rinses, because I want to prevent any further dental issues or complications that may manifest themselves due to the radiation damage sustained by my jaw bones in 2004.

Of course, I also continue to not utilize tobacco of any type (never have), and I still don't drink any alcoholic beverages. I know – all pretty boring stuff, but basically, I'm now doing the same types of things to take care of myself that I did prior to my freak Cancer occurrence. The difference this time around, though, is that I am not taking great care of my body merely as a ***lifestyle choice.*** Actually, I'm doing what I do now, because, it's a ***life choice.*** That is – quite truthfully, my post-Cancer life depends upon me being ever-vigilant with my body and my health. I can definitely relate to Woody Allen when he said, *"I'm not afraid of death; I just don't want to be there when it happens."* So, like Mr. Allen, I am doing my best to elude the *Bid D* (and the *Big C* for that matter), and I attempt to do this by maintaining the status quo with my good health so that it doesn't fall by the wayside. However, even though I am steadfast in doing all of the "right" things—health and fitness wise—and, although all of my Aftercare exams have, fortunately, been favorable, I will admit that the process hasn't been without a few scary moments along the way.

Lions and Tigers and Scares – Oh My!

During the last five years—from 2008 to this day—I will say that my body's *Symptom Sensors* have *activated* a few times out of the clear blue, and, the warnings or feelings have troubled me to the point where I've chosen to seek medical intervention, just in case. It was either realize that, or suffer physically, and then worry myself to death, emotionally, about the potentiality of a Cancer recurrence or, God-forbid, a brand new Cancer. One of the prospective Late Side Effects in Cancer patients who have received Radiation Therapy for their Cancer (such as me) is – you guessed it – *the development of a second Cancer sometime later in their life.* So, being the life-loving person that I am, whenever something has felt out of whack with my body, I've opted to do the logical thing and put my health concerns in the hands of professionals. In all such cases, if the physicians that I've visited weren't already conscious that I was a Cancer survivor, I informed them of my status, up-front, so that they would know to be much more attentive in carrying out their diagnostic due diligence.

Following are a few examples of activities and outcomes that have taken place during the last 5+ years when I've set out to see a doctor because my body’s *“Check Engine”* light had, all of a sudden, *lit up,* and *stayed on* for an unusually long and worrisome time:

- ***Unexplained Gut-Wrenching Episodes***

In 2008, the first year of me living again in my home State of New Mexico after moving from Virginia, I experienced a condition, that, out of nowhere one night while I was sleeping, quickly doubled me over with some of the most severe, unrelenting pain—abdominal or otherwise—that I have ever experienced during my life (and that includes my nearly unendurable Cancer-treatment-related mouth and throat pain; passing two horrible Kidney Stones; and, sitting through an IRS audit!). But seriously, from the first unbearable episode that night, and for about a month after, I had over a dozen such flare-ups, which required five trips to the Emergency Room (ER), a week-long admission to the hospital, and me seeing one physician after another, including a Gastrointestinal (GI) Specialist. Also, during this time, I submitted to every diagnostic test under the sun (together with many conducted by the GI Specialist whose job it is to know and identify such things), and, I’d been given God-knows-how-much Morphine during my many hospital visits to help relieve the excruciating pain.

During this four-week-long hellish nightmare, I could only work at my job sporadically, I couldn’t sleep well at night, and I lost almost 25 lbs. of bodyweight due to the continuous bouts of diarrhea and vomiting (sorry for that graphic) that hit me day and night. But, the hardest pill of all for me to swallow (pun intended), is that after an entire month of intense medical care, seeing over a dozen doctors including a GI Specialist, and submitting to one diagnostic test after another, I received plenty of medical *opinions* – but, absolutely *no diagnosis or cure*. Then, to add insult to injury, one of the “doctors” who delivered absolutely no beneficial or definitive solutions for my problem, did provide me with some extremely non-helpful feedback as I lay in bed during my disastrous, one-week marathon stay in the hospital. This doctor pompously told me, *“I’ve got to hand it to you – you are definitely a Medical Enigma.”* Translation: *“Sorry Pal – despite my numerous, intense years of medical school and residency, and, in spite of my many illustrious years of experience as a highly-skilled physician, I don’t have a single clue what’s wrong with you. You’re on your own, but, best of luck to you, though.”* Yeah, thanks.

My biggest concern during the entire ordeal, of course, was that my abdominal condition was being prompted by some form of Cancer (my Grandmother on my Mom's side passed from Pancreatic Cancer), or, if not that, at a basic minimum, my condition might be compromising my Immune System to the point where the despicable "C" could find conditions in my body to its liking and then put down roots once again. An undermined Immune System is all that Cancer cells need to "stake out their territory" in the body if there are other contributing risk factors that will permit that takeover to take place. Thankfully for me, however, after I had been jabbed, prodded, and scanned no-telling how many times during that atrocious month, the doctors were, ultimately, able to tell me what my medical condition ***wasn't.*** In other words, the physicians didn't know what my medical issue was, mind you, but they did know what it was not – ***as in, they knew that it was not Cancer.*** Obviously, this appreciative news did bring me considerable relief from my concerns about the possibility of another Cancer occurrence. But, even with the outcomes of those extremely welcome reports, it's still almost like someone saying to you, *"Okay, the good news is, we captured the Lion. The bad news is, the Tiger's still on the loose."* Thanks, Doc, but no thanks.

Because my GI problems continued to wreak havoc with me, and, since the medical establishment did not have any idea what was wrong with me, I took to the Internet and Googled, and I researched every medical site that I could find in the hopes of determining what might be causing my unremitting abdominal pain issues. Finally, on the ever-helpful www.pubmed.com, while looking at many medical case histories, I came across an article curiously titled, *"Eosinophilic Enteritis – a Diagnostic Dilemma."* I concluded at the time that that description seemed serendipitous, as it appeared to be an ideal match with the *"Medical Enigma"* label that the haughty doctor had stuck on me in the hospital. Not wanting this coincidental opportunity to slip past me, I decided to combine the two mysteries together as one, hoping that something helpful might come out of the pairing. And, thank God that I did, because, after numerous minutes of reading the patient case histories and comparing the actual, referenced patients' symptoms with mine, I realized that *all* of their descriptions *matched identically* with what I was going through. At that exciting moment, I ***knew*** that that ***had*** to be my problem, and that my next goal would be to get the information to a doctor who would do something about it. I was so thrilled about my late-night discovery that I called and woke up my brother, Buz, to share the fantastic news with him.

I discovered in analyzing the pubmed.com case histories that Eosinophilic Enteritis is an Auto-Immune condition (usually brought on by harsh allergies) in which an individual's White Blood Cells—*Eosinophils*—assault healthy tissues in the linings of the Esophagus, Stomach, and Upper Intestinal Tract. In so-doing, the condition can cause the most extreme, piercing pain that, admittedly, only several CCs of Morphine prescribed in the hospital were able to take care of whenever I experienced a gut-wrenching episode. The ultimate cure-all for Eosinophilic Enteritis—which is the prescription medication, Prednisone®—was also depicted in the pubmed.com patient medical histories, together with explanations of the overwhelming successes that have been experienced with the drug in relieving and preventing the symptoms of this devastating condition. Having the vital Internet article in my hand was one thing; it would be quite another matter to convince a physician that I—*a mere mortal patient*—had found both the diagnosis *and* the cure for my condition. And, it would be still another for them to actually prescribe the panacea: Prednisone®.

Nevertheless, to that end, I instantaneously printed the article with the intention of scheduling an appointment with my GI clinic to seek a doctor's help. Unfortunately, the very night that I located the article on the Internet, I had another incredibly painful flare-up, and called 911 to have an ambulance take me to the hospital. I folded up the pubmed.com information, stuck it in my pants pocket, and took it with me on the ambulance drive to the ER. Eventually, after two excruciating hours of waiting in the ER without pain medication, the physician saw me. I explained my health situation to the doctor and requested a painkiller which, thankfully, she ordered and the nurses delivered. The doctor then took the time to tell me, *"I'm from India and we fix people."* which I thought was a strange thing for a doctor to say, but, I realized that her conceited claim was just the opening I needed. I thought to myself, "*This is perfect – a doctor who can help me!"* However, when I took the printed information from my pocket and unfolded it to show and tell her about the Eosinophilic Enteritis and the Predinosone®, she blew me off with her response. She told me, *"I'm too busy, and I don't have time to read that information."* And then, just like that, she left the room. *WTF?!* First, the "doctor" brags that she "fixes people," and then, one minute later, after I give her the perfect opportunity to "fix" me by, literally, handing to her ***both*** the diagnosis ***and*** the cure for my condition, she tells me that she's too busy to help me and then she bolts out of the room. I don't know about in India, but I do know in the U.S. that that is the polar opposite of fixing people; that is shitty, disgusting medical practice.

In any event, when I eventually returned home from the ER the next day, I got ahold of the GI clinic to schedule an appointment. Unfortunately, but not surprisingly, their office could not fit me into their busy schedule right away, and the earliest appointment I could get was two weeks away. So, finally, after two *really long* weeks of waiting (and enduring three more horrifying flare-ups in the interim, including one *at* the GI Clinic), I got to see a GI doctor. Thankfully, my standard GI doctor (who had no clue about my condition, but *did* have terrible, condescending, and arrogant *bedside manners*) was on vacation, so I was able to see a younger and more modest physician. This doctor, who, coincidentally, had performed the Colonoscopy on me during my week-long hospital debacle, actually remembered me from that procedure. Realizing the pure hell that I had been suffering through since that exam, he decided to sit down and listen to me as I read the pubmed.com *Eosinophilic Enteritis* case histories to him.

After a few minutes of me reading, and us talking, about my problem, he ultimately became convinced by the medical findings in the peer-reviewed articles, my earnest "sales pitch," and, likely, the look in my distressed, but hopeful, eyes. The doctor nodded and told me, *"Mr. Sickler, I think that you may be on to something."* He then instantly wrote me that priceless prescription for Prednisone® that I had been dreaming of for over two weeks. He also scheduled me for Biopsy Surgery the following day so that he could try to determine, beyond a shadow of a doubt, what was responsible for my recurring abdominal problems. After tearfully thanking him for bigheartedly listening to me, and for the prescription, I took off straight from his office to the pharmacy to purchase the Prednisone® The Pharmacist had no sooner handed the prescription bottle to me than I found the nearest drinking fountain and instantly took two of the pills.

Bright and early the next day, the GI specialist performed the Biopsy Surgeries on me and extracted some tissue samples from my stomach walls and my upper intestines. He also ordered some Blood Tests in an effort to evaluate my Eosinophil count. Later that day, he called me with the outcomes of both tests, which confirmed that ***my diagnosis was correct.*** He pointed out to me that I did, in fact, have *Eosinophilic Enteritis.* The physician further validated this by telling me that my Blood Tests, alone, revealed a level of Eosinophils ***FAR*** above the normal, tolerable amount. That news, of course, begs the question: *How did all of the doctors in the ER and the hospital, and my original GI Specialist, not notice my incredibly high amounts of Eosinophils when I had my blood drawn no less than a dozen times during my month-long ordeal?* I mean, the lab results have a huge, bold "H," which stands for "High" right next to the Eosinophil level.

But, be that as it may, phenomenally, within two days of me swallowing my first dose of Prednisone®, *my Eosinophilic Enteritis symptoms were completely gone!* 100% vanquished in two days on my own, after a month of complete dead-ends with doctors, and God only knows how much money wasted by my Insurance (and on *my* Co-pays!) with absolutely nothing to show for it. Because I had *both diagnosed and cured myself using the Internet* after multiple doctors had failed to do so with numerous fancy tests and exams, the humble GI Specialist said to me during a follow-up visit, *"Mr. Sickler, what you did was remarkable. You are amazing."* Thanks for your help, Doc, and, by the way, I'm still Cancer-free, to be more exact.

Since that rude awakening in 2008, I've experienced quite a number of other health scares that—from a potential "C" perspective—have disturbed me sufficiently, physically and mentally, for me to request medical attention – again, *just in case.* These instances include:

- ***Unexplained Neck, Shoulder, and Chest Pain and Numbness***

In 2010, out of clear blue (isn't that always the way it takes place?) I started experiencing inexplicable numbness and continuous pain in the area on the left side of my neck, my upper left chest, and my left shoulder, for two to three days. It wasn't muscular pain that would've been caused by the bench press or another exercise injury (believe me, I *DO* know how those feel!), but, was a deeper, sharper, achy-type of sensation that radiated from my left shoulder, to the left side of my neck, and down my chest on the left region of my body. After I entered my symptoms into the *Symptom Checkers* on some medical websites, I got the big, bold red warnings that instructed me to *"obtain medical help immediately"* as my pain *"could be due to a cardiac condition."* I did feel certain that *that* was not the problem, but, what *really* disturbed me were the additional references on that website—among other possible causes—that what I was feeling may be referred pain, being caused by, of all things, Lung Cancer. ***Lung Cancer?*** – you have got to be kidding me! That is the exact form of Secondary Cancer that I dread most because it is a known metastasis location for my form of Base of Tongue Cancer in later Stages.

Of course, that dreaded "C" word brought my worst fears to mind, so, once again, erring on the side of caution, I drove myself in to the ER. I had no sooner checked in and explained my symptoms to the nurse when she briskly whisked me away and had me hooked up to the EKG machine. Their job-one was to substantiate whether or not I was having any cardiac events. Thankfully, my EKG came back squeaky clean, as did the images from the ensuing CT Scans of my chest area that the ER physician had ordered. While these test results confirmed that I did not have any heart problems, of greatest importance is that it was positively verified that I did not have Lung Cancer. This was extraordinary news on both counts. However, not unlike the Eosinophilic Enteritis debacle I described previously, the physicians had absolutely no idea what was responsible for my chest and upper left shoulder and neck pain, or for the numbing sensation. Once again, though, they did know what *was not* causing it: Cancer.

As sorry as it may seem that I could not receive a diagnosis regarding the discomfort in my chest, the *non-diagnosis of Cancer* was good enough for me. The fact that Cancer was not the problem was a fabulous blessing, which I excitedly let the ER staff know as I departed the hospital. They all looked at me like I was crazy *(all in a day's work for them!),* but I presume that a person would have to be a Cancer survivor to fully comprehend just how terrific it is to dodge such bullets – "false alarms" though they may be. The unexplained chest, shoulder, and neck pain, as well as numbness in those areas, still do bug me every day. I honestly think that they may be a Late Side Effect caused by my Radiation Therapy over nine years before.

- ***Unexplained Pain on the Left Side of My Throat***

This one hit me suddenly, and right where it counts – smack-dab in the eye of the storm. Yes, in 2011, I woke up from sleep one night with a nasty sore throat that was paradoxically located only on the ***left side of my neck. That rings a bell!*** This was precisely in the same location where I suffered the throat pain back in 2004, and is exactly where my Primary Tumor had been located. I didn't need to be reminded of the cause of the insistent agony at *that* time, and, the scary similarities between that known perpetrator, and this unknown cause, were not lost on me – not for a split second. Had this identical thing occurred in the *pre-Cancer me*, or, if I had been suffering from a Cold or the Flu at that time in 2011 and could have attributed the symptoms to a *genuine* sore throat, I, probably would have taken the obligatory over-the-counter remedies in an effort to deaden the pain without giving it a second thought. But, I had not been unwell *this* time, and when I attempted to quash the latest discomfort with pain-deadening throat spray and by gargling with salt water, the soreness on the left side of my throat just would not go away – at least not to my liking. If it looks like a duck, quacks like a duck, and walks like a duck, it's probably a duck. Probably…but, not definitely.

Subsequent to my thankful Cancer-free recovery a few years prior, I began living a *"New Normal"* way of life in which I do not take anything regarding my health for granted. This new throat pain in 2011 represented déjà vu of the nastiest kind, in that it dredged up some extremely horrifying memories of a very tough time in my life when I could have lost my life. Going over the options in my mind on that recent throat scare, I just prayed that it was not my time for a repeat performance. I mean, one Cancer for me is more than enough, thank you very much! But, acting on my worst fears, I contacted my Ear, Nose, and Throat (ENT) doctor's office, explained my concerns and symptoms, and asked if them if they may possibly work me into their crammed appointment schedule as quickly as possible.

At my present ENT office, appointments generally must be scheduled approximately six months in advance due to an extremely unbalanced doctor-to-patient ratio. However, with some juggling of appointments the office was able to schedule a time within four days of my phone call. When all was said and done following my urgent check-up, the ENT physician was confounded as to what could have prompted my throat pain. His very thorough physical examination of my throat and Base of Tongue found nothing untoward. But, most importantly, his exam revealed that I did not have any indications of a new Cancer Tumor, or, of any unusual Lymph Node activity. This news overjoyed me to no end, of course, and I thanked the ENT for fitting me in. He assured me, *"It's better to be safe than sorry – you did the right thing."* Ultimately, a few days later, almost as quickly as the throat pain arose, it went away, never to be heard from again. I sometimes wonder if God gives us "pop-quizzes" just to see if we are paying attention. If that's the case, I'm glad I passed *this* test.

- ***Unexplained Lower Right Rib-Cage Pain***

Another example of an *oh crap!* moment I had in which my body's *early warning system alarms* went off occurred in mid-2013, actually, just a few months prior to this being written. This particular medical conundrum involved the region of my lower rib cage on the right side, which one day, out of nowhere (there I go again), decided to start throbbing. The unforeseen pain was pretty intense, especially when I put any pressure on the ribs, themselves, and, I honestly did not have a clue as to what might be causing the discomfort. I do lift weights every day, and, with one exercise in my workouts, I perform daily weighted Side Bends, which strengthen the muscles located on the sides of the body, including the vicinity near the ribs. I've been doing this same movement for many years with the same poundages, so I know that I did not injure myself performing that exercise.

Notwithstanding that, though, I, honestly, could not think of anything else that I may have done to cause the nagging pain. I have hurt my ribs and connective tissues before, and I've pulled muscles during sports, workouts, or while doing manual labor. But, *this* pain was quite disconcerting because it seemed to radiate beneath, above, and around the rib bone, itself. Not only that, but, the hurting did not go away after three or four days, as do most minor muscle pulls or strains. Taking all of this under consideration, I decided that it was time to fire up the Internet and start Googling to see what the *cyber-doctors* had to say about this inexplicable and unrelenting pain.

Taking a direct approach, I Googled *"pain on lower right rib cage,"* and, to my amazement, I was rewarded with 417,000 results. I did not expect that, but up popped website after website of articles, blogs, and commentary on the subject of pain in the lower right ribs. Although nowhere as common as a Google search for *"broken leg"* (63 million results), or for the ever-popular *"flatulence"* (4.8 million results), I was very surprised that such a large number of people had experienced the same type of pain as me in the same area of the ribs. I also found it slightly peculiar that this form of pain actually had its own term—***Lower Right Rib*** *pain*—and its own description, as well as its own abbreviation: *LRR.* Who would have thunk it?

Having obviously hit the *LRR* mother lode, I started clicking on websites, reading patient testimonials and physician commentary, and researching these quasi-common symptoms. Preliminarily, what I found out was that there are several issues that can be responsible for discomfort in the LRR area, including, by the way, a bad case of gas (*hello flatulence!)*. Unfortunately, however, many of the medical websites had to go and completely ruin my day by pointing out that LRR pain can also be caused by that worst of all "C" words: Cancer. And, not just one type or two, mind you, but *three* different forms of the nasty disease: Lung, Liver, and Bone. ***Lung, Liver, and Bone*** – hmmmm, sounds like a good name for a Law Firm, doesn't it?

At any rate, I thought – *not again!* Is there *any* condition in the body, besides an Ingrown Toenail, a Leg Cramp, or a bad case of Hemorrhoids, that doesn't have some type of Cancer associated with it? With over 200 known forms of Cancer and the entire body being susceptible to their ways and means, they, absolutely, do get around. In any event, after reading on several medical websites regarding the potential culprits for LRR pain, and, being the due-diligent person I am, I hopped in the car and drove myself into the ER - *again.* After checking in and explaining my reason for being there (and that I am a Cancer survivor), the ER staff punctually assigned me to an exam room, where I soon saw a Nurse Practitioner (NP). I discussed with her the pain-related symptoms that I had been feeling, and that I was concerned because they had lasted for a few days, and that I didn't know what their cause(s) might be. I told her that my worst worries would be that the discomfort I was feeling might be some variety of referred pain being caused by one of the Cancers or another serious condition that I had found profiled on the many medical websites.

The NP was very sympathetic and she totally understood my qualms. She, subsequently, had several tubes of my blood drawn and tested, and then had me participate in CT Scans of my abdomen and chest. Some time later, the NP entered the room with the outcome of my Blood Tests and CT Scans and, she enthusiastically informed me that I did not have an extreme condition such as Cancer. *"Perhaps,"* she said, *"you may have somehow caused damage and inflammation of the cartilage joining your ribs on the right side."* But, she didn't know for definite. I didn't have a clue how or when it happened, but, in any event, I thanked her profusely for the great news. Once again, I received a medical opinion, but no clear diagnosis of the condition. That's okay, though, because at least I knew what the pain *was not: the big C.* A few days later, thank God, the mystery pain went away.

- ***A Summary of My Medical "False Alarms"***

Okay, so now let's summarize all of those False Alarms that I have experienced with my health between 2008 and 2013: During that period, I have had four (4) somewhat scary health conditions for which I have requested medical assistance due to my concerns that something serious, such as Cancer, might be the problem. In all four cases, thankfully, Cancer was explicitly ruled out as the culprit, but, in only one of the four situations was there a definite diagnosis made regarding the condition. In that one case, coincidentally, it was *me* who made the diagnosis and also determined a cure, not a physician. The medical establishment, with its skilled professionals and various diagnostic tools and tests at their disposal, was not able to determine the exact cause of my symptomatic pain in all four instances.

Slightly ironic, to say the least, but, even so, some significant take-aways have come out of these experiences, which are: 1) Most importantly and appreciatively, that I am still ***Cancer-free!;*** 2) that Medicine is not an exact science, but doctors, nurses, and associated health care professionals do the best they can to fix what ails us; 3) that the Internet can be both a blessing and a curse for many reasons, but, for health-related assistance, the online information *might* be an extremely helpful tool when used together with professional, reliable medical care; and, finally, that, obviously, I *am a Medical Enigma,* just as the bigheaded doctor said. That's one thing he *did* get right!

The News…the Damn News

When I was going through an agonizing depressive state and attending Psychotherapy sessions for a couple of years in 2005 and 2006 after my Cancer treatments ended in 2004, I made a conscious judgment to swear off of listening to, watching, or reading the news in all formats: Online, magazines, TV, radio, newspapers, etc. This, because, let's face it, news is predominately bad, and, unfortunately, it's the bad news that sells and receives all of the press. Life can be challenging enough during and after Cancer treatments and recovery without adding to that despair with sensationalized reports regarding murder, political corruption and malfeasance, religious hypocrisy, corporate greed, military cover-ups, and horrible natural disasters, to name but a few. During my deep, dark Depression, I felt so terrible, mentally, that bad news was the last thing that I wanted to see, hear, and read. Sometimes in life, no news *literally is* good news, and, for me, the lengthy period of my Cancer Recovery was one of them.

Somewhere around the 2007 timeframe, however, after I was finally able to successfully break free of my anxiety and Depression, I, once again, found myself able to stomach the news (or *some* news – I still have a very difficult time with political uselessness). In the last couple of years, though, I must admit that one particular type of news has given me pause, and has made me poignantly conscious of information that, at least in my personal opinion, is much worse than a juicy, sex scandal involving a religious politician and his mistress. That is, it seems that not one week goes by when there isn't a report about an actor, a musician, an author, an artist, a singer, or another special, famous person, that has just passed away because of Cancer.

Unfortunately, I am extremely well aware (especially while writing this Book), of the numbers of men, women, teens, and young children in the U.S. and in the world that succumb to this despicable disease on an annual basis. Not to discourage or frighten the Reader with gloomy Cancer statistics, but, in the U.S., over 550,000 valiant people—and, worldwide, over 7.6 million courageous individuals—

lose their hard-fought battles with Cancer every year. While all of these "private" individual losses are definitely felt and mourned by the respective loved ones, family members and friends of the Cancer warriors, the general population probably doesn't learn much about most of these lesser-known, fallen heroes of the Cancer Wars. But, when the Cancer victim happens to be a distinguished celebrity, or is famous for whatever reason, we *do* find out about it. And, it is these ever-present, sporadic news reminders of Cancer's ruthless lethality that, I, as a Cancer survivor, find extremely disheartening.

Recently, it occurred to me that an inconceivable number of well-known men and women had been passing away, based on news accounts that I had read regarding many individuals. So, in an effort to satisfy my own curiosities of the causes of their respective deaths (knowing full-well what I might find), in 2013, I conducted a small "study" on the internet of about twenty-five *house-hold-name* actors, actresses, musicians, and other entertainers who had perished during the preceding year. Many of these individuals were men and women just about my age *with whom I had grown up* during the 1950s, 60s, and 70s, while several were older, and some were younger. But, in any event, of all of those unfortunate people that I researched (where the causes of their respective mortalities were mentioned in the news articles), my calculations found that around 90% of these individuals died from some form of Cancer. Just think about this: 9 out of 10 of these celebrated men and women passed on because of Cancer—or, from complications related to the malicious disease. And do keep in mind that most of these individuals had the money and the means to receive the finest medical treatment possible. As you have probably figured out by reading this Book, Cancer doesn't give a damn about how wealthy, how good looking, how healthy, how "powerful," or, how young or old a person is. If Cancer gets your number, that's the way it is. Thankfully, however, according to recent statistics, about 80% of all Cancer victims, combined, will survive their disease.

For all Cancer victims, and for those few famous people who don't make it, however, I am extremely sad, and also for the families of the celebrities who lost their lives to this disease. Being a Cancer survivor myself, I, perceptibly, am very well aware of the potential, not-so-good consequences that may come with a Cancer occurrence. What I find very distressing, though, is the reality that these eminent people— whether they were respected actors, musicians, politicians, artists, authors, or, members or other professions in the public eye— are no longer around to inspire us, to entertain us, to make us laugh, to teach us, and to grace our lives. But, perhaps, the most disquieting actuality of all, is the reason that these well-known people have sung their final song, danced their final dance, or given their final speech, is all because of one unacceptable and unforgiveable cause: ***Cancer.*** Certainly, it is sad, and it is what it is. But, the disappointing reality of these distinguished, bigger-than-life people taking their *final bow* in life with many potentially good years ahead of them would make any individual—and particularly a Cancer survivor such as myself— think twice about their *own life*, and, about how long their *own run* will last. Hopefully, I, and all Cancer survivors, will still have many more lively songs and encores to go before *our* final curtain falls.

Life Insurance – Get it While the Gettin's Good

God knows there are a lot of things in life that can ruin one's day, but, I'm extremely certain that a person receiving a diagnosis of Cancer is right at the apex of that list. I'll absolutely give it my vote! With an occurrence of Cancer, there are just so many factors to cope with and consider: The chilling, potential lethality of the disease; the dreaded (but necessary) Cancer-killing Treatments; the discouraging and generally uncomfortable treatment-related Side Effects and Late Effects; the virtually jammed schedule of medical commitments; the associated impacts on families, friends, work, school, and play-time; and, obviously, all of the physical pain and emotional suffering that comes with that complete package. Talk about having a lot on one's plate! Well, while we're on that subject, let's add one more Cancer-related morsel to the mix: The difficulty (or impossibility) of buying Life Insurance as a Cancer survivor, and, especially if the person is a survivor of advanced, Stage III or IV Cancer. Yes, unfortunately, it is true – as a Cancer Survivor, one might as well be walking around with a *Scarlet "C"* on their forehead – at least insofar as the greedy and uncompassionate Life Insurance companies are concerned.

I discovered exactly how *persona non grata* I am to the Life Insurance companies when, in 2012, I started cold-calling around to inquire about taking out a Life Insurance policy on myself, eight-ish years after my Cancer diagnosis. Jayni and I thought it would be a sensible idea for me to acquire such a policy to cover her financially, should, God forbid, something not-so-good happen to me. Well, it was an excellent idea *until* I started speaking to the insurance agents. The second I mentioned the words, *"I'm a Cancer survivor."* a hush would fall on our conversation, almost as though I were standing by myself in the barrenness of Death Valley (no suppositions intended). Typically, the first words out of the agents' collective mouths were, *"What form of Cancer did you have?"* Reciting from a script, they next corralled me with, *"What Stage was your Cancer?" "Did your Cancer metastasize and to where?"* and, *"How long have you been out of Cancer treatment?"* Oh yeah, they also asked me my age.

With every answer that I provided to the insurance agents, I found myself descending farther and farther into a bottomless abyss. Before I started calling around to the insurers, I Googled the topic of *"Cancer Survivor and Life Insurance"* and, based on what I read on many sites about the severed relationships between Cancer survivors and insurance companies, I figured that the two would probably mix like oil and water. It turns out I was correct, but, I had *no* idea that I would be subjected to a *Grand Inquisition* when I actually contacted the insurance corporations in-person. It was almost as though I was being put on trial for the "crime" of having survived Cancer. This is one *"Late Side Effect"* of Cancer that I never dreamt of having.

In short, to a person, the insurance folks did not like the fact that I had had Cancer at the Base of the Tongue. This is because, over 75% of the time, my particular Cancer is caused by tobacco or alcohol usage, and the survivability and mortality statistics for those risk factors are, well, not the finest. However, I used neither tobacco nor alcohol, and, in fact, the form of Base of Tongue Cancer I had—which most likely was precipitated by Humanpapillomavirus (HPV) during unprotected sex—has an average *90% survival rate.* Despite these blatant, scientifically-proven differences between the causative factors and relative prognoses for this form of Cancer, however, and, in spite of me pointing out all these inconsistencies to the insurance companies, they did not care. This is because the Actuarial Tables they use—which are all based on the U.S. National Cancer Institute (www.cancer.gov) SEER data that is very similar to the survivability information that I profiled in Chapter 10 of this Book—are carved in stone. In other words, Base of Tongue Cancer is Base of Tongue Cancer – period. *Score:* Insurance companies:1, Cancer survivors: 0.

The insurance agents on the phone also balked at the fact that my Cancer was graded a Stage IV, which, as I've stated many times within this Book, is the most advanced, and, in general, is the most entrenched in the body and requires the most intensive treatment to eliminate. And, because of that, advanced Stage Cancers (III and IV) also present the greatest risk for some survivors experiencing…how should I gently put this…an earlier than anticipated demise. For that reason alone, as one can readily presume, most insurers won't touch such Cancer survivors with a 10-foot pole. The *Score*, now, if you're keeping track, is Insurance companies: 2, Cancer survivors: 0. Then, there's that question regarding whether or not the Cancer had spread or metastasized to the Lymph Nodes, or other areas within the body. If the answer to that is, *"Yes,"* as it is in my case, that's another big, fat reason for rejection of a policy. The Cancer Stage and metastasis (or lack thereof) go hand-in-hand, meaning that the higher the Stage, the more likely the spread of Cancer within the body, and visa-versa. So, if you've got one, you've also got the other, and Life Insurance companies don't like that "risky" combination one little bit.

During my research about this love-hate relationship, I found out that the Cancer survivors that limited Life Insurance companies ***will consider insuring*** are those that had Prostate or Breast Cancer, ***but only*** if their Primary Tumor was localized, completely removed, had not metastasized within the body, was graded Stage I, and, if the patient/survivor has no other health conditions that might place them in the "high-risk" category. Even at that, premiums are considerably higher for the Cancer survivor than they would be for a person of the same age in superior health that has never had Cancer. Nevertheless, my Cancer *did* metastasize to my Lymph Nodes, and, even though all traces of Cancer were gotten rid of from both my Nodes and my Tongue and have never relapsed, the truth that Cancer *did spread* to my Lymph Nodes from my Tongue "blew me out of the water" from the get-go. *Score* – Insurance companies: 3, Cancer survivors: 0.

Regarding the significant, *"How long have you been out of Cancer treatment?"* question, theoretically, if you are a longer-term survivor—which, based on my research on this topic, is "five years or greater," per the Life Insurance industry—you are more suitably looked upon by the insurers. Any Cancer survivors with fewer than five years of survivability under their belt are still considered a high-risk by the insurers, even if they had a lower-Staged Cancer with no additional complications. In any case, based on the 5-year criteria, I would have anticipated that my 8 years of survivorship at the time I called the insurance companies would, theoretically, give me a point in the "Win" column, and, perhaps, get my big toe in the door. Nice try, but, unfortunately, even being a "veteran," longer-term survivor such as me won't get *anything* in the door, ***IF*** you have other strikes against you, such as a riskier form of Cancer, according to the SEER prognosis data (which mine was), and/or, an advanced Stage Cancer with Lymph Node Metastasis (which mine was). Also, the insurers take the survivor's age into consideration, meaning, the younger the better (again, per Actuarial life expectancy data - that's a no-brainer) for any prospective insured Cancer survivors. So, with me being 60 years old when I called the insurers, my age was yet another smudge against me, despite the facts that I was in terrific health and fantastic physical shape – *especially for a 60-year old.* Well, 0 out of 5 sucks, and the *Final Score* of this game is: Insurance companies: 5, Me: 0.

99% of the insurance companies I called to query about the possibility of obtaining a Life Insurance policy as a Cancer survivor, essentially, disqualified me over the phone when I responded to their interrogations. However, one insurance company did decide to give me the benefit of the doubt and arranged for me to obtain a physical exam. I also had to sign no fewer than five medical release forms so that the insurer could request all of my medical records from those physicians who treated my Cancer many years ago, and, from those doctors whom I have been seeing for my subsequent follow-up care. Thankfully, I did pass my physical exam with flying colors, but, the ***medical records portion took forever.*** This was simply because the Hospital Records Offices, being, well, Hospital Records Offices, did not make this one of their highest priorities. In fact, this was even lower than their lowest priority. Nevertheless, several months later, when the requisite medical records *finally* did arrive at the insurance company, I was told that they were evaluated by a "medical doctor" working for the Life Insurance company (and fully responsible for protecting that valuable *bottom line*). Following that evaluation, the insurance company representative contacted us and shared with me and Jayni, the foreseeable: *"We had to decline your request for Life Insurance because your Cancer was a higher Stage and had spread to your Lymph Nodes."* Well yeaahh…just like I said to you during my original phone call. But, thanks for the free medical exam…

With all of this being said, the overarching moral of the story here is: *If the Reader is young-ish and married, and whether or not they have children, if they want to make certain that their loved ones are taken care of financially should they meet an untimely passing,* ***DO NOT WAIT to purchase Life Insurance! Buy Life Insurance at an earlier age and before Cancer or any other medical maladies have had an occasion to attack one's body, wreak havoc with one's health, or worse.*** Insurers of all varieties loathe pre-existing medical conditions in potential customers. But, those companies writing Life Insurance policies will high-tail it from Cancer survivors (especially we advanced-Stage survivors) faster than you can say, *"billion dollar profits."* As we all know, the Actuaries and Physicians (who make the determination to rebuff or approve Life Insurance coverage) that work for the insurance companies are all perfect physical specimens, and they, personally, never have any medical tribulations from their birth through their death. This places them in a faultless position to play "God," and to judge others' health predicaments. Please excuse me for my clear sarcasm, but, hopefully, the Reader gets my point.

It's difficult enough for a person to cope with an undeserved malignant Cancer diagnosis to begin with, and, it's definitely not an easy thing for any individual to battle and survive their disease. But, when a Cancer survivor then has to suffer rejection of Life Insurance coverage by insurance companies…well…that simply adds insult to injury – *literally.* I understand from a business perspective that it's all about multi-million dollar CEO bonuses, billion dollar corporate profits, and keeping the Shareholders happy. But, bad things happen to good people, including Cancer survivors and their families, and they deserve a fair shake too. At the very least, Cancer survivors—including those with advanced Stage Cancers who have been given a favorable prognosis (>75%+ survival rate)—should be offered Life Insurance products of some sort regardless of what the SEER tables say. And, at the very most, Cancer survivors should not have to pay the price for the insurance industry's lack of compassion, or for their unconstrained and ostentatious worship of the *almighty bottom line.*

Every Cancer patient / survivor is different from one another, as are the circumstances of each patient's and survivor's Cancer risk factors and causes, their therapy outcomes, and *how they are living their lives after Cancer – either healthfully or not.* Consequently, for these reasons, all Cancer patients and survivors should be examined ***individually*** by the insurance industry, and should never be pigeon-holed into some statistical spreadsheet as though they are all carbon copies of each other. This will never occur, however, because ***their loyalty is to money*** – not the afflicted. In any case, Dear Reader, try to avoid this exasperation. If possible (and if it is not too late), plan ahead for the worst while you have the chance, as all "pre-existing" conditions have to start in someone, sometime. In other words, buy Life Insurance for your family ***before*** *"the shit hits the fan."*

Writing: The Best Medicine (At Least for Me)

A reasonable individual could rationally ask the question, *"If a Cancer survivor doesn't like what Cancer will do to men, women, and children (who does?); does not like a mere mention of the word, "Cancer;" and, did not like what Cancer did to their own body and life, why would they voluntarily put themselves through the anguish of writing an entire book about it?"* That's a fair question, but, from *my* perspective, the answer is actually, relatively simple: *I* wrote ***this Book*** about Cancer *because of* those precise reasons, and because, I wanted to address those exact questions. In other words, I did it for my own therapeutic motives, and, I did it, hopefully, for the benefit of others touched in some way by this atrocious disease. The iconic story-teller, Ernest Hemingway, once proffered, *"There is nothing to writing. All you do is sit down at a typewriter and bleed."* I'm not certain if Mr. Hemingway was speaking in a literal or in a figurative sense, but, I have found my arduous-yet-victorious Cancer ordeal to be the perfect opportunity for me to allow my figurative blood—that is, my many thoughts and stories—to flow from my heart and soul (and my typewriter-esque PC) onto the written page. In the profound words of poet and memoirist, Maya Angelou, *"There is no greater agony than bearing an untold story inside you."* Bleed, baby, bleed.

I have mentioned a few times within this Book that I kept a Cancer journal every day for over three years in which I documented anything of significance that took place during my challenging, but ultimately triumphant, Cancer journey. I found the entire journaling experience to be super-beneficial and therapeutic in itself, because, my daily note-taking relieved my already stressed-out brain cells (at least, those cells that were still remaining post-Chemo!) from having to remember the inexhaustible accounts of both the minutia and the magnitude that can accompany such an unanticipated roller-coaster ride. But, perhaps, most importantly, my journaling efforts allowed me an opportunity to not only release my frustrations and anguish in response to the physical and emotional pain that I endured much of the time, but, it also served as a sounding board from which I could celebrate my sporadic successes, no matter their scale. It was those copious journaling notes, together with material given to me by my Medical Team physicians as well as the outcomes of my persevering research, which, ultimately, became the fodder for this Book.

In addition to my journaling efforts, and my authoring of this Book to tell my Cancer story, I also put *Writing* to beneficial uses in additional modes during the Recovery Phase of my Cancer journey. Specifically, in 2005, I finally took the time to write and consolidate my poetry into two volumes that I had intended for most of my life to accomplish. I have written rhyming verse ever since I was about twelve years old, and I had accumulated several dozen of my poems, limericks, and other musings throughout my life. My Mom's Mom, Ellen (or Nana, as we called her), had always urged me to include all of my poetry within a book. Inevitably, however, I always managed to come up with one reason or another for never accomplishing that goal. With my Cancer occurrence, however, all of that changed—as did my views about life in general—and I decided to *finally allot the time* to achieve what Nana had encouraged me for many years to do.

In 2005, to help keep my brain gainfully occupied while my body was recovering from my Cancer Treatments and Side Effects, I attained my dream by publishing two books of my poetry, namely: *A Time for Rhyme, Part I – The Early Years, and, Part II – The Middle Years*. Subsequently, during my Cancer Recovery, I attended Psychotherapy to help me get past my dire post-Cancer Depression. At that time, I began a writing project to assist me with better coping with my pent up feelings, and I recorded daily notes of my thoughts, good and bad, happy and sad, which I discussed with my Therapist during our weekly sessions. Over several months, I accumulated so many thoughts, opinions, and quotations I had written that I decided to build a book around them. That resulting book, *Out of My Mind, From my Heart, and Off My Chest!,* was published in 2009. Without a doubt, I found that the actual writing of that book, joined with the mental/physical process of "getting things off of my chest" and onto paper, were very useful tools in helping me get past my anxieties.

Although it's been many years since I conquered my Cancer-related anxieties, I have found the authoring of this Book, *Cancer Is One Big Pain-In-The-Neck!,* to be an equally beneficial release of so much I have contained over the last nine years that I have wanted to contribute to others. With all of that being said, as I put the finishing touches on the closing Chapter of this Book, I will confess that I am feeling somewhat pensive—and even a little bit down—about typing the final word and tying a bow on this weighty creation. I can relate to our friend, Ernest Hemingway, when he confessed, *"After writing a story I was always empty and both sad and happy, as though I had made love."* On second thought, I'll just say I can *partially* relate to Mr. Hemingway's expression. While I will agree that completion of this compendium on Cancer does leave me with bittersweet feelings, its conclusion isn't quite of the post-lovemaking sort with which I'm familiar. But, in all seriousness, the writing of this Book—all 650+ pages of it—has been a *labor of love* that, for the last few years, has kept my mind occupied, my heart consoled, and, during more recent times, has kept me out of Jayni's hair around the house.

Having this Book—this virtual friend—waiting for me when Jayni and I were not off doing something together, or, when I wasn't engaged in other activities, has helped me keep busy during the cold winter months, and has helped to fill countless hours after work and on weekends with the delights of successfully capturing my thoughts and research within these pages, amid my sporadic frustrations with *Writer's Block.* Now, with my computer-generated confidante about to become "physical," I'll be left with uncharacteristic spaces in my days and nights that I'll have to fill with another writing project that inspires my brain and satisfies my soul. Nothing, however, will ever be able to compare with this exceptional experience. I am blessed to be alive nine+ years after my Cancer diagnosis, and I am honored to have been able to share with others what I've learned along the way.

Epilogue

There is a very good possibility that many Readers of this Book, including you, may remember during their childhood reading a book titled, ***The Little Engine That Could.*** That children's book, very popular to this day, was first published in 1930 in America, and has been used for decades to teach children the benefits of optimism, determination, hope, hard work, and, planning and achieving one's goals. The inspiring story of the strong and courageous Little Engine has been retold countless times over the years, but, no matter how or when it is conveyed, the underlying theme always remains the same:

> A stranded train is not able to find an engine—including the larger and very powerful ones situated in the railroad yard—that is willing to pull the heavy train cars up a vertical grade and over a mountain to complete its expedition. Only a shiny Little Engine is disposed to try. So, the hopeful Little Engine is coupled to the hefty load and, though it struggles, it finally begins its lengthy journey. As it starts its slow ascent up the mountain, the Little Engine continuously repeats to itself, *"I think I can, I think I can, I think I can!"* Slowly, but surely, the Little Engine inches along the rails with its cumbersome cargo in-tow, until, finally, the engine and the complete train make it successfully over the top of the mountain, and begin the slow descent to the final destination in the valley below. Having overcome an almost seemingly unattainable task, the triumphant Little Engine modestly keeps repeating to itself, *"I thought I could, I thought I could, I thought I could."*

And, so this uplifting and heart-warming story goes – a story that is realistically brought to life by immeasurable Cancer patients throughout the world on a daily basis. These dauntless men, women, and children find themselves coupled, literally, to the heavy burden of a disease with which they must contend over "dangerous terrain," and many ups, downs, and scary, jagged curves, for weeks, months, or, perhaps, even years, on-end. Ultimately, while these brave souls keep encouraging themselves, *"I think I can, I think I can, I think I can,"* most will survive their strenuous journeys and will reach their well-earned and intended destinations: ***Cancer-Free,*** *or* ***Cancer-in-Remission*** outcomes. Having attained their ambitions, these Cancer-patients-turned-Survivors, will, from time-to-time, modestly remind themselves, *"I thought I could, I thought I could, I thought I could."*

If you, or, one of your family members or friends have been diagnosed with Cancer, and, if any one of these individuals may find themselves in the same predicament as the valiant Little Engine, the patient must look at their Cancer occurrence as an opportunity. Not an opportunity to hang back in the "railroad yard" thinking negative, pessimistic, or discouraging thoughts about things that *they can't do.* But, a very important and life-saving opportunity to never stop being determined, optimistic, and focused about things that *they can do* to successfully overcome both their long, wearisome journey, and their encumbering Cancer. Once safely at their destination on the "valley floor," these courageous Cancer Survivors will sometimes look back at the mountain they conquered with a feeling of relief. But, more often than not, they surely will look ahead at the positive, wonderful world that awaits them as they reclaim their lives. And, these brave, strong souls will keep chugging, and chugging, and chugging along.

May you always have hope, always look for the silver linings among the dark clouds, and always keep telling yourself, *"I think I can, I think I can, I think I can!"* Then, despite the uphill climb and the cumbersome load that you may be bearing, you will conquer the challenges and make it safely to your magnificent and well-deserved destination on the other side. And, when you finally do arrive, don't forget to keep reminding yourself that, *you thought you could!*

My best to you on *your* journey,

Butch Sickler
www.headandneckcancerbook.com

Hope Wins

©

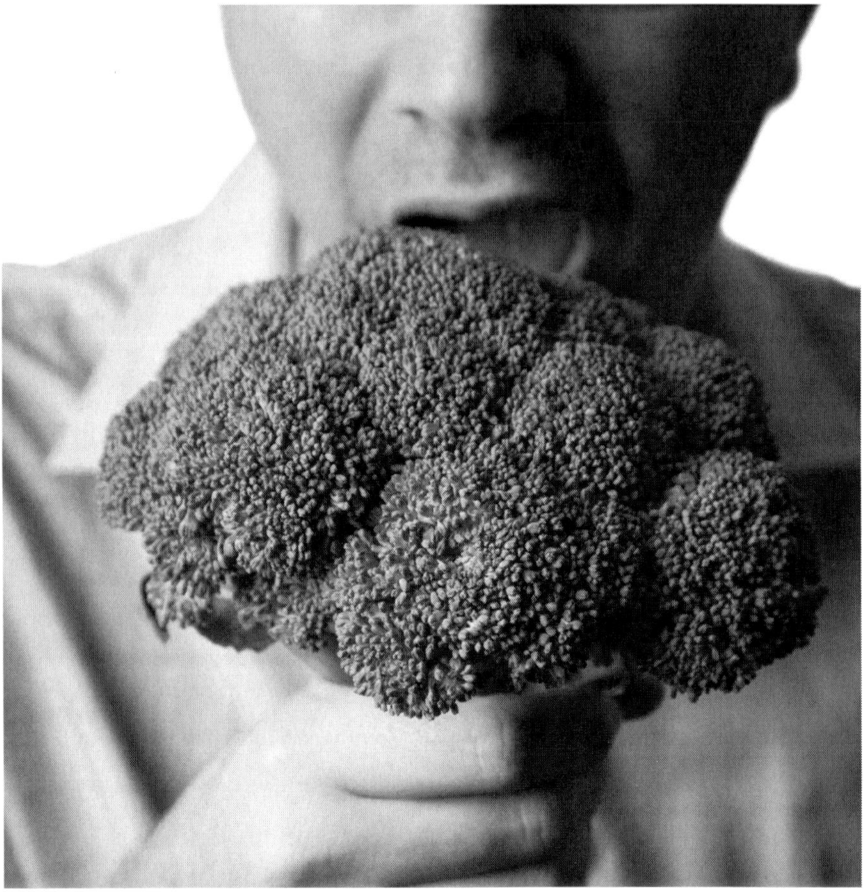

"I ate Broccoli two times a day for years, and I still got Cancer. No doubt the Broccoli Industry would attribute this anomaly to 'Operator Error.'"

-- Butch Sickler

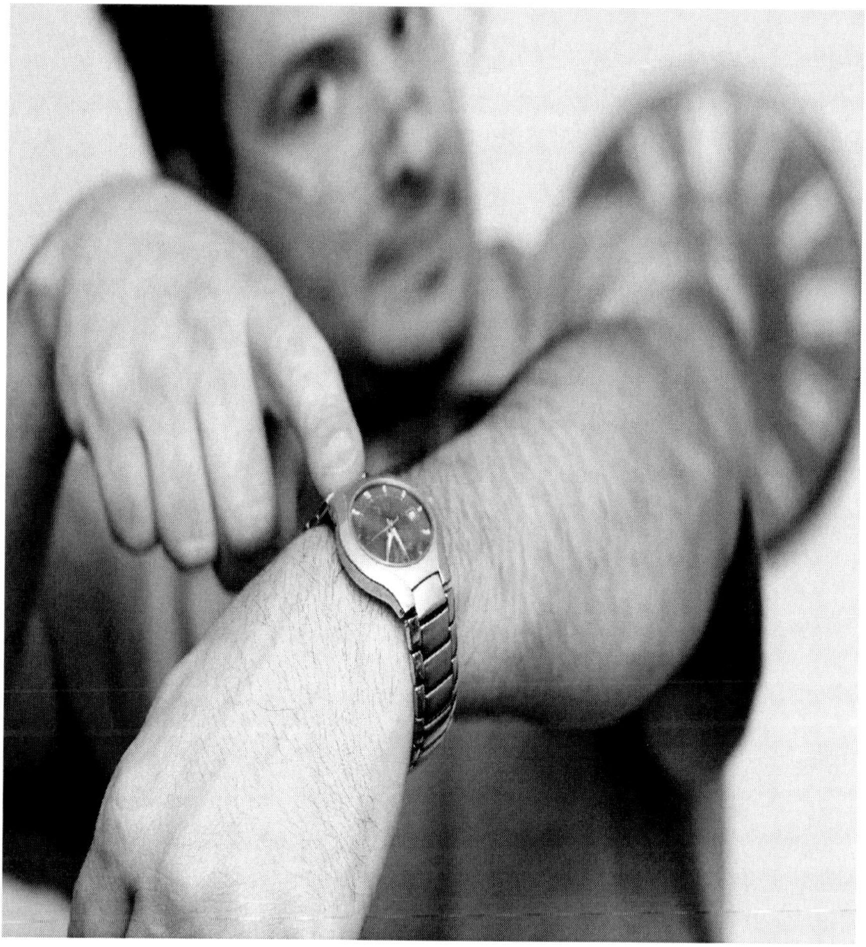

"If you are writing a book about your Cancer Experience and your Editor gives you a 'Drop-Dead' date, you may want to find a different Publisher."

-- Butch Sickler

I Miss You, Mom, Vik, Angel, & Arnie

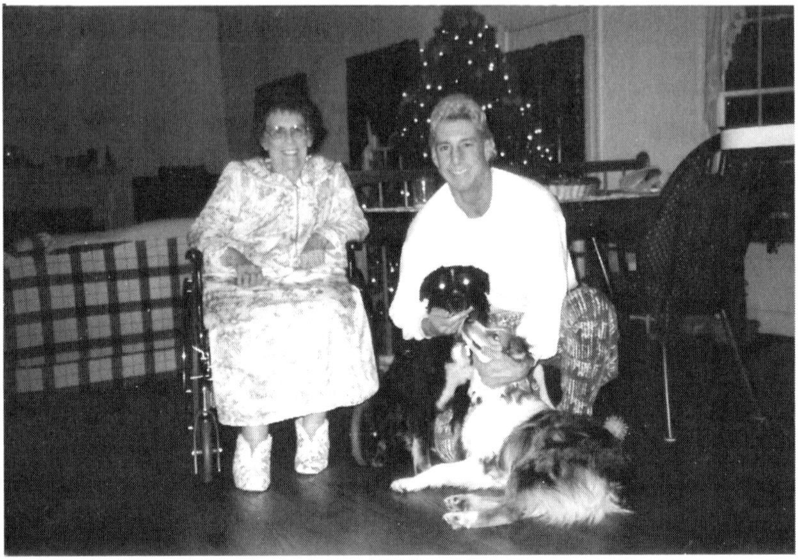

Over the last few years, many things have taken place in the world, in my family's life, and in my own life. Thankfully, countless of these circumstances have been heartening and hopeful, and have brought happiness, laughter, and encouragement to most of those concerned. But, sadly, there also have been a few happenings that have induced sorrow, tears, and discontentment to those so-affected. Specifically, in my own world, our Mom, Betty, and my pups, Angel and Arnie—pictured in the above photo I took in 1999 when Mom visited me at my farm in Virginia—brought me so much joy, and God-knows-how-much-amusement for so many years. Just as Mom had always been there for me throughout my childhood and adult life, so, too, had my two devoted and protective furry companions shared with me their unconditional love for over the last fourteen years. However, as we all know, one of the ironies of living is our inevitable passing. It was on June 3, 2005, that we lost our beautiful Sister, Vikki, and, it was a very sad day on April 13, 2012, that our lovely Mom passed away. More recently, my brave, bright, and loving Angel (the white, multi-colored pup above) went to Doggie Heaven in July 2013, and Arnie, a big goofball and Angel's lifelong Buddy, passed-on in September 2013. Each of these selfless Beings were so supportive of me during my Cancer ordeal, and I will always miss the joy that they brought to my life. I'm comforted knowing they're all in a much better place.

Index

Author-Specific Information